Concepts of Physical Fitness

ACTIVE LIFESTYLES FOR WELLNESS

Concepts of Physical Fitness

Fitness

ACTIVE LIFESTYLES FOR WELLNESS
Thirteenth Edition

Charles B. Corbin
Arizona State University—East

Gregory J. Welk
Iowa State University

William R. Corbin
Yale University

Karen A. Welk
Mary Greeley Medical Center
Ames, Iowa

Boston   Burr Ridge, IL   Dubuque, IA   Madison, WI   New York   San Francisco   St. Louis
Bangkok   Bogotá   Caracas   Kuala Lumpur   Lisbon   London   Madrid   Mexico City
Milan   Montreal   New Delhi   Santiago   Seoul   Singapore   Sydney   Taipei   Toronto

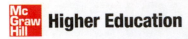

Higher Education

CONCEPTS OF PHYSICAL FITNESS: ACTIVE LIFESTYLES FOR WELLNESS, THIRTEENTH EDITION

1 2 3 4 5 6 7 8 9 0 DOW/DOW 0 9 8 7 6 5

ISBN 0-07-302853-3

Publisher: *William Glass*
Executive editor: *Nicholas R. Barrett*
Director of development: *Kathleen Engelberg*
Senior developmental editor: *Michelle Turenne*
Executive marketing manager: *Pamela S. Cooper*
Editorial and marketing coordinator: *Nancy Null*
Media producer: *Lance Gerhart*
Technology developmental editor: *Julia D. Ersery*
Senior project manager: *Jill Moline-Eccher*
Senior production supervisor: *Richard DeVitto*
Designer: *Preston Thomas*
Media supplement producer: *Ron Nelms, Jr.*
Senior photo research coordinator: *Alexandra B. Ambrose*
Art editor: *Emma Ghiselli*
Freelance photo researchers: *David & Emily Tietz*
Art director: *Robin Mouat*
Cover design: *Preston Thomas*
Interior design: *Ellen Pettengill*
Typeface: *10/12 Janson*
Compositor: *Precision Graphics*
Printer: *RR Donnelley*

Cover image: © *Lori Adamski Peek/Getty Images/Stone*

The credits section for this book begins on page C-1 and is considered an extension of the copyright page.

Library of Congress Cataloging-in-Publication Data

Concepts of physical fitness : active lifestyles for wellness / Charles B. Corbin . . . [et al.].—13th ed.
    p. cm.
Includes bibliographical references and index.
ISBN 0-07-302853-3 (softcover : alk. paper)
    1. Exercise. 2. Physical fitness. 3. Physical fitness—Problems, exercises, etc.
RA781.C58 2006
613.7--dc22   2004063187

www.mhhe.com

Brief Contents

Contents

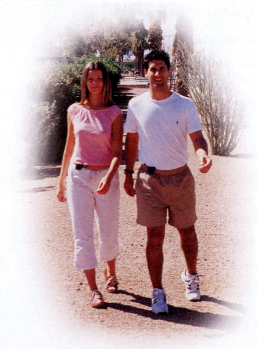

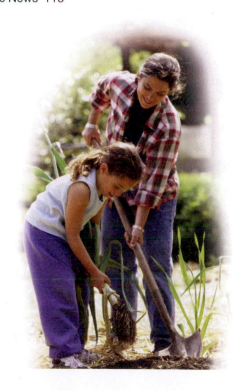

Section IV

Physical Activity: Special Considerations 207

Section V
Nutrition and Body Composition 273

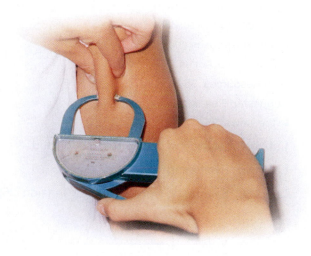

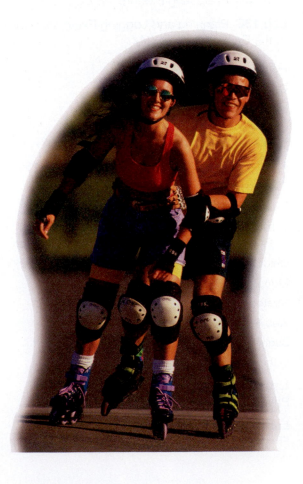

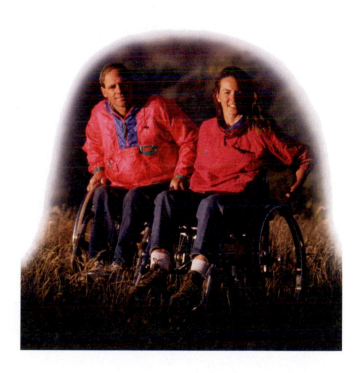

Preface

Lucky Thirteen!

We consider this thirteenth edition of *Concepts of Physical Fitness: Active Lifestyles for Wellness* to be a lucky charm. At the time of the publication of this edition it will be nearly 40 years since the first edition of the book was published. This edition features the new design and new pedagogical features introduced in the twelfth edition. With the retirement of Ruth Lindsey (see box), Greg Welk (Iowa State University) becomes second author and takes on additional author duties. Will Corbin (Yale University), a clinical psychologist and specialist in substance abuse, destructive behaviors, and stress management is the third author. Karen Welk, a physical therapist (Mary Greeley Medical center in Ames, Iowa) takes over the role as fourth author.

The content in this edition continues to evolve as we learn more about fitness, wellness, and healthy lifestyles. In our early editions, we focused on trying to get people fit and well. To be sure, fitness is an important product, as is wellness, another product of healthy lifestyle change. But scientific advances have shown that health, wellness, and fitness (all products) are not things you can "do" to people. You have to help people help themselves. Educating them and giving them the self-management skills that help them adopt healthy lifestyles can do this.

The focus of the new millennium is on the *process*. Healthy lifestyles, or what a person does, rather than what a person can do, constitute process. If a person does the process (i.e., adopt a healthy lifestyle), positive changes will occur to the extent that change is possible for that specific person. As noted in the first concept of

Dedication

The authors wish to dedicate this book in loving memory of **Charles Samuel "Charlie" Corbin** (April 22, 2004–July 18, 2004), son of Will and Suzi Corbin, grandson of Cathie and Chuck Corbin and **Alyson Welk** (April 30, 1995–June 2, 2003), daughter of Karen and Greg Welk.

A Tribute to Ruth Lindsey

Retiring Author

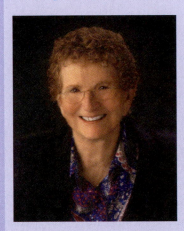

Dr. Ruth Lindsey, professor emeritus at California State University–Long Beach, is a recognized national leader in physical activity and fitness with a special expertise in biomechanics, kinesiology, questionable exercises, nutrition, and physical activity for senior adults. She is the author of more than a dozen books, including *Body Mechanics, The Ultimate Fitness Book, Concepts of Fitness and Wellness,* and *Concepts of Physical Fitness*. Her early books in biomechanics pioneered the field and provided the basis for much of what we currently know about safe versus questionable exercises. Dr. Lindsey's writings on back care are considered classics.

Dr. Lindsey was one of the original authors of *Concepts of Physical Education,* the predecessor of the twelfth edition of this book. Over the years, she has served numerous national organizations as an officer or a committee person, has presented numerous lectures, and is regularly cited in health and fitness publications. She received her doctorate from Indiana University and served on the faculties of Oklahoma State University and the University of Utah before her extended stay on the faculty at California State University at Long Beach.

Over the years, hundreds of thousands of students have been exposed to Dr. Lindsey's writings. On behalf of those students and their teachers, the co-authors of this book honor Dr. Lindsey for her many contributions related to the areas of fitness, health, and wellness. Ruth Lindsey, enjoy your retirement!

the book, lifestyles are the most important factors, influencing health, wellness, and fitness. Healthy lifestyles (the processes) are also within a person's individual control. *Any person* can benefit from lifestyle change, and any person can change a lifestyle. These lifestyle changes will make a difference in health, fitness, and wellness for all people.

The emphasis on lifestyle change in the twelfth edition is consistent with the focus of national health objectives for the new millennium. Though the principal national health goals are to increase years and quality of life (products) for all people, the methods of accomplishing these goals focus on changing lifestyles. As we move into the new century, we must adopt a new way of thinking to help all people change their lifestyles to promote health, fitness, and wellness.

Our Basic Philosophy

The HELP Philosophy

Over time, the features of our book evolve. However, the HELP philosophy on which the book is based remains sound. We believe that the "new way of thinking" based on the HELP philosophy serves us, the faculty who choose our book, and the students who use it. **H** is for *health*. Health and its positive component—wellness—are central to the philosophy. Health, fitness, and wellness are for all people. **E** is for *everyone*. **L** is for *lifetime lifestyle change*, and **P** is for *personal*. The goal is to HELP all people to make personal lifetime lifestyle changes that promote health, fitness, and wellness.

To assure that the book is consistent with the HELP philosophy and to be sure it is useful to everyone, we include discussions to adapt healthy lifestyles based on personal needs. Separate sections are *not* included for specific groups, such as older people, women, ethnic groups, or those with special needs. Rather, we focus on healthy lifestyles *for all people* throughout the book.

Meeting Higher-Order Objectives

The "new way of thinking" based on the HELP philosophy suggests that each person must make decisions about healthy lifetime lifestyles if the goals of longevity and quality of life are to be achieved. What one person chooses may be quite different from what another chooses. Accordingly, our goal in preparing this edition is to help readers become good problem solvers and decision makers. Rather than focusing on telling them what to do, we offer information to help readers make informed choices about lifestyles. The stairway to lifetime fitness and wellness that we present helps readers understand the importance of "higher-order objectives" devoted to problem solving and decision making.

New Content

The thirteenth edition is one year earlier than would typically be the case. This early revision was done so that this edition of *Concepts of Physical Fitness* will be in cycle with other books in the *Concepts* series. A summary of new content that builds on the new features of the twelfth edition follows.

- The new design that first appeared in the twelfth edition (featuring new pedagogical features such as Technology Updates, Study Resources, Strategies for Action and In the News) has been updated and is enhanced with new photos and figures.
- Statistics, web addresses, and suggested readings for all concepts have been updated. Among the more prominent new statistic are those for life expectancy, causes of death, and health disparities.
- New labs on factors influencing health, wellness and fitness and evaluating fast food options (new in 12th ed.).
- The most recent statistics concerning participation in physical activity guidelines from several organizations including ACSM. Information is also included concerning the new President's Challenge program for promoting lifetime physical activity.
- New national blood pressure standards are included as well as new information on deep vein thrombosis.
- New information on maximum heart rate formula, dose response, blood indicators of heart disease, swim test, range of motion information, muscle fitness exercises and illustrations, body fatness rating chart, and on posture and back care is included.
- New information on wind-chill (a new chart), warm-up, self-management skills, autonomous social support, walking and pedometers, exercise balls, and exercises for core fitness is included.
- New information on micronutrients, glycemic index, food supplements and fast foods is included.
- Concept 21 contains a new comprehensive model of healthy lifestyle planning that provides additional coverage of spirituality; the new model integrates physical, social, intellectual, work, and spiritual environments with suggestions for prayer, meditation, and support. Also new information concerning cities with the best emergency medical systems is included.

Enhanced Pedagogically Sound Design

The new design introduced in the twelfth edition has been enhanced with new figures and photos. The features of the enhanced design were created to make the book more attractive and pleasing to the eye while also adding pedagogical features that enhance student learning. Examples include the color tabs to help identify special features. specially colored pages unique to each book feature, icons for identifying special features, and revised concept headers. The tear-out labs can be easily identified by their unique color and numbered tabs.

Online Labs

The popular labs are now available online. To access the labs, Visit the Online Learning Center at **www.mhhe.com/ corbin13e.**

New Tables, Figures, and Photos

More than eighty-five new tables, figures, and photos are included since the implementation of the new design. Some of the figures and photos are done with a special treatment called text wrapping. This allows pictures to be integrated in the text. This method also helps us present complex information in an easy-to-understand way. Several new anatomical illustrations have been added.

Technology Update Features

Each concept contains a technology feature. These features describe technological advances relating to health, wellness, and fitness lifestyles. Examples include global positioning systems and heart rate watches.

In the News Features

These features include information that is so current that much of it was added right before the book went to press.

New Web Materials

Over the years, we have prided ourselves on being current. We have provided Web icons in the book that allow students to access current information exclusively related to our book, as well as more generic information. Access to Web materials has been made easier by including the book Web address for the accompanying Online Learning Center at the top of each left-hand page. As in the past, specific URLs appear in the body of the text as well as at the end of each concept.

Expanded Coverage for North America

New statistics for all of North America have been added to those typically presented for the United States. Several Canadian websites have been included, as have been new statistics, and a color version of the Canadian food guide is included.

Factual Updates

As is true with all of our new editions, facts, statistics, references, and other information are updated throughout.

Deleted Content

One of the problems that we have encountered over time has been the lengthening of the book because of the expansion of knowledge related to health, wellness, and fitness. In this edition, we made a conscious effort to cut words to save space and to allow new material to be added without lengthening the book. Also, the new design is more efficient, allowing us to add new information.

Popular Continuing Features

The thirteenth edition retains many of the popular features that made the previous editions so successful. Some of these features are as follows:

Pedagogically Sound Organization

Planning and self-management strategies are presented early to familiarize students with basic principles and guidelines that will be used in later planning. Preparation strategies and basic activity principles follow. Each type of health-related fitness and the type of activity that promotes each component of fitness are included in the next section. This section is organized around the physical activity pyramid. Special considerations—including safe exercise, care of the back and neck, posture, and performance—are included in the next section. Other priority healthy lifestyles are the focus of nutrition, body composition, and stress-management sections. The final section is designed to help students become good health, wellness, and fitness consumers.

Strategies for Action

At the end of each concept, *strategies for action* are provided. These are suggestions for putting content into action. Many of these strategies require readers to perform or practice self-assessment or other self-management techniques.

Magazine Format

The attractive new design supports student reading and studying with an appealing magazine format. This format has been shown to be educationally effective and has been well received by users.

Activity Features

Exercises for each part of physical fitness are illustrated and described in easy to locate tables. Opportunities to perform the exercises are provided in the labs.

Web Icons

The Web icons unique to this book allow learners to locate (at point of use) additional pictures, tables, and figures that illustrate concepts presented in the book. Web addresses to supplemental resource materials, such as a self-study guide, sample exam questions, and definitions of terms, as well as other enrichment materials, are also provided on the Online Learning Center and in the *Web Resources* section at the end of each concept. The Web address for the Online Learning Center (**www.mhhe. com/corbin13e**) is included as a header at the top of each left-facing page.

Attractive and Easy-to-Use Labs

The attractive and popular labs are designed to get users involved in practicing self-management skills that will promote healthy lifestyle change. The labs are in a bright, attractive, and educationally effective format. They are easy to find and easy to use. In many cases, lab resource materials that aid the student in performing lab activities precede them. These resources are retained in the book even when the labs are torn out. This allows future use of such materials as fitness self-assessments. The physical activity labs are designed to get people active early in the course and ultimately to allow each user to plan his or her own personal activity program.

Focus on Self-Management Skills

The educational effectiveness of a book depends on more than just presenting information. If lifestyle changes are to be implemented, there must be opportunities to learn how to make these changes. Research suggests that learning self-management skills is important to lifestyle change. A section on self-management skills is included early in the book, and additional discussions of how to practice and implement these skills is included throughout the book.

Health Goals for the Year 2010

The health goals are based on the health goals for the new millennium (Health Goals for the Year 2010). These goals are provided at the beginning of each concept to help readers relate content to goals.

What's in This for You?

This student guide follows the Preface and is designed to help students use the features of the book more effectively. Instructors are encouraged to urge students to read this section prior to using the book.

Terms at Point-of-Use

It greatly pleased us that the *Surgeon General's Report on Physical Activity and Health* adopted our physical fitness definitions. Just as we have led the way in defining fitness, we now include state-of-the-art definitions related to wellness and quality of life. These—and all other definitions—are now included at the first point-of-use to make them easier to locate.

Continued Use of Conceptual Format

We use concepts rather than chapters, and each concept contains factual statements that follow concise informational paragraphs. This tried-and-true method has proven to be educationally sound and well received by students and instructors.

Pedagogical Aids

Web Resources

Located at the end of every concept, additional websites are listed to provide students with additional online resources that supplements the content just learned.

Suggested Readings

Because students want to know more about a particular topic, a list of readings is given at the end of each chapter. Most suggested readings are readily available at bookstores or public libraries.

Appendices

Concepts of Physical Fitness: Active Lifestyles for Wellness, thirteenth edition, includes six appendices that are valuable resources for the student. The metric conversion chart; metric conversions of selected charts and tables; calorie guide to common foods; calories of protein, carbohydrates, and fats in foods; calorie, fat, saturated fat, cholesterol, and sodium content of selected fast-food items; and Canada's food guide to healthy eating are included for your use.

Ancillaries

A Note for Instructors

As with past editions, you will see that we have updated this edition with the most recent scientific information. We have designed experiences to promote higher-order thinking. There is another consideration we think to be important. As usual, we have worked to keep the price of the book low.

As always with our *Concepts* books, an extensive list of ancillary materials is available to help you provide the most effective instruction. Brief descriptions of these materials follow.

Instructor's Resource Materials

Instructor's Resource CD

Course Integrator Guide

This includes all the features of a useful instructor's manual, such as learning objectives, suggested lecture outlines, suggested activities, media resources, and Web links. It also integrates the text with all the health resources McGraw-Hill offers, such as the Online Learning Center, Image Presentation PowerPoint™, HealthQuest CD-ROM, *Healthy Living* Video Clips CD-ROM, and the Health and Human Performances website. The guide also includes references to relevant print and broadcast media. Instructors can access the guide at www.mhhe.com/corbin13e.

Computerized Test Bank

McGraw-Hill's EZ Test is a flexible and easy-to-use electronic testing program available in higher education. The program allows instructors to create tests from book specific items. It accommodates a wide range of question types and instructors may add their own questions. Multiple versions of the test can be created and any test can be exported for use with course management systems such as WebCT, BlackBoard or PageOut. The program is available for Windows and Macintosh environments.

Image Presentation PowerPoint™

The Image Presentation is an electronic library of visual resources. It comprises images from the text displayed in PowerPoint™, which allows the user to view, sort, search, use, and print catalog images. It also includes a complete, ready-to-use PowerPoint™ presentation, which allows users to play chapter-specific slideshows.

Student Self-Assessment Material

Dietary Analysis Software

Available for Windows and Macintosh computers, this user-friendly diet analysis software allows students to track their food intake over a period of days and generate a variety of easy-to-read reports and graphs. The program tracks over 30 nutrient categories. Students can choose from nearly 8,000 foods or add their own to the database. Other features include a weight management function and a website devoted to diet analysis–related resources.

Internet Resources

Online Learning Center

www.mhhe.com/corbin13e This website offers resources to students and instructors. It includes downloadable ancillaries, Web links, student quizzes, additional information on topics of interest, and more. Resources for the instructor include

- Course Integrator Guide
- Downloadable PowerPoint™ presentations
- Lecture outlines
- Discussion questions
- Concept summaries

Resources for the student include

- Flashcards
- Online labs
- Interactive quizzes

Interactive CD-ROM

HealthQuest CD-ROM

HealthQuest is designed to help students explore the behavioral aspects of personal health and wellness through a state-of-the-art interactive CD-ROM. Your students will be able to assess their current health and wellness status, determine their health risks, and explore options and make decisions to improve the behaviors that impact their health. Adopters of this text can obtain more information from your local McGraw-Hill sales representative.

Print Publications

Daily Fitness and Nutrition Journal by McGraw-Hill

This logbook helps students keep track of their diet and exercise programs, and it serves as a diary to help students log their behaviors.

Acknowledgments

The evolution of this book would not have been possible without the input of those who have used the book and those who have provided us with reviews. At the risk of inadvertently failing to mention someone, we want to acknowledge the following people for their role in the development of this book.

First, we would like to acknowledge a few people who have made special contributions over the years. Linus Dowell, Carl Landiss, and Homer Tolson, all of Texas A & M University, were involved in the development of the first *Concepts* book, and their contributions were also important as we helped start the fitness movement in the 1960s.

Other pioneers were Jimmy Jones of Henderson State University, who started one of the first *Concepts* classes in 1970 and has led the way in teaching fitness in the years that have followed; Charles Erickson, who started a quality program at Missouri Western; and Al Lesiter, a leader in the East at Mercer Community College in New Jersey. David Laurie and Barbara Gench at Kansas State University, as well as others on that faculty, were instrumental in developing a prototype concepts program, which research has shown to be successful.

A special thanks is extended to Andy Herrick and Jim Whitehead, who have contributed to much of the development of various editions of the book, including excellent suggestions for change. Mark Ahn, Keri Chesney, Chris MacCrate, Guy Mullins, Stephen Hustedde, Greg Nigh, Doreen Mauro, Marc vanHorne, along with other employees of the Consortium for Instructional Innovation and the Micro Computer Resource Facility at Arizona State University, and Betty Craft, Ken Rudich, and Fred Huff and other employees at the Distance Learning Technology Program at Arizona State University, deserve special recognition.

Second, we wish to extend thanks to the following people who provided comments for the current editions of our *Concepts* books: Eugene B. Blackwell, Surry Community College (NC); Joseph W. Bubenas, Hofstra University and Queensborough Community College; Dawn Ketterman-Benner, Moravian College (PA); R. Cody McMurtry, Newberry College (SC); and Jan Sholes, Frederick Community College (MD).

Third, we want to acknowledge the following people who have aided us in the preparation of past editions: Debra Atkinson, Iowa State University; Rose Schmitz, Texas A & M University; Dixie Stanforth, University of Texas at Austin; Kenneth R. Turley, Harding University; and James R. Whitehead, University of North Dakota; Virginia L. Hicks, University of Wisconsin at Whitewater; Jon Kolb, University of Calgary; J. Dirk Nelson, LeTourneau University (TX); Patricia A. Zezula, Huntington College (IN); Craig Koppelman, University of Central Arkansas; Robert W. Rausch, Jr., Westfield State College; Amy P. Richardson, University of Central Arkansas; Terry R. Tabor, University of North Florida; Sharon Rifkin, Broward Community College; William B. Karper, University of North Carolina at Greensboro; Larry E. Knuth, Rio Hondo College; Maridy Troy, University of Alabama at Tuscaloosa; Kenneth L. Cameron, United States Military Academy at West Point; Thomas E. Temples, North Georgia College & State University; Bridget Cobb, Armstrong Atlantic State University; Tillman (Chuck) Williams, Southwest Missouri State University; Mary Jeanne Kuhar, Central Oregon Community College; Jennifer L. H. Lechner, St. Petersburg Junior College; Laura Switzer, Southwestern Oklahoma State University; Robert L. Slevin, Towson University; Karen (Pea) Poole, University of North Carolina at Greensboro; Paul Downing, Towson University; David Horton, Liberty University; Lindy S. Pickard, Broward Community College; Laura L. Borsdorf, Ursinus College; Frederick C. Surgent, Frostsburg State University; James A. Gemar, Moorhead State University; Vincent Angotti, Towson University; Judi Phillips, Del Mar College; Joseph Donnelly, Montclair State University; Harold L. Rainwater, Asbury College; Candi D. Ashley, University of South Florida; Dennis Docheff, United States Military Academy; Robin Hoppenworth, Wartburg College; Linda Farver, Liberty University; Peter Rehor, Montana State University; Martin W. Johnson, Mayville State University; Keri Lewis, North Carolina State University; J. D. Parsley, University of St. Thomas; Marika Botha, Lewis-Clark State College; Robert J. Mravetz, University of

Akron; Debra A. Beal, Northern Essex Community College; Roger Bishop, Wartburg College; David S. Brewster, Indiana State University; Ronnie Carda, University of Wisconsin–Madison; Curt W. Cattau, Concordia University; Cindy Ekstedt Connelley, Catawaba College; J. Ellen Eason, Towson State University; Bridgit A. Finley, Oklahoma City Community College; Diane Sanders Flickner, Bethel College; Judy Fox, Indiana Wesleyan University; Earlene Hannah, Hendrix College; Carole J. Hanson, University of Northern Iowa; John Merriman, Valdosta State College; Beverly F. Mitchell, Kennesaw State College; George Perkins, Northwestern State University; James J. Sheehan, Fitchburg State College; Mary Slaughter, University of Illinois; Paul H. Todd, Polk Community College; Susan M. Todd, Vancouver Community College–Langara Campus; Kenneth E. Weatherman, Floyd College; Newton Wilkes, Bridget Cobb, John Dippel, and Todd Kleinfelter, Northwestern State University of Louisiana; and John R. Webster, Central Connecticut State University. A special thanks is extended to Patty Williams, Ann Woodard, Laurel Smith, Bill Carr (Polk Community College), James Angel, Jeanne Ashley, Stanley Brown, Ronnie Carda, Robert Clayton, Melvin Ezell, Jr., Brigit Finley, Pay Floyd, Carole Hanson, James Harvey, John Hayes, David Horton, Sister Janice Iverson, Tony Jadin, Richard Krejei, Ron Lawman, James Marett, Pat McSwegin, Betty McVaigh, John Merriman, Beverly Mitchell, Sandra Morgan, Robert Pugh, Larry Reagan, Mary Rice, Roberts Stokes, Paul Tood, Susan Todd, Marjorie Avery Willard, Karen Cookson, Dawn Strout, Earlene Hannah, Ken Weatherman, J. Ellen Eason, William Podoll, John Webster, James Shebban, David Brewster, Kelly Adam, Lisa Hibbard, Roger Bishop, Mary Slaughter, Jack Clayton Stovall, Karen Watkins, Ruth Cohoon, Mark Bailey, Nena Amundson, Bruce Wilson, Sarah Collie, Carl Beal, George Perkins, Stan Rettew, Ragene Gwin, Judy Fox, Diane Flickner, Cindy Connelley, Curt Cattau, Don Torok, and Dennis Wilson.

Finally, we want to acknowledge others who have contributed, including Virginia Atkins, Charles Cicciarella, Donna Landers, Susan Miller, Robert Pangrazi, Karen Ward, Darl Waterman, and Weimo Zhu. Among other important contributors are former graduate students who have contributed ideas, made corrections, and contributed in other untold ways to the success of these books. We wish to acknowledge Jeff Boone, Laura Borsdorf, Lisa Chase, Tom Cuddihy, Darren Dale, Bo Fernhall, Ken Fox, Connie Fye, Louie Garcia, Steve Feyrer-Melk, Sarah Keup, Guy LeMasurier, Kirk Rose, Jack Rutherford, Cara Sidman, Scott Slava, Dave Thomas, Min Qui Wang, Jim Whitehead, Bridgette Wilde, and Ashley Woodcock.

Author Acknowledgments

A very special thanks goes to David E. Corbin of the University of Nebraska at Omaha and Jodi Hickman LeMasurier. Dr. Corbin is a health educator who has provided valuable assistance. Jodi spent many hours researching photos for this book and developed the index. We especially appreciate the Spanish translation of vocabulary terms by Julio Morales from Lamar University, as well as the thorough and excellent proofreading by Bob Widen for this edition. We also want to thank Cara Sidman for developing the current test bank materials and for her excellent assistance in so many other ways. Finally we want to thank Ron Hager and Lynda Ransdell for their assistance with the development of the Web resources and the development of the test bank materials for past editions.

Finally, we would like to thank all past editors (there have been many) and our current editors, Michelle Turenne, Jill Moline-Eccher, and Nick Barrett who do the tedious jobs that make these excellent books possible.

What's in This for You?

Students, are you looking for health, wellness, and fitness information online? Working hard to get in shape? Trying to improve your grade? All the features in *Concepts of Physical Fitness: Active Lifestyles for Wellness* will help you do this and more! Take a look.

Concept Statement

A concept statement is included at the beginning of each concept. The content elaborates and expands on each concept statement.

Health Goals

The content of each concept is designed to help you meet national health goals outlined in *Healthy People 2010*.

Technology Update

The *Technology Update* features include information about a technological innovation that is related to the content of the concept.

Good health, wellness, fitness, and healthy lifestyles are important for all people.

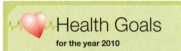

Health Goals
for the year 2010

- Increase quality and years of healthy life.
- Eliminate health disparities.
- Increase incidence of people reporting "healthy days."
- Increase access to health information and services for all people.

National Health Goals

At the beginning of each concept in this book is a section containing abbreviated statements of the national health goals from the document *Healthy People 2010: National Health Promotion and Disease Prevention Objectives*. These statements, established by expert groups representing more than 350 national organizations, are intended as realistic national health goals to be achieved by the year 2010. These objectives for the first decade of the new millennium are intended to improve the health of those in the United States, but they seem important for all people in North America and in other industrialized cultures throughout the world. The health objectives are designed to contribute to the current World Health Organization strategy of "Health for All." This book is written with the achievement of these important health goals in mind.

Introduction

www.mhhe.com/phys_fit/web01 Click 01. The first national health goals were developed in 1979 to be accomplished by the year 1990. The focus of those objectives was on reduction in the death rate among infants, children, adolescents, young adults, and adults. Except for reducing death rates among adolescents, those goals were met and the average life expectancy was increased by more than 2 years by the 1990s. Those first national health objectives gave way to the *Healthy People 2000* objectives, designed to be accomplished by the turn of the century. The emphasis in these objectives shifted from reduction in premature death to disease prevention and health promotion. While many of these objectives have been achieved, others have yet to be accomplished.

For *Healthy People 2010*, achieving the vision of "healthy people in healthy communities" is paramount. Two central goals have been established. First, the goals emphasize quality of life, well-being, and functional capacity—all important wellness considerations. This emphasis is based on the World Health Organization's focus on quality of life and its efforts to break down the artificial divisions between physical and mental well-being. Second, the national health goals for 2010 take the "bold step" of trying to "eliminate" health disparities as opposed to reducing them. Consistent with national health goals for the new millennium, this book is designed to aid all people in adopting healthy lifestyles that will allow them to achieve lifetime health, wellness, and fitness.

Technology Update
Internet Access

This book provides a number of ways to help you access reliable health and wellness information from the Internet. The *On the Web* icons throughout the book include URLs that provide additional information and links to informative sites on the Internet. The list of *Web Resources* at the end of each concept provide URLs for various organizations that provide high-quality health information. The *On the Web* and *Web Resources* features can be accessed electronically (without typing the URL) by visiting the Online Learning Center address that is featured at the top of every even-numbered page of the book. This site also includes a number of study aids, including concept outlines, concept terms, and sample quiz questions to help you apply the information in the book.

Health and Wellness

Good health is of primary importance to adults in our society. When polled about important social values, 99 percent of adults in the United States identified "being in good **health**" as one of their major concerns. The two other concerns expressed most often were good family life and good self-image. The 1 percent who did not identify good health as an important concern had no opinion on any social issues. Among those polled, none

---

Illness The ill feeling and/or symptoms associated with a disease or circumstances that upset homeostasis.

Wellness The integration of many different components (social, emotional-mental, spiritual, and physical) that expand one's potential to live (quality of life) and work effectively and to make a significant contribution to society. Wellness reflects how one feels (a sense of well-being) about life as well as one's ability to function effectively. Wellness, as opposed to illness (a negative), is sometimes described as the positive component of good health.

Quality of Life A term used to describe wellness. An individual with quality of life can enjoyably do the activities of life with little or no limitation and can function independently. Individual quality of life requires a pleasant and supportive community.

Lifestyles Patterns of behavior or ways an individual typically lives.

Definition Boxes

All terms that are bold in your book are defined in an accompanying definition box to reinforce this information.

In the News

This feature is located at the end of each concept. *In the News* is designed to provide very current information about health, wellness, and fitness.

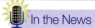 In the News

Changes in Use of Hormone Replacement Therapies May Have Implications for Osteoporosis

Doctors have routinely prescribed hormone replacement therapy (HRT) for women to reduce risks for heart disease and osteoporosis following menopause. Over 6 million women were reported to be taking this type of regimen, but these patterns were dramatically altered when a major National Institutes of Health study reported increased risks for cardiovascular events and breast cancer in those taking HRT. The result caused the clinical trial on HRT to be halted and has caused doctors to recommend that women stop taking HRT. This change in medical practice could have major implications for other health risks in women, particularly for osteoporosis. The National Osteoporosis Foundation (www.nof.org) reports that over half of all women over the age of fifty will have an osteoporotic fracture sometime in their lifetime. Experts have predicted the prevalence of osteoporosis to increase. Participation in regular weight-bearing exercise is the most important preventive measures that women (and men) can take to maintain their bone mass and prevent osteoporosis later in life.

Tables of Exercises

Many concepts include illustrations of exercises that you can use to develop health-related fitness, to care for the back and neck, or to improve posture. These exercises are included in tables at the end of the concepts. Complete descriptions of proper technique are included with the illustrations.

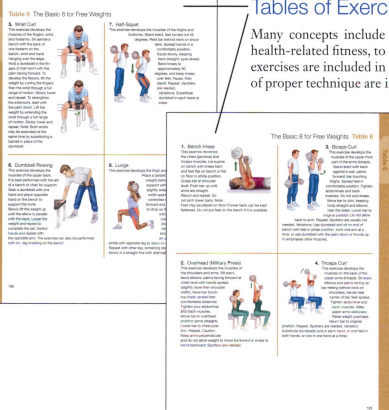

Lab Resource Materials

Many concepts include self-assessments. These concepts have a *Lab Resource Materials* section on the pages preceding the labs for that concept. They are designed to help the reader perform the self-assessments properly. They are included on non-tear out pages so that they can be used for repeat self-assessments.

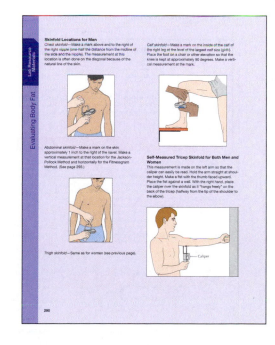

Tear-Out Labs

These are located at the end of each concept, and are designed to help you self-assess, self-monitor, and self-plan healthy lifestyles.

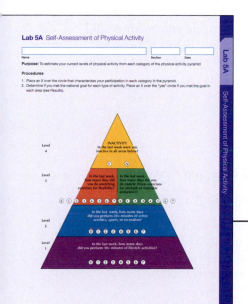

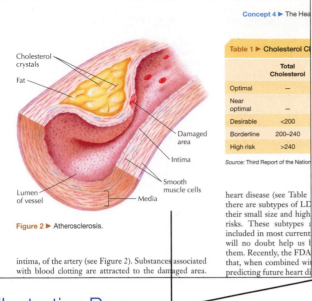

Cholesterol crystals

Fat

Damaged area

Intima

Smooth muscle cells

Lumen of vessel

Media

Figure 2 ▶ Atherosclerosis.

intima, of the artery (see Figure 2). Substances associated with blood clotting are attracted to the damaged area.

Table 1 ▶ Cholesterol C	
	Total Cholesterol
Optimal	—
Near optimal	—
Desirable	<200
Borderline	200–240
High risk	>240

Source: Third Report of the Natio

heart disease (see Table
there are subtypes of LD
their small size and high
risks. These subtypes a
included in most current
will no doubt help us b
them. Recently, the FDA
that, when combined wi
predicting future heart di

ally reached in the twenties
th age. Though muscular
re, it is not as dramatic as
gth. As people grow older,
th and muscular endurance
o train than people who do
ressive resistance training is
ring.

nalize the weaker person.
e endurance (the number of
nated number of pounds), a
antage. However, if you are
endurance (the number of
ated percentage of your max-
er person does not have an
hen and women can compete
cular endurance activities. In
ks, women have done as well
xample, the women at the
my do as well as the men on
endurance.

related to cardiovascular
e same thing. Cardiovascu-
h the efficiency of the heart
and respiratory system. It is
t stress these systems, such as
ming. Muscular endurance
of the local skeletal muscles
them. Most forms of cardio-

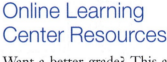
www.mhhe.com/corbin13e

When the thigh muscles (quadriceps) extend the knee they are the agonist (hamstrings = antagonist)

When the muscles on the back of thigh (hamstrings) flex the knee they are the agonist (quadriceps = antagonist)

Figure 2 ▶ Agonist and antagonist muscles.

the antagonist. If the quadriceps become too strong relative to the antagonist hamstring muscles, the risk for
injury increases (see Figure 2).

Illustration Program

Instructional full-color illustrations and photo-graphs here and throughout the book enhance learning with an exciting visual appeal.

On the Web

Web icons appear to indicate supplemental materials that are available on the Web. Look for the icons throughout your book. To access the information, sim-ply type the Web address provided next to the icon and you will be taken directly to the supplementary information.

Online Learning Center Resources

Want a better grade? This address appears throughout to remind you about the study aids and other resources available at our *Online Learning Center.*

Too much activity can lead to hyperkinetic conditions. The information presented in this con-cept points out the health benefits of physical activity performed in appropriate amounts. When done in excess or incorrectly, physical activity can result in **hyperkinetic conditions.** The most common hyper-

kinetic condition is overuse injury to muscles, connec-tive tissue, and bones. Recently, anorexia nervosa and body neurosis have been identified as conditions asso-ciated with inappropriate amounts of physical activity. These conditions will be discussed in the concept on performance.

Strategies for Action

A self-assessment of risk factors can help you modify your lifestyle to reduce risk for heart disease. www.mhhe.com/phys_fit/web04 Click 10. The Heart Disease Risk Factor Questionnaire in Lab 4A will help you assess your personal risk for heart disease. The questionnaire helps you to become aware of each of the risk factors for heart disease described in this concept. Although the questionnaire is educationally useful in making you aware of risk factors, it is not a substitute for a regular med-ical exam. When you have your regular physical exam, it would be wise to ask for a blood test, especially as you grow older or if your score on the questionnaire is high.

Selecting physical activities from the physical activity pyramid can help you achieve the health benefits described in this concept. The physical activity pyramid provides a conceptual model of the rela-tive importance of different types of physical activity. Subsequent concepts in the book will cover the different components of health-related fitness and the type and amount of activity needed to improve these components. The lab activities in each of these concepts and the cul-minating lab activity at the end of the book are designed to help you plan for lifelong physical activity.

Study Resources

Check out additional online study resources for this concept in the Student Edition of the Online Learning Center at www.mhhe.com/corbin13e.

Web Resources

American Cancer Society www.cancer.org
American Diabetes Association www.diabetes.org
American Heart Association www.americanheart.org
Canadian Diabetes Association www.diabetes.ca
Centers for Disease Control and Prevention www.cdc.gov
Healthy People 2010 www.health.gov/healthypeople
National Stroke Association www.stroke.org
National Osteoporosis Foundation www.nof.org

Suggested Readings

Additional reference materials for Concept 4 are available at www.mhhe.com/phys_fit/web04 Click 11.

Bassuk, S. S, and Manson, J. E. 2003. Physical activity and cardiovascular disease prevention in women: How much is good enough? *Exercise and Sport Sciences Reviews* 31(4):176–181.

Booth, F. W., and M. W. Chakravarthy. 2002. Cost and consequences of sedentary living: New battleground for an old enemy. *President's Council on Physical Fitness and Sports Research Digest* 3(16):1–8.
Brown, D. W., et al. 2004. Associations between physical activity dose and health-related quality of life. *Medi-cine and Science in Sports and Exercise* 36(5):890–896.
Carnethon, M. R., et al. 2003. Cardiorespiratory fitness of young adults and the development of cardiovascular disease risk factors. *Journal of the American Medical Association* 290(23):3092–3100.
Chintanadilok, J., and D. T. Lowenthal. 2002. Exercise in treating hypertension. *The Physician and Sportsmedi-cine* 30(3):11–28.
Cotman, C. W., and C. Engesser-Cesar. 2002. Exercise enhances and protects brain function. *Exercise and Sport Sciences Reviews* 30(2):75–79.
Drezner, J. A., and S. A. Herring. 2001. Managing low back pain. *Physician and Sportsmedicine* 29(8):37–43.
Dziura, J., et al. 2004. Physical activity reduces Type 2 dia-betes risk in aging independent of body weight change. *Journal of Physical Activity and Health* 1(1):19–28.

Hyperkinetic Conditions Diseases/illnesses or health conditions caused by, or contributed, to by too much physical activity.

Strategies for Action

Located toward the end of each concept, these strategies provide information and suggest labs that can help promote self-management skills to achieve your healthy lifestyle goals.

Web Resources and Suggested Readings

At the end of each concept, URLs help you find quality online resources. Recent references are provided to help you read more about current topics.

Health, Wellness, Fitness, and Healthy Lifestyles: An Introduction

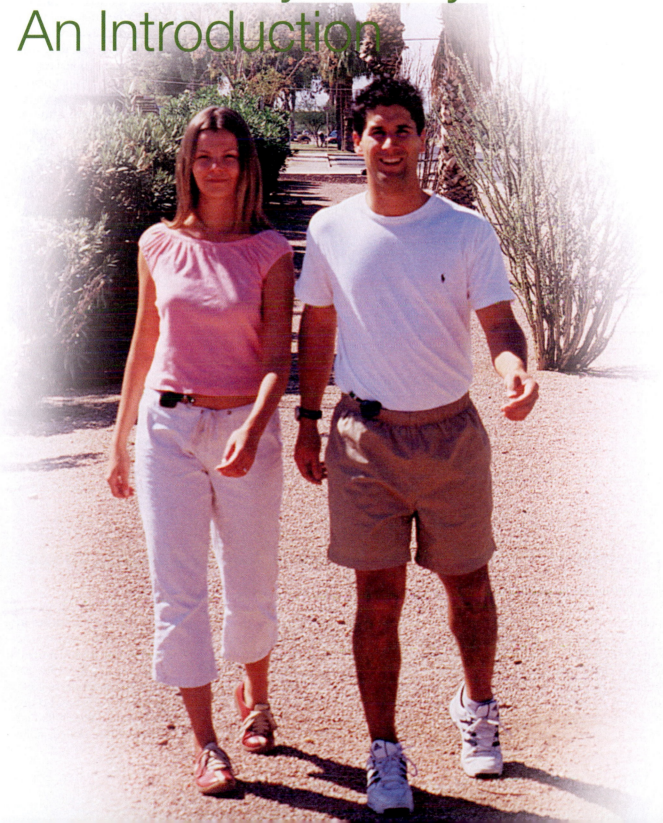

Good health, wellness, fitness, and healthy lifestyles are important for all people.

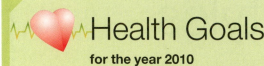

Health Goals
for the year 2010

- Increase quality and years of healthy life.
- Eliminate health disparities.
- Increase incidence of people reporting "healthy days."
- Increase access to health information and services for all people.

National Health Goals

At the beginning of each concept in this book is a section containing abbreviated statements of the national health goals from the document *Healthy People 2010: National Health Promotion and Disease Prevention Objectives*. These statements, established by expert groups representing more than 350 national organizations, are intended as realistic national health goals to be achieved by the year 2010. These objectives for the first decade of the new millennium are intended to improve the health of those in the United States, but they seem important for all people in North America and in other industrialized cultures throughout the world. The health objectives are designed to contribute to the current World Health Organization strategy of "Health for All." This book is written with the achievement of these important health goals in mind.

Introduction

 www.mhhe.com/phys_fit/web01 Click 01. The first national health goals were developed in 1979 to be accomplished by the year 1990. The focus of those objectives was on reduction in the death rate among infants, children, adolescents, young adults, and adults. Except for reducing death rates among adolescents, those goals were met and the average life expectancy was increased by more than 2 years by the 1990s. Those first national health objectives gave way to the *Healthy People 2000* objectives, designed to be accomplished by the turn of

the century. The emphasis in these objectives shifted from reduction in premature death to disease prevention and health promotion. While many of these objectives have been achieved, others have yet to be accomplished.

For *Healthy People 2010*, achieving the vision of "healthy people in healthy communities" is paramount. Two central goals have been established. First, the goals emphasize quality of life, well-being, and functional capacity—all important wellness considerations. This emphasis is based on the World Health Organization's focus on quality of life and its efforts to break down the artificial divisions between physical and mental well-being. Second, the national health goals for 2010 take the "bold step" of trying to "eliminate" health disparities as opposed to reducing them. Consistent with national health goals for the new millennium, this book is designed to aid all people in adopting healthy lifestyles that will allow them to achieve lifetime health, wellness, and fitness.

Technology Update
Internet Access

This book provides a number of ways to help you access reliable health and wellness information from the Internet. The *On the Web* icons throughout the book include URLs that provide additional information and links to informative sites on the Internet. The list of *Web Resources* at the end of each concept provide URLs for various organizations that provide high-quality health information. The *On the Web* and *Web Resources* features can be accessed electronically (without typing the URL) by visiting the Online Learning Center address that is featured at the top of every even-numbered page of the book. This site also includes a number of study aids, including concept outlines, concept terms, and sample quiz questions to help you apply the information in the book.

Health and Wellness

Good health is of primary importance to adults in our society. When polled about important social values, 99 percent of adults in the United States identified "being in good **health**" as one of their major concerns. The two other concerns expressed most often were good family life and good self-image. The 1 percent who did not identify good health as an important concern had no opinion on any social issues. Among those polled, none

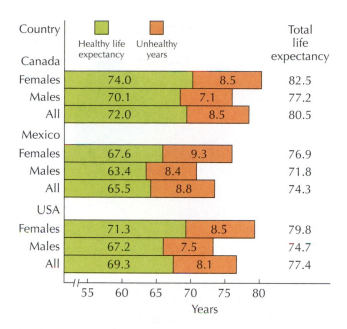

Figure 1 ▶ Healthy life expectancy for North America.

Sources: World Health Organization and National Center for Health Statistics.

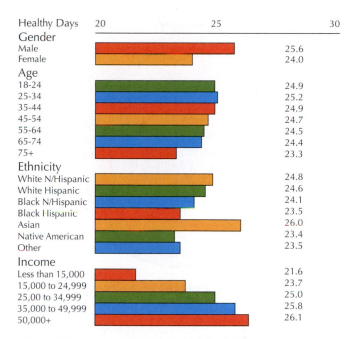

Figure 2 ▶ Healthy days from the past 30 by gender, age, income, and ethnicity.

Source: U.S. Department of Health and Human Services.

felt that good health was unimportant. Results of surveys in Canada and other Western nations show similar commitments to good health.

Increasing the span of healthy life is a principal health goal. www.mhhe.com/phys_fit/web01 Click 02.

The principal public health goal of Western nations is to increase the healthy life span of all individuals. Over the past 100 years the life expectancy for the average person has increased by 60 percent. Currently, life expectancy is at a record high of 77.4 for people in the United States. Increasing healthy life span means more than just living longer. It also means having fewer unhealthy years. Unhealthy years include those with illness, impaired function, and/or significantly reduced quality of life. Over the past decade the number of unhealthy years has decreased considerably from near 10 to approximately 8 years. African Americans, Hispanics, and Native Americans have a lower life expectancy and a greater number of unhealthy years than white non-Hispanics. As illustrated in Figure 1, life expectancy in North America is related to the country in which you live, with Canadians living the longest and those from Mexico having the lowest life expectancy. In all three countries, women have a greater life expectancy than men, though men typically have fewer unhealthy years.

Health varies greatly with income, gender, age, and ethnicity. Eliminating health disparities is the second major health goal as outlined in *Healthy People 2010*. One way to determine if health disparities exist is to compare groups based on the number of **healthy days** they experience each month. As illustrated in Figure 2, females, older

people, minority groups, and those with low income are likely to have relatively low numbers of healthy days. The relatively higher number of unhealthy days for women is, at least in part, because they live longer and for this reason have more unhealthy years late in life. Unhealthy days takes its biggest drop after age 75. Low income is one likely reason for health disparities among ethnic groups. Both physical and mental health problems are the most frequent reasons for unhealthy days. Physical illness, pain, depression, anxiety, sleeplessness, and limitations in ability to function or perform enjoyable activities are problems most frequently reported.

Health is more than freedom from illness and disease. Over 50 years ago, the World Health Organization defined health as more than freedom from illness, disease, and debilitating conditions. Prior to that time, you were considered to be "healthy" if you were not sick. In recent years, health experts have expanded the definition of

Health Optimal well-being that contributes to one's quality of life. It is more than freedom from disease and illness, though freedom from disease is important to good health. Optimal health includes high-level mental, social, emotional, spiritual, and physical wellness within the limits of one's heredity and personal abilities.

Healthy Days A self-rating of the number of days (per week or month) a person considers himself or herself to be in good or better than good health.

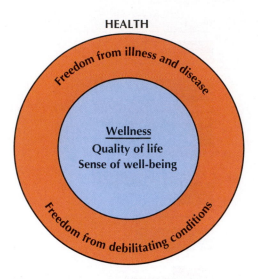

HEALTH

Freedom from illness and disease

Wellness
Quality of life
Sense of well-being

Freedom from debilitating conditions

Figure 3 ▶ A model of optimal health, including wellness.

health to include wellness as exemplified by "quality of life" and "a sense of well-being."

Figure 3 illustrates the modern concept of health. This general state of being is characterized by freedom from disease and debilitating conditions (outer circle) as well as wellness (center circle).

Wellness is the positive component of optimal health. Death, disease, **illness,** and debilitating conditions are negative components that detract from optimal health. Death is the ultimate opposite of optimal health. Disease, illness, and debilitating conditions obviously detract from optimal health. **Wellness** has been recognized as the positive component of optimal health, as evidenced by a sense of well-being reflected in optimal functioning, health-related **quality of life,** meaningful work, and a contribution to society. Wellness allows the expansion of one's potential to live and work effectively and to make a significant contribution to society. Healthy People 2010 objectives use the term health-related quality of life to describe a general sense of happiness and satisfaction with life.

Health and wellness are personal. Each individual is different from all others. Health and wellness depend on each person's individual characteristics. Making comparisons to other people on specific individual characteristics may produce feelings of inadequacy that detract from one's profile of total health and wellness. Each of us has personal limitations and personal strengths. Focusing on strengths and learning to accommodate weaknesses are essential keys to optimal health and wellness.

Health and wellness are multidimensional. The dimensions of health and wellness include the emotional (mental), intellectual, social, spiritual, and physical. Figure 4 illustrates the importance of each dimension to total wellness. Some people include environmental and voca-

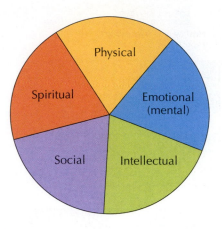

Figure 4 ▶ The dimensions of health and wellness.

tional dimensions in addition to the five described in Figure 4. In this book, health and wellness are considered to be personal factors. Environmental factors, including the factors in the vocational (work) environment, are considered to be factors that influence the five dimensions of personal wellness, rather than dimensions of personal wellness. For this reason, they are not included in Figure 4. Environmental factors do contribute significantly to personal health, wellness, and fitness and are discussed in detail in the final concept of this book. Throughout this book, references will be made to these wellness dimensions (see Tables 1 and 2) to help reinforce their importance.

Wellness reflects how one feels about life as well as one's ability to function effectively. A positive total outlook on life is essential to wellness and each of the wellness dimensions. A "well" person is satisfied in work, is spiritually fulfilled, enjoys leisure time, is physically fit, is socially involved, and has a positive emotional-mental outlook. This person is happy and fulfilled. Many experts believe that a positive total outlook is a key to wellness (see Table 2).

The way one perceives each of the dimensions of wellness affects total outlook. Researchers use the term *self-perceptions* to describe these feelings. Many researchers believe that self-perceptions about wellness are more important than actual ability. For example, a person who has an important job may find less meaning and job satisfaction than another person with a much less important job. Apparently, one of the important factors for a person who has achieved high-level wellness and a positive outlook on life is the ability to reward himself/herself. Some people, however, seem unable to give themselves credit for their successes. The development of a system that allows a person to perceive the self positively is important. Of course, the adoption of positive **lifestyles** that encourage improved self-perceptions is also important. The questionnaire in Lab 1A will help you assess your self-perceptions of the various wellness dimensions. For optimal wellness, it is important to find positive feelings about each dimension.

Table 1 ▶ Definitions of Health and Wellness Dimensions

Emotional-mental health—A person with emotional health (1) is free from emotional/mental illnesses or debilitating conditions, such as clinical depression, and (2) possesses emotional wellness. The goals for the nation's health refer to mental rather than emotional health and wellness. In this book, mental health and wellness are considered to be the same as emotional health and wellness.

Emotional/mental wellness—Emotional wellness is a person's ability to cope with daily circumstances and to deal with personal feelings in a positive, optimistic, and constructive manner. A person with emotional wellness is generally characterized as happy instead of depressed.

Intellectual health—A person with intellectual health is free from illnesses that invade the brain and other systems that allow learning. A person with intellectual health also possesses intellectual wellness.

Intellectual wellness—Intellectual wellness is a person's ability to learn and to use information to enhance the quality of daily living and optimal functioning. A person with intellectual wellness is generally characterized as informed instead of ignorant.

Physical health—A person with physical health is free from illnesses that affect the physiological systems of the body, such as the heart and the nervous system. A person with physical health possesses an adequate level of physical fitness and physical wellness.

Physical wellness—Physical wellness is a person's ability to function effectively in meeting the demands of the day's work and to use free time effectively. Physical wellness includes good physical fitness and the possession of useful motor skills. A person with physical wellness is generally characterized as fit instead of unfit.

Social health—A person with social health is free from illnesses or conditions that severely limit functioning in society, including antisocial pathologies.

Social wellness—Social wellness is a person's ability to interact with others successfully and to establish meaningful relationships that enhance the quality of life for all people involved in the interaction (including self). A person with social wellness is generally characterized as involved instead of lonely.

Spiritual health—Spiritual health is the one component of health that is totally comprised of the wellness dimension; for this reason, spiritual health is considered to be synonymous with spiritual wellness.

Spiritual wellness—Spiritual wellness is a person's ability to establish a values system and act on the system of beliefs, as well as to establish and carry out meaningful and constructive lifetime goals. Spiritual wellness is often based on a belief in a force greater than the individual that helps one contribute to an improved quality of life for all people. A person with spiritual wellness is generally characterized as fulfilled instead of unfulfilled.

P = Physical   I = Intellectual   Sp = Spiritual
S = Social   E = Emotional

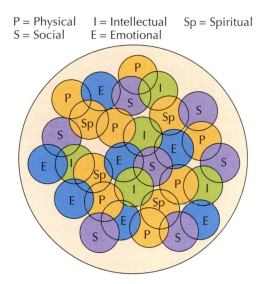

Figure 5 ▶ The integration of wellness dimensions.

Table 2 ▶ The Dimensions of Wellness

–	Wellness Dimensions	+
Depressed	Emotional-mental	Happy
Ignorant	Intellectual	Informed
Unfit	Physical	Fit
Lonely	Social	Involved
Unfulfilled	Spiritual	Fulfilled
Negative	Total outlook	Positive

Illness The ill feeling and/or symptoms associated with a disease or circumstances that upset homeostasis.

Wellness The integration of many different components (social, emotional-mental, spiritual, and physical) that expand one's potential to live (quality of life) and work effectively and to make a significant contribution to society. Wellness reflects how one feels (a sense of well-being) about life as well as one's ability to function effectively. Wellness, as opposed to illness (a negative), is sometimes described as the positive component of good health.

Quality of Life A term used to describe wellness. An individual with quality of life can enjoyably do the activities of life with little or no limitation and can function independently. Individual quality of life requires a pleasant and supportive community.

Lifestyles Patterns of behavior or ways an individual typically lives.

Health and wellness are integrated states of being.
The segmented pictures of health and wellness shown in Figure 4 and Tables 1 and 2 are used only to illustrate the multidimensional nature of health and wellness. In reality, health, and its positive component (wellness), is an integrated state of being that is best depicted as many threads that can be woven together to produce a larger, integrated fabric. Each specific dimension relates to each of the others and overlaps all others. The overlap is so frequent and so great that the specific contribution of each thread is almost indistinguishable when looking at the total (Figure 5). The total is clearly greater than the sum of the parts.

It is possible to possess health and wellness while being ill or possessing a debilitating condition. Many illnesses are curable and may have only a temporary effect on health. Others, such as Type I diabetes, are not curable but can be managed with proper eating, physical activity, and sound medical treatment. Those with manageable conditions may, however, be at risk for other health problems. For example, unmanaged diabetes is associated with a high risk for heart disease and other health problems.

Debilitating conditions, such as the loss of a limb or loss of function in a body part, can contribute to a lower level of functioning or an increased risk for illness and thus to poor health. On the other hand, such conditions need not necessarily limit one's wellness. As will be explained later in this concept, a person with a debilitating condition who has a positive outlook on life may have better overall health than a person with a poor outlook on life but with no debilitating condition.

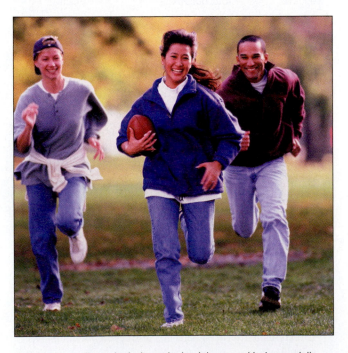

Possessing wellness includes enjoying leisure and being socially involved.

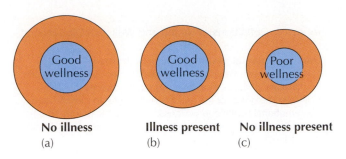

Figure 6 ▶ Wellness need not be limited by illness.

Just as wellness is possible among those with illness and disability, evidence is accumulating to indicate that people with a positive outlook are better able to resist the progress of disease and illness than are those with a negative outlook. Thinking positive thoughts has been associated with enhanced results from various medical treatments and better results from surgical procedures.

Figure 6 illustrates the fact that the most desirable condition is buoyant health (*a*), including freedom from illness and a high level of wellness. However, a person with a physical illness but who possesses a good wellness (*b*) has a better overall health status than a person with no illness but poor wellness (*c*).

Wellness is a useful term that may be used by quacks as well as experts. www.mhhe.com/phys_fit/web01 Click 03. Unfortunately, some individuals and groups have tried to identify wellness with products and services that promise benefits that cannot be documented. Because well-being is a subjective feeling it is easy for quacks to make claims of improved wellness for their product or service without facts to back them up.

Holistic health is a term that is similarly abused. Optimal health includes many areas; thus, the term *holistic* (total) is appropriate. In fact, the word *health* originates from a root word meaning "wholeness." Unfortunately, many quacks include their questionable health practices under the guise of holistic health. Care should be used when considering services and products that make claims of wellness and/or holistic health to be sure that they are legitimate.

Physical Fitness

Physical fitness is a multidimensional state of being. **Physical fitness** is the body's ability to function efficiently and effectively. It is a state of being that consists of at least five health-related and six skill-related physical fitness components, each of which contributes to total quality of life. Physical fitness is associated with a person's ability to work effectively, enjoy leisure time, be healthy, resist **hypokinetic diseases or conditions**, and meet emergency situations. It is related to, but different from, health and wellness. Although the development of physical fitness is the result of many things, optimal physical fitness is not possible without regular physical activity.

The health-related components of physical fitness are directly associated with good health. The five components of health-related physical fitness are body composition, cardiovascular fitness, flexibility, muscular endurance, and strength (see Figure 7). Each health-related fitness characteristic has a direct relationship to good health and reduced risk for hypokinetic disease. It is for this reason that the five health-related physical fitness components are emphasized in this book.

Possessing a moderate amount of each component of health-related fitness is essential to disease prevention and health promotion, but it is not essential to have exceptionally high levels of fitness to achieve health benefits. High levels of health-related fitness relate more to performance than to health benefits. For example, moderate amounts of strength are necessary to prevent back and posture problems, whereas high levels of strength contribute most to improved performance in activities such as football and jobs involving heavy lifting.

The skill-related components of physical fitness are more associated with performance than with good health. The components of skill-related physical fitness are agility, balance, coordination, power, reaction time, and speed (see Figure 8). They are called skill-related because people who possess them find it easy to achieve high levels of performance in motor skills, such as those required in sports and in specific types of jobs. Power is sometimes referred to as a combined component of fitness, since it requires both strength (a health-related component) and speed (a skill-related component). Because power is considered by most experts to be more associated with performance than with good health, it is classified as a skill-related component of fitness in this book. Skill-related fitness is sometimes called sports fitness or motor fitness.

There is little doubt that other abilities could be classified as skill-related fitness components. Also, each part of skill-related fitness is multidimensional. For example, coordination could be hand-eye coordination, such as batting a ball; foot-eye coordination, such as kicking a ball; or any of many other possibilities. The six parts of skill-related fitness identified here are those commonly associated with successful sports and work performance. It should be noted that each could be measured in ways other than those presented in this book. Measurements are provided to help you understand the nature of total physical fitness and to help you make important decisions about lifetime physical activity.

Metabolic fitness is a nonperformance component of total fitness. Physical activity can provide health benefits that are independent of changes in traditional health-related fitness measures. Physical activity promotes good **metabolic fitness;** a state associated with reduced risk for many chronic diseases. It is characterized by healthy blood fat levels, blood pressure, and blood sugar and insulin levels, as well as healthy body fatness. Individuals with poor metabolic fitness tend to exhibit high LDL (bad cholesterol), low HDL (good cholesterol), high triglycerides, high blood pressure, high blood sugar levels, and a large waist girth. The tendency of these risks to cluster together has led scientists to refer to this condition as the *metabolic syndrome* (also known as Syndrome X, or insulin resistance syndrome). Because physical inactivity is related to all of these conditions, some experts include it as part of the metabolic syndrome.

Bone integrity is often considered to be a nonperformance measure of fitness. Traditional definitions do not include **bone integrity** as a part of physical fitness, but

Physical Fitness The body's ability to function efficiently and effectively. It consists of health-related physical fitness and skill-related physical fitness, which have at least eleven components, each of which contributes to total quality of life. Physical fitness also includes metabolic fitness and bone integrity. Physical fitness is associated with a person's ability to work effectively, enjoy leisure time, be healthy, resist hypokinetic diseases, and meet emergency situations. It is related to, but different from, health, wellness, and the psychological, sociological, emotional, and spiritual components of fitness. Although the development of physical fitness is the result of many things, optimal physical fitness is not possible without regular exercise.

Hypokinetic Diseases or Conditions *Hypo-* means "under" or "too little," and *-kinetic* means "movement" or "activity." Thus, *hypokinetic* means "too little activity." A hypokinetic disease or condition is one associated with lack of physical activity or too little regular exercise. Examples include heart disease, low back pain, adult-onset diabetes, and obesity.

Metabolic Fitness Metabolic fitness is a positive state of the physiological systems commonly associated with reduced risk for chronic diseases such as diabetes and heart disease. Metabolic fitness is evidenced by healthy blood fat (lipid) profiles, healthy blood pressure, healthy blood sugar and insulin levels, and other nonperformance measures.

Bone Integrity Soundness of the bones is associated with high density and absence of symptoms of deterioration.

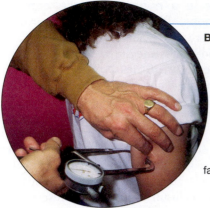

Body composition— The relative percentage of muscle, fat, bone, and other tissues that comprise the body. A fit person has a relatively low, but not too low, percentage of body fat (body fatness).

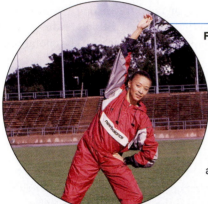

Flexibility—The range of motion available in a joint. It is affected by muscle length, joint structure, and other factors. A fit person can move the body joints through a full range of motion in work and in play.

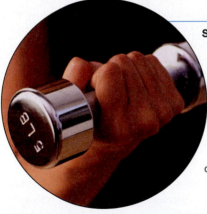

Strength—The ability of the muscles to exert an external force or to lift a heavy weight. A fit person can do work or play that involves exerting force, such as lifting or controlling one's own body weight.

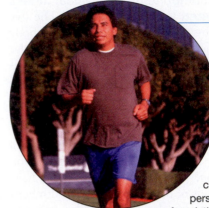

Cardiovascular fitness—The ability of the heart, blood vessels, blood, and respiratory system to supply fuel and oxygen to the muscles and the ability of the muscles to utilize fuel to allow sustained exercise. A fit person can persist in physical activity for relatively long periods without undue stress.

Muscular endurance—The ability of the muscles to exert themselves repeatedly. A fit person can repeat movements for a long period without undue fatigue.

Figure 7 ▶ Components of health-related physical fitness.

some experts feel that it should be. Like metabolic fitness, bone integrity cannot be assessed with performance measures as can most health-related fitness parts. Regardless of whether it is considered as a part of fitness or a component of health, there is little doubt that strong, healthy bones are important to optimal health and are associated with regular physical activity and sound diet.

The many components of physical fitness are specific but are also interrelated. Physical fitness is a combination of several aspects, rather than a single char-

acteristic. A fit person possesses at least adequate levels of each of the health-related, skill-related, and metabolic fitness components. People who possess one aspect of physical fitness do not necessarily possess the other aspects.

Some relationships exist among different fitness characteristics, but each of the components of physical fitness is separate and different from the others. For example, people who possess exceptional strength do not necessarily have good cardiovascular fitness, and those who have good coordination do not necessarily possess good flexibility. Lab 1B is designed to help you distinguish among the different parts of health-related and skill-related physical fitness. A separate questionnaire helps you estimate your current fitness levels.

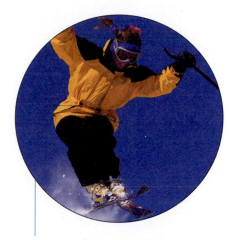

Agility—The ability to rapidly and accurately change the direction of the movement of the entire body in space. Skiing and wrestling are examples of activities that require exceptional agility.

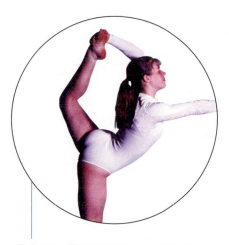

Balance—The maintenance of equilibrium while stationary or while moving. Water skiing, performing on the balance beam, or working as a riveter on a high-rise building are activities that require exceptional balance.

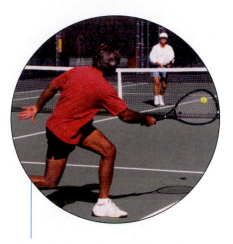

Coordination—The ability to use the senses with the body parts to perform motor tasks smoothly and accurately. Juggling, hitting a tennis ball, batting a baseball, or kicking a ball are examples of activities requiring good coordination.

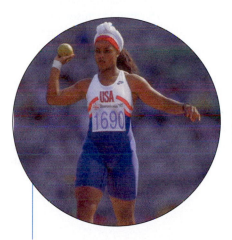

Power—The ability to transfer energy into force at a fast rate. Throwing the discus and putting the shot are activities that require considerable power.

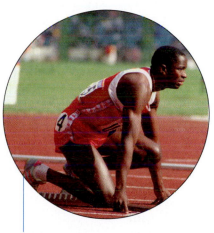

Reaction time—The time elapsed between stimulation and the beginning of reaction to that stimulation. Driving a racing car and starting a sprint race require good reaction time.

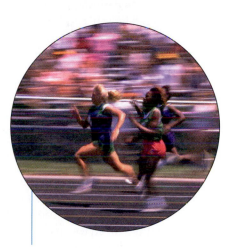

Speed—The ability to perform a movement in a short period of time. A runner on a track team or a wide receiver on a football team needs good foot and leg speed.

Figure 8 ▶ Components of skill-related physical fitness.

Good physical fitness is important, but it is not the same as physical health and wellness. Good physical fitness contributes directly to the physical component of good health and wellness and indirectly to the other four components. Good fitness has been shown to be associated with reduced risk for chronic diseases, such as heart disease, and has been shown to reduce the consequences of many debilitating conditions. In addition, good fitness contributes to wellness by helping us look our best, feel good, and enjoy life. Other physical factors can also influence health and wellness. For example, having good physical skills enhances quality of life by allowing us to participate in enjoyable activities, such as tennis, golf, and bowling. Although fitness can assist in performing these activities, regular practice is also necessary. Another example is the ability to fight off viral and bacterial infections. Although fitness can promote a strong immune system, other physical factors can influence our susceptibility to these and other conditions.

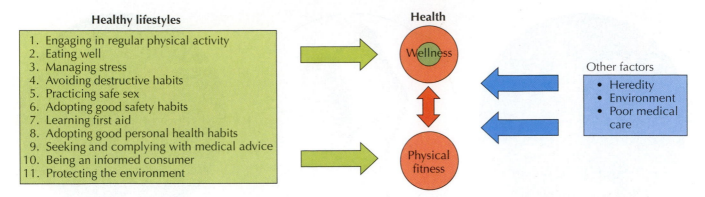

Figure 9 ▶ Factors influencing health, wellness, and physical fitness.

For optimal health and wellness, it is important to have good physical fitness *and* physical wellness. It is also important to strive for good emotional-mental, social, spiritual, and intellectual health and wellness. Each of the healthy lifestyles described in Figure 9 will be discussed in greater detail later in this book.

Healthy Lifestyles

🌐 **Lifestyle change, more than any other factor, is considered to be the best way of preventing illness and early death in our society.** www.mhhe.com/phys_fit/web01 Click 04. When people in Western society die before the age of sixty-five, the death is considered to be premature. The most important factors contributing to early death are unhealthy lifestyles. Based on the "leading health indicators" in *Healthy People 2010*, eleven healthy lifestyles have been associated with reduced disease risk and increased wellness. As shown in Figure 9, these lifestyles affect health, wellness, and physical fitness. The double-headed arrow between health/wellness and physical fitness illustrates the interaction between these factors. Physical fitness is important to health and wellness development and vice versa. Other factors, some not as much in your control as healthy lifestyles, also affect your health, fitness, and wellness. These factors include environmental factors (e.g., pollution, contaminants in the workplace), human biology (inherited conditions), and inadequacies in the health-care system, to name but a few.

🌐 **The major causes of early death have shifted from infectious diseases to chronic lifestyle-related conditions.** www.mhhe.com/phys_fit/web01 Click 05. Scientific advances and improvements in medicine and health care have dramatically reduced the incidence of infectious diseases over the past 100 years (see Table 3). Diptheria and polio, both major causes of death in the 20th century, have been virtually eliminated in Western culture. Smallpox was globally eradicated in 1977.

Infectious diseases have been replaced with chronic lifestyle-related conditions as the major causes of death. Four of the top six (heart disease, cancer, stroke, and diabetes) fall into this category. The good news is that there were significant reductions in death rates from the top three causes of death over the past decade. HIV/AIDS, formerly in the top ten, has dropped well down the list, primarily because of the development of treatments to increase the life expectancy of those infected. Many among the top 10 are referred to as chronic lifestyle-related conditions because alteration of lifestyles can result in reduced risk for these conditions.

Table 3 ▶ Major Causes of Death

Current Rank	Cause	1900 Rank	Cause
1.	Heart disease	1.	Pneumonia
2.	Cancer	2.	Tuberculosis
3.	Stroke	3.	Diarrhea/enteritis
4.	Bronchitis/emphysema	4.	Heart disease
5.	Injuries/accidents	5.	Stroke
6.	Diabetes	6.	Liver disease
7.	Pneumonia/influenza	7.	Injuries
8.	Alzheimer's disease	8.	Cancer
9.	Kidney disease	9.	Senility
10.	Septicemia	10.	Diphtheria

Source: National Center for Health Statistics.

Healthy lifestyles are critical to wellness. Just as unhealthy lifestyles are the principal causes of modern-day illnesses, such as heart disease, cancer, and diabetes, healthy lifestyles can result in an improved feeling of wellness that is critical to optimal health. In recognizing the importance of "years of healthy life," the Public Health Service also recognizes what it calls "measures of well-being." This well-being, or wellness, is associated with social, mental, spiritual, and physical functioning. Being physically active and eating well are two examples of healthy lifestyles that can improve well-being and add years of quality living. Many of the healthy lifestyles associated with good physical fitness and optimal wellness will be discussed in detail later in this book. The Healthy Lifestyle Questionnaire at the end of this concept gives you the opportunity to assess your current lifestyles.

Regular physical activity, sound nutrition, and stress management are considered to be priority healthy lifestyles. Three of the lifestyles listed in Figure 9 are considered to be priority healthy lifestyles. These are engaging in regular **physical activity** or **exercise,** eating well, and managing stress. There are several reasons for placing priority on these lifestyles. First, they affect the lives of all people. Second, they are lifestyles in which large numbers of people can make improvement. Finally, modest changes in these behaviors can make dramatic improvements in individual and public health. For example, statistics suggest that modest changes in physical activity patterns and nutrition can prevent more than 400,000 deaths annually. Stress also has a major impact on drug, alcohol, and smoking behavior, so managing stress can help individuals minimize or avoid those behaviors.

The other healthy lifestyles shown in Figure 9 are also very important for good health. The reason that they are not emphasized as priority lifestyles is that not all people have problems in these areas. Many healthy lifestyles will be discussed in this book, but the focus is on the priority healthy lifestyles because virtually all people can achieve positive wellness benefits if they adopt them.

The "actual causes" of most deaths are due to unhealthy lifestyles. Many of the leading causes of death listed in Table 3 can be attributed, in large part, to unhealthy lifestyles. Public health experts have used epidemiological statistics to provide listings of the "actual causes of death" (factors that lead to the direct causes). Tobacco is the leading cause of actual death but inactivity and poor diet account for the next largest percentage of deaths (see Table 4). The actual percentage of deaths attributed to inactivity and poor diet have recently been questioned but their overall influence on health is indisputable. The information presented throughout this book is designed to help you change behaviors to reduce

Table 4 ▶ Actual Causes of Death in the United States		
Rank	**Actual Cause**	**Percent of Deaths**
1.	Tobacco use	18.1
2.	Inactivity/poor diet	16.6
3.	Alcohol consumption	3.5
4.	Microbial agents (flu, pneumonia)	3.1
5.	Toxic agents	2.3
6.	Motor vehicles	1.8
7.	Firearms	1.2
8.	Sexual behavior	0.8
9.	Illicit drug use	0.7
10.	Other	<0.5

Source: Mokdad, et al., 2004.

risk for early death from the actual causes outlined in Table 4.

The HELP Philosophy

The HELP philosophy can provide a basis for making healthy lifestyle change possible. The four-letter acronym *HELP* summarizes the overall philosophy used in the book. Each letter in the word *HELP* characterizes an important part of the philosophy (*Health* is available to *Everyone* for a *Lifetime*—and it's *Personal*). The concepts in the book provide important principles and guidelines that help you adopt positive lifestyles. The lab experiences provide experiences that build the behavioral skills needed to learn and maintain these lifestyles.

A personal philosophy that emphasizes health can lead to behaviors that promote it. The *H* in HELP stands for *health.* One theory that has been extensively tested indicates that people who believe in the benefits of healthy lifestyles are more likely to

Physical Activity Generally considered to be a broad term used to describe all forms of large muscle movements, including sports, dance, games, work, lifestyle activities, and exercise for fitness. In this book, exercise and physical activity will often be used interchangeably to make reading less repetitive and more interesting.

Exercise Physical activity done for the purpose of getting physically fit.

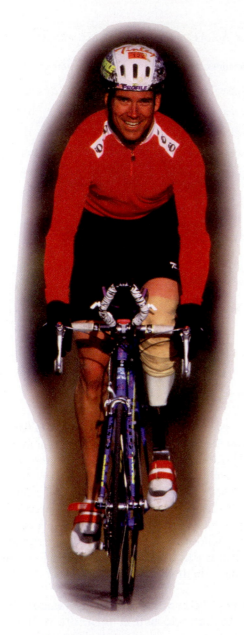

Physical activity is for everyone.

engage in healthy behaviors. The theory also suggests that people who state intentions to put their beliefs in action are likely to adopt behaviors that lead to health, wellness, and fitness.

Everyone can benefit from healthy lifestyles. The *E* in HELP stands for *everyone*. Accepting the fact that anyone can change a behavior or lifestyle means that *you* are included. Nevertheless, many adults feel ineffective in making lifestyle changes. Physical activity is not just for athletes—it is for all people. Eating well is not just for other people—you can do it, too. All people can learn stress-management techniques. Healthy lifestyles can be practiced by everyone. As noted earlier in this concept, important health goals include eliminating health disparities and promoting "Health for All."

Healthy behaviors are most effective when practiced for a lifetime. The *L* in HELP stands for *lifetime*. Young people sometimes feel immortal because the harmful effects of unhealthy lifestyles are often not immediate. As we grow older, we begin to realize that we are not immortal and that unhealthy lifestyles have cumulative negative effects. Starting early in life to emphasize healthy behaviors results in long-term health, wellness, and fitness benefits. One study showed that, the longer healthy lifestyles are practiced, the greater the beneficial effects. This study also demonstrated that long-term healthy lifestyles can even overcome hereditary predisposition to illness and disease.

Healthy lifestyles should be based on personal needs. The *P* in HELP stands for *personal*. No two people are exactly alike. Just as no single pill cures all illnesses, no single lifestyle prescription exists for good health, wellness, and fitness. Each person must assess personal needs and make lifestyle changes based on those needs.

 Strategies for Action

Self-assessments of lifestyles will help you determine areas in which you may need changes to promote optimal health, wellness, and fitness. As you begin your study of health, wellness, fitness, and healthy lifestyles, it is wise to make a self-assessment of your current behaviors. The Healthy Lifestyle Questionnaire in the lab resource materials will allow you to assess your current lifestyle behaviors to determine if they are contributing positively to your health, wellness, and fitness. Because this questionnaire contains some very personal

information, answering all the questions honestly will help you get an accurate assessment. As you continue your study, you may want to refer back to this questionnaire to see if your lifestyles have changed.

Initial self-assessments of wellness and fitness will provide information for self-comparison. www.mhhe.com/phys_fit/web01 Click 06. The Healthy Lifestyle Questionnaire allows you to assess your lifestyles or behaviors. It is also important to assess your wellness and fitness at an early stage. These early assessments will only be estimates. As you continue your study, you will have the opportunity to do more comprehensive self-assessments that will allow you to see how accurate your early estimates were.

In Lab 1A, you will estimate your wellness using a Wellness Self-Perceptions Questionnaire, which assesses five wellness dimensions. Remember, wellness is a state of being that is influenced by healthy lifestyles. Because other factors such as heredity, environment, and health care affect wellness, it is possible to have good wellness scores even if you do not do well on the lifestyle questionnaire. However, over a lifetime, unhealthy lifestyles will catch up with you and have an influence on your wellness and fitness.

Lab 1B allows you to get a better understanding of the components of health-related and skill-related physical fitness. You will perform some simple stunts to help you distinguish among the different fitness parts. You can use these as a basis for estimating your current fitness levels. Later, you will use more accurate tests to get a good

assessment of your fitness. Like wellness, fitness is a state of being that is influenced by healthy lifestyles, especially regular physical activity. Some young people have relatively good fitness—especially skill-related fitness—even if they have not been doing regular activity. Over a lifetime, inactivity greatly influences your fitness.

The World Health Organization (WHO) has developed a wellness instrument called the WHO Quality of Life Assessment (WHOQOL). There is a long version, with 100 items, and a shorter, 16-item version that assess physical, psychological, social, and spiritual factors, as well as general quality of life status. Some of the factors in the assessment include energy and fatigue, pain and comfort, sleep and rest, self-esteem, work capacity, effective daily living, personal relationships, and spirituality. You can learn more about this assessment by accessing the WHO website (see *Web Resources*) and searching for WHOQOL. You can also access it directly through the "On the Web" resource (www.mhhe.com/phys_fit/web01 Click 06).

Study Resources

Check out additional online study resources for this concept in the Student Edition of the Online Learning Center at www.mhhe.com/corbin13e.

Web Resources

American Medical Association (AMA) **www.ama-assn.org**
Centers for Disease Control and Prevention (CDC)
   www.cdc.gov
Health Canada **www.healthcanada.ca**
Healthfinder **www.healthfinder.gov**
Healthy People 2010 **www.health.gov/healthypeople**
National Center for Chronic Disease Prevention and Health Promotion Publications **www.cdc.gov/nccdphp/publicat.htm**
National Center for Health Statistics **www.cdc.gov/nchs/**
President's Council on Physical Fitness and Sports
   www.fitness.gov
World Health Organization **www.who.int**

Suggested Readings

Additional reference materials for Concept 1 are available at **www.mhhe.com/phys_fit/web01 Click 07.**

Blair, S. N., et al. 2001. *Active Living Every Day.* Champaign, IL: Human Kinetics.

*Booth, F. W., and M. V. Chakravarthy. 2002. Cost and consequences of sedentary living: New battleground

for an old enemy. *President's Council on Physical Fitness and Sports Research Digest* 3(16):1–8.

Brown, D. W., et al. Associations between physical activity dose and health-related quality of life. *Medicine and Science in Sports and Exercise* 36(5):890–896.

Centers for Disease Control and Prevention. 2000. *Measuring Healthy Days.* Atlanta: CDC.

Centers for Disease Control and Prevention. 2000. Ten great public health accomplishments—United States. *Morbidity and Mortality Weekly Reports* 48(12): 241–243. Also available at **www.cdc.gov.**

*Corbin, C. B., and R. P. Pangrazi. 2001. Toward a uniform definition of wellness: A commentary. *President's Council on Physical Fitness and Sports Research Digest* 3(15):1–8.

*Corbin, C. B., R. P. Pangrazi, and B. D. Franks. 2000. Definitions: Health, fitness, and physical activity. *President's Council on Physical Fitness and Sports Research Digest* 3(9):1–8.

Lakka, T. A., et al. 2003. Sedentary lifestyle, poor cardiorespiratory fitness, and the metabolic syndrome. *Medicine and Science in Sports and Exercise* 35(8):1279–1286.

Mokdad, A. H., et al. 2004. Actual causes of death in the United States. *Journal of the American Medical Association* 291(10):1238–1246.

Noonan, P. J. 2004. Do you suffer from Syndrome X? *USA Weekend* (April):23–35.

Payne, W. A., and D. B. Hahn. 2005. *Understanding Your Health.* 8th ed. St. Louis: McGraw-Hill.

Ropeik, D., and G. Gray. 2002. *Risk: A Practical Guide for Deciding What's Really Safe and What's Really Dangerous in the World around Us.* Boston: Houghton Mifflin.

Sanmartin, C., et al. 2004. *Joint Canada/United States Survey of Health, 2002–2003.* Atlanta, GA: Centers for Disease Control and Prevention.

U.S. Department of Health and Human Services. 1996. *Physical Activity and Health: A Report of the Surgeon General.* Atlanta: U.S. Department of Health and Human Services.

U.S. Department of Health and Human Services. Nov. 2000. *Healthy People 2010.* 2nd ed. With *Understanding and Improving Health* and *Objectives for Improving Health.* 2 vols. Washington, DC: U.S. Government Printing Office.

Valois, R. F., et al. 2004. Physical activity behaviors and perceived life satisfaction among public high school adolescents. *Journal of School Health* 74(2):59–65.

World Health Organization. 2003. *Poverty and Health.* Geneva, Switzerland: WHO.

World Health Organization. 2004. *World Health Report 2003: Shaping the Future.* Geneva: WHO (available on the web at http://www.who.int/whr/2003/en/).

*Also available at www.fitness.gov.

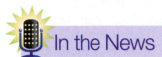

In the News

Health, Wellness, and Fitness: The Good News

Reports of bad news are common in the media. The tragic events of September 11, 2001; the horrors of ongoing wars; and the continuing threat of terrorism have added considerable stress to our lives. These events also cause us all to pause and consider what is truly important in our lives. The importance of family, friends, good health, and personal safety are certainly high on most people's list of priorities. It is our hope that the information in this book will help you to focus on wellness and quality of life issues that are important to you, your friends, and your loved ones.

The reports of bad news in the media may lead some people to conclude that events are out of our personal control. However, information from a variety of recent studies indicates that there is considerable good news about health, wellness, and fitness. In particular, it is clear that adopting healthy lifestyles can make a major difference in health and contribute to a higher quality of life. One recent study (see Brown et al., 2004) demonstrated that adults meeting the recommended guidelines for physical activity were more likely to report fewer unhealthy days and to have higher health-related quality of life, compared with people not meeting the guidelines. A similar study on adolescents (see Valois et al., 2004) indicated that youth that were not actively involved in physical activity had reduced life satisfaction (assessed through a validated survey known as the Student Life Satisfaction Scale). These results confirm that an active lifestyle is associated with a higher health-related quality of life. The following are some other positive trends in health and health care.

- Life expectancy is currently at an all-time high (see Figure 2).
- Most people in the United States (85 percent) and Canada (88 percent) report having good, very good, or excellent health. One in four reports having excellent health in both countries.
- The incidence of major killers has decreased in the past five years including heart disease (–3 percent), cancer (–1 percent), stroke (–3 percent), accidents (–2 percent), and HIV (–2 percent).
- Medical care, for those who seek it and can afford it, is better than at any time in history.
- More adults have had exams, such as mammograms, than in previous decades.
- Death rates from automobile injuries have fallen primarily because new cars are safer than ever before and more people wear seat belts than in the past.
- Infant mortality rates have fallen by 75 percent since 1950.
- Youth deaths (12 months to 24 years) have decreased 50 percent since 1950.
- Eighty-one percent of adults rate their personal health as good or excellent.
- More than 78 percent of adults are satisfied with their standard of living.
- Health and fitness club membership increased 100 percent from 1980 to 1990 and 63 percent to the present.
- Over 50 percent of all adults own home exercise equipment.
- We have more vacation time than previous generations.
- Smoking has decreased by 50 percent over the past five decades.

The 20th century produced many great achievements in health. The Centers for Disease Control and Prevention (CDC) recently identified ten major achievements, including vaccinations, safer workplaces, safer and healthier foods, and decline in heart disease deaths to name but a few. Evidence suggests many similar positive developments will occur this new century.

This "good news" provides optimism that we can overcome threats to our safety and health and make progress in meeting national health goals outlined in this book. We have placed special emphasis on the *Healthy People 2010* vision of helping "us all to make healthy lifestyle choices for ourselves and our families." For more details see "On the Web" feature for this concept (www.mhhe.com/phys_fit/web01 Click 02).

Lab Resource Materials: The Healthy Lifestyle Questionnaire

The purpose of this questionnaire is to help you analyze your lifestyle behaviors and to help you make decisions concerning good health and wellness for the future. Information on this Healthy Lifestyle Questionnaire is of a personal nature. For this reason, this questionnaire is not designed to be submitted to your instructor. It is for your information only. Answer each question as honestly as possible and use the scoring information to help you assess your lifestyle.

Directions: Place an X over the "yes" circle to answer yes. If you answer "no," make no mark. Score the questionnaire using the procedures that follow.

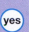 1. I accumulate 30 minutes of moderate physical activity most days of the week (brisk walking, stair climbing, yard work, or home chores).

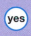 2. I do vigorous activity that elevates my heart rate for 20 minutes at least 3 days a week.

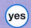 3. I do exercises for flexibility at least 3 days a week.

 4. I do exercises for muscle fitness at least 2 days a week.

 5. I eat three regular meals each day.

 6. I select appropriate servings from the food guide pyramid each day.

 7. I restrict the amount of fat in my diet.

 8. I consume only as many calories as I expend each day.

 9. I am able to identify situations in daily life that cause stress.

 10. I take time out during the day to relax and recover from daily stress.

 11. I find time for family, friends, and things I especially enjoy doing.

 12. I regularly perform exercises designed to relieve tension.

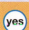 13. I do not smoke or use other tobacco products.

 14. I do not abuse alcohol.

 15. I do not abuse drugs (prescription or illegal).

 16. I take over-the-counter drugs sparingly and use them only according to directions.

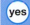 17. I abstain from sex or limit sexual activity to a safe partner.

 18. I practice safe procedures for avoiding sexually transmitted diseases (STDs).

 19. I use seat belts and adhere to the speed limit when I drive.

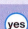 20. I have a smoke detector in my house and check it regularly to see that it is working.

 21. I have had training to perform CPR if called on in an emergency.

 22. I can perform the Heimlich maneuver effectively if called on in an emergency.

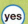 23. I brush my teeth at least two times a day and floss at least once a day.

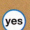 24. I get an adequate amount of sleep each night.

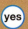 25. I do regular self-exams, have regular medical checkups, and seek medical advice when symptoms are present.

 26. When I receive advice and/or medication from a physician, I follow the advice and take the medication as prescribed.

 27. I read product labels and investigate their effectiveness before I buy them.

 28. I avoid using products that have not been shown by research to be effective.

 29. I recycle paper, glass, and aluminum.

30. I practice environmental protection, such as carpooling and energy conservation.

 Overall Score—Total Yes Answers

Scoring: Give yourself 1 point for each yes answer. Add your scores for each of the lifestyle behaviors. To calculate your overall score, sum the totals for all lifestyles.

Physical Activity	Nutrition	Managing Stress	Avoiding Destructive Habits	Practicing Safe Sex	Adopting Safety Habits
1. ☐	5. ☐	9. ☐	13. ☐	17. ☐	19. ☐
2. ☐	6. ☐	10. ☐	14. ☐	18. ☐	20. ☐
3. ☐	7. ☐	11. ☐	15. ☐		
4. ☐	8. ☐	12. ☐	16. ☐		
☐ Total +	☐ Total +	☐ Total +	☐ Total +	☐ Total +	☐

Knowing First Aid	Personal Health Habits	Using Medical Advice	Being an Informed Customer	Protecting the Environment	Sum All Totals for Overall Score
21. ☐	23. ☐	25. ☐	27. ☐	29. ☐	
22. ☐	24. ☐	26. ☐	28. ☐	30. ☐	
☐ Total +	☐ Total +	☐ Total +	☐ Total +	☐ Total =	☐

Interpreting Scores: Scores of 3 or 4 on the four-item scales are indicative of generally positive lifestyles. For the two-item scales, a score of 2 indicates the presence of positive lifestyles. An overall score of 26 or more is a good indicator of healthy lifestyle behaviors. It is important to consider the following special note when interpreting scores.

Special Note: Your scores on the Healthy Lifestyle Questionnaire should be interpreted with caution. There are several reasons for this. First, all lifestyle behaviors do not pose the same risks. For example, using tobacco or abusing drugs has immediate negative effects on health and wellness, whereas others, such as knowing first aid, may have only occasional use. Second, you may score well on one item in a scale but not on another. If one item indicates an unhealthy lifestyle in an area that poses a serious health risk, your lifestyle may appear to be healthier than it really is. For example, you could get a score of 3 on the destructive habits scale and be a regular smoker. For this reason, the overall score can be particularly deceiving.

Strategies for Change: In the space below, you may want to make some notes concerning the healthy lifestyle areas in which you could make some changes. You can refer to these notes later to see if you have made progress.

Lab 1A Wellness Self-Perceptions

Name	**Section**	**Date**

Purpose: To assess self-perceptions of wellness

Procedures

1. Place an X over the appropriate circle for each question (4 = strongly agree, 3 = agree, 2 = disagree, 1 = strongly disagree).
2. Write the number found in that circle in the box to the right.
3. Sum the three boxes for each wellness dimension to get your wellness dimension totals.
4. Sum all wellness dimension totals to get your comprehensive wellness total.
5. Use the rating chart to rate each wellness area.
6. Complete the Results section and the Conclusions and Implications section.

Question	Strongly Agree	Agree	Disagree	Strongly Disagree	Score
1. I am happy most of the time.	4	3	2	1	
2. I have good self-esteem.	4	3	2	1	
3. I do not generally feel stressed.	4	3	2	1	
			Emotional Wellness Total	**=**	
4. I am well informed about current events.	4	3	2	1	
5. I am comfortable expressing my views and opinions.	4	3	2	1	
6. I am interested in my career development.	4	3	2	1	
			Intellectual Wellness Total	**=**	
7. I am physically fit.	4	3	2	1	
8. I am able to perform the physical tasks of my work.	4	3	2	1	
9. I am physically able to perform leisure activities.	4	3	2	1	
			Physical Wellness Total	**=**	
10. I have many friends and am involved socially.	4	3	2	1	
11. I have close ties with my family.	4	3	2	1	
12. I am confident in social situations.	4	3	2	1	
			Social Wellness Total	**=**	
13. I am fulfilled spiritually.	4	3	2	1	
14. I feel connected to the world around me.	4	3	2	1	
15. I have a sense of purpose in my life.	4	3	2	1	
			Spiritual Wellness Total	**=**	
			Comprehensive Wellness (Sum of 5 wellness scores)		

In the results below record your scores from the previous page, then determine your ratings for each score using the Wellness Rating Chart. Record your ratings in the Results section.

Results

Wellness Dimension	Score	Rating
Emotional		
Intellectual		
Physical		
Social		
Spiritual		
Comprehensive		

Wellness Rating Chart

Rating	Wellness Dimension Scores	Comprehensive Wellness Score
High-level wellness	10–12	50–60
Good wellness	8–9	40–49
Marginal wellness	6–7	30–39
Low-level wellness	Below 6	Below 30

Conclusions and Implications: In the space provided below, use several paragraphs to describe your current state of wellness. Do you think the ratings are indicative of your true state of wellness? Are there areas in which there is room for improvement?

Lab 1B Fitness Stunts and Fitness Estimates

Name		Section	Date

Purpose: To help you better understand each of the eleven components of health-related and skill-related physical fitness and to help you estimate your current levels of physical fitness

Special Note: The stunts performed in the lab are **not intended as valid tests of physical fitness.** It is hoped that the performance of the stunts will help you better understand each component of fitness, so that you can estimate your current fitness levels. You should not rely primarily on the results of the stunts to make your estimates. Rather, you should rely on previous fitness tests you have taken and your own best judgment of your current fitness. Later in this book, you will learn how to perform accurate assessments of each fitness component and determine the accuracy of your estimates.

Procedures

1. Perform each of the stunts described in Chart 1 on page 20.
2. Use past fitness test performances and your own judgment to estimate your current levels for each of the health-related and skill-related physical fitness parts. Low Fitness = improvement definitely needed, Marginal Fitness = some improvement necessary, Good fitness = adequate for healthy daily living.
3. Place an X in the appropriate circle for your fitness estimate in the Results section.

Results

Fitness Component	Low Fitness	Marginal Fitness	Good Fitness
Body composition	◯	◯	◯
Cardiovascular fitness	◯	◯	◯
Flexibility	◯	◯	◯
Muscular endurance	◯	◯	◯
Strength	◯	◯	◯
Agility	◯	◯	◯
Balance	◯	◯	◯
Coordination	◯	◯	◯
Power	◯	◯	◯
Reaction time	◯	◯	◯
Speed	◯	◯	◯

Conclusions and Implications: In several sentences, discuss the information you used to make your estimates of physical fitness. How confident are you that these estimates are accurate?

19

Directions: Attempt each of the stunts in Chart 1. Place an X in the circle next to each component of physical fitness to indicate that you have attempted the stunt.

Chart 1 ▶ Physical Fitness Stunts

Balance

1. *One-foot balance.* Stand on one foot; press up so that the weight is on the ball of the foot with the heel off the floor. Hold the hands and the other leg straight out in front for ten seconds.

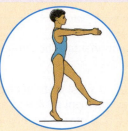

Power

2. *Standing long jump.* Stand with the toes behind a line. Using no run or hop step, jump as far as possible. Men must jump their height plus 6 inches. Women must jump their height only.

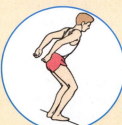

Agility

3. *Paper ball pickup.* Place two wadded paper balls on the floor 5 feet away. Run until both feet cross the line, pick up the first ball, and return both feet behind the starting line. Repeat with the second ball. Finish in five seconds.

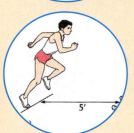

Reaction Time

4. *Paper drop.* Have a partner hold a sheet of notebook paper so that the side edge is between your thumb and index finger, about the width of your hand from the top of the page. When your partner drops the paper, catch it before it slips through the thumb and finger. Do not lower your hand to catch the paper.

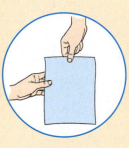

Speed

5. *Double-heel click.* With the feet apart, jump up and tap the heels together twice before you hit the ground. You must land with your feet at least 3 inches apart.

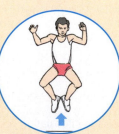

Coordination

6. *Paper ball bounce.* Wad up a sheet of notebook paper into a ball. Bounce the ball back and forth between the right and left hands. Keep the hands open and palms up. Bounce the ball three times with each hand (six times total), alternating hands for each bounce.

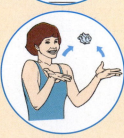

Cardiovascular Fitness

7. *Run in place.* Run in place for one-and-a-half minutes (120 steps per minute). Rest for one minute and count the heart rate for 30 seconds. A heart rate of 60 (for 30 sec.) or lower passes. A step is counted each time the right foot hits the floor.

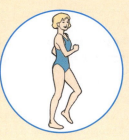

Flexibility

8. *Backsaver toe touch.* Sit on the floor with one foot against a wall. Bend the other knee. Bend forward at the hips. After three warm-up trials, reach forward and touch your closed fists to the wall. Bend forward slowly; do not bounce. Repeat with the other leg straight. Pass if fists touch the wall with each leg straight.

   Note: This is a stunt, not an exercise.

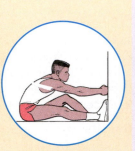

Body Composition

9. *The pinch.* Have a partner pinch a fold of fat on the back of your upper arm (body fatness), halfway between the tip of the elbow and the tip of the shoulder.

   Men: No greater than 3/4 of an inch.

   Women: No greater than 1 inch.

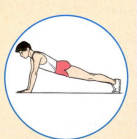

Strength

10. *Push-up.* Lie face down on the floor. Place the hands under the shoulders. Keeping the legs and body straight, press off the floor until the arms are fully extended. Women repeat once; men, three times.

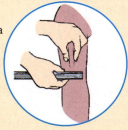

Muscular Endurance

11. *Side leg raise.* Lie on the floor on your side. Lift your leg up and to the side of the body until your feet are 24 to 36 inches apart. Keep the knee and pelvis facing forward. Do not rotate so that the knees face the ceiling. Perform ten with each leg.

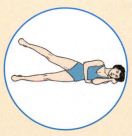

Using Self-Management Skills to Adhere to Healthy Lifestyle Behaviors

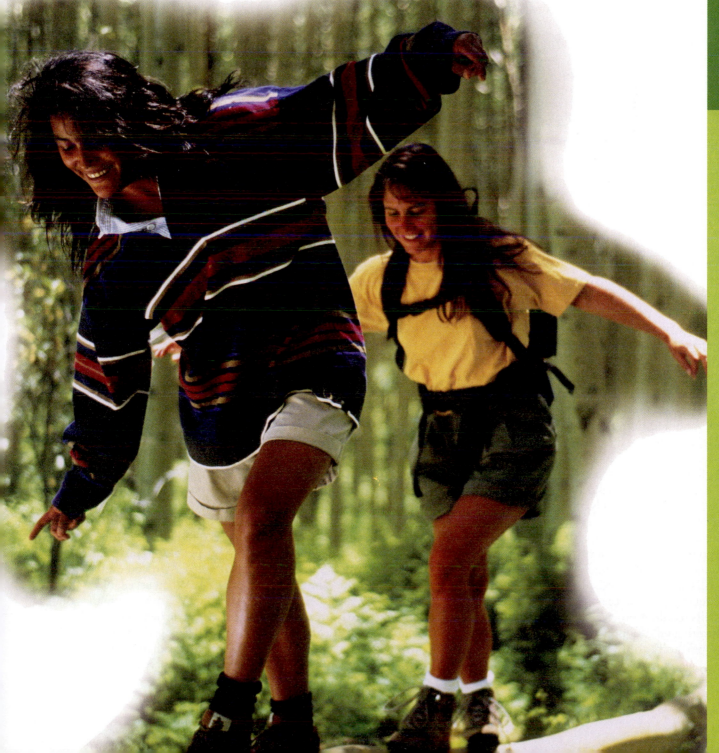

Learning and regularly using self-management skills can help you adopt and maintain healthy lifestyles throughout life.

Health Goals

for the year 2010

- Increase quality and years of healthy life.
- Increase incidence of people reporting "healthy days."
- Increase adoption and maintenance of daily physical activity.
- Increase proportion of all people who eat well.
- Decrease personal stress levels and mental health problems.
- Modify determinants of good health.

Reducing illness and debilitating conditions and promoting wellness and fitness are important public health goals. Experts in health promotion have begun to emphasize the use of social-ecological models that target environmental and policy changes to promote positive health behaviors. Adopting positive lifestyles still depend on personal responsibility but evidence suggests that most people are not effectively making lifestyle changes, even when they want to do so. Experts have determined that people who practice healthy lifestyles possess certain characteristics. These characteristics can be modified to improve the health behaviors of all people. Researchers have also identified several special skills, referred to as self-management skills, that can be useful in helping you alter factors related to adherence and ultimately help you make lifestyle changes. Like any skill, self-management skills must be practiced if they are to be useful. The factors relating to adherence and the self-management skills described in this Concept can be applied to a wide variety of healthy lifestyles. In early sections of this book, the focus is on using self-management skills to become and stay active throughout life. In the later sections of the book, the focus is on using these skills to adopt other healthy lifestyles that promote good health and wellness. In the final section, you get an opportunity to use the skills to make informed choices and plan for healthy living.

Making Lifestyle Changes

Many adults want to make lifestyle changes but are unable to do so. The majority of adults (66 percent) would prefer to alter their diet to improve health rather than take medicine. Nine out of ten people indicate that regular physical activity is important to their health. Approximately two-thirds of adults feel "great stress" at least 1 day a week and would like to reduce their stress levels. In spite of these statistics, those who profess interest in dietary change are often unsuccessful in making lasting changes. Those who say they value physical activity often fail to adhere to even modest activity schedules. Though stress reduction is important, nearly half of all adults still feel that there is a stigma associated with seeking help for an emotional problem. Changes in other lifestyles are frequently desired but often not accomplished.

Practicing one healthy lifestyle does not mean you will practice another, though adopting one healthy behavior often leads to the adoption of another. College students are more likely to participate in regular physical activity than older adults. However, they are also much more likely to eat poorly and abuse alcohol. Many young women adopt low-fat diets to avoid weight gain and smoke because they have the mistaken belief that smoking will contribute to long-term weight maintenance. These examples illustrate the fact that practicing one healthy lifestyle does not ensure **adherence** to another. However, there is evidence that making one lifestyle change often makes it easier to make other changes. For example, smokers who have started regular physical activity programs often see improvements in fitness and general well-being and decide to stop smoking.

People do not make lifestyle changes overnight. Rather, people progress forward and backward through several stages of change. www.mhhe.com/phys_fit/web02 Click 01. When asked about a specific healthy lifestyle, people commonly respond with yes or no answers. If asked, "Do you exercise regularly?" the answer is yes or no. When asked, "Do you eat well?" the answer is yes or no. We now know that there are many different stages of lifestyle behavior.

Prochaska and colleagues developed a model for classifying **stage of change** as part of their transtheoretical model. They suggest that lifestyle changes occur in at

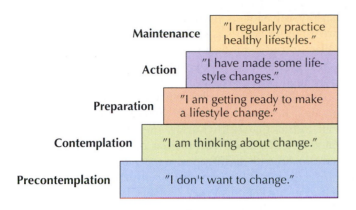

Figure 1 ▶ Stages of lifestyle change.

least five different stages. These stages are illustrated in Figure 1. The stages were originally developed to help clarify negative lifestyles. Smokers were among the first studied. Smokers who are not considering stopping are at the stage of precontemplation. Those who are thinking about stopping are classified in the contemplation stage. Those who have bought a nicotine patch or a book about smoking cessation are classified in the preparation stage. They have moved beyond contemplation and are preparing to take action. The action stage occurs when the smoker makes a change in behavior, even a small one. Cutting back on the number of cigarettes smoked is an example. The fifth stage is maintenance. When a person finally stops smoking for a relatively long period of time (e.g., 6 months), this stage has been reached.

The stages of change model (as illustrated in Figure 1) has been applied to positive lifestyles as well as negative ones. Those who are totally sedentary are considered to be in the precontemplation stage. Contemplators are thinking about becoming active. A person at the preparation stage may have bought a pair of walking shoes and appropriate clothing for activity. Those who have started activity, even if infrequent, are considered to be at the stage of action. Those who have been exercising regularly for at least 6 months are at the stage of maintenance.

Whether the lifestyle is positive or negative, people move from one stage to another in an upward or a downward direction. Individuals in action may move on to maintenance or revert back to contemplation. Smokers who succeed in quitting permanently report having stopped and started dozens of times before reaching lifetime maintenance. Similarly, those attempting to adopt positive lifestyles, such as eating well, often move back and forth from one stage to another, depending on their life circumstances.

Once maintenance is attained, relapse is less likely to occur. Although it is possible to relapse completely, it is generally less likely after the maintenance stage is reached. At this point, the behavior has been integrated into a personal lifestyle and it becomes easier to sustain. For example, a person who has been active for years does not have to undergo the same thought processes as a beginning exerciser—the behavior becomes automatic and habitual. Similarly, a nonsmoker is not tempted to smoke in the same way as a person who is trying to quit. Some people have termed the end of this behavior change process as termination.

Factors That Promote Lifestyle Change

There are many factors associated with achieving advanced stages of healthy behavior. The ultimate goal for any health behavior is to reach the stage of maintenance (see Figure 1). *Healthy People 2010* refers to these factors as **determinants,** which are factors that determine health behaviors. In fact, the national strategy is to help people change these factors, so that an increased number of adults will reach and stay at the level of maintenance. These factors relate equally well to stages of change for other healthy lifestyles. For ease of understanding, they are classified as **personal, predisposing, enabling,** and **reinforcing factors.** Predisposing factors help precontemplators get going—to move them toward contemplation or even preparation. Enabling factors help those in contemplation or preparation take the step toward action. Reinforcing factors move people from action to maintenance and help those in maintenance stay there.

Adherence Adopting and sticking with healthy behaviors such as regular physical activity or sound nutrition as part of your lifestyle.

Stage of Change The level of motivational readiness to adopt a specific health behavior.

Determinants Factors identified by health experts as responsible for healthy and unhealthy behaviors.

Personal Factors Factors, such as age or gender, related to healthy lifestyle adherence but not typically under personal control.

Predisposing Factors Factors that make you more likely to decide that you should make a healthy lifestyle, such as regular physical activity, a part of your normal routine.

Enabling Factors Factors that help you carry out your healthy lifestyle plan.

Reinforcing Factors Factors that provide encouragement to maintain healthy lifestyles, such as physical activity, for a lifetime.

Personal factors affect health behaviors but are often out of your personal control. Your age, gender, heredity, social status, and current health and fitness levels are all personal factors that affect your health behaviors. For example, there are significant differences in health behaviors among people of various ages. According to one survey, young adults between the ages of eighteen and thirty-four are more likely to smoke (30 percent) than those sixty-five and older (13 percent). On the other hand, young adults are much more likely to be physically active than older adults.

Gender differences are illustrated by the fact that women use health services more often than men. Women are more likely than men to have identified a primary care doctor and are more likely to participate in regular health screenings. As you will discover in more detail later in this book, heredity plays a role in health behaviors. For example, some people have a hereditary predisposition to gain weight, and this may affect their eating behaviors.

Age, gender, and heredity are factors you cannot control. Other personal factors that relate to health behaviors include social status and current health and fitness status. Evidence indicates that people of lower socioeconomic status and those with poor health and fitness are less likely to contemplate or participate in activity and other healthy behaviors. No matter what personal characteristics you have, you can change your health behaviors. If you have several personal factors that do not favor healthy lifestyles, it is important to do something to change your behaviors. Making an effort to modify the factors that predispose, enable, and reinforce healthy lifestyles is essential.

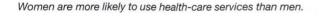

Women are more likely to use health-care services than men.

Predisposing factors are important in getting you started with the process of change. There are many predisposing factors that help you move from contemplation to preparation and taking action with regard to healthy behavior. A person who possesses many of the predisposing factors is said to have self-motivation (also called intrinsic motivation). If you are self-motivated, you will answer positively to two basic questions: "Am I able?" and "Is it worth it?"

"Am I able to do regular activity?" "Am I able to change my diet or to stop smoking?" Figure 2 includes a list of four factors that help you say, "Yes, I am able." Two of these factors are **self-confidence** and **self-efficacy.** Both have to do with having positive perceptions about your own ability. People with positive self-perceptions are more self-motivated and feel they are capable of making behavior changes for health improvement. Other factors that help you feel you are able to do a healthy behavior include easy access and a safe environment. For example, people who have easy access to exercise equipment at home or the workplace or who have a place to exercise within 10 minutes of home are more likely to be active than those who do not. A safe environment, such as safe neighborhoods or parks, increases the chances that a person will be active.

"Is it worth it?" People who say yes to this question are willing to make an effort to change their behaviors. Predisposing factors that make it worth it to change behaviors include enjoying the activity, balancing attitudes, believing in the benefits of a behavior, and having knowledge of the health benefits of a behavior (see Figure 2). If you enjoy something and feel good about it (have positive attitudes and beliefs), you will be self-motivated to do it. It will be worth it. Taking steps to change the predisposing factors will help you become self-motivated and move toward effectively changing your health behaviors.

Enabling factors are important in moving you from the beginning stages of change to action and maintenance. Enabling factors include a variety of skills that help people follow through with decisions to make changes in behaviors. Eight of these most important skills are listed in Figure 2. A few examples of the skills that enable healthy lifestyle change include goal setting, self-assessment, and self-monitoring.

Reinforcing factors are important in adhering to lifestyle changes. Once a person has reached the action or maintenance stage, it is important to stay at this high level. Reinforcing factors help people stick with a behavior change (see Figure 2).

As illustrated in Figure 2, perhaps the most important reinforcing factor is success. If you change a behavior and have success, it makes you want to keep doing the behavior. If you fail, you may conclude that the behavior does not work and give up on it. Planning for success is essential for adhering to healthy lifestyle changes. Using the self-management skills described in this concept and throughout this book can help you plan effectively and achieve success.

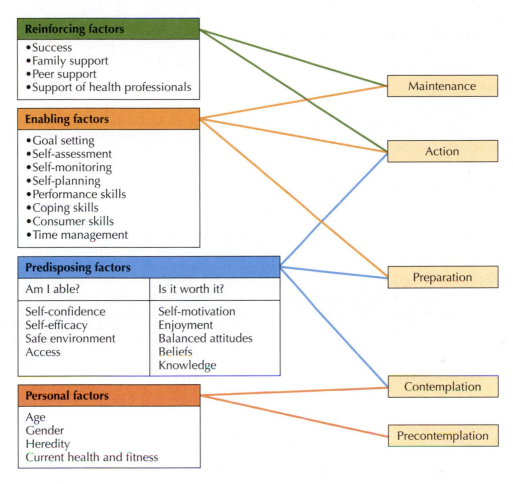

Figure 2 ▶ Factors that influence change in healthy behaviors.

Social support from family, peers, and health professionals can also be reinforcing. There are, however, different kinds of support and some are more helpful than others. Support for well-informed personal choices is referred to as support of autonomy. One example is the encouragement of family, friends, or a doctor for starting and sticking to a nutritious diet. The supporting person might ask, "How can I help you meet your goals?" One of the goals of this book is to help you take responsible control of your own behaviors concerning your personal health, fitness, and wellness.

Not all feedback is perceived as reinforcing and supportive. Although the people providing the feedback may feel that they are being helpful and supportive, some feedback may be perceived as applying pressure or as an attempt to control behavior. For example, scolding a person for not sticking to his or her diet, or even offering the suggestion that "you are not going to get anywhere if you don't stick to your diet," will often be perceived as applying pressure. Research suggests that support of autonomy, providing support for personal choices, is most effective in enabling and reinforcing behavior change. Those who want to help friends and family make behavior changes should be careful to avoid applying pressure and should make attempts to provide positive support for well-informed choices.

Self-Management Skills

Learning self-management skills can help you alter factors that lead to healthy lifestyle change. Personal, predisposing, enabling, and reinforcing factors influence the way you live. These factors are of little practical significance, however, unless they can be altered to promote healthy lifestyles. Learning **self-management skills**

Self-Confidence The belief that you can be successful at something (for example, the belief that you can be successful in sports and physical activities and can improve your physical fitness).

Self-Efficacy Confidence that you can perform a specific task. (A type of specific self-confidence.)

Self-Management Skills Skills that you can learn to help you change to and adhere to healthy lifestyles such as regular physical activity and good nutrition (see Tables 1, 2, and 3 for examples).

Table 1 ▶ Self-Management Skills for Changing Predisposing Factors

Self-Management Skill	How Is It Useful?
Overcoming Barriers	**Lifestyle Example**
This involves developing skills that allow you to overcome problems, such as lack of facilities, lack of equipment, and inconvenience. People who develop skills to overcome barriers can learn to rearrange schedules and acquire personal equipment and other skills to overcome these barriers.	People at work are often exposed to snack foods high in empty calories. For this reason, their nutrition is not what it could be. Skills in overcoming barriers include planning, preparing, and selecting good foods.
Building Self-Confidence and Motivation	**Lifestyle Example**
This involves taking small steps that allow success. With each small step, confidence and motivation increase and you develop the feeling "I can do that."	A person says, "I would like to be more active, but I have never been good at physical activities." Starting with a 10-minute walk, the person sees that "I can do it." Over time, the person becomes confident and motivated to do more physical activity.
Balancing Attitudes	**Lifestyle Example**
This involves learning to balance positive and negative attitudes. To adhere to a healthy lifestyle, it is important to develop positive attitudes and reduce the negative attitudes.	A person does not do activity because he or she lacks support from friends, has no equipment, and does not like to get sweaty. These are negatives. Shifting the balance to positive things such as fun, good health, and good appearance, can help promote activity.
Building Knowledge and Changing Beliefs	**Lifestyle Example**
An educated person knows the truth and builds his or her beliefs on sound information. Knowledge does not always change beliefs, but awareness of the facts can play an important role in achieving good health.	A person says, "I don't think what I eat has much to do with my health and wellness." Acquiring knowledge is fundamental to being an educated person. Studying the facts about nutrition can provide the basis for changes in beliefs and lifestyles.

 Technology Update

Personal Digital Assistant

Many adults underestimate the number of calories they consume and overestimate the activity they perform each day. One important self-management skill that can help people be more realistic is self-monitoring. The development of hand-held computers can now make self-monitoring easier. These computers are also called personal digital assistants (PDAs). Software is now available for PDAs that allow you to record and analyze calories consumed in food and expended in activity. To see the features of this type of software program visit **www.vivonic.com**.

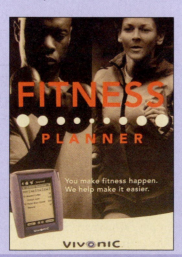

(sometimes called self-regulation skills) can help you change the predisposing, enabling, and reinforcing factors described in Tables 1, 2, and 3. In fact, some of the enabling factors are self-management skills. It takes practice to learn these skills, but with effort anyone can learn them. There are many opportunities to learn self-management skills in this book. Many of the labs allow you to practice these skills.

It takes time to change unhealthy lifestyles. People in Western cultures are used to seeing things happen quickly. We flip a switch, and the lights come on. We want food quickly, and thousands of fast-food restaurants provide it. The expectation that we should have what we want when we want it has led us to expect instantaneous changes in health, wellness, and fitness. Unfortunately, there is no quick way to health. There is no pill that can reverse the effects of a lifetime of sedentary living, poor eating, or tobacco abuse. Changing your lifestyle is the key. But lifestyles that have been practiced for years are not easy to change. As you progress through this book, you will have the opportunity to learn how to implement self-management skills. Learning these skills is the surest way to make permanent lifestyle changes.

Table 2 ▶ Self-Management Skills for Changing Enabling Factors

Self-Management Skill	How Is It Useful?
Goal-Setting Skills	**Lifestyle Example**
This involves learning how to establish things that you want to achieve in the future. It is important that goals be realistic and achievable. Learning to set goals for behavior change is especially important for beginners.	A person wants to lose body fat. If he or she sets a goal of losing 50 pounds, success is unlikely. Setting a process goal of restricting 200 calories a day or expending 200 more a day for several weeks makes success more likely.
Self-Assessment Skills	**Lifestyle Example**
This involves how to assess your own fitness, health, and wellness. In addition, it requires you to learn to interpret your own self-assessment results. It takes practice to become good at doing self-assessments.	A person wants to know his or her health strengths and weaknesses. The best procedure is to select good tests and self-administer them. Practicing the assessments in this book will help you become good at self-assessment.
Self-Monitoring Skills	**Lifestyle Example**
This involves monitoring behavior and record keeping. Many people think that they adhere to healthy lifestyles, but they do not. They have a distorted view of what they actually do. Self-monitoring helps give you a true picture of your own behavior and progress.	A person can't understand why he or she is not losing weight, even though he or she is restricting calories. Keeping records may show that the person is eating more than he or she thinks. Learning to keep records of progress is also important to adherence.
Self-Planning Skills	**Lifestyle Example**
This involves learning how to plan for yourself rather than having others do all the planning for you. Knowledge and practice in planning can help you develop these skills.	A person wants to be more active, to eat better, and to manage stress. Self-planning skills will help him or her plan a personal activity, nutrition, or stress-management program.
Performance Skills	**Lifestyle Example**
This involves learning the skills necessary for performing specific tasks, such as sports or relaxation. These skills can help you feel confident and enjoy activities.	A person avoids physical activity because he or she does not have the physical skills equal to peers'. Learning sports or other motor skills allows this person to choose to be active, anyway.
Coping Skills	**Lifestyle Example**
This involves developing a new way of thinking about things. People with this skill can see situations in more than one way and learn to think more positively about life situations.	A person is stressed and frequently anxious. Learning stress-management skills, such as relaxation, can help a person cope. Like all skills, stress-management skills must be practiced to be effective.
Consumer Skills	**Lifestyle Example**
This involves gaining knowledge about products and services. It also may require rethinking untrue beliefs that may lead to poor consumer decisions.	A person avoids seeking medical help when sick. Instead, the person takes an unproven remedy. Learning consumer skills provides knowledge for making sound medical decisions.
Time-Management Skills	**Lifestyle Example**
This involves recordkeeping similar to self-monitoring. It relates to total time use rather than the monitoring of specific behaviors. Skillful monitoring of time can help you plan and adhere to healthy lifestyles.	A person wants more quality time with family and friends. Monitoring time can help a person reallocate time to spend it in ways that are more consistent with personal priorities.

Table 3 ▶ Self-Management Skills for Changing Reinforcing Factors

Self-Management Skill	How Is It Useful?
Social Support	**Lifestyle Example**
This involves learning how to get the support of others for healthy lifestyles. You learn how to get support from family and friends for your autonomous decisions. Support of a doctor can help.	A person has gradually developed a plan to be active. Friends and loved ones encourage activity and help the person develop a schedule that will allow and encourage regular activity.
Relapse Prevention	**Lifestyle Example**
This involves staying with a healthy behavior once you have adopted it. It is sometimes easy to relapse to an unhealthy lifestyle. There are skills such as avoiding high-risk situations and learning how to say "no" that can help you avoid relapse.	A person stops smoking. To stay at maintenance, the person can learn to avoid situations where there is pressure to smoke. The person can learn methods of saying "no" to those who offer tobacco.

Strategies for Action

Many people feel that factors influencing health and wellness are out of their control. www.mhhe.com/phys_fit/web02 Click 02. A recent poll indicates that 91 percent of adults would like to change their lifestyles to make their lives more enjoyable and to change factors associated with wellness. Unfortunately, many people feel that they do not have personal control over good health and wellness. For example, one survey suggests that most of the lifestyle changes deemed important in our society remain in the realm of fantasies, just beyond realization. Experts have shown that people who feel that health is beyond personal control express such ideas as "Bad things [illness] can't happen to me and good things [wellness] are beyond my reach."

Many people can benefit from a new way of thinking about health, wellness, and fitness. Many people have unrealistic expectations about health and fitness. They compare their fitness with that of athletes and their appearance with that of models and movie stars, often setting standards for themselves that are impossible to achieve. Some say, "I could never do that," when considering becoming physically active, altering eating pat-

terns, or learning to manage stress. Many lack information about what is really possible concerning healthy lifestyles. Those who feel a lack of control set unrealistic standards for themselves and lack confidence in their own abilities to change.

Adopting a new way of thinking can have dramatic implications. A major purpose of this text is to help you adopt a new way of thinking toward health behaviors. This new way of thinking acknowledges that many of the factors that influence health, wellness, and fitness are largely within your control. Learning and practicing self-management skills can help you develop this new way of thinking.

With practice, you can improve self-management skills that lead to acquiring and maintaining healthy lifestyles. Many opportunities are provided in this book for you to practice and learn self-management skills. Table 4 refers you to labs in the text designed to enhance specific self-management skills.

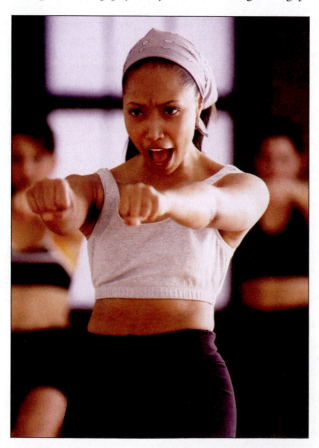

A new way of thinking can help you adopt healthy lifestyles.

Table 4 ▶ Opportunities for Learning Self-Management Skills

Self-Management Skill	Lab Number
Overcoming barriers	19C, 20A, 20B
Building self-confidence and motivation	1A, 6A
Balancing attitudes	6A
Building knowledge and beliefs	3B, 4A, 6A, 8A, 12A, 20A, 20B
Goal setting	7A, 10B, 11C, 11D, 13C, 17A, 21C
Self-assessment	1A, 1B, 2A, 3A, 4A, 5A, 8A, 10A, 11A, 11B, 13A, 13B, 14A, 15A, 15B, 15C, 16A, 16B, 18A, 18B, 18C, 19B, 21A,
Self-monitoring	7A, 9B, 10B, 11C, 11D, 13C, 16A, 16B, 17B, 21B, 21C
Self-planning	7A, 9B, 10B, 11C, 11D, 13C, 21B, 21C
Performance skills	3B, 9A, 12A, 19B, 19C
Adopting coping skills	19A, 19D
Learning consumer skills	16B, 25A, 25B
Managing time	19C
Finding social support	19B
Preventing relapse	17A, 21B, 21C

Table 5 ▶ Theories and Models Associated with Healthy Lifestyle Adoption

Transtheoretical Model

This model is also referred to as the stages of change model. This model suggests five stages of change that characterize various health behaviors. The model suggests that doing the correct things (processes) at the right time (stage of change) is important to self-change in health behaviors.

Social Cognitive Theory

Social cognitive theory is also referred to as social learning theory. Central to this theory are self-efficacy and positive expectations about behavior change. Also, the theory suggests that a person must value the outcomes of a behavior if he or she is likely to do that behavior.

Health Beliefs Model

This model suggests that a person's health behavior is related to the following five factors: the belief that a health problem will have harmful effects, the belief that a person is susceptible to the problem, the perceived benefits of changing a lifestyle to prevent the problem, the perceived barriers to overcoming the problem, and the confidence that he or she can do what is necessary to prevent it.

Theory of Planned Behavior

This theory is often combined with the theory for reasoned action. It has the same basic tenets but adds the concept of "perceived control" over the environment. The person must believe that he or she has some control over the factors that allow the performance of that behavior. Perceived control is in many ways similar to self-efficacy in social cognitive theory.

Social Ecological Model

The social ecological model is based on the notion that health behavior change is influenced by the interactions of intrapersonal, social, cultural, and physical environmental factors. For example, when people smoke, they affect the environment, which in turn affects the health of others in the environment. While this model does not focus on individual behavior change, it is included here to emphasize the importance of a multitude of social and environmental factors on public health.

Self-Determination Theory

Central to self-determination theory is the importance of choice in a person's life (autonomy). Perceptions of competence at mastering life's tasks are also critical to the theory. Making personal choices in an attempt to master the tasks of daily living are emphasized rather than making choices based on external pressures to comply. Self-determination theory and cognitive evaluation theory (its subtheory) emphasize intrinsic motivation. The intrinsic motivation inherent in behaviors that are exciting and/or fulfilling is important in making activity choices.

Theory of Reasoned Action

This theory suggests that a person's behavior is most associated with the person's intention to do the behavior. The two factors most likely to influence a person's intentions are attitudes (beliefs) and the social environment (opinions of others).

Assessing self-management skills that influence healthy lifestyles provides a basis for changing your health, wellness, or fitness. Lab 2A allows you to assess predisposing, enabling, and reinforcing factors associated with regular physical activity. Lab 2B provides you with an opportunity to assess your current self-management skills for physical activity. In subsequent concepts, you will practice the self-management skills relating to a variety of healthy lifestyles.

🌐 **You can benefit from a critical analysis of the theories and models that help us understand the factors that lead to healthy living.** www. mhhe.com/phys_fit/web02 Click 03. Much of the information presented in this concept is based on theories and models used by researchers to study the factors associated with healthy living. Table 5 provides brief descriptions of several of the most widely accepted theories and models. You do not have to have a thorough understanding of health behavior theory to use the self-management skills (see Tables 1–3). The brief descriptions in Table 5 are intended to give you a brief overview, rather than a comprehensive understanding, of the theories and models. These brief descriptions, as well as the suggested readings at the end of the concept, should be useful to those seeking more information concerning health behavior change theory.

Study Resources

Check out additional online study resources for this concept in the Student Edition of the Online Learning Center at www.mhhe.com/corbin13e.

Web Resources

ACSM's Fit Society Page **www.acsm.org/health+fitness/fit_society.htm**
ACSM's Health and Fitness Journal
www.acsm.org/publications/health_fitness_journal.htm

Journal of Sport and Exercise Psychology www.humankinetics. com/products/journals/journal.cfm?id=JSEP

The Sport Psychologist www.humankinetics.com/products/ journals/journal.cfm?id=TSP

Suggested Readings

 Additional reference materials for Concept 2 are available at www.mhhe.com/phys_fit/web02 Click 04.

Bandura, A. 2004. Health promotion by social cognitive means. *Health Education and Behavior* 31(2):143–164.

Bandura, A. 1986. *Social Foundations of Thought and Action: A Social-Cognitive Theory.* Englewood Cliffs, NJ: Prentice-Hall.

Deci, E. L., and R. M. Ryan (eds.). 2002. *Handbook of Self-Determination Research.* Rochester, NY: University of Rochester Press.

Janz, N. K., et al. 2002. The health belief model. In K. Glanz et al. (eds.). *Health Behavior and Health Education: Theory, Research and Practice.* 3rd ed. San Francisco: Jossey-Bass.

Levy, S. S. 2004. Effects of a self-determination theory-based mail-mediated intervention on adults' exercise behavior. *American Journal of Health Promotion* 18(5):345–349.

Maddux, J. E. 2002. Self-efficacy: The power of believing you can. In C. R. Snyder and S. J. Lopez (eds.). *Handbook of Positive Psychology.* Oxford, UK: Oxford University Press.

Marcus, B. H., and B. A. Lewis. 2003. Physical activity and the stages of change motivational readiness for change model. *President's Council on Physical Fitness and Sports Research Digest* 4(1):1–8.

Montano, D. E., and D. Kasperzyk. 2002. The theory of reasoned action and theory of planned behavior. In K. Glanz et al. (eds.). *Health Behavior and Health Education: Theory, Research and Practice.* 3rd ed. San Francisco: Jossey-Bass.

Prochaska, J. O., et al. 2002. The transtheoretical model and stages of change. In K. Glanz et al. (eds.). *Health Behavior and Health Education: Theory, Research and Practice.* 3rd ed. San Francisco: Jossey-Bass.

Rhodes, R. E., et al. 2002. Extending the theory of planned behavior to the exercise domain. *Research Quarterly for Exercise and Sport* 73(2):193–199.

Ryan, R. M., and E. L. Deci. 2000. Self-determination theory and the facilitation of intrinsic motivation, social development, and well-being. *American Psychologist* 55:68–78.

Sallis, J. F., and N. Owen. 2002. Ecological models. In K. Glanz et al. (eds.). *Health Behavior and Health Education: Theory, Research and Practice.* 3rd ed. San Francisco: Jossey-Bass.

Stewart, D. E. 2004. What about men's health? Women's perspectives of men's health and gender medicine. *Journal of Men's Health and Gender* 1(1):20–21.

Stone, W. J., and D. A. Klein. 2004. Long-term exercisers: What can we learn from them? *ACSM's Health and Fitness Journal* 8(2):11–14.

Taylor, S. 2003. *Health Psychology.* 5th ed. St Louis: McGraw-Hill.

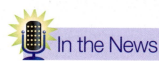 **In the News**

Who Sees a Doctor Regularly?

Not all people are equally likely to use self-management skills to improve their health. For example, it has been well established that women are more likely than men to focus on health concerns. In the past it has been assumed that the shorter life expectancy of men is determined by hormonal and genetic factors. New evidence suggests that men can improve their health and reduce their risk for premature death by avoiding unnecessary risks that contribute to accidents, by adopting healthier lifestyles (eating better, not smoking, exercising), and by seeking regular medical consultation.

Gender comparisons on health and health care indicate that men are much less likely than women to have a regular physician. Surveys indicate that more than 50 percent of young men have no regular doctor and that three times as many men as women have not visited a doctor in the past year. Other interesting findings include

- Fewer than one in five men visit a doctor in the first few days of sickness.

- Forty percent wait at least 1 week or as long as possible.
- Many men do not know whom to see if a problem arises.
- Men often fail to get important health screenings (e.g., prostate, testicular, and blood lipids).

Reasons men avoid seeing a physician:

- Sickness is seen as a weakness, seen as unmanly.
- Pain is considered normal, not a symptom of a problem.
- Men may deny possible illness.
- They think, "I don't have time. I will do it later."

Reasons women are more willing to see a doctor:

- They have established a relationship with physicians early because of family health care or childbearing.
- They are aware of health issues from the media.
- They are more open to health discussions with friends.

Married men seek help more than single men because wives prompt them.

Source: Commonwealth Fund and American Medical News.

Lab 2A The Physical Activity Adherence Questionnaire

Name	Section	Date

Purpose: To help you understand the factors that influence physical activity adherence and to see which factors you might change to improve your chances of achieving the action or maintenance level for physical activity

Procedures

1. The factors that predispose, enable, and reinforce adherence to physically active living are listed below. Read each statement. Place an X in the circle under the most appropriate response for you: very true, somewhat true, or not true.
2. When you have answered all of the items, determine a score by summing the four numbers for each type of factor. Then sum the three scores (predisposing, enabling, reinforcing) to get your total score.
3. Record your scores in the Results section and answer the questions in the Conclusions and Implications section.

	Very True	Somewhat True	Not True	
Predisposing Factors				
1. I am very knowledgeable about physical activity.	3	2	1	
2. I have a strong belief that physical activity is good for me.	3	2	1	
3. I enjoy doing regular exercise and physical activity.	3	2	1	
4. I am confident of my abilities in sports, exercise, and other physical activities.	3	2	1	
		Predisposing Score	**=**	
Enabling Factors				
5. I possess good sports skills.	3	2	1	
6. I know how to plan my own physical activity program.	3	2	1	
7. I have a place to do physical activity near my home or work.	3	2	1	
8. I have the equipment I need to do physical activities I enjoy.	3	2	1	
		Enabling Score	**=**	
Reinforcing Factors				
9. I have the support of my family for doing my regular physical activity.	3	2	1	
10. I have many friends who enjoy the same kinds of physical activities that I do.	3	2	1	
11. I have the support of my boss and my colleagues for participation in activity.	3	2	1	
12. I have a doctor and/or an employer who encourages me to exercise.	3	2	1	
		Reinforcing Score	**=**	
		Total Score (Sum 3 Scores)	**=**	

Results: Record your scores in the "score" column. Use your score and the Physical Activity Adherence Rating Chart to determine your ratings. Record your ratings in the "rating" column below.

Physical Activity Adherence Ratings

Adherence Category	Score	Rating
Predisposing		
Enabling		
Reinforcing		
Total		

Physical Activity Adherence Ratings Chart

Classification	Predisposing Score	Enabling Score	Reinforcing Score	Total Score
Adherence likely	11–12	11–12	11–12	33–36
Adherence possible	9–10	9–10	9–10	25–32
Adherence unlikely	<9	<9	<9	<25

Conclusions and Implications: In several sentences, discuss your ratings from this questionnaire. Also discuss the predisposing, enabling, and reinforcing factors that you may need to alter or increase your prospects for lifetime activity.

In several sentences, speculate about adherence factors for other healthy lifestyles, such as eating well and managing stress. Do you think you need more, or less, work in these areas, as compared with physically active living?

Lab 2B The Self-Management Skills Questionnaire

Name	Section	Date

Purpose: To help you assess your self-management skills that are important to adhering to physically active lifestyles

Procedures

1. Each question reflects one of the self-management skills described in the text. Read each statement. After each statement, place an X over the circle indicating whether you think the item is very true, somewhat true, or not true.
2. When you have answered all of the items, score the questionnaire using the information in the Results section. Determine your ratings and answer the questions in the Conclusions and Implications section.

	Very True	Somewhat True	Not True	Score
1. I regularly assess my health-related fitness and rate my fitness test results using health-fitness standards.	3	2	1	
2. I keep regular physical activity logs to monitor current physical activity levels.	3	2	1	
3. I set realistic and attainable fitness and activity goals and monitor progress in meeting these goals.	3	2	1	
4. I have planned a personal program that includes activities for all parts of fitness and for optimal health benefits.	3	2	1	
5. I have the motor skills necessary to perform several physical activities on a regular basis.	3	2	1	
6. I have more positive than negative attitudes about physical activity.	3	2	1	
7. I find a way to do my activity even when the weather is bad or my time is limited.	3	2	1	
8. I know how to identify fitness misinformation and quackery.	3	2	1	
9. I know how to get others to do exercise with me and to get the support of others for doing my own activity program.	3	2	1	
10. I know and use strategies to stick with it especially when I have not been active for a while.	3	2	1	
11. I participate in activities that I am not very good at because I am able to enjoy them even if I don't excel.	3	2	1	
12. I manage my time to allow regular performance of my physical activity program.	3	2	1	
Total Score (Sum 12 Scores)				

Self-Management Skills Ratings Chart

Rating	Individual Scores	Total Score
Good	3	30–36
Marginal	2	24–29
Needs improvement	1	< 24

Results: Record your score for each skill in the chart below. There is one question for each self-management skill. Your score for each self-management skill is the number inside the circle for that question (see previous page). The number of the question for each skill is noted in the chart below. To get your total score, sum the scores for all of the self-management skills. Determine your rating for each skill and for your total score using the Self-Management Skills Rating Chart on the previous page.

Self-Management Skills Results

Self-Management Skill	Item	Score	Rating
Self-assessment	1		
Self-monitoring	2		
Goal setting	3		
Self-planning	4		
Performance skills	5		
Balancing attitudes	6		
Overcoming barriers	7		
Learning consumer skills	8		
Finding social support	9		
Preventing relapse	10		
Adopting coping strategies	11		
Time management	12		
Total			

Conclusions and Implications: In several sentences, discuss your ratings regarding self-management skills. In which areas do you think you need to learn more to be able to be a better self-manager?

In several sentences, speculate about your self-management skills for other healthy lifestyles, such as eating well and managing stress. Do you think you need more or less work in these areas, as compared with managing for physically active living?

Preparing for Physical Activity

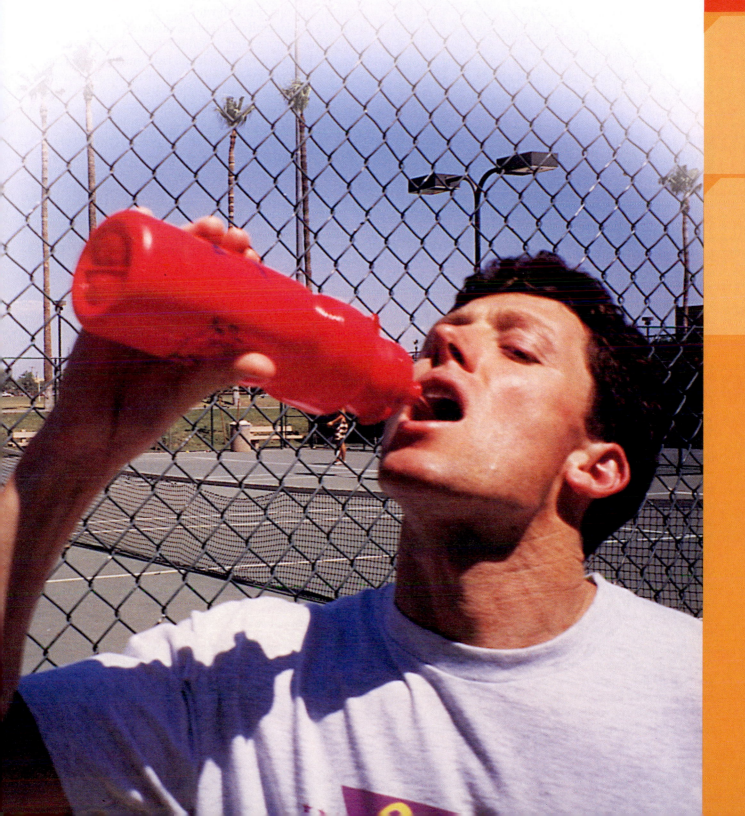

Proper preparation can help make physical activity enjoyable, effective, and safe.

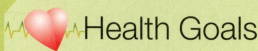

Health Goals

for the year 2010

- Improve health, fitness, and quality of life through daily physical activity.

- Increase leisure-time physical activity.

For people just beginning a physical activity program, adequate preparation may be the key to persistence. For those who have been regularly active for some time, sound preparation can help reduce risk of injury and make activity more enjoyable. It is hoped that a person armed with good information about preparation will become involved and stay involved in physical activity for a lifetime. For long-term maintenance, physical activity must be something that is a part of a person's normal lifestyle. Some factors that will help you prepare for and make physical activity a part of your normal routine are presented in this concept.

Factors to Consider before Beginning Physical Activity

 Before beginning regular physical activity, it is important to establish medical readiness. www.mhhe.com/phys_fit/web03 Click 01. Physical activity requires the cardiovascular system to work harder. While this level of stress can promote positive adaptations, the stress on the heart can be unsafe and dangerous for certain individuals. The British Columbia (Canada) Ministry of Health conducted extensive research to devise a procedure that would help people know when it was advisable to seek medical consultation prior to beginning or altering an exercise program. The goal was to prevent unnecessary medical examinations, while helping people to be reasonably assured that regular exercise was appropriate. The research resulted in the development of the Physical Activity Readiness Questionnaire **(PAR-Q).** The most recent revision of the PAR-Q consists of seven simple questions you can ask yourself to determine if medical consultation is necessary prior to exercise involvement.

The American College of Sports Medicine (ACSM) has developed additional guidelines to help determine if medical consultation or a **clinical exercise test** is necessary prior to participation in physical activity programs. The ACSM divides people into three general categories (see Table 1). Young adults classified as apparently healthy with low risk, and who give no yes answers to the PAR-Q, are generally cleared for moderate and vigorous physical activity without a medical exam or clinical exercise test. For those with moderate risk, moderate exercise is generally appropriate without a medical exam or an exercise test, but both are recommended prior to undertaking vigorous physical activity. For those in the category high risk, a medical exam and exercise testing are recommended for moderate and vigorous activity. When resuming physical activity after an injury or illness, consultation with a physician is always wise, no matter what your age or medical condition.

Table 1 ▶ American College of Sports Medicine Risk Stratification Categories and Criteria

Stratification Category	Criteria
Low risk	Younger people (less than forty-five for men and fifty-five for women) are considered at low risk when they have no heart disease symptoms and have no more than one of the risk factors listed below.
Moderate risk	People without heart disease symptoms but who are older (men forty-five or more and women fifty-five and older) OR who have two or more of the risk factors listed below.
High risk	People with one or more of the signs or symptoms listed below OR who have known cardiovascular, pulmonary, or metabolic disease.

Risk Factors

Family history of heart disease; smoker; high blood pressure (hypertension); high cholesterol; abnormal blood glucose levels; obesity (BMI of > 30 or waist girth of > 100 cm); sedentary lifestyle; low HDL cholesterol level.

Signs and Symptoms

Chest, neck, or jaw pain from lack of oxygen to the heart; shortness of breath at rest or in mild exercise; dizziness or fainting; difficult or labored breathing when lying, sitting, or standing; ankle swelling; fast heartbeat or heart palpitations; pain in the legs from poor circulation; heart murmur; unusual fatigue or shortness of breath with usual activities.

Source: American College of Sports Medicine.

Technology Update

Automated External Defibrillator

Ideally it would be possible to screen all exercisers to assure that they are free from cardiovascular disease risk. Inevitably, however, there will be those for whom disease goes undetected, resulting in heart problems during or after exercise. One form of new technology for saving lives is the automated external defibrillator (AED). After identifying cardiac arrest and performing CPR, if ventricular fibrillation (chaotic electrical activity to heart muscle) occurs, it may be necessary to "shock" the heart back to a normal rhythm. The

AED has a heart rhythm analysis system, which advises the operator when a "shock" is appropriate. The operator must then take final action to deliver the shock. A recent position statement of the American College of Sports Medicine and the American Heart Association advises health and fitness clubs—especially those that have a large member base, those with older members, and those with members known to have disease—to have the AED system available. The AED should be used as part of an emergency plan that includes training of all exercise personnel. Federal law and "Good Samaritan Laws" in forty-seven states extend protection to AED users.

Table 2 ▶ Dressing for Activity

Clothing

- Avoid clothing that is too tight or that restricts movement.
- Material in contact with skin should be porous.
- Clothing should protect against wind and rain but allow for heat loss and evaporation—e.g., Gortex.
- Wear layers so that a layer can be removed if not needed.
- Wear socks for most activities to prevent blisters, abrasions, odor, and excessive shoe wear.
- Socks should be absorbent and fit properly (too tight causes ingrown toenails; too loose causes blisters).
- Do not use nonporous clothing that traps sweat in an attempt to lose weight; these garments prevent evaporation and cooling.

Special Clothing

- Women should consider an exercise bra.
- Men should consider an athletic supporter.
- Wear helmets and padding for activities with risk of falling such as biking or inline skating.
- Wear reflective clothing for night activities.
- Wear water shoes for some aquatic activities.
- Consider lace-up ankle braces to prevent injury.
- Consider a mouthpiece for basketball and other contact sports.

Shoes

- A heel counter can provide stability and movement control.
- A heel notch can protect Achilles tendon.
- Adequate heel width is important for stability and to prevent ankle injury.
- Some cushion prevents shock to the foot; too much cushion inhibits the reflexes that protect the foot.
- Lightweight shoes reduce energy cost in activity.
- Use soles (Out and Mid) with good traction to reduce risk of falling.
- Wear shoes of adequate size (about one-half size larger than normal).
- The toe box should have adequate room to wiggle toes and to allow space if you wear two pairs of socks.
- Replace shoes periodically if heels and soles break down—even if the fabric is still good.
- Wear shoes made of material that can breathe, such as nylon mesh, to help sweat evaporation and reduce shoe weight gain.
- Consider high tops for basketball.
- Cross trainers are the best all-purpose choice.

There is no way to be absolutely sure that you are medically sound to begin a physical activity program. Even a thorough exam by a physician cannot guarantee that a person does not have some limitations that may cause a problem during exercise. Use of the PAR-Q and adherence to the ACSM guidelines are advised to help minimize the risk while preventing unnecessary medical cost. However, if you are unsure about your readiness for activity, a medical exam and a clinical exercise test are the surest ways to make certain that you are ready to participate.

Those who plan to do intensive training (particularly for sports) may want to answer some additional questions concerning whether a medical exam is necessary before beginning (see Lab 3A).

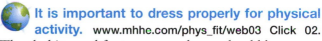

It is important to dress properly for physical activity. www.mhhe.com/phys_fit/web03 Click 02. The clothing and footwear you choose should be appropriate for the specific activity you plan to perform. Comfort is more important than looks. Table 2 provides guidelines for dressing for activity, and Figure 1 shows the characteristics of a good activity shoe.

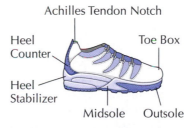

Figure 1 ▶ Characteristics of a good activity shoe.

PAR-Q An acronym for Physical Activity Readiness Questionnaire; designed to help determine if you are medically suited to begin an exercise program.

Clinical Exercise Test A test, typically administered on a treadmill, in which exercise is gradually increased in intensity while the heart is monitored by an EKG. Symptoms not present at rest, such as an abnormal EKG, may be present in an exercise test.

Factors to Consider during Daily Physical Activity

There are three components of the daily activity program: the warm-up exercise, the workout, and the cool-down exercise. The key component of a fitness program is the daily workout. Experts agree, however, that the workout should be preceded by a warm-up and followed by a cool-down. The **warm-up** prepares the body for physical activity, and the **cool-down** returns the body to rest and promotes effective recovery by aiding the return of blood from the working muscles to the heart (see Figure 2).

The cardiovascular warm-up prior to the workout is recommended to prepare the muscles and heart for the workout. www.mhhe.com/phys_fit/web03 Click 03. There are two reasons for warming up prior to activity. The first is to prepare the heart muscle and circulatory system. When you start physical activity, blood flow is not immediately available to the heart and muscles. A proper warm-up decreases the risk of irregular heartbeats associated with poor coronary circulation. A proper warm-up can also improve performance, since it minimizes the premature formation of **lactic acid** at the start of physical activity (for more information see Concept 14). Research suggests that 2 minutes of walking, jogging, or mild exercise is adequate for moderate activities; however, some experts recommend 5 minutes or more of moderate activity as a warm-up for vigorous activity.

The second reason for a warm-up is to stretch the skeletal muscles. This phase of the warm-up includes exercises that stretch the muscles and tendons. Advocates of this type of warm-up suggest that stretching can make the muscles more elastic and extensible, thus reducing risk of injury and enhancing performance. However, recent research casts doubt on the benefit of a stretching warm-up in reducing injury. Also, evidence suggests that stretching immediately before activities requiring strength and power may actually reduce force production, resulting in poorer rather than improved performances. Additional research is necessary to answer all questions associated with the stretching warm-up. In the meantime, most experts suggest that a static stretching warm-up before physical activity, especially when performed after a general cardiovascular warm-up, is prudent.

A warm-up that is suitable for walking, jogging, running, cycling, and even basketball is illustrated in Figure 3. This warm-up can be used for other activities, provided stretching exercises for the major muscle groups involved in the activities are added. Additional exercises, appropriate for inclusion in a stretching warm-up, are illustrated in the flexibility concept. The cardiovascular warm-up is suitable for most activities, but other mild exercise (such as a slow swim for swimmers or a slow ride for cyclists) can be substituted.

In summary, there is good evidence that a general cardiovascular warm-up of 2 to 5 minutes is important before performing vigorous physical activity. If you choose to perform a stretching warm-up, make certain that you use gentle, static stretch. The stretching warm-up is not intended to substitute for a regular program of stretching exercises designed to improve flexibility (see Concept 10).

A cool-down after the workout is important to promote an effective recovery from physical activity. The cool-down is done immediately after the workout. Like the warm-up, there are two principal components of a cool-down: static muscle stretching and an activity for the cardiovascular system. Although not all experts agree, some believe that static muscle stretching *after* the workout is more important than stretching before because it may help relieve spasms in fatigued muscles. Stretching as part of the cool-down may be more effective for lengthening the muscles than stretching at other times because the muscle temperature is elevated and, therefore, the stretching is more likely to produce optimal flexibility improvements.

A cardiovascular portion of the cool-down is also important. During physical activity, the heart pumps a large

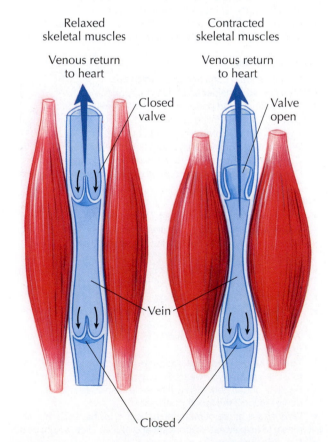

Figure 2 ▶ Muscle contractions aid the veins in returning blood to the heart.

The exercises shown here can be used before a moderate workout as a warm-up, or after a workout as a cool-down. Perform these exercises slowly, preferably after completing a cardiovascular warm-up. Do not bounce or jerk against the muscle. Hold each stretch for at least 15-30 seconds. Perform each exercise at least once and up to three times. Other stretching exercises are presented in the concept on flexibility that can be used in a warm-up or cool-down.

Cardiovascular Exercise

Before you perform a vigorous work-out, walk or jog slowly for 2 minutes or more. After exercise, do the same. Do this portion of the warm-up prior to muscle stretching.

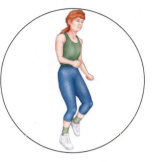

Leg Hug

This exercise stretches the hip and back extensor muscles. Lie on your back. Bend one leg and grasp your thigh under the knee. Hug it to your chest. Keep the other leg straight and on the floor. Hold. Repeat with the opposite leg.

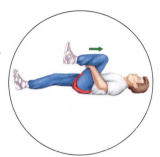

Calf Stretcher

This exercise stretches the calf muscles (gastrocnemius and soleus). Face a wall with your feet 2 or 3 feet away. Step forward on left foot to allow both hands to touch the wall. Keep the heel of your right foot on the ground, toe turned in slightly, knee straight, and buttocks tucked in. Lean forward by bending your front knee and arms and allowing your head to move nearer the wall. Hold. Repeat with the other leg.

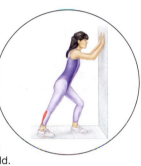

Seated Side Stretch

This exercise stretches the muscles of the trunk. Begin in a seated position with the legs crossed. Stretch the left arm over the head to the right. Bend at the waist (to right), reaching as far as possible to the left with the right arm. Hold. Do not let the trunk rotate. Repeat to the opposite side. For less stretch the overhead arm may be bent. This exercise can be done in the standing position but is less effective.

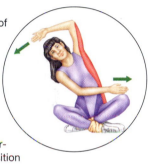

Hamstring Stretcher

This exercise stretches the muscles of the back of the upper leg (hamstrings) as well as those of the hip, knee, and ankle. Lie on your back. Bring the right knee to your chest and grasp the toes with the right hand. Place the left hand on the back of the right thigh. Pull the knee toward the chest, push the heel toward the ceiling, and pull the toes toward the shin. Attempt to straighten the knee. Stretch and hold. Repeat with the other leg.

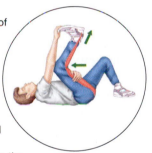

Zipper

This exercise stretches the muscle on the back of the arm (triceps) and the lower chest muscles (pecs). Lift right arm and reach behind head and down the spine (as if pulling up a zipper). With the left hand, push down on right elbow and hold. Reverse arm position and repeat.

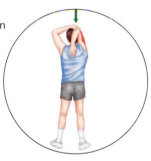

Figure 3 ▶ Sample warm-up and cool-down exercises.

amount of blood to supply the working muscles with the oxygen necessary to keep moving. The muscles squeeze the veins (see Figure 2), which forces the blood back to the heart. Valves in the veins prevent the blood from flowing backward. As long as exercise continues, the blood is moved by the muscles back to the heart, where it is once again pumped to the body. If exercise is stopped abruptly, the blood is left in the area of the working muscles and has no way to get back to the heart. In the case of the runner, the blood pools in the legs. Because the heart has less blood to pump, blood pressure may drop. This can result in dizziness and can even cause a person to pass out. The best way to prevent this problem is to taper off or slow down gradually after exercise. A cardiovascular cool-down should include 2 or more minutes of walking, slow jogging, or any nonvigorous activity that uses the muscles involved in the workout.

Warm-Up Light to moderate activity done prior to the workout. Its purpose is to reduce the risk of injury and soreness and possibly improve performance in a physical activity.

Cool-Down Light to moderate activity done after a workout to help the body recover; often consisting of the same exercises used in the warm-up.

Lactic Acid A by-product of the metabolic processes that occurs during vigorous physical activity; a cause of muscle fatigue.

Physical Activity in the Heat

Physical activity in hot and humid environments challenges the body's heat loss mechanisms. www.mhhe.com/phys_fit/web03 Click 04. During vigorous activity the body produces heat that must be dissipated to regulate body temperature. The body has several ways to dissipate heat. *Conduction* is the transfer of heat from a hot body to a cold body. *Convection* is the transfer of heat through the air or any other medium. Fans and wind can facilitate heat loss by convection and help regulate temperature. The primary method of cooling is through *evaporation* of sweat. The chemical process involved in evaporation transfers heat from the body and reduces the body temperature. When conditions are humid, the effectiveness of evaporation is reduced, since the air is already saturated with moisture. This is why it is difficult to regulate body temperature when conditions are hot and humid.

Heat-related illness can occur if proper hydration is not maintained. Maximum sweat rates during physical activity in the heat can approach 1–2 liters per hour. If this fluid is not replaced, **dehydration** can occur. If dehydration is not corrected with water or other fluid-replacement drinks, it becomes increasingly more difficult for the body to maintain normal body temperatures. At some point, the rate of sweating decreases as the body begins to conserve its remaining water. It shunts blood to the skin to transfer excess heat directly to the environment, but this is less effective than evaporation. **Hyperthermia** and associated heat-related problems can result (see Table 3).

One way to monitor the amount of fluid loss is to monitor the color of your urine. The American College of Sports Medicine indicates that clear (almost colorless) urine produced in large volumes indicates that you are hydrated. Dark yellow urine is a good indicator of dehydration and need for fluid replacement. Dietary supplements that contain amphetamine derivatives and/or creatine may contribute to undetected dehydration among some individuals.

Table 3 ▶ Types of Heat-Related Problems

Problem	Symptoms	Severity
Heat cramps	Muscle cramps, especially in muscles most used in exercise	Least severe
Heat exhaustion	Muscle cramps, weakness, dizziness, headache, nausea, clammy skin, paleness	Moderately severe
Heat stroke	Hot, flushed skin, dry skin (lack of sweating), dizziness, fast pulse, unconsciousness, high temperature	Extremely severe

Acclimatization improves the body's tolerance in the heat. Individuals with good fitness will respond better to activity in the heat than individuals with poor fitness. With regular exposure, the body adapts to the heat. The majority of the adaptation to hot environments occurs in 7 to 14 days but complete acclimatization can take up to 30 days. As you adapt to the heat, your body becomes conditioned to sweat earlier, to sweat more profusely, and to distribute the sweat more effectively around the body, and the composition of sweat is altered. This process makes it easier for your body to maintain a safe body temperature.

When doing physical activity in hot and humid environments, special precautions should be taken to prevent heat-related problems. www.mhhe.com/phys_fit/ web03 Click 05.

- Limit or avoid physical activity in hot or humid environments. The **apparent temperature** (also referred to as the heat index) is an index that combines temperature and humidity. Physical activity is safe when the apparent temperature is below 80°F (26.7°C). Above this temperature, there are four zones (see Table 4) that illustrate the danger of doing physical activity when the apparent temperature is high. When apparent temperatures reach the danger zones, activity should be limited or canceled. With extreme care, experienced exercisers who have become acclimatized to the heat may be able to perform at higher apparent temperatures than those who are less experienced. However, care should be used by all people who perform physical activity in hot and humid environments.
- Drink fluids before, during, and after activity. Guidelines suggest about 2 cups before activity and about 1 cup for each 15–20 minutes during activity. After activity, drink about 2 cups for each pound of weight lost. The thirst mechanism lags behind the body's actual need for fluid, so drink even if you don't feel thirsty. Fluid-replacement beverages (e.g., Gatorade, Power-Aid) are designed to provide added energy (from carbohydrates) without impeding hydration. If you choose to use one of these beverages, select one that contains electrolytes and no more than 4 to 8 percent carbohydrates.
- Gradually expose yourself to physical activity in hot and humid environments to facilitate acclimatization.
- If possible, exercise in the morning or evening.
- Dress properly for exercise in the heat and humidity. Wear white or light colors that reflect rather than absorb heat. Select wickable clothes instead of cotton to aid evaporative cooling. Rubber, plastic, or other nonporous clothing is especially dangerous. A porous hat or cap can help when exercising in direct sunlight.
- Rest at regular intervals, preferably in the shade.
- Watch for signs of heat stress. If signs are present, stop immediately.

Table 4 ▶ Exercise in the Heat (Apparent Temperatures)

To read the table, find air temperature on the top; then find the humidity on the left. Find the apparent temperature where the columns meet.

Relative Humidity (%)	Air Temperature (Degrees F)										
	70	75	80	85	90	95	100	105	110	115	120
100	72	80	91	108	132						
95	71	79	89	105	128						
90	71	79	88	102	122						
85	71	78	87	99	117	141					
80	71	78	86	97	113	136					
75	70	77	86	95	109	130					
70	70	77	85	93	106	124	144				
65	70	76	83	91	102	119	138				
60	70	76	82	90	100	114	132	149			
55	69	75	81	89	98	110	126	142			
50	69	75	81	88	96	107	120	135	150		
45	68	74	80	87	95	104	115	129	143		
40	68	74	79	86	93	101	110	123	137	151	
35	67	73	79	85	91	98	107	118	130	143	
30	67	73	78	84	90	96	104	113	123	135	148
25	66	72	77	83	88	94	101	109	117	127	139
20	66	72	77	82	87	93	99	105	112	120	130
15	65	71	76	81	86	91	97	102	108	115	123
10	65	70	75	80	85	90	95	100	105	111	116
5	64	69	74	79	84	88	93	97	102	107	111
0	64	69	73	78	83	87	91	95	99	103	107

"Apparent Temperatures"
(Heat Index)

- = Exreme danger zone
- = Danger zone
- = Extreme caution zone
- = Caution zone
- = Safe

Source: Data from National Oceanic and Atmospheric Administration.

If overheating occurs, take immediate steps to cool the body. Take these steps: Stop physical activity, get out of the heat and into the shade, remove excess clothing, drink cool water, and immerse the body in cool water. If symptoms of heat stroke are present, seek immediate medical attention; statically stretch cramped muscles.

quently, cognitive functions decrease, speech and movement become impaired, and bizarre behavior may occur. Frostbite results from water crystallizing in the tissues causing cell destruction.

Physical Activity in Other Environments

Physical activity in exceptionally cold and windy weather can be dangerous. www.mhhe.com/phys_fit/web03 Click 06. Physical activity in the cold presents the opposite problems as exercise in the heat. In the cold, the primary goal is to retain the body's heat and avoid **hypothermia** and frostbite. Early signs of hypothermia include shivering and cold extremities caused by blood shunted to the body core to conserve heat. As the core temperature continues to drop, heart rate, respiration, and reflexes are depressed. Subse-

Dehydration Excessive loss of water from the body, usually through perspiration, urination, or evaporation.

Hyperthermia Excessively high body temperature caused by excessive heat production or impaired heat loss capacity. Heat stroke is a hyperthermic condition.

Apparent Temperature A combination of temperature and humidity, used to determine if it is dangerous to perform physical activity (also called heat index).

Hypothermia Excessively low body temperature (less than 95°F) characterized by uncontrollable shivering, loss of coordination, and mental confusion.

A combination of cold and wind (windchill) poses the greatest danger. Recent research conducted in Canada, in cooperation with the U.S. National Weather Service, produced new tables for determining **windchill factor** and the time of exposure necessary to get frostbite (see Table 5). The old method of measurement overestimated the impact of cold weather. Consider the following guidelines for performing physical activity in cold and wind:

- Limit or cancel activity if the windchill factor reaches the danger zone (see Table 5).
- Dress properly in the wind and cold. Wear light clothing in several layers rather than one heavy garment. The layer of clothing closest to the body should transfer (wick) moisture away from the skin to a second, more absorbent layer. Polypropylene and capilene are examples of wickable fabrics. A porous windbreaker will keep wind from cooling the body and will allow the release of body heat. The hands, feet, nose, and ears are most susceptible to frostbite, so they should be covered. Wear a hat or cap, mask, and mittens. Mittens are warmer than gloves. A light coating of petroleum jelly on exposed body parts can be helpful.
- Keep from getting wet in cold weather.

High altitude may limit performance and require adaptation of normal physical activity.
www.mhhe.com/phys_fit/web03 Click 07. The ability to do vigorous physical tasks is diminished as altitude increases. Breathing rate and heart rates are more elevated at high altitude. With proper acclimation (gradual exposure), the body adjusts to the lower oxygen pressure found at high altitude, and performance improves. Nevertheless, performance ability at high altitudes, especially for activities requiring cardiovascular fitness, is usually less than would be expected at sea level. At extremely high altitudes, the ability to perform vigorous physical activity may be impossible without an extra oxygen supply. When moving from sea level to a high altitude, vigorous exercise should be done with caution. Acclimation to high altitudes requires a minimum of 2 weeks and may not be complete for several months. Care should be taken to drink adequate water at high altitude.

Exposure to air pollution should be limited.
www.mhhe.com/phys_fit/web03 Click 08. Various pollutants can also cause poor physical performance, and in some cases health problems. Ozone, a pollutant produced primarily by the sun's reaction to car exhaust, can cause symptoms, including headache, coughing, and eye irritation. Similar symptoms result from exposure to carbon monoxide, a tasteless and odorless gas, caused by combustion of oil, gasoline, and/or cigarette smoke. Most news media in metropolitan areas now provide updates on ozone and carbon monoxide levels in their weather reports. When levels of these pollutants reach moderate levels, some people may need to modify their exercise. When levels are high, some may need to postpone exercise. Exercisers wishing to avoid ozone and

Table 5 ▶ Windchill Factor Chart

Actual Temperature Reading (Degrees F)	Estimated Wind Speed (mph)									Minutes to frostbite
	Calm	5	10	15	20	25	30	35	40	
40	40	36	34	32	30	29	28	27	27	
30	30	25	21	19	17	16	15	14	13	
20	20	13	9	6	4	3	1	0	-1	
10	10	1	-4	-7	-9	-11	-12	-14	-15	
0	0	-11	-16	-19	-22	-24	-26	-27	-29	30
-10	-10	-22	-28	-32	-35	-37	-39	-41	-43	10
-20	-20	-34	-41	-45	-48	-51	-53	-55	-57	5
-30	-30	-46	-53	-58	-61	-64	-67	-69	-71	
-40	-40	-57	-66	-71	-74	-78	-80	-82	-84	

Source: National Weather Service, 2001.

carbon monoxide may want to exercise indoors early in the morning or later in the evening. It is wise to avoid areas with a high concentration of traffic.

Pollens from certain plants may cause allergic reactions for certain people. Some people are allergic to dust or other particulates in the air. Weather reports of pollens and particulates may help exercisers determine the best times for their activities and when to avoid vigorous activities.

Soreness and Injury

Understanding soreness can help you persist in physical activity and avoid problems. www.mhhe.com/phys_fit/web03 Click 09. Some people avoid physical activity because they remember earlier experiences, such as team practices or training for special events, that caused soreness 24 to 48 hours after the intense exercise. They feel that all activity will make them sore, and they want to avoid this unpleasant experience. It is true that intense exercise, especially to muscle groups that are not normally exercised, can cause what is called delayed-onset muscle soreness (**DOMS**). Some people mistakenly believe that lactic acid is the cause of muscle soreness. Lactic acid, however, returns to normal levels 30 minutes after exercise, whereas DOMS occurs at least 24 hours following exercise. DOMS results from microscopic muscle tears, not a build-up of lactic acid. In some cases, DOMS is accompanied by swelling and pain, but in general the condition has no long-term consequences.

To reduce the likelihood of DOMS, it is important to progress your program gradually. Lengthening (eccentric) contractions are more likely to cause DOMS than shortening (concentric) contractions, so limit downhill running. Doing moderate exercise when you have soreness does not seem to put you at risk for muscle injury. Fortunately, DOMS lasts only a day or two and is uncommon for those who exercise regularly and consistently.

Being able to treat minor injuries will help reduce their negative effects. www.mhhe.com/phys_fit/web03 Click 10. Minor injuries, such as muscle sprains and strains, are common to those who are persistent in their exercise. If a serious injury should occur or, if symptoms persist, it is important to get immediate medical attention. However, for minor injuries, following the **RICE** formula will help you reduce the pain and speed recovery. In this acronym, *R* stands for *rest*. Muscle sprains and strains heal best if rested. Rest helps you avoid further damage to the muscle. *I* stands for *ice*. The quick application of cold (ice or ice water) to a minor injury minimizes swelling and speeds recovery. Cold should be applied to as large a surface area as possible (soaking is best). If ice is used, it should be wrapped to avoid direct contact with the skin. Apply cold for 20–30 minutes, three times a day for several days. *C* stands for *compression*. Wrapping or compressing the injured area also helps minimize swelling and speeds recovery. Elastic bandages are good for applying compression. For a sprained ankle, wearing a tied high top shoe until a bandage can be located provides good compression. Elastic socks may also be useful. Care should be taken to avoid wrapping an injury too tightly because this can result in loss of circulation to the area. *E* stands for *elevation*. Keeping the injured area elevated (above the level of the heart) is effective in minimizing swelling. If pain or swelling persists, or if there is any doubt about the seriousness of an injury, seek medical help.

Taking over-the-counter pain remedies can help reduce the pain of muscle strains and sprains. Aspirin and ibuprofen (e.g., Excedrin, Motrin) have anti-inflammatory properties. However, acetaminophen (e.g., Tylenol) does not have anti-inflammatory properties. It may reduce the pain but will not reduce inflammation.

The most common injuries incurred in physical activity are sprains and strains. A strain occurs when the fibers in a muscle are injured. Common activity-related injuries are hamstring strains that occur after a vigorous sprint. Other commonly strained muscles include the muscles in the front of the thigh, the low back, and the calf. A sprain is an injury to a ligament—the connective tissue that connects bones to bones. The most common sprain is to the ankle; frequently, the ankle is rolled to the outside when jumping or running. Evidence suggests that lace-up ankle braces made of nonelastic material are effective in reducing ankle sprains. Other common sprains are to the knee, the shoulder, and the wrist.

Tendonitis is an inflammation of the tendon and is most often a result of overuse rather than trauma. Tendonitis can be painful but often does not swell to the extent that sprains do. For this reason, elevation and compression are not as effective as ice and rest.

Windchill Factor An index that uses air temperature and wind speed to determine the chilling effect of the environment on humans.

DOMS An acronym for delayed-onset muscle soreness, a common malady that follows relatively vigorous activity, especially among beginners.

RICE An acronym for rest, ice, compression, and elevation; a method of treating minor injuries.

Muscle cramps can be relieved by statically stretching a muscle. Muscle cramps are pains in the large muscles that result when the muscles contract vigorously for a continued period of time. Muscle cramps are usually not considered to be an injury, but they are painful and may seem like an injury. They are usually short in duration and can often be relieved with proper treatment.

Cramps can result from lack of fluid replacement (dehydration), from fatigue, and from a blow directly to a muscle. Static stretching can help relieve some cramps. For example, the calf muscle, which often cramps among runners and other sports participants, can be relieved using the calf stretcher exercise, which is part of the warm-up in this concept.

Strategies for Action

Screening for risks can help make activity safer. Athletes in competitive sports often undergo physical examinations to screen for potential cardiac arrhythmias or conditions known to increase risks during exercise. Recreational athletes may not take the same precautions. The best advice is to get a physical prior to beginning serious training. This is especially critical if you have a family history of heart problems. The PAR-Q assessment in Lab 3A will provide a basic screen to determine if you should consult a physician.

A proper warm-up and cool-down can make activity more effective and more enjoyable. A proper warm-up can prepare your body for activity and a gradual cool-down can improve recovery. Lab 3B provides a sample flexibility-based warm-up and cool-down routine that may be helpful. Determine what works best for your personal needs.

Study Resources

Check out additional online study resources for this concept in the Student Edition of the Online Learning Center at www.mhhe.com/corbin13e.

Web Resources

ACSM's Fit Society Page **www.acsm.org/health+fitness/ fit_society.htm**
ACSM's Health and Fitness Journal
    www.acsm.org/publications/health_fitness_journal.htm
American College of Sports Medicine **www.acsm.org**
National Athletic Trainers Association **www.nata.org**
Med Watch **www.fda.gov/medwatch**
The Physician and Sportsmedicine **www.physsportsmed.com**

Suggested Readings

 Additional reference materials for Concept 3 are available at **www.mhhe.com/phys_fit/web03 Click 11.**

American College of Sports Medicine. 2000. *ACSM's Guidelines for Exercise Testing and Prescription.* 6th ed. Philadelphia: Lippincott, Williams and Wilkins.

American College of Sports Medicine and American Heart Association. 2002. Automated external defibrillators in health/fitness facilities. *Medicine and Science in Sports and Exercise* 34(3):561–564.

Bailes, J. E., et al. 2002. The neurosurgeon in sport: Awareness of the risks of heatstroke and dietary supplements. *Neurosurgery* 51(2):283–288.

Bracko, M. R. 2002. Can stretching prior to exercise and sports improve performance and prevent injury? *ACSM's Health and Fitness Journal* 6(5):17–22.

Hootman, J. M., et al. 2002. Epidemiology of musculoskeletal injuries among sedentary and physically active adults. *Medicine and Science in Sports and Exercise* 34(5):838–844.

Inter-Association Task Force on Exertional Heat Illnesses. 2003. Inter-Association Task Force on Exertional Heat Illnesses consensus statement. *National Athletic Trainers Association Newsletter* June:24–29. Also available online at **www.nata.org.**

Weaver, W. D., and M. A. Peberty. 2002. Perspective: Defibrillators in public places: One step closer to home. *New England Journal of Medicine* 347(16):1223–1224.

In the News

The Benefits of Defibrillators

The recent evidence concerning the effectiveness of public access defibrillation (PAD) using automated external defibrillators (AED) has created new needs in the field. The American Heart Association has developed a course, called Heartsaver, that covers CPR and techniques for using an AED (see **www.americanheart.org**). Home defibrillators are also becoming more common (see **www.heartsathome.com**).

Lab 3A Readiness for Physical Activity

Name	Section	Date

Purpose: To help you determine your physical readiness for participation in a program of regular exercise

Procedures

1. Read the directions on the "PAR-Q & You" on page 46.
2. Answer each of the seven questions on the form.
3. If you answered "yes" to one or more of the questions, follow the directions just below the PAR-Q questions regarding medical consultation.
4. If you answered "no" to all seven questions, follow the directions at the lower left-hand corner of the PAR-Q.
5. Answer the five questions about physical readiness for sports or vigorous training in Chart 1 below.
6. Record your score below and answer the question in the Conclusions and Implications section.

Results

Chart 1 ▶ Physical Readiness for Sports or Vigorous Training

Answer the PAR-Q before using this chart. If your answer to any of these questions is "yes," then you should consult with your personal physician by telephone or in person to determine if you have a potential problem with sports or vigorous training.

Yes **No**

☐ ☐ 1. Do you plan to participate on an organized team that will play intense competitive sports (e.g., varsity team, professional team)?

☐ ☐ 2. If you plan to participate in a collision sport (even on a less organized basis), such as football, boxing, rugby, or ice hockey, have you been knocked unconscious more than one time?

☐ ☐ 3. Do you currently have symptoms from a previous muscle injury?

☐ ☐ 4. Do you currently have symptoms from a previous back injury, or do you experience back pain as a result of involvement in physical activity?

☐ ☐ 5. Do you have any other symptoms during physical activity that give you reason to be concerned about your health?

Determine your PAR-Q score. Place an X over the circle that includes the number of yes answers that you had for the PAR-Q (see page 46).

0 1 2 3 4 5 6 7

Determine your readiness for sports or rigorous training (see Chart 1 above). Place an X over the number of yes answers that you had for the Physical Readiness for Sports or Vigorous Training chart.

0 1 2 3 4 5

Conclusions and Implications: In several sentences, discuss your readiness for physical activity. Base your comments on your questionnaire results and the types of physical activities you plan to perform in the future.

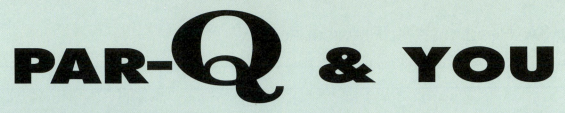

Regular physical activity is fun and healthy, and increasingly more people are starting to become more active every day. Being more active is very safe for most people. However, some people should check with their doctor before they start becoming much more physically active.

If you are planning to become much more physically active than you are now, start by answering the seven questions in the box below. If you are between the ages of fifteen and sixty-nine, the PAR-Q will tell you if you should check with your doctor before you start. If you are over sixty-nine years of age, and you are not used to being very active, check with your doctor.

Common sense is your best guide when you answer these questions. Please read the questions carefully and answer each one honestly: check YES or NO.

YES	NO	
☐	☐	1. Has your doctor ever said that you have a heart condition <u>and</u> that you should only do physical activity recommended by a doctor?
☐	☐	2. Do you feel pain in your chest when you do physical activity?
☐	☐	3. In the past month, have you had chest pain when you were not doing physical activity?
☐	☐	4. Do you lose your balance because of dizziness or do you ever lose consciousness?
☐	☐	5. Do you have a bone or joint problem that could be made worse by a change in your physical activity?
☐	☐	6. Is your doctor currently prescribing drugs (for example, water pills) for your blood pressure or heart condition?
☐	☐	7. Do you know of <u>any other reason</u> you should not do physical activity?

If
you
answered

Yes

No

YES to one or more questions

Talk with your doctor by phone or in person BEFORE you start becoming much more physically active or BEFORE you have a fitness appraisal. Tell your doctor about the PAR-Q and which questions you answered YES.

- You may be able to do any activity you want—as long as you start slowly and build up gradually. Or you may need to restrict your activities to those that are safe for you. Talk with your doctor about the kinds of activities you wish to participate in and follow his or her advice.
- Find out which community programs are safe and helpful for you.

NO to all questions

If you answered NO honestly to <u>all</u> PAR-Q questions, you can be reasonably sure that you can

- Start becoming much more physically active—begin slowly and build up gradually. This is the safest and easiest way to go.
- Take part in a fitness appraisal—this is an excellent way to determine your basic fitness so that you can plan the best way for you to live actively.

DELAY BECOMING MUCH MORE ACTIVE:

- If you are not feeling well because of a temporary illness, such as a cold or a fever—wait until you feel better or
- If you are or may be pregnant—talk to your doctor before you start becoming more active.

Please note: If your health changes so that you then answer YES to any of the above questions, tell your fitness or health professional. Ask whether you should change your physical activity plan.

<u>Informed Use of the PAR-Q:</u> The Canadian Society for Exercise Physiology, Health Canada, and their agents assume no liability for persons who undertake physical activity, and if in doubt after completing this questionnaire, consult your doctor prior to physical activity.

You are encouraged to copy the PAR-Q but only if you use the entire form

*Developed by the British Columbia Ministry of Health.

Produced by the British Columbia Ministry of Health and the Department of National Health & Welfare

Physical Activity Readiness
Questionnaire • PAR-Q
(revised 2002)

Note: It is important that you answer all questions honestly. The PAR-Q is a scientifically and medically researched pre-exercise selection device. It complements exercise programs, exercise testing procedures, and the liability considerations attendant with such programs and testing procedures. PAR-Q, like any other preexercise screening device, will misclassify a small percentage of prospective participants, but no preexercise screening method can entirely avoid this problem.

Lab 3B The Warm-Up and Cool-Down

Name   **Section**   **Date**

Purpose: To familiarize you with a sample group of warm-up or cool-down exercises

Procedures

1. Perform a 2- to 5-minute cardiovascular warm-up (walk, jog, slow jump rope, swim).
2. Perform the exercises in Chart 1 on the back of this lab page three times each. Hold the stretch for 15 to 30 seconds.
3. Complete the Results section below and answer the questions in the Conclusions and Implications section.

Results: In the following, put an X over the circle that represents the amount of tightness you felt when performing each of the stretching warm-up and cool-down exercises. Tightness indicates that you may have shortness of a specific muscle group and that stretching exercises at times other than the warm-up or cool-down are needed.

	None	Moderate	Severe
Calf stretcher	○	○	○
Hamstring stretcher	○	○	○
Leg hug	○	○	○
Sitting side stretch	○	○	○
Zipper	○	○	○

Conclusions and Implications: In several sentences, discuss the warm-up and cool-down. Include in the discussion your feelings about the adequacy of the warm-up and cool-down for you personally. Those who plan to do vigorous sports will need to supplement this group of exercises.

Chart 1 ▶ Sample warm-up and cool-down exercises.

The exercises shown here can be used before a moderate workout as a warm-up or after a workout as a cool-down. Perform these exercises slowly, preferably after completing a cardiovascular warm-up. Do not bounce or jerk against the muscle. Hold each stretch for at least 15-30 seconds. Perform each exercise at least once and up to three times. Other stretching exercises are presented in the concept on flexibility and they can be used in a warm-up or cool-down.

Cardiovascular Exercise

Before you perform a vigorous work-out, walk or jog slowly for two minutes or more. After exercise, do the same. Do this portion of the warm-up prior to muscle stretching.

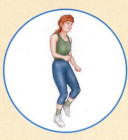

Leg Hug

This exercise stretches the hip and back extensor muscles. Lie on your back. Bend one leg and grasp your thigh under the knee. Hug it to your chest. Keep the other leg straight and on the floor. Hold. Repeat with the opposite leg.

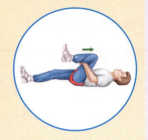

Calf Stretcher

This exercise stretches the calf muscles (gastrocnemius and soleus). Face a wall with your feet 2 or 3 feet away. Step forward on left foot to allow both hands to touch the wall. Keep the heel of your right foot on the ground, toe turned in slightly, knee straight, and buttocks tucked in. Lean forward by bending your front knee and arms and allowing your head to move nearer the wall. Hold. Repeat with the other leg.

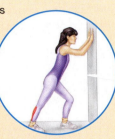

Seated Side Stretch

This exercise stretches the muscles of the trunk. Begin in a seated position with the legs crossed. Stretch the left arm over the head to the right. Bend at the waist (to right), reaching as far as possible to the left with the right arm. Hold. Do not let the trunk rotate. Repeat to the opposite side. For less stretch the overhead arm may be bent. This exercise can be done in the standing position but is less effective.

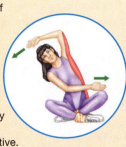

Hamstring Stretcher

This exercise stretches the muscles of the back of the upper leg (hamstrings) as well as those of the hip, knee, and ankle. Lie on your back. Bring the right knee to your chest and grasp the toes with the right hand. Place the left hand on the back of the right thigh. Pull the knee toward the chest, push the heel toward the ceiling, and pull the toes toward the shin. Attempt to straighten the knee. Stretch and hold. Repeat with the other leg.

Zipper

This exercise stretches the muscle on the back of the arm (triceps) and the lower chest muscles (pecs). Lift right arm and reach behind head and down the spine (as if pulling up a zipper). With the left hand, push down on right elbow and hold. Reverse arm position and repeat.

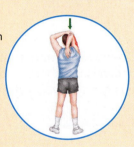

The Health Benefits of Physical Activity

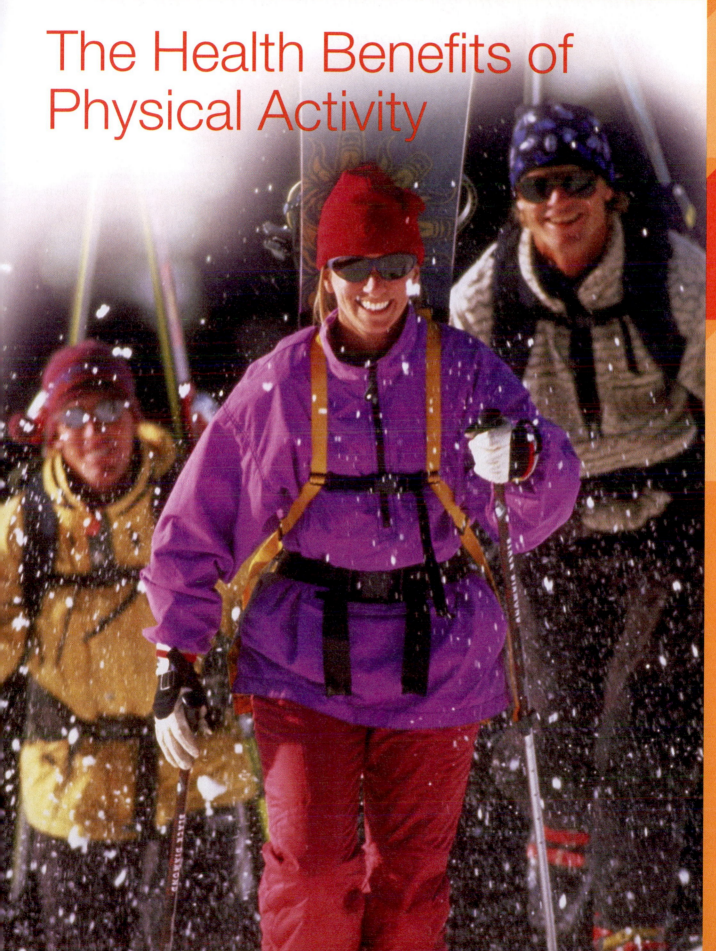

Physical activity and good physical fitness can reduce risk of illness and contribute to optimal health and wellness.

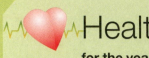

Health Goals

for the year 2010

- Increase quality and years of healthy life.

- Increase incidence of "healthy days."

- Increase daily physical activity.

- Increase prevalence of a healthy weight and reduce prevalence of overweight.

- Reduce days with pain for those with arthritis, osteoporosis, and chronic back problems.

- Reduce activity limitations, especially among older adults.

- Reduce incidence of and deaths from cancer.

- Increase diagnosis of and reduce incidence of Type II diabetes.

- Decrease incidence of depression.

- Decrease incidence of heart diseases, including stroke and high blood pressure.

- Decrease incidence of high cholesterol levels among adults.

The *Surgeon General's Report on Physical Activity and Health* was an especially important document that informed the general public of the risks of sedentary living and the health benefits of physical activity. Since that document was published, more evidence has accumulated supporting the health benefits of an active lifestyle. One recent study has shown that physical fitness measured using a treadmill test is a more powerful predictor of longevity than any other risk factor, including smoking, heart problems, high blood pressure, high cholesterol, and diabetes. The evidence has led to reports, such as *Healthy People 2010* in the United States and *Achieving Health for All* in Canada, that establish health goals designed to promote active healthy living in the 21st century. In this concept, the health benefits of regular physical activity will be summarized.

Physical Activity and Hypokinetic Diseases

Regular physical activity and good fitness can promote good health, help prevent disease, and be a part of disease treatment. www.mhhe.com/phys_fit/web04 Click 01. There are three major ways in which regular physical activity and good fitness can contribute to optimal health and wellness. First, they can aid in disease/illness prevention. There is considerable evidence that the risk of **hypokinetic diseases or conditions** can be greatly reduced among people who do regular physical activity and achieve good physical fitness. Virtually all **chronic diseases** that plague society are considered to be hypokinetic, though some relate more to inactivity than others. Nearly three-quarters of all deaths among those eighteen and older are a result of chronic diseases. Leading public health officials have suggested that physical activity reduces the risk for several of these diseases. Physical activity also stimulates positive changes with respect to other risk factors and may produce a shortcut for the control of chronic diseases, much as immunization controls infectious diseases.

Second, physical activity and fitness can be significant contributors to disease/illness treatment. Even with the best disease prevention practices, some people will become ill. Regular exercise and good fitness have been shown to be effective in alleviating symptoms and aiding rehabilitation after illness for such hypokinetic conditions as diabetes, heart disease, and back pain.

Finally, physical activity and fitness are methods of health and wellness promotion. They contribute to quality living associated with wellness, the positive component of good health. In the process, they aid in meeting many of the nation's health goals.

 Too many adults suffer from hypokinetic disease and the economic cost is high. www.mhhe. com/phys_fit/web04 Click 02. In 1961, Kraus and Raab coined the term *hypokinetic disease* to describe health problems associated with lack of physical activity. They showed how sedentary living, or, as they called it "take it easy" living, contributes to the leading killer diseases in our society. For example four of the major causes of death are considered to be hypokinetic; heart disease, cancer, stroke, and diabetes. Some experts have differentiated between hypokinetic diseases such as those listed and hypokinetic conditions such as back pain and obesity. Although experts agree that these are hypokinetic conditions, there is no universal agreement that conditions such as these are diseases.

Lack of physical activity is associated with the clinical condition known as metabolic syndrome. Metabolic syndrome, or Syndrome X, was briefly discussed in Concept 1. Experts have recently outlined specific characteristics of this condition and it is now a recognized medical condition. A person is considered to have metabolic syndrome if three or more of the following are present: high waist girth (>40 inches), high blood triglycerides (>150), low HDL (>40), high blood pressure (>135/85), and high fasting blood glucose (>100). Because the condition is so inextricably linked with sedentary living, some experts have suggested that the condition should really be known as *inactivity syndrome*. A public health advocacy group has coined the related term **sedentary death syndrome (SeDS)** to more fully characterize the health implications of sedentary living. Greater awareness in the medical community about the negative consequences of inactivity should lead to more emphasis on prevention and more funding for physical activity programs.

Regular physical activity over a lifetime may overcome the effects of inherited risk. Some people with a family history of disease may conclude they can do nothing because their heredity works against them. There is no doubt that heredity significantly affects risk for early death from hypokinetic diseases. New studies of twins, however, suggest that active people are less likely to die early than inactive people with similar genes. This suggests that long-term adherence to physical activity can overcome other risk factors, such as heredity.

Hypokinetic diseases and conditions have many causes. Regular physical activity and good physical fitness are only two of the preventive factors associated with the conditions described in this concept as hypokinetic diseases. Other healthy lifestyle factors, such as nutrition and stress management, cannot be overlooked.

Physical Activity and Cardiovascular Diseases

The many types of cardiovascular diseases are the leading killers in automated societies. There are many forms of **cardiovascular disease (CVD)**. Some are classified as **coronary heart disease (CHD)** because they affect the heart muscle and the blood vessels inside the heart. **Coronary occlusion** (heart attack) is a type of CHD. **Atherosclerosis** and **arteriosclerosis** are two conditions that increase risk for heart attack and are considered to be types of CHD. **Angina pectoris** (chest or arm pain), which occurs when the oxygen supply to the heart muscle is diminished, is sometimes considered to be a type of CHD, though it is really a symptom of poor circulation.

Hypertension (high blood pressure), **stroke** (brain attack), **peripheral vascular disease,** and **congestive heart failure** are other forms of CVD. Inactivity relates in some way to each of these types of disease.

In the United States, CHD accounts for approximately 31 percent of all premature deaths. Stroke accounts for an

Hypokinetic Diseases or Conditions *Hypo-* means "under" or "too little" and *-kinetic* means "movement" or "activity." Thus, *hypokinetic* means "too little activity." A hypokinetic disease or condition is associated with lack of physical activity or too little regular exercise. Examples include heart disease, low back pain, and adult-onset diabetes.

Chronic Diseases Disease or illnesses associated with lifestyle or environmental factors, as opposed to infectious diseases; hypokinetic diseases are considered to be chronic diseases.

Sedentary Death Syndrome (SeDS) A group of symptoms associated with sedentary living, including low health-related fitness (low cardiovascular fitness and weak muscles), low bone density, and the presence of metabolic syndrome (poor metabolic fitness).

Cardiovascular Disease (CVD) A broad classification of diseases of the heart and blood vessels that includes CHD, as well as high blood pressure, stroke, and peripheral vascular disease.

Coronary Heart Disease (CHD) Diseases of the heart muscle and the blood vessels that supply it with oxygen, including heart attack.

Coronary Occlusion The blocking of the coronary blood vessels; sometimes called heart attack.

Atherosclerosis The deposition of materials along the arterial walls; a type of arteriosclerosis.

Arteriosclerosis Hardening of the arteries due to conditions that cause the arterial walls to become thick, hard, and nonelastic.

Angina Pectoris Chest or arm pain resulting from reduced oxygen supply to the heart muscle.

Hypertension High blood pressure.

Stroke A condition in which the brain, or part of the brain, receives insufficient oxygen as a result of diminished blood supply; sometimes called apoplexy or cerebrovascular accident (CVA)

Peripheral Vascular Disease Lack of oxygen supply to the working muscles and tissues of the arms and legs, resulting from decreased blood flow.

Congestive Heart Failure The inability of the heart muscle to pump the blood at a life-sustaining rate.

additional 7 percent. Men are more likely to suffer from heart disease than women. African American, Hispanic, and Native American populations are at higher than normal risk. Heart disease and stroke death rates are similar in the United States, Canada, Great Britain, Australia, and other automated societies.

There is a wealth of statistical evidence that physical inactivity is a primary risk factor for CHD. Much of the research relating inactivity to heart disease has come from occupational studies that show a high incidence of heart disease in people involved only in sedentary work. Even with the limitations inherent in these types of studies, the findings of more and more occupational studies present convincing evidence that the inactive individual has an increased risk for coronary heart disease. A study summarizing all of the important occupational studies shows a 90 percent reduced risk for coronary heart disease for those in active versus inactive occupations.

Studies also indicate that adults who expend a significant number of calories per week in strenuous sports and other activities have reduced risk for coronary heart disease. In fact, improving activity levels is among the best ways to reduce the risk for heart disease among adults.

The American Heart Association, after carefully examining the research literature, elevated sedentary living from a secondary to a primary risk factor, comparable to high blood pressure, high blood cholesterol, obesity, and cigarette smoke. The reason for this change is that inactivity increases risk in multiple ways and large numbers of adults are sedentary and vulnerable to these risks. After reviewing hundreds of studies on exercise and heart disease, the *Surgeon General's Report on Physical Activity and Health* concluded that "physical inactivity is causally linked to atherosclerosis and coronary heart disease."

Physical Activity and the Healthy Heart

Regular physical activity will increase the ability of the heart muscle to pump blood as well as oxygen. A fit heart muscle can handle extra demands placed on it. Through regular exercise, the heart muscle gets stronger, contracts more forcefully, and therefore pumps more blood with each beat. This results in a slower heart rate (especially during physical activity) and greater heart efficiency. The heart is just like any other muscle—it must be exercised regularly to stay fit. The fit heart has open, clear arteries free of atherosclerosis (see Figure 1).

The hypothetical "normal" resting heart rate is said to be 72 beats per minute (bpm). However, resting rates of 50 to 85 bpm are common. People who regularly do physical activity will typically have lower resting heart

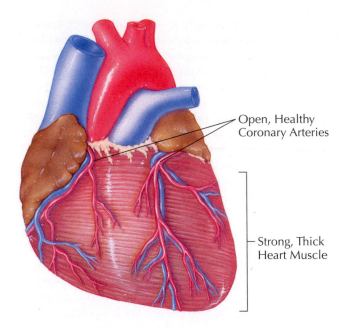

Open, Healthy
Coronary Arteries

Strong, Thick
Heart Muscle

Figure 1 ▶ The fit heart muscle.

rates than people who do no regular activity. Some endurance athletes have heart rates in the 30 and 40 bpm range, which is considered healthy or normal. Although resting heart rate is *not* considered to be a good measure of health or fitness, decreases in individual heart rate following training reflect positive adaptations. Low heart rates in response to a standard amount of physical activity *are* a good indicator of fitness. The bicycle and step tests presented later in this book use your heart rate response to a standard amount of exercise to estimate your cardiovascular fitness.

Physical Activity and Atherosclerosis

 Atherosclerosis, which begins early in life, is implicated in many cardiovascular diseases. www.mhhe.com/phys_fit/web04 Click 03. Atherosclerosis is a condition that contributes to heart attack, stroke, hypertension, angina pectoris, and peripheral vascular disease. Deposits on the walls of arteries restrict blood flow and oxygen supply to the tissues. Atherosclerosis of the coronary arteries, the vessels that supply the heart muscle with oxygen, is particularly harmful. If these arteries become narrowed, the blood supply to the heart muscle is diminished, and angina pectoris may occur. Atherosclerosis increases the risk of heart attack because a fibrous clot is more likely to obstruct a narrowed artery than a healthy, open one.

Current theory suggests that atherosclerosis begins when damage occurs to the cells of the inner wall, or

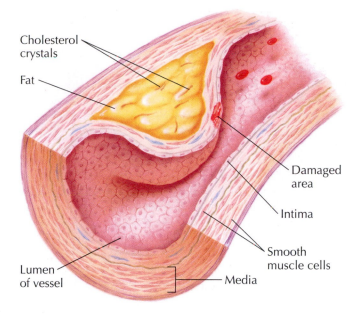

Cholesterol crystals

Fat

Damaged area

Intima

Smooth muscle cells

Lumen of vessel

Media

Figure 2 ▶ Atherosclerosis.

Table 1 ▶ Cholesterol Classifications (mg/dL)				
	Total Cholesterol	LDL-C	HDL-C	TC/HDL-C
Optimal	—	<100	—	3.5 or less
Near optimal	—	100–129	—	—
Desirable	<200	—	>60	—
Borderline	200–240	130–160	39–59	3.6–5.0
High risk	>240	>160	40	5.0+

Source: Third Report of the National Cholesterol Education Program.

intima, of the artery (see Figure 2). Substances associated with blood clotting are attracted to the damaged area. These substances seem to cause the migration of smooth muscle cells, commonly found only in the middle wall of the artery (media), to the intima. In the later stages, fats (including cholesterol) and other substances are thought to be deposited, forming plaques, or protrusions, that diminish the internal diameter of the artery. Research indicates that the first signs of atherosclerosis begin in early childhood.

 Regular physical activity can help prevent atherosclerosis by lowering blood lipid levels. www.mhhe. com/phys_fit/web04 Click 04. There are several kinds of **lipids** (fats) in the bloodstream, including **lipoproteins,** phospholipids, triglycerides, and cholesterol. Cholesterol is the most well known, but it is not the only culprit. Many blood fats are manufactured by the body itself, whereas others are ingested in high-fat foods, particularly saturated fats. Saturated fats are fats that are solid at room temperature.

As noted earlier, blood lipids are thought to contribute to the development of atherosclerotic deposits on the inner walls of the artery. One substance, called **low-density lipoprotein (LDL),** is considered to be a major culprit in the development of atherosclerosis. LDL is basically a core of cholesterol surrounded by protein and another substance that makes it water soluble. The benefit of regular exercise is that it can reduce blood lipid levels, including LDL-C (the cholesterol core of LDL). People with high total cholesterol and LDL-C levels have been shown to have a higher than normal risk for

heart disease (see Table 1). New evidence indicates that there are subtypes of LDL cholesterol (characterized by their small size and high density) that pose even greater risks. These subtypes are hard to measure and not included in most current blood tests, but future research will no doubt help us better understand and measure them. Recently, the FDA approved a skin cholesterol test that, when combined with traditional tests, may help in predicting future heart disease.

Triglycerides are another type of blood lipid. Elevated levels of triglycerides are positively related to heart disease. Triglycerides lose some of their ability to predict heart disease with the presence of other risk factors, so high levels are more difficult to interpret than other blood lipids. Normal levels are considered to be 150 mg/dL or less. Values of 151 to 199 are borderline, 200 to 499 are high, and above 500 are very high. It would be wise to include triglycerides in a blood lipid profile. Physical activity is often prescribed as part of a treatment for high triglyceride levels.

Whereas LDLs carry a core of cholesterol that is involved in the development of atherosclerosis, **high-density lipoprotein (HDL)** picks up cholesterol (HDL-C) and carries it to the liver, where it is eliminated from the body.

Lipids All fats and fatty substances.

Lipoproteins Fat-carrying proteins in the blood.

Low-Density Lipoprotein (LDL) A core of cholesterol surrounded by protein; the core is often called "bad cholesterol."

Triglycerides A type of blood fat associated with increased risk for heart disease.

High-Density Lipoprotein (HDL) A blood substance that picks up cholesterol and helps remove it from the body; often called "good cholesterol."

Regular physical activity can help prevent atherosclerosis by increasing HDL in the blood. For this reason, it is often called the "good cholesterol." High levels of HDL are considered to be desirable. When you have a blood test, it is wise to ask for information about total cholesterol, LDL, and HDL levels. A recent report has provided new information about healthy levels for each (see Table 1). Individuals who do regular physical activity have lower total cholesterol, lower LDL, and higher HDL levels. For this reason a total blood lipid profile should be considered rather than using a single indicator when calculating risk.

Regular physical activity can help prevent atherosclerosis by reducing blood coagulents. **Fibrin** and platelets (types of cells involved in blood coagulation) deposit at the site of an injury on the wall of the artery, contributing to the process of plaque build-up, or atherosclerosis. Regular physical activity has been shown to reduce fibrin levels in the blood. The breakdown of fibrin seems to reduce platelet adhesiveness and the concentration of platelets in the blood.

Indicators of inflammation of the arteries are predictive of atherosclerosis. Recently, other constituents of the blood have been shown to be associated with risk for cardiovascular disease. C-reactive protein (CRP) was identified in the 1930s but only recently has it been shown, in combination with LDL and HDL levels, to be a predictor of heart disease and stroke. Triggered by an inflammation in the arteries, levels of CRP in the blood increase. Preliminary standards suggest that below 1 milligram per liter of blood is low, between 1 and 3 mg/L is moderate and above 3 mg/L is high. At least one study has shown that high-fit people have lower CRP levels than low-fit people.

High levels of the amino acid homocysteine have also been associated with increased risk for heart disease, though the American Heart Association says it is too early to begin screening for it. Tentative fasting values have been established at 5 to 15 millimoles per liter of blood for the normal range, 16 to 30 as moderate, 31 to 100 as intermediate, and above 100 as high. Adequate levels of folic acid, vitamin B_6, and B_{12} help prevent high blood homocysteine levels, so eating foods that ensure adequate daily intake of these vitamins is recommended.

MPO, interleukin-6, and Cp-HSP60 (chlamydia pneumonia heat shock protein) are other blood constituents that are related to heart disease. All are associated with inflammations that damage the arterial wall and promote build-up of atherosclerosis. More research is necessary before these indicators will be used in medical risk profiles.

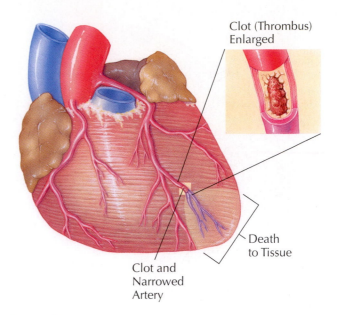

Clot (Thrombus) Enlarged

Death to Tissue

Clot and Narrowed Artery

Figure 3 ▶ Heart attack.

Physical Activity and Heart Attack

Regular physical activity reduces the risk for heart attack, the most prevalent and serious of all cardiovascular diseases. www.mhhe.com/phys_fit/web04 Click 05. A heart attack (coronary occlusion) occurs when a coronary artery is blocked (see Figure 3). A clot, or thrombus, is the most common cause, reducing or cutting off blood flow and oxygen to the heart muscle. If the blocked coronary artery supplies a major portion of the heart muscle, death will occur within minutes. Occlusions of lesser arteries may result in angina pectoris or a nonfatal heart attack.

People who perform regular sports and physical activity have half the risk for a first heart attack, compared with those who are sedentary. Possible reasons are less atherosclerosis, greater diameter of arteries, and less chance of a clot forming.

Regular exercise can improve coronary circulation and, thus, reduce the chances of a heart attack or dying from one. Within the heart, many tiny branches extend from the major coronary arteries. All of these vessels supply blood to the heart muscle. Healthy arteries can supply blood to any region of the heart as it is needed. Active people are likely to have greater blood-carrying capacity in these vessels, probably because the vessels are larger and more elastic. Also, the active person may have a more profuse distribution of arteries within the heart muscle (see Figure 4), which results in greater blood flow. A few studies show that physical activity may promote the growth of "extra" blood vessels, which are thought to open up to provide the heart muscle with the necessary

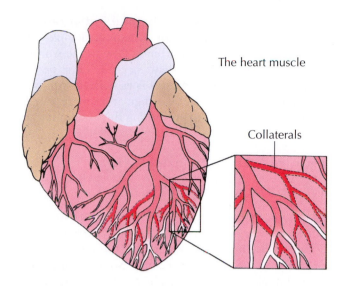

The heart muscle

Collaterals

Figure 4 ▶ Coronary collateral circulation.

blood and oxygen when the oxygen supply is diminished, as in a heart attack. Blood flow from extra blood vessels is referred to as **coronary collateral circulation.**

Improved coronary circulation may provide protection against a heart attack because a larger artery would require more atherosclerosis to occlude it. In addition, the development of collateral blood vessels supplying the heart may diminish the effects of a heart attack if one does occur. These extra (or collateral) blood vessels may take over the function of regular blood vessels during a heart attack.

The heart of the inactive person is less able to resist stress and is more susceptible to an emotional storm that may precipitate a heart attack. The heart is rendered inefficient by one or more of the following circumstances: high heart rate, high blood pressure, and excessive stimulation. All of these conditions require the heart to use more oxygen than is normal and decrease its ability to adapt to stressful situations.

The inefficient heart is one that beats rapidly because it is dominated by the **sympathetic nervous system,** which speeds up the heart rate. Thus, the heart continuously beats rapidly, even at rest, and never has a true rest period. High blood pressure also makes the heart work harder and contributes to its inefficiency.

Research indicates five things concerning physical activity and the inefficient heart:

1. Regular activity leads to dominance of the **parasympathetic nervous system,** which slows heart rate and helps the heart work efficiently.
2. Regular activity helps the heart rate return to normal faster after emotional stress.

3. Regular activity strengthens the heart muscle, making it better able to weather an **emotional storm.**
4. Regular activity reduces hormonal effects on the heart, thus lessening the chances of the circulatory problems that accompany this state.
5. Regular activity reduces the risk of sudden death from ventricular fibrillation (arrhythmic heartbeat).

Regular physical activity is one effective means of rehabilitation for a person who has coronary heart disease or who has had a heart attack. Not only does regular physical activity seem to reduce the risk of developing coronary heart disease, but those who already have the condition may reduce the symptoms of the disease through regular exercise. For people who have had heart attacks, regular and progressive exercise can be an effective prescription when carried out under the supervision of a physician. Remember, however, that exercise is not the treatment of preference for all heart attack victims. In some cases, it may be harmful.

Physical Activity and Other Cardiovascular Diseases

Regular physical activity is associated with a reduced risk for high blood pressure (hypertension). Approximately 30 percent of adults have borderline or high-risk hypertension. More men than women are likely to be hypertensive, as are more Blacks than Whites. Native Americans and Hispanics have a higher than normal incidence of hypertension, and the incidence for all groups increases as people grow older. A recent research summary indicates that the effects of physical activity on blood pressure are more dramatic

Fibrin A sticky, threadlike substance that, in combination with blood cells, forms a blood clot.

Coronary Collateral Circulation Circulation of blood to the heart muscle associated with the blood-carrying capacity of a specific vessel or development of collateral vessels (extra blood vessels).

Sympathetic Nervous System The branch of the autonomic nervous system that prepares the body for activity by speeding up the heart rate.

Parasympathetic Nervous System The branch of the autonomic nervous system that slows the heart rate.

Emotional Storm A traumatic emotional experience that is likely to affect the human organism physiologically.

than previously thought and are independent of age, body fatness, and other factors. Inactive, less fit individuals have a 30 to 50 percent greater chance of being hypertensive than active, fit people. Regular physical activity can also be one effective method of reducing blood pressure for those with hypertension. Physical inactivity in middle age is associated with risk for high blood pressure later in life. The most plausible reason is a reduction in resistance to blood flow in the blood vessels, probably resulting from dilation of the vessels.

The hypothetical "goal" blood pressure is 120 mm Hg (**systolic blood pressure**) over 80 mm Hg (**diastolic blood pressure**). However, systolic pressures as low as 100 mm Hg and up to 130 mm Hg are considered in the normal range. Diastolic pressures of 60 to 85 mm Hg are also considered to be in the normal range. Exceptionally low blood pressures (below 100 systolic and 60 diastolic) do not pose the same risks to health as high blood pressure but can cause dizziness, fainting, and lack of tolerance to change in body positions. Classifications for blood pressure are shown in Table 2. Stage 1 hypertension is sometimes called "mild," Stage 2 "moderate," and Stage 3 "severe." Some experts do not like these terms because people with "mild" or "moderate" hypertension may not feel the need to seek medical help. All stages of hypertension should be taken seriously.

Regular physical activity can help reduce the risk for stroke. Stroke is a major killer of adults. People with high blood pressure and atherosclerosis are susceptible to stroke. Since regular exercise and good fitness are important to the prevention of high blood pressure and atherosclerosis, exercise and fitness are considered helpful in the prevention of stroke.

Regular physical activity is helpful in the prevention of peripheral vascular disease. People who exercise regularly have better blood flow to the working muscles and other tissues than inactive, unfit people. Since peripheral vascular disease is associated with poor circulation to the extremities, regular exercise can be considered one method of preventing this condition.

Physical Activity and Other Hypokinetic Conditions

Physical activity reduces the risk of some forms of cancer. www.mhhe.com/phys_fit/web04 Click 06. Cancer is the second leading cause of death in the United States. According to the American Cancer Society, cancer is a group of diseases characterized by uncontrollable growth and spread of abnormal cells. The first editions of this book did not include any form of cancer as a hypokinetic disease. We now know, however, that overall death rates from cancer are lower among active people than those who are sedentary (50 to 250 percent) and that some specific forms of cancer are related to sedentary living. These cancers are described in Table 3 with possible reasons for the cancer/inactivity link (if known). The entries in Table 3 are listed in order based on the strength of evidence supporting the cancer/inactivity link.

The American Cancer Society recently released guidelines designed to help reduce risk for cancer as a result of eating well and doing regular activity. The document places a special emphasis on maintaining a healthy body fatness level as one method of reducing cancer risk. Physical activity is also considered to be important to the wellness of the cancer patient. Patients can benefit from activity in many ways, including improved quality of life,

Table 2 ▶ Blood Pressure Classifications for Adults*

Category	Systolic Blood Pressure (mm Hg)	Diastolic Blood Pressure (mm Hg)
Goal	<120	<80
Normal	<130	<85
High normal	130–139	85–89
Stage 1 hypertension	140–159	90–99
Stage 2 hypertension	160–179	100–109
Stage 3 hypertension	≥180	≥110

Source: National Institutes of Health.

*Not taking antihypertensive drugs and not acutely ill. When the systolic and diastolic blood pressure categories vary, the higher reading determines the blood pressure classification.

Table 3 ▶ Cancer and Sedentary Living

Cancer Type	Link to Sedentary Living
Colon	Exercise speeds movement of food and cancer-causing substances through the digestive system.
Breast	Exercise decreases the amount of exposure of breast tissue to circulating estrogen. Lower body fat is also associated with lower estrogen levels. Early life activity is deemed important for both reasons.
Rectal	Similar to colon cancer
Prostate	Limited evidence, no established link
Testicular	Limited evidence, no established link
Pancreatic	Limited evidence, no established link

physical functioning, and self-esteem, as well as less dependence on others and reduced risk for other diseases.

 Physical activity plays an important role in the management and treatment of diabetes. www.mhhe.com/phys_fit/web04 Click 07. Diabetes mellitus (diabetes) is a group of disorders that results when there is too much sugar in the blood. It occurs when the body does not make enough **insulin** or when the body is not able to use insulin effectively. Diabetes is the seventh leading cause of death among people over forty. It accounts for at least 10 percent of all short-term hospital stays and has a major impact on health-care costs in Western society. According to the American Diabetes Association (ADA), there are 17 million people in the United States who have diabetes. Unfortunately, 5.9 million of those don't know it. An estimated additional 10 million are pre-diabetic; they have metabolic profiles characteristic of those with diabetes (see *Web Resources*, ADA or Canadian Diabetes Association, for more statistics).

Type I diabetes, or insulin-dependent diabetes, accounts for a relatively small number of the diabetes cases and is not considered to be a hypokinetic condition. Type II diabetes (often not insulin-dependent) was formerly called "adult-onset diabetes." In recent years, Type II diabetes has become common in children and is associated with high levels of body fat.

People who perform regular physical activity are less likely to suffer from Type II diabetes than sedentary people. For people with Type II diabetes, regular physical activity can help reduce body fatness, decrease **insulin resistance,** improve **insulin sensitivity,** and improve the body's ability to clear sugar from the blood in a reasonable time. All of these factors contribute to controlling the disease. With sound nutritional habits and proper medication, physical activity can be useful in the management of both types of diabetes.

 Regular physical activity is important to maintaining bone density and decreasing risk for osteoporosis. www.mhhe.com/phys_fit/web04 Click 08. As noted in Concept 1, bone integrity is considered by some experts as a health-related component of physical fitness. Healthy bones are dense and strong. When bones lose calcium and become less dense, they become porous and are at risk for fracture. The bones of young children are not especially dense, but during adolescence (see Figure 5) bone density increases to a level higher than at any other time in life (peak bone density). Though bone density often begins to decrease in young adulthood, it is not until older adulthood that bone loss becomes dramatic. As illustrated in Figure 5, many older adults have lost enough bone density to have a condition called **osteoporosis** (when bone density drops below the osteoporosis threshold). Some will have crossed the fracture threshold,

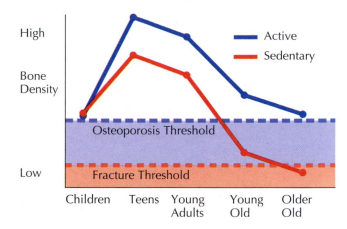

Figure 5 ▶ Changes in bone density with age.

putting them at risk for fractures especially to the hip, vertebrae, and other "soft" or "spongy" bones of the skeletal system. Active people have a higher peak bone mass and are more resistant to osteoporosis (see blue line in Figure 5) than sedentary people (see red line in Figure 5).

Women, especially postmenopausal women, have a higher risk of osteoporosis than men. Males typically have a higher peak bone mass than females and for this reason can lose more bone density over time without reaching the osteoporosis or fracture threshold. More women reach the osteoporosis and fracture thresholds at earlier ages than men. Other risk factors for osteoporosis are northern European ancestry, smoking, caffeine use,

Systolic Blood Pressure The upper blood pressure number, often called working blood pressure. It represents the pressure in the arteries at its highest level just after the heart beats.

Diastolic Blood Pressure The lower blood pressure number, often called "resting pressure." It is the pressure in the arteries at its lowest level occurring just before the next beat of the heart.

Insulin A hormone secreted by the pancreas that regulates levels of sugar in the blood.

Insulin Resistance A condition that occurs when insulin becomes ineffective or less effective than necessary to regulate sugar levels in the blood.

Insulin Sensitivity A person with insulin resistance (see previous definition) is said to have decreased insulin sensitivity. The body's cells are not sensitive to insulin so they resist it and sugar levels are not regulated effectively.

Osteoporosis A condition associated with low bone density and subsequent bone fragility, leading to high risk for fracture.

alcohol use, current or previous eating disorders, early menstruation, low dietary calcium intake, low body fat, amenorrhea, and extended bed rest.

Guidelines for building bone integrity and preventing osteoporosis include the following:

- Do regular weight-bearing exercise and resistance training that stresses the bones of the body. The load bearing and pull of the muscles in these types of exercises build bone density.
- Eat a diet rich in calcium. Calcium is necessary to build strong bones. At-risk groups should consider a calcium supplement.
- Postmenopausal women, after consultation with a physician, should consider a calcium supplement and medications, such as raloxifene (sold as Evista) and alendronate (sold as Fosomax), that help prevent bone loss. Another drug, zoledronic acid, which was originally approved to stop calcium loss from the bones of cancer patients, shows promise for treatment of osteoporosis in the future.
- Hormone replacement therapy (HRT), also called estrogen replacement therapy (ERT), has been shown to reduce risk for osteoporosis among postmenopausal women. However, results of a long-term study (Women's Health Initiative) suggest that HRT can increase risk for breast cancer, stroke, and heart disease. Many women, and their doctors, are reevaluating their medication based on this evidence.
- Start early in life to build strong bones because peak bone mass is developed in the teen years.
- It is never too late to start. Following these guidelines has been shown to help people of all ages, including those eighty and over.
- Older people with osteoporosis should consider protective pads, shown to prevent fractures from falls.

Active people who possess good muscle fitness are less likely to have back and musculoskeletal problems than inactive, unfit people. Because few people die from it, back pain does not receive the attention given to such medical problems as heart disease and cancer. But back pain is considered to be the second leading medical complaint in the United States, second only to headaches. Only the common cold and the flu cause more days lost from work. At some point in our lives, approximately 80 percent of all adults will experience back pain that limits their ability to function normally. In National Safety Council data, the back was the most frequently injured of all body parts, and the injury rate was double that of any other part of the body.

Many years ago, medical doctors began to associate back problems with the lack of physical fitness. It is now known that the great majority of back ailments are the result of poor muscle strength, low levels of endurance, and poor flexibility. Tests on patients with back problems show weakness and lack of flexibility in key muscle groups.

Though lack of fitness is probably the leading reason for back pain in Western society, there are many other factors that increase the risk of back ailments, including poor posture, improper lifting and work habits, heredity, and disease states, such as scoliosis and arthritis.

Physical activity is important in maintaining a healthy body weight and avoiding the numerous health conditions associated with obesity. Recently, the surgeon general issued a *Call to Action to Prevent and Decrease Overweight and Obesity*. This report notes that one-third of adults are obese and 61 percent are classified as overweight based on the body mass index. Approximately 13 percent of children and 14 percent of teens are classified as obese, dramatically up from 20 years ago. Obesity is not a disease state in itself but is a hypokinetic condition associated with a multitude of far-reaching complications. Research has shown that fat people who are fit are not at especially high risk for early death. However, when high body fatness is accompanied by low cardiovascular and low metabolic fitness, risk for early death increases substantially. Obesity contributes to sedentary death syndrome, described earlier in this concept.

Physical activity reduces the risk and severity of a variety of common mental (emotional) health disorders. Such disorders can be considered hypokinetic conditions. Some mental (emotional) health conditions are prevalent in modern society. Nearly one-half of adult Americans will report having a mental health disorder at some point in life. A recent summary of studies revealed that there are several emotional/mental disorders that are associated with inactive lifestyles.

Depression is a stress-related condition experienced by many adults. Thirty-three percent of inactive adults report that they often feel depressed. For some, depression is a serious disorder that physical activity alone will not cure; however, recent research does indicate that activity, combined with other forms of therapy, can be effective.

Anxiety is an emotional condition characterized by worry, self-doubt, and apprehension. More than a few studies have shown that symptoms of anxiety can be reduced by regular activity. Low-fit people who do regular aerobic activity seem to benefit the most. In one study, one-third of active people felt that regular activity helped them to better cope with life's pressures.

Physical activity is also associated with better and more restful sleep. People with insomnia (the inability to sleep) seem to benefit from regular activity if it is not done too vigorously right before going to bed. A recent study indicates that 52 percent of the population feel that physical activity helps them sleep better. Regular aerobic activity is associated with reduced brain activation, which can result in greater ability to relax or fall asleep.

Even more common than depression and insomnia is the condition called Type A behavior. Type A personalities are stress-prone individuals with a greater than normal incidence of diseases. A Type A person is tense, overcompetitive, and worried about meeting time schedules. Apparently, all Type A personalities are not equally stressed. It has been suggested that aggressive Type A personalities are most likely to be prone to negative consequences of stress. Regular physical activity can benefit the Type A person, especially the aggressive Type A. Noncompetitive activities are best for this personality type.

A final benefit of regular exercise is increased self-esteem. Improvements in fitness, appearance, and the ability to perform new tasks can improve self-confidence and self-esteem.

Physical activity can help the immune system fight illness. Until recently, infectious disease and other diseases of the immune system were not considered to be hypokinetic. Recent evidence indicates that regular moderate to vigorous activity can actually aid the immune system in fighting disease. Each of us is born with "an innate immune system," which includes anatomical and physiological barriers, such as skin, mucous membranes, body temperature, and chemical mediators, that help prevent and resist disease. We also develop an "acquired immune system" in the form of special disease-fighting cells that help us resist disease. Figure 6 shows a J-shaped curve that illustrates the benefits of exercise to acquired immune function. Sedentary people have more risk than those who do moderate activity, but with very high and sustained vigorous activity, such as extended high performance training, immune system function actually decreases.

Regular moderate and reasonable amounts of vigorous activity have been shown to reduce incidence of colds and days of sickness from infection. The immune system

benefit may extend to other immune system disorders as well. There is evidence that regular physical activity for immune disorders such as HIV can enhance quality of life. However, as Figure 6 indicates, too much exercise may cause problems rather than solve them.

Regular physical activity can have positive effects on some nonhypokinetic conditions. Some nonhypokinetic conditions that can benefit from physical activity are

- *Arthritis.* Many, if not most, arthritics are in a deconditioned state resulting from a lack of activity. The traditional advice that arthritics should avoid physical activity is now being modified in view of the findings that carefully prescribed exercise can improve general fitness and, in some cases, reduce the symptoms of the disease.
- *Asthma.* Asthmatics often have physical activity limitations. New evidence suggests that, with proper management, activity can be part of their daily life. In fact, when done properly, activity can reduce airway reactivity and medication use. Because exercise can trigger bronchial constriction, it is important to choose appropriate types of activity and to use inhaled medications to prevent bronchial constriction caused by exercise or other triggers, such as cold weather. Asthmatics should avoid cold weather exercise.
- *Premenstrual syndrome (PMS).* PMS, a mixture of physical and emotional symptoms that occurs prior to menstruation, has many causes. However, current evidence suggests that changes in lifestyle, including regular exercise, may be effective in relieving PMS symptoms.
- *Other conditions.* Low- to moderate-intensity aerobic activity and resistance training are currently being prescribed for some people who have chronic pain (persistent pain without relief) and/or fibromyalgia (chronic muscle pain). Evidence also suggests that active people have a 30 percent less chance of having gallstones than inactive people, and activity may decrease risk of impotence.

Physical Activity and Aging

 Regular physical activity can improve fitness and improve functioning among older adults. www.mhhe.com/phys_fit/web04 Click 09. Approximately 30 percent of adults age seventy and over have difficulty with one or more activities of daily living. Women have more limitations than men, and low-income groups have more limitations than higher-income groups. Nearly one-half get no assistance with the activity in which they are limited.

The inability to function effectively as you grow older is associated with lack of fitness and inactive lifestyles. This loss of function is sometimes referred to as "acquired aging," as opposed to "time-dependent" aging. Because so

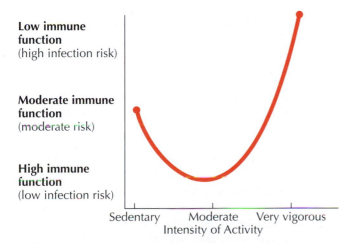

Low immune function
(high infection risk)

Moderate immune function
(moderate risk)

High immune function
(low infection risk)

Sedentary   Moderate   Very vigorous
Intensity of Activity

Figure 6 ► Physical activity and immune function.

many people experience limitations in daily activities and often find it difficult to get assistance, it is especially important for older people to stay active and fit. In Africa, Asia, and South America, where older adults maintain an active lifestyle, individuals do not acquire many of the characteristics commonly associated with aging in North America.

In general, older adults become much less active than younger adults. Losses in muscle fitness are associated with loss of balance, greater risk of falling, and less ability to function independently. Studies also show that exercise can enhance cognitive functioning and perhaps reduce risk for dementia. Though the amount of activity performed must be adapted as people grow older, fitness benefits discussed in the next section and throughout this book apply to people of all ages.

Regular physical activity can compress illness into a shorter period of our life. An important national health goal is to increase the years of healthy life. Living longer is important, but being able to function effectively during all years of life is equally—if not more—important. *Compression* refers to shortening the total number of years that illnesses and disabilities occur. Compressing the illness means dramatically decreasing the years of illness. Healthy lifestyles, including regular physical activity, have been shown to compress illness and increase years of effective functioning.

Health, Wellness, and Fitness Promotion

Good health-related physical fitness and regular physical activity are important to health promotion and feeling well. Regular physical activity and good fitness not only help prevent illness (see Table 4) and disease but also promote quality of life and wellness. Good health-related physical fitness can help you look good, feel good, and enjoy life. Some of the specific benefits of wellness that are associated with good fitness are the following:

- *Good physical fitness can help an individual enjoy leisure time.* A person who is lean, has no back problems, does not have high blood pressure, and has reasonable skills in a lifetime of sports is more likely to get involved and stay regularly involved in leisure-time activities than one who does not have these characteristics. Enjoying your leisure time may not add years to your life but can add life to your years.
- *Good physical fitness can help an individual work effectively and efficiently.* A person who can resist fatigue, muscle soreness, back problems, and other symptoms associated with poor health-related fitness is capable of working productively and having energy left over at the end of the day. Surveys of employees who are involved with employee fitness programs indicate that 75 percent have

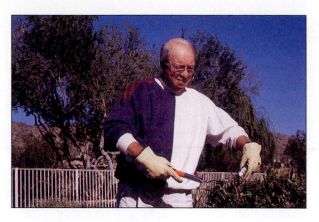

Fitness improves work efficiency.

an improved sense of well-being. Employers indicate that absenteeism decreases by up to 50 percent among program participants. People with good skill-related fitness may be more effective and efficient in performing specific motor skills required for certain jobs.

- *Good physical fitness is essential to effective living.* Although the need for each component of physical fitness is specific to each individual, every person requires enough fitness to perform normal daily activities without undue fatigue. Whether it be walking, performing household chores, or merely feeling good and enjoying the simple things in life without pain or fear of injury, good fitness is important to all people.
- *Physical fitness is the basis for dynamic and creative activity.* Though the following quotation by former President John F. Kennedy is more than 30 years old, it clearly points out the importance of physical fitness:

The relationship between the soundness of the body and the activity of the mind is subtle and complex. Much is not yet understood, but we know what the Greeks knew: that intelligence and skill can only function at the peak of their capacity when the body is healthy and strong, and that hardy spirits and tough minds usually inhabit sound bodies. Physical fitness is the basis of all activities in our society; if our bodies grow soft and inactive, if we fail to encourage physical development and prowess, we will undermine our capacity for thought, for work, and for the use of those skills vital to an expanding and complex America.

President Kennedy's belief that activity and fitness are associated with intellectual functioning has now been backed up with research. A recent research summary suggests that, though modest, the effect of activity and fitness on intellectual functioning is positive. One study shows activity to foster new brain cell growth. Time taken to be active during the day has been shown to help children learn more, even though less time is spent in intellectual pursuits.

- *Good physical fitness may help you function safely and assist you in meeting unexpected emergencies.* Emergencies are

Table 4 ▶ Health and Wellness Benefits of Physical Activity and Fitness

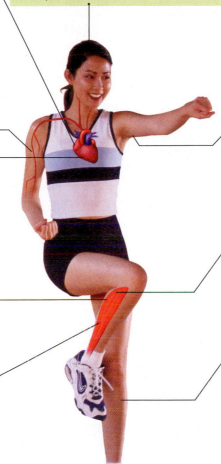

Improved Cardiovascular
- Stronger heart muscle fitness and health
- Lower heart rate
- Better electric stability of heart
- Decreased sympathetic control of heart
- Increased O₂ to brain
- Reduced blood fat, including low-density lipoproteins (LDLs)
- Increased protective high-density lipoproteins (HDLs)
- Delayed development of atherosclerosis
- Increased work capacity
- Improved peripheral circulation
- Improved coronary circulation
- Resistance to "emotional storm"
- Reduced risk for heart attack
- Reduced risk for stroke
- Reduced risk for hypertension
- Greater chance of surviving a heart attack
- Increased oxygen-carrying capacity of the blood

Improved Strength and Muscular Endurance
- Greater work efficiency
- Less chance for muscle injury
- Reduced risk for low back problems
- Improved performance in sports
- Quicker recovery after hard work
- Improved ability to meet emergencies

Resistance to Fatigue
- Ability to enjoy leisure
- Improved quality of life
- Improved ability to meet some stressors

Other Health Benefits
- Decreased diabetes risk
- Quality of life for diabetics
- Improved metabolic fitness
- Extended life
- Decrease in dysfunctional years
- Aids for some people who have arthritis, PMS, asthma, chronic pain, fibromyalgia, or impotence
- Improved immune system

Enhanced Mental Health and Function
- Relief of depression
- Improved sleep habits
- Fewer stress symptoms
- Ability to enjoy leisure and work
- Improved brain function

Improved Wellness
- Improved quality of life
- Leisure-time enjoyment
- Improved work capacity
- Ability to meet emergencies
- Improved creative capacity

Opportunity for Successful Experience and Social Interactions
- Improved self-concept
- Opportunity to recognize and accept personal limitations
- Improved sense of well-being
- Enjoyment of life and fun
- Improved quality of life

Improved Appearance
- Better figure/physique
- Better posture
- Fat control

Greater Lean Body Mass and Less Body Fat
- Greater work efficiency
- Less susceptibility to disease
- Improved appearance
- Less incidence of self-concept problems related to obesity

Improved Flexibility
- Greater work efficiency
- Less chance of muscle injury
- Less chance of joint injury
- Decreased chance of developing low back problems
- Improved sports performance

Bone Development
- Greater peak bone density
- Less chance of developing osteoporosis

Reduced Cancer Risk
- Reduced risk for colon and breast cancer
- Possible reduced risk for rectal, testicular, prostate, and pancreatic cancers

Reduced Effect of Acquired Aging
- Improved ability to function in daily life
- Better short-term memory
- Fewer illnesses
- Greater mobility
- Greater independence
- Greater ability to operate an automobile
- Lower risk for dementia

never expected, but, when they do arise, they often demand performance that requires good fitness. For example, flood victims may need to fill sandbags for hours without rest, and accident victims may be required to walk or run long distances for help. Also, good fitness is required for such simple tasks as safely changing a spare tire or loading a moving van without injury.

Many economic benefits are associated with employee physical activity. A comprehensive review of the literature indicates that worksite physical activity programs can improve health, wellness, and fitness; reduce health-care costs; and decrease absenteeism. The costs associated with providing physical activity for employees more than offsets the cost of medical care and

Table 5 ▶ Hypokinetic Disease Risk Factors

Factors That Cannot Be Altered

1. *Age*—As you grow older, your risk of contracting hypokinetic diseases increases. For example, the risk for heart disease is approximately three times as great after sixty as before. The risk of back pain is considerably greater after forty.

2. *Heredity*—People who have a family history of hypokinetic disease are more likely to develop a hypokinetic condition such as heart disease, hypertension, back problems, obesity, high blood lipid levels, and other problems. African Americans are 45 percent more likely to have high blood pressure than Caucasians; therefore, they suffer strokes at an earlier age with more severe consequences.

3. *Gender*—Men have a higher incidence of many hypokinetic conditions than women. However, differences between men and women have decreased recently. This is especially true for heart disease, the leading cause of death for both men and women. Postmenopausal women have a higher heart disease risk than premenopausal women.

Factors That Can Be Altered

4. *Regular physical activity*—As noted throughout this book, regular exercise can help reduce the risk for hypokinetic disease.

5. *Diet*—A clear association exists between hypokinetic disease and certain types of diets. The excessive intake of saturated fats, such as animal fats, is linked to atherosclerosis and other forms of heart disease. Excessive salt in the diet is associated with high blood pressure.

6. *Stress*—People who are subject to excessive stress are predisposed to various hypokinetic diseases, including heart disease and back pain. Statistics indicate that hypokinetic conditions are common among those in certain high-stress jobs and those having Type A personality profiles.

7. *Tobacco use*—Smokers have five times the risk of heart attack as nonsmokers. Most striking is the difference in risk between older women smokers and nonsmokers. Tobacco use is also associated with the increased risk for high blood pressure, cancer, and several other medical conditions. Apparently, the more you use, the greater the risk. Stopping tobacco use even after many years can significantly reduce the hypokinetic disease risk.

8. *Body (fatness)*—Having too much body fat is now a primary risk factor for heart disease and is a risk factor for other hypokinetic conditions as well. For example, loss of fat can result in relief from symptoms of Type II diabetes, can reduce problems associated with certain types of back pain, and can reduce the risks of surgery.

9. *Blood lipids, blood glucose, and blood pressure levels*—High scores on these factors are associated with health problems, such as heart disease and diabetes. Risk increases considerably when several of these measures are high.

10. *Diseases*—People who have one hypokinetic disease are more likely to develop a second or even a third condition. For example, if you have diabetes,* your risk of having a heart attack or stroke increases dramatically. Although you may not be entirely able to alter the extent to which you develop certain diseases and conditions, reducing your risk and following your doctor's advice can improve your odds significantly.

*Some types of diabetes cannot be altered.

lost days of work associated with inactivity. Nearly one-half of worksites offer some type of program. A national goal is to increase this to 75 percent.

Hypokinetic Disease Risk Factors

There are many different positive lifestyles that can reduce the risk for disease. Many of the factors that contribute to optimal health and quality of life are also considered risk factors. Changing these risk factors can dramatically reduce the risk for hypokinetic diseases. Inactivity, poor nutrition, smoking, and inability to cope with stress are all risk factors associated with various diseases (see Table 5).

Not all risk factors are under your personal control. Some factors that can contribute to the increased risk for disease are not under your personal control. Three uncontrollable risk factors are age, heredity, and gender. These factors that cannot be altered by lifestyle changes are presented in Table 5.

Altering risk factors can help reduce the risk for more than one adverse condition at the same time. By altering the controllable risk factors, you can reduce the risk for several hypokinetic conditions. For example, controlling body fatness reduces the risk for diabetes, hypertension, and back problems. Altering your diet can reduce the chances of developing high levels of blood lipids and reduce the risk for atherosclerosis.

Risk reduction does not guarantee freedom from disease. Reducing risk alters the probability of disease but does not assure disease immunity.

 ## Technology Update

Angioplasty, Pacemakers, and Plaque Busters

Many recent technological advances have contributed to the recent 3 percent drop in heart disease deaths. Examples include

- *Angioplasty for the brain.* This procedure, formerly used only in the heart, uses a catheter with a balloon to clear an artery in the brain and a wire mesh cylinder (stent) to keep the artery open.
- *Dual-chamber pacemakers.* A device with two electrodes is placed in the heart muscle to synchronize the two halves of a failing heart. The device reduces death rates.
- *Statins and plaque busters.* Statins are a class of drugs that improve lipid profiles. Plaque busters, (referred to as "liquid Drano" for the heart) have even greater potential for clearing clogged arteries.

Too much activity can lead to hyperkinetic conditions. The information presented in this concept points out the health benefits of physical activity performed in appropriate amounts. When done in excess or incorrectly, physical activity can result in **hyperkinetic conditions.** The most common hyper-kinetic condition is overuse injury to muscles, connective tissue, and bones. Recently, anorexia nervosa and body neurosis have been identified as conditions associated with inappropriate amounts of physical activity. These conditions will be discussed in the concept on performance.

Strategies for Action

 A self-assessment of risk factors can help you modify your lifestyle to reduce risk for heart disease. www.mhhe.com/phys_fit/web04 Click 10. The Heart Disease Risk Factor Questionnaire in Lab 4A will help you assess your personal risk for heart disease. The questionnaire helps you to become aware of each of the risk factors for heart disease described in this concept. Although the questionnaire is educationally useful in making you aware of risk factors, it is not a substitute for a regular medical exam. When you have your regular physical exam, it would be wise to ask for a blood test, especially as you grow older or if your score on the questionnaire is high.

Selecting physical activities from the physical activity pyramid can help you achieve the health benefits described in this concept. The physical activity pyramid provides a conceptual model of the relative importance of different types of physical activity. Subsequent concepts in the book will cover the different components of health-related fitness and the type and amount of activity needed to improve these components. The lab activities in each of these concepts and the culminating lab activity at the end of the book are designed to help you plan for lifelong physical activity.

Study Resources

Check out additional online study resources for this concept in the Student Edition of the Online Learning Center at www.mhhe.com/corbin13e.

Web Resources

American Cancer Society **www.cancer.org**
American Diabetes Association **www.diabetes.org**
American Heart Association **www.americanheart.org**
Canadian Diabetes Association **www.diabetes.ca**
Centers for Disease Control and Prevention **www.cdc.gov**
Healthy People 2010 **www.health.gov/healthypeople**
National Osteoporosis Foundation **www.nof.org**
National Stroke Association **www.stroke.org**

Suggested Readings

 Additional reference materials for Concept 4 are available at **www.mhhe.com/phys_fit/web04** Click 11.

Bassuk, S. S., and Manson, J. E. 2003. Physical activity and cardiovascular disease prevention in women: How much is good enough? *Exercise and Sport Sciences Reviews* 31(4):176–181.

Booth, F. W., and M. W. Chakravarthy. 2002. Cost and consequences of sedentary living: New battleground for an old enemy. *President's Council on Physical Fitness and Sports Research Digest* 3(16):1–8.

Brown, D. W., et al. 2004. Associations between physical activity dose and health-related quality of life. *Medicine and Science in Sports and Exercise* 36(5):890–896.

Carnethon, M. R., et al. 2003. Cardiorespiratory fitness of young adults and the development of cardiovascular disease risk factors. *Journal of the American Medical Association* 290(23):3092–3100.

Chintanadilok, J., and D. T. Lowenthal. 2002. Exercise in treating hypertension. *The Physician and Sportsmedicine* 30(3):11–28.

Cotman, C. W., and C. Engesser-Cesar. 2002. Exercise enhances and protects brain function. *Exercise and Sport Sciences Reviews* 30(2):75–79.

Drezner, J. A., and S. A. Herring. 2001. Managing low back pain. *Physician and Sportsmedicine* 29(8):37–43.

Dziura, J., et al. 2004. Physical activity reduces Type 2 diabetes risk in aging independent of body weight change. *Journal of Physical Activity and Health* 1(1):19–28.

Hyperkinetic Conditions Diseases/illnesses or health conditions caused by, or contributed, to by too much physical activity.

Fitzgerald, S. J., et al. 2004. Muscular fitness and all-cause mortality: Prospective observations. *Journal of Physical Activity and Health* 1(1):7–18.

Genest, J., and T. R. Pedersen. 2003. Prevention of cardiovascular ischemic events: High-risk and secondary prevention. *Circulation* 107(15):2059–2065.

Ivey, F. M., et al. 2003. A single bout of walking exercise enhances endogenous fibrinolysis in stroke patients. *MSSE* 35(1):193–199.

Lee, I-Min. 2003. Physical activity and cancer prevention: Data from epidemiological studies. *Medicine and Science in Sports and Exercise* 35(11):1823–1827.

Lee, I. M., and S. N. Blair. 2002. Cardiorespiratory fitness and stroke mortality in men. *Medicine and Science in Sports and Exercise* 34(4):592–595.

Lee, I., and R. S. Paffenbarger. 2001. Preventing coronary heart disease: The role of physical activity. *The Physician and Sportsmedicine* 29(2):37–52.

McGill, S. M. 2001. Low back stability. *Exercise and Sports Sciences Reviews* 29(1):26–31.

Modlesky, C. M., and R. D. Lewis. 2002. Does exercise during growth have a long-term effect on bone health? *Exercise and Sport Sciences Reviews* 30(4):171–176.

National Cholesterol Education Program. 2001. Executive summary of the third report of the national cholesterol education program expert panel on detection, evaluation, and treatment of high blood cholesterol in adults. *Journal of the American Medical Association* 285:2486–2497.

National Institutes of Health. 2002. Osteoporosis prevention, diagnosis, and therapy. *NIH Consensus Statements* 17(1):1–45.

Nieman, D. C. 2001. Does exercise alter immune function and respiratory infections? *President's Council on Physical Fitness and Sports Research Digest* 3(13):1–8.

Pearson, T. A., et al. 2003. Markers of inflammation and cardiovascular disease: Application to clinical and public health practice: Statement for healthcare professionals from the Centers for Disease Control and Prevention and the American Heart Association. *Circulation* 107(3):499–511.

Short, K. R., and M. J. Joyner. 2002. Activity, obesity, and Type II diabetes *Exercise and Sport Sciences Reviews* 30(2):51–52.

Slattery, M. L., and J. D. Potter. 2002. Physical activity and colon cancer. *Medicine and Science in Sports and Exercise* 34(6):913–919.

Turner, C. H., and A. G. Robling. 2003. Designing exercise regimens to increase bone strength. *Exercise and Sports Sciences Reviews* 31(1):40–44.

U.S. Department of Health and Human Services. 1996. *Physical Activity and Health: A Report of the Surgeon General.* Atlanta: U.S. Department of Health and Human Services.

World Health Organization. 2004. *World Health Report 2003: Shaping the Future.* Geneva: WHO (available at http://www.who.int/whr/2003/en/).

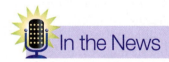 In the News

Health Promotion Initiatives

Recent estimates suggest that over 75 percent of the $1.8 trillion the U.S. spends annually on health care is associated with chronic diseases, yet only 2 percent of annual health-care spending goes toward prevention. Politicians are beginning to take notice of the economic and social burden associated with unhealthy lifestyles and have released new legislation intended to improve the health of Americans:

- The HeLP America Act is a broad piece of legislation intended to improve the quality and quantity of health promotion programming in schools and communities. Another section of the bill provides funding for reimbursements of expenses for preventive care and expands the provision of these preventive services programs in the health-care system.

- The Great Outdoors Act (also known as the GO bill) is a bipartisan proposal that would establish a multibillion-dollar trust fund to support a broad array of recreation, conservation, and park maintenance programs. The legislation would provide a permanent funding source to help build and maintain trails, parks, wild lands, ball fields, courts, and playgrounds across the country. These settings are critical for active recreation, so the GO bill can have a major impact on physical activity patterns in the country.

These pieces of legislation are currently in consideration. Contact your local and state representatives to support these important health promotion initiatives.

Lab 4A Assessing Heart Disease Risk Factors

Name	**Section**	**Date**

Purpose: To assess your risk of developing coronary heart disease

Heart Disease Risk Factor Questionnaire

Risk Points

	① 1	② 2	③ 3	④ 4	Score
Unalterable Factors					
1. How old are you?	30 or less	31–40	41–54	55+	
2. Do you have a history of heart disease in your family?	None	Grandparent with heart disease	Parent with heart disease	More than one with heart disease	
3. What is your gender?	Female		Male		
			Total Unalterable Risk Score		
Alterable Factors					
4. Do you get regular physical activity?	4–5 days a week	3 days a week	Less than 3 days a week	No	
5. Do you have a high-fat diet?	No	Slightly high in fat	Above normal in fat	Eat a lot of meat and fried and fatty foods	
6. Are you under much stress?	Less than normal	Normal	Slightly above normal	Quite high	
7. Do you use tobacco?	No	Cigar or pipe	Less than 1/2 pack a day or use smokeless tobacco	More than 1/2 pack a day	
8. What is your percent of body fat?	F = 17–28% M = 10–20%	29–31% 21–23%	32–35% 24–30%	35+% 30+%	
9. What is the systolic number in your blood pressure?	120	121–140	141–160	160+	
10. Do you have other diseases?	No	Ulcer	Diabetes*	Both	

Extra Points: Add points for as many of the following test results as you have available: 1 point for CRP above 3, 1 point for homocysteine above 100, 3 points for LDL above 130, 3 points for TC/HDL-C above 4. If only total cholesterol is available, add 1 point for a score of 200 to 240 or 3 points for scores above 240.

Total Alterable Risk Score	
Extra Points	
Grand Total Risk Score	

Adapted from CAD Risk Assessor, William J. Stone. Reprinted by permission.

*Diabetes is a risk factor that is often not alterable.

Procedures

1. Complete the ten questions and the extra points, if available, on the Heart Disease Risk Factor Questionnaire by circling the answer that is most appropriate for *you* (see front of this lab).
2. Look at the top of the column for each of your answers. In the box provided at the right of each question, write down the number of risk points for that answer.
3. Determine your unalterable risk score by adding the risk points for questions 1, 2, and 3.
4. Determine your alterable risk score by adding the risk points for questions 4 through 10.
5. Determine your total heart disease risk score by adding the scores obtained in steps 3 and 4.
6. Look up your risk ratings on the Heart Disease Risk Rating Scale and record them in the Results section. Answer the questions in the Conclusions and Implications section.

Results: Write your risk scores and risk ratings in the appropriate boxes below.

Heart Disease Risk Scores and Ratings

	Score	Rating
Unalterable risk		
Alterable risk		
Total heart disease risk		

Heart Disease Risk Rating Chart

Rating	Unalterable Score	Alterable Score	Total Score
Very high	9 or more	21 or more	31 or more
High	7–8	15–20	26–30
Average	5–6	11–14	16–25
Low	4 or less	10 or less	15 or less

Conclusions and Implications: The higher your score on the Heart Disease Risk Factor Questionnaire, the greater your heart disease risk. In several sentences, discuss your risk for heart disease. Which of the risk factors do you need to control to reduce your risk for heart disease? Why?

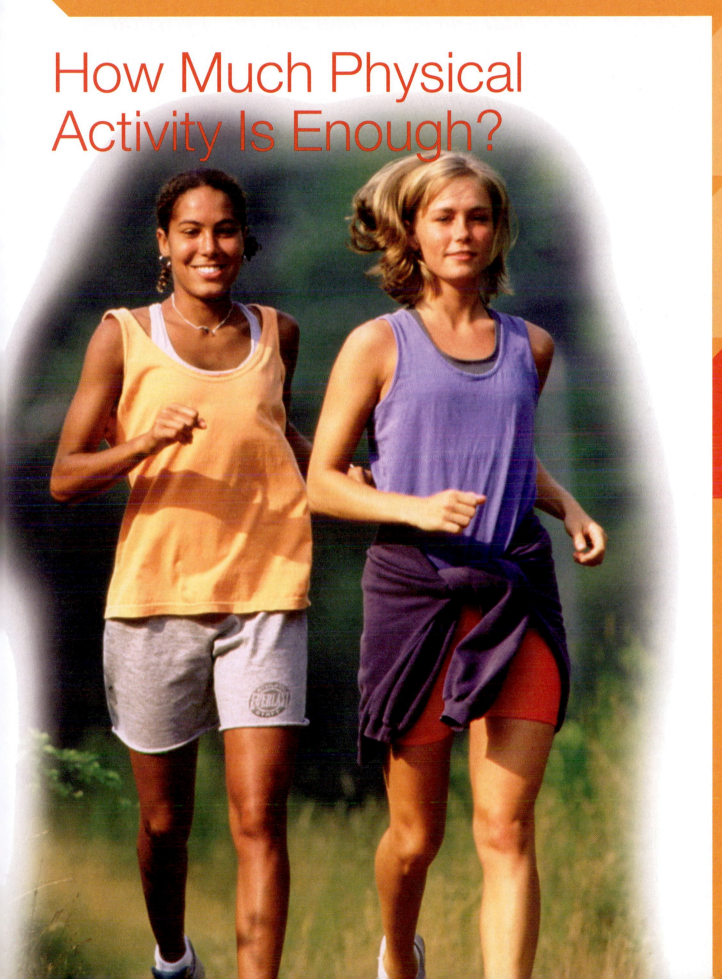

How Much Physical Activity Is Enough?

There is a minimal and an optimal amount of physical activity necessary for developing and maintaining good health, wellness, and fitness.

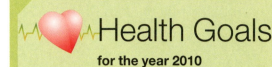

Health Goals

for the year 2010

- Improve health, fitness, and quality of life of all people through the adoption and maintenance of regular, daily physical activity.

- Increase proportion of people who do moderate daily activity for 30 minutes.

- Increase proportion of people who do vigorous physical activity 3 days a week.

- Increase proportion of people who do regular exercises for muscle fitness.

- Increase proportion of people who do regular exercise for flexibility.

Just as there is a correct dosage of medicine for treating an illness, there is a correct dosage of physical activity for promoting health benefits and developing physical fitness. Several important principles of physical activity provide the basis for determining the correct dose or amount of physical activity. In this concept, a formula for implementing the important physical activity principles will be presented. This formula and the concepts of "threshold of training" and "target zones" will be described to help you determine how much physical activity is enough. New evidence indicates that the amount of physical activity necessary for developing metabolic fitness, and its associated health benefits, is different from the amount of physical activity necessary for developing health-related fitness and other performance benefits. Research also shows that the amount of activity or exercise necessary for maintaining fitness may differ from the amount needed to develop it. The guidelines presented in this concept, and throughout this book, are consistent with the most recent guidelines of the American College of Sports Medicine (see *Suggested Readings*). The guidelines were developed over time by many experts. However, the research and writings of Dr. Michael L. Pollock (1936–1998) were instrumental in the creation and evolution of the guidelines. The authors of

this book would like to acknowledge Dr. Pollock's contribution to our knowledge and understanding of the amount of physical activity necessary for good health, fitness, and wellness.

The Principles of Physical Activity

Overload is necessary to achieve health, wellness, and fitness benefits of physical activity. The **overload principle** is the most basic of all physical activity principles. This principle indicates that doing "more than normal" is necessary if benefits are to occur. In order for a muscle (including the heart muscle) to get stronger, it must be overloaded, or worked against a load greater than normal. To increase flexibility, a muscle must be stretched longer than is normal. To increase muscular endurance, muscles must be exposed to sustained exercise for a longer than normal period. The health benefits associated with metabolic fitness seem to require less overload than for health-related fitness improvement, but overload is required just the same.

Physical activity should be increased progressively for safe and effective results. The **principle of progression** indicates that overload should not be increased too slowly or too rapidly if benefits are to result. A simple example relates to working with your hands. If you have not done anything for a while and you do too much work with your hands, you develop blisters. You are less able to work the next day. A day or more of recovery may be necessary before you are back to normal. If, however, you begin gradually and increase the work you do each day, you develop calluses. The calluses make your hands tougher, and you are able to work long, or longer without injury or soreness. The benefits of all forms of physical activity are best when you gradually increase overload. Doing too much too soon is counterproductive.

The benefits of physical activity are specific to the form of activity performed. The **principle of specificity** states that to benefit from physical activity, you must overload specifically for that benefit. For example, strength-building exercises may do little for developing cardiovascular fitness, and stretching exercises may do little for altering body composition or metabolic fitness.

Overload is specific to each component of fitness and each health or wellness benefit desired. Overload is also specific to each body part. If you exercise the legs, you build fitness of the legs. If you exercise the arms, you build fitness of the arms. For this reason, some people can have disproportionate fitness development. Some gymnasts, for example, have good upper body development but poor leg development, whereas some soccer players have well-developed legs but lack upper body development.

Specificity is important in designing your warm-up, workout, and cool-down programs for specific activities. Training is most effective when it closely resembles the activity for which you are preparing. For example, if your goal is to improve your skill in putting the shot, it is not enough to strengthen the arm muscles. You should perform a training activity requiring overload that closely resembles the motion you use in the actual sport.

The benefits achieved from overload last only as long as overload continues. The **principle of reversibility** is basically the overload principle in reverse. To put it simply, if you don't use it, you will lose it. It is an important principle because some people have the mistaken impression that, if they achieve a health or fitness benefit, it will last forever. This, of course, is not true. There is evidence that you can maintain health benefits with less physical activity than it took to achieve them. Still, if you do not adhere to regular physical activity, any benefits attained will gradually erode away.

🌐 **In general, the more physical activity you do, the more benefits you receive. However, there are exceptions to this rule.** www.mhhe.com/phys_fit/ **web05 Click 01.** A recent report of an international symposium (see *Medicine and Science in Sports and Exercise, Suggested Readings*) provides evidence to suggest that, the larger the dose of physical activity, the greater the benefits (response). This is called the **dose-response** relationship. This relationship is illustrated by the fact that people who do moderate amounts of regular activity (a moderate dose) have a lower overall death rate, compared with those who are sedentary (who do no doses of activity). People who do vigorous activity or moderate activity of longer duration (a bigger dose) have an even greater reduction in risk for early death.

In general, the evidence supports a dose-response relationship

Doing lifestyle activities can benefit your health.

for physical activity. It is important, however, to recognize that more is not always better. As the principle of progression indicates, beginners will benefit most from small doses of activity. For them, doing too much too soon is a bad idea. Also, the **principle of diminishing returns** indicates that, as you get fitter and fitter, you may not get as big a benefit for each additional amount of activity that you perform. When improvements become more difficult and performance levels off, maintenance may become most important. In some cases, excessive amounts of activity can be counterproductive.

Health, wellness, and fitness benefits occur as you increase your physical activity. But it is important to understand that, if you keep increasing physical activity by equal increments, each additional amount of activity will yield less benefit. At some point, improvements will plateau and, if activity is overdone, may actually decrease.

The FIT Formula

The acronym FIT can help you remember the three important variables for applying the overload principle and its corollaries. For physical activity to be effective, it must be done with enough frequency and intensity and for a long enough time. The first letter

---

Overload Principle The basic principle that specifies that you must perform physical activity in greater than normal amounts (overload) to get an improvement in physical fitness or health benefits.

Principle of Progression The corollary of the overload principle that indicates the need to gradually increase overload to achieve optimal benefits.

Principle of Specificity The corollary of the overload principle that indicates a need for a specific type of exercise to improve each fitness component or fitness of a specific part of the body.

Principle of Reversibility The corollary of the overload principle that indicates that disuse or inactivity results in loss of benefits achieved as a result of overload.

Dose-Response A term adopted from medicine. With medicine it is important to know what response (benefit) will occur from taking a specific dose. When studying physical activity, it is important to know what dose provides the best response (most benefits). The contents of this book are designed to help you choose the best doses of activity for the responses (benefits) you desire.

Principle of Diminishing Returns The corollary of the overload principle indicating that, the more benefits you gain as a result of activity, the harder additional benefits are to achieve.

from these three words spells **FIT** and can be considered as the formula for achieving health, wellness, and fitness benefits:

*F*requency (how often)—Physical activity must be performed regularly to be effective. The number of days a person does activity in a week is used to determine frequency. Most benefits require at least 3 days and up to 6 days of activity per week, but frequency ultimately depends on the specific benefit desired.

*I*ntensity (how hard)—Physical activity must be intense enough to require more exertion (overload) than normal to produce benefits. The method for determining appropriate intensity varies with the desired benefit. For example, metabolic fitness and associated health benefits require only moderate intensity; cardiovascular fitness for high-level performance requires vigorous activity that elevates the heart rate well above normal.

*T*ime (how long)—Physical activity must be done for an adequate length of time to be effective. The length of the activity session depends on the type of activity and the expected benefit (see various levels of Figure 1).

Some people add a second *T* to create the acronym FITT. This is done to illustrate the fact that there is a FIT formula for each different *Type*, or mode, of physical activity. In this book, the acronym FIT formula will be used to describe the amount of activity necessary to produce benefits for each type of activity from the physical activity pyramid described later in this concept. The FIT formula provides a practical means of applying the overload principle progressively for each specific type of activity and for each of the specific benefits expected.

The threshold of training and target zone concepts help you use the FIT formula. The **threshold of training** is the minimum amount of activity (frequency, intensity, and time) necessary to produce benefits. Depending on the benefit expected, slightly more than normal activity may not be enough to promote health, wellness, or fitness benefits. The **target zone** begins at the threshold of training and stops at the point where the activity becomes counterproductive. Figure 1 illustrates the threshold of training and target zone concepts.

Some people incorrectly associate the concepts of threshold of training and target zones with only cardiovascular fitness. As the principle of specificity suggests, each component of fitness, including metabolic fitness, has its own FIT formula and its own threshold and target zone. The target and threshold levels for **health benefits** are different from those for achieving **performance benefits** associated with high levels of physical fitness. Details of the different FIT formula, threshold levels, and target zones for the various benefits of activity are presented later in this book.

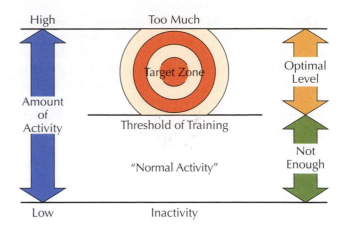

Figure 1 ▶ Physical activity target zone.

🌐 **It takes time for physical activity to produce health, wellness, and fitness benefits, even when the FIT formula is properly applied.** www.mhhe.com/phys_fit/web05 Click 02. Sometimes people just beginning a physical activity program expect to see immediate results. They expect to see large losses in body fat or great increases in muscle strength in just a few days. Evidence shows, however, that improvements in health-related physical fitness and the associated health benefits take several weeks to become apparent. Though some people report psychological benefits, such as "feeling better" and a "sense of personal accomplishment" almost immediately after beginning regular exercise, the physiological changes will take considerably longer to be realized. Proper preparation for physical activity includes learning not to expect too much too soon and not to do too much too soon. Attempts to overdo it and to try to get fit fast will probably be counterproductive, resulting in soreness and even injury. The key is to start slowly, stay with it, and enjoy yourself. Benefits will come to those who persist.

The Physical Activity Pyramid

The physical activity pyramid classifies activities by type and associated benefits. The **physical activity pyramid** (see Figure 2) is a good way to illustrate different types of activities and how each contributes to the development of health, wellness, and physical fitness. The pyramid evolved from a pyramid of activity emphasis developed more than 20 years ago and from the food guide pyramid developed by the U.S. Department of Agriculture to help people understand appropriate servings of foods. Like the food guide pyramid, the physical activity pyramid has four levels. Each level includes one or two types of activity and characterizes the "portions" of physical activity necessary to produce different health, wellness, and fitness benefits.

The four levels of the pyramid are based on the beneficial health outcomes associated with regular physical activity. Activities having broad general health and wellness benefits for the largest number of people are placed at the base of the pyramid. Significant national health and economic benefits will occur if we can get inactive people, especially those who are totally sedentary, to do some type of activity. The activities at the lower levels can provide these benefits, and because they are relatively low in intensity, they may appeal to the large number of people who can most benefit from beginning an activity program. The activities at the lower levels of the pyramid typically require greater frequency than those at higher levels.

🌐 Lifestyle activities are at the base of the physical activity pyramid. www.mhhe.com/phys_fit/web05 Click 03.

Lifestyle physical activity is encouraged as a part of everyday living and can contribute significantly to good health, wellness, and fitness. Lifestyle activities include walking to or from work, climbing the stairs rather than taking an elevator, working in the yard, and doing any other type of exercise as part of your normal daily activities. The *Surgeon General's Report on Physical Activity and Health* suggests the accumulation of 30 minutes of physical activity equal to brisk walking on most, if not all, days of the week (see Figure 2, level 1).

Research has clearly documented that lifestyle activities can yield important health benefits even if the person does no other forms of activity. For example, studies have demonstrated that individuals with active jobs have reduced risks for many chronic conditions. Individuals who use active commuting (biking or walking) to get to work or to run errands have also been found to have better health profiles. The regular accumulation of activity as a part of one's lifestyle is sufficient to promote positive improvements in metabolic fitness, and these improvements can positively impact health. Additional activity from the other layers of the pyramid are strongly recommended, and additional benefits occur from involvement in these activities. Lifestyle activity can be viewed as the baseline, or minimal, activity that should be performed. A summary of the FIT formula for this type of activity is illustrated in level 1 of Figure 2.

Active aerobics and sports and recreation are at the second level of the pyramid.

Aerobic activities (level 2) include those that are of such an intensity that they can be performed for relatively long periods of time without stopping but that also elevate the heart rate significantly. Lifestyle activities (level 1), also known as **moderate activity,** are technically aerobic but are not especially vigorous and are, therefore, not considered to be "active aerobics." More **vigorous activities,** such as

jogging, biking, and aerobic dance, are commonly classified as "active aerobic" activities. This type of activity is included in the second level of the pyramid because benefits can be accomplished in as few as 3 days a week and is especially good for building cardiovascular fitness and helping to control body fat. This type of activity can provide metabolic fitness and health benefits similar to lifestyle activities.

Active sports and recreation are also included at level 2 of the pyramid. Examples of active sports include basketball, tennis, and racquetball, and active recreation includes hiking, backpacking, skiing, and rock climbing. Many of these activities involve short and intense bursts of physical activity followed by intermittent rest. They are typically performed longer than the continuous forms of active aerobic activities and can provide similar benefits. Some sports, such as golfing, may be better classified as a lifestyle activity, since it is done at a lower intensity and typically not for aerobic benefits. In general, activities at level 2 of the pyramid may substitute for activities at level 1 if done according to the FIT formula, but many experts encourage activities from both levels. They reason that people who develop active lifestyles from level 1 will be more likely to stay

FIT A formula used to describe the frequency, intensity, and length of time for physical activity to produce benefits. (When "FITT" is used, the second *T* refers to the type of physical activity you perform.)

Threshold of Training The minimum amount of physical activity that will produce benefits.

Target Zone Amounts of physical activity that produce optimal benefits.

Health Benefits The results of physical activity that provide protection from hypokinetic disease or early death.

Performance Benefits The results of physical activity that improve physical fitness and physical performance capabilities.

Physical Activity Pyramid Pyramid that illustrates how different types of activities contribute to the development of health and physical fitness. Activities lower in the pyramid require more frequent participation, whereas activities higher in the pyramid require less frequency.

Moderate Activity For the purposes of this book, activity equal in intensity to a brisk walk. Level 1 activities from the activity pyramid are included in this category.

Vigorous Activities For the purposes of this book, activities that elevate the heart rate and are greater in intensity than brisk walking; also referred to as moderate to vigorous activities. Those activities from level 2 of the pyramid are included in this category.

active later in life when they are less likely to participate in activities from level 2. Others argue that, if you are active at level 2, you will be fit enough to continue active aerobics and sports as you grow older. A summary of the FIT formula for level 2 activities is included in Figure 2.

Flexibility and muscle fitness exercises are at level 3 of the pyramid. Flexibility (stretching) exercises are a type of physical activity that is planned specifically to develop flexibility. This type of exercise is necessary because activities lower in the pyramid often do not contribute to flexibility development. The muscle fitness category includes exercises that are planned specifically to build strength and muscular endurance. This type of exercise is necessary because activities lower in the pyramid often do not contribute to these parts of fitness. A general description of the FIT formula for level 3 exercises is included in Figure 2.

Some rest is necessary but, with the exception of sleep, long periods of inactivity are discouraged. Rest or inactivity can be important to good health. Some time off just to relax is important to us all, and, of course, proper amounts of rest and 8 hours of uninterrupted sleep help

us recuperate. But sedentary living (too much inactivity) results in low fitness as well as poor health and wellness. Rest and inactivity are placed at the top of the pyramid (see Figure 2) because they should be done sparingly, compared with other types of activity in the pyramid.

🌐 **There are multiple sets of guidelines for physical activity, each designed to help you achieve specific benefits.** www.mhhe.com/phys_fit/web05 Click 04. A recent headline in one of the nation's leading newspapers declared, "Health guidelines: It's tough keeping up." It is true that it is easy to be confused when there are many seemingly different sources of information available. Unfortunately, the aforementioned article contributes to confusion rather than to clarification. The article, and several others like it, suggests that the basic physical activity recommendation of 30 minutes of moderate physical activity on most days of the week has been changed. The article suggested that the federal government's "new set of standards has raised the bar to 60 minutes a day." This statement is incorrect. The 30-minute recommendation of the surgeon general, supported by the CDC and the American College of Sports Medicine, was first presented in 1996 and remains the current recommendation for providing the basic health benefits of physical activity. The

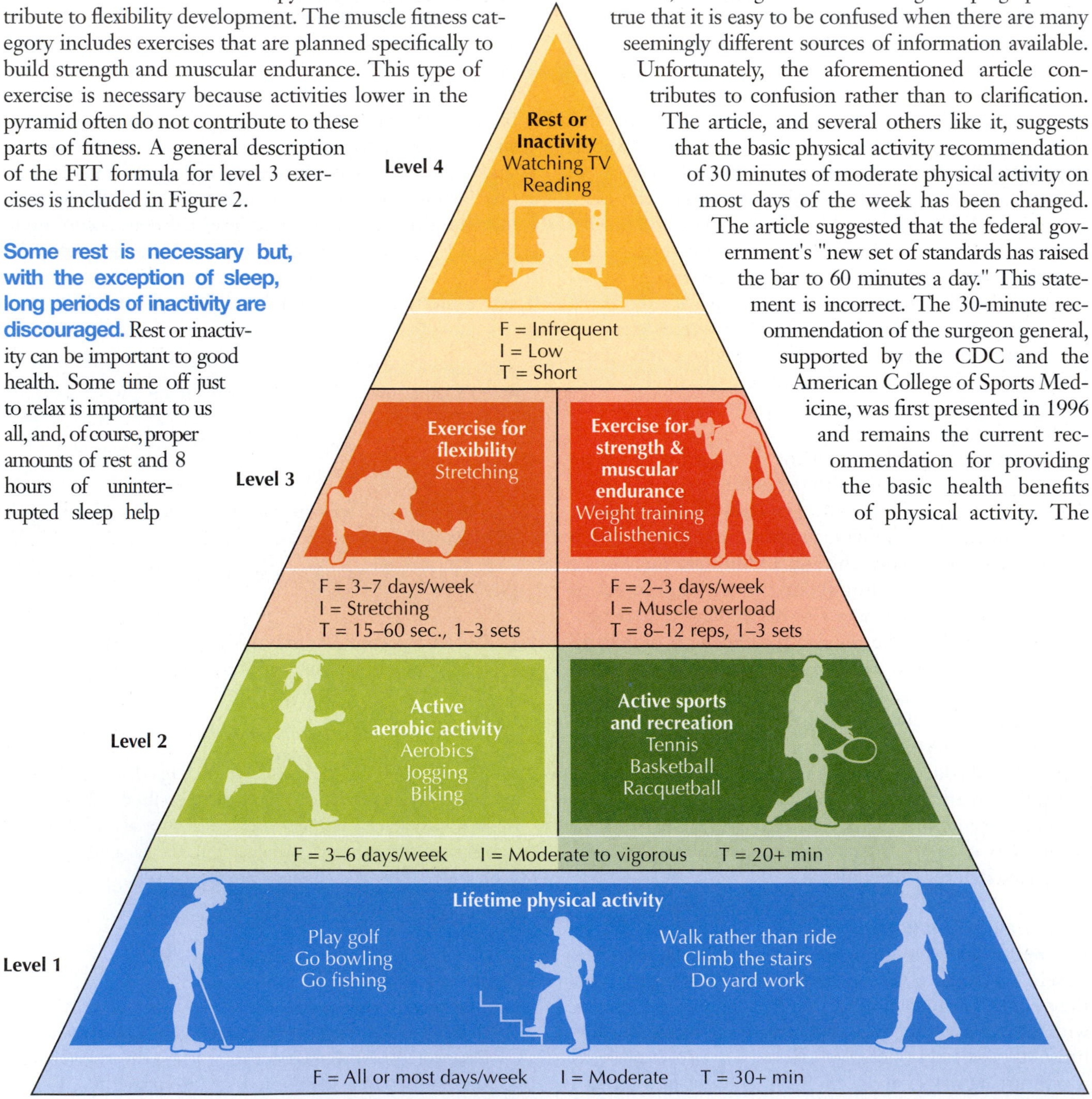

Level 4

Rest or Inactivity
Watching TV
Reading

F = Infrequent
I = Low
T = Short

Level 3

Exercise for flexibility
Stretching

Exercise for strength & muscular endurance
Weight training
Calisthenics

F = 3–7 days/week
I = Stretching
T = 15–60 sec., 1–3 sets

F = 2–3 days/week
I = Muscle overload
T = 8–12 reps, 1–3 sets

Level 2

Active aerobic activity
Aerobics
Jogging
Biking

Active sports and recreation
Tennis
Basketball
Racquetball

F = 3–6 days/week   I = Moderate to vigorous   T = 20+ min

Level 1

Lifetime physical activity

Play golf
Go bowling
Go fishing

Walk rather than ride
Climb the stairs
Do yard work

F = All or most days/week   I = Moderate   T = 30+ min

Figure 2 ▶ The physical activity pyramid.

60-minute recommendation was proposed by the Foods and Nutrition Board of the Institute of Medicine (IOM), not the Surgeon General's Office. The IOM is a private organization and its recommendation is designed as a guideline for the amount of physical activity necessary to result in body weight maintenance. It is important to understand that there can be different guidelines that are correct, each designed to accomplish a different goal. But not all guidelines you read about are accurate.

Ask yourself the following questions when you interpret news or information about physical activity:

- *Is the organization/agency that is making the recommendation credible?* Not all organizations are equal. Organizations such as the CDC and the Surgeon General's Office are governmental agencies charged with making health recommendations. Professional organizations such as the American College of Sports Medicine and the American Alliance for Health, Physical Education, and Recreation have expertise in physical activity and use boards of experts to make recommendations.

- *What benefits can be expected if the guidelines are followed?* As you learned on the previous pages of this book, there are different guidelines for each of the different types of activities in the physical activity pyramid. Each type of activity and each type of fitness has its own FIT formula. Level 1 activities are associated primarily with the general health benefits described in Concept 4. Other levels provide different benefits, including enhanced performance, reduced risk for injury, and improvement of different aspects of health, wellness, and fitness (see Concepts 7–11). Overall calorie expenditure from all levels of the pyramid contributes to the maintenance of a healthy body composition.

- *What is the mission or purpose of the recommending group?* There are many credible organizations, but their missions vary. The Surgeon General's Office is especially interested in reducing risk for chronic disease among the general population, and its 30-minute recommendation is based on this mission. The Food and Nutrition Board of the IOM is charged with making a recommendation for the intake of nutrients and maintenance of a healthy body weight. Its recommendation is based accordingly. Do not conclude that the recommendations of one group supercedes the recommendations of another group. In this case, the recommendations are complementary, pursuing different purposes.

- *For what groups or types of people are the guidelines intended?* In some cases, more than one group will make recommendations for different groups of people. For example, the National Association for Sport and Physical Activity has prepared physical activity guidelines for children. These are different from the guidelines recommended for adults.

There is no doubt that physical activity guidelines and recommendations will be modified in the future. Recommendations by groups such as the Surgeon General's Office will change as new scientific evidence is presented. In the meantime, there will no doubt be additional recommendations from different groups for different purposes. It is hoped that answering the preceding questions will help you make decisions concerning guidelines most appropriate for meeting your specific need.

Some important factors should be considered when using the physical activity pyramid. The physical activity pyramid is a useful model for describing different types of activity and their benefits. The pyramid is also useful in summarizing the FIT formula for each of the different benefits of activity. But as the American College of Sports Medicine pointed out, physical activity guidelines ". . . cannot be implemented in an overly rigid fashion . . . and . . . recommendations presented should be used with careful attention to the goals of the individual." This important point should be considered when using the pyramid. The following guidelines for using the pyramid should also be considered:

- *No single activity provides all of the benefits.* Many people have asked the question "What is the perfect form of physical activity?" It is now evident that there is no single activity that can provide all of the health, wellness, and fitness benefits. For optimal benefits to occur, it is desirable to perform activities from all levels of the pyramid because each type of activity has quite different benefits. As other guidelines will indicate, care should be used not to overgeneralize this recommendation.

- *In some cases, one type of activity can substitute for another.* Activities in level 1 of the pyramid provide general health benefits, such as reduced risk for heart disease, cancer, and other chronic conditions. Activities in level 2 provide many of the same benefits as well as the added health and performance benefits (see Concept 9). For this reason, a person who meets the FIT formula for level 2 activities does not necessarily need to perform activities at level 1. Nevertheless, many experts recommend regular lifestyle activity from level 1 for those who do regular vigorous level 2 activities. The rationale is that people who develop habits of regular lifestyle activity when they are young will continue to perform them later in life, when vigorous activity is less likely. Also, performing activities from all levels of the pyramid provides variety that may aid adherence.

- *Something is better than nothing.* Some people may look at the pyramid and say, "I just don't have time to do all of these activities." This could lead some to throw up their hands in despair, resulting in the conclusion "I just won't do anything at all." The best evidence indicates that something is better than nothing. If you do nothing or feel that you can't do it all, performing a lifestyle physical activity is a good start. Additional activities from different levels of the pyramid can be added as time allows.

- *Activities from level 3 are useful even if you are limited in performing activities at other levels.* Though flexibility and muscle fitness exercises do not produce all of the benefits associated with regular physical activity, they will produce benefits even if you are unable to perform as much activity from other levels as you like.
- *Good planning will allow you to schedule activities from all levels in a reasonable amount of time.* In subsequent concepts, you will learn more about each level of the pyramid, as well as more information about planning a total physical activity program.

When healthful levels of fitness and activity have been achieved, maintenance is a worthy goal. Goals for improvement are recommended for individuals who don't achieve the good fitness zones for all parts of fitness or those who do not meet guidelines for physical activity. After establishing healthy levels of physical fitness and establishing regular patterns of activity, maintaining these levels is a more important goal than continued improvement.

Physical Activity Patterns

 The proportion of adults meeting national health goals varies with activity type and gender. www.mhhe.com/phys_fit/web05 Click 05. National health goals have been established for each of the types of activity illustrated in the physical activity pyramid. The proportion of adults eighteen and over who meet national health goals for moderate activity (at least 5 days a week), vigorous activity (at least 3 days a week), muscle fitness exercise (no frequency specified), and flexibility (at least 3 days a week) are presented in Table 1. Also presented in Table 1 are proportions of people who are totally inactive (no leisure-time bouts of activity of at least 10 minutes) and proportions of people who meet one or both of the moderate or vigorous standards.

A higher proportion of people reach the vigorous physical activity than the moderate activity criteria. With the exception of flexibility activity, the proportion of males achieving the various activity criteria is higher for males than for females. Only 14 percent of adults meet the moderate activity standard (equal to the surgeon general's recommendation). However, 30.6 percent can be considered "active enough" because they meet either the moderate or the vigorous standard. Unfortunately, 38.3 percent of all adults not only fail to get enough exercise but also get no leisure activity of any kind.

Technology Update
Physical Activity Information

Advances in technology have made it easier for public health officials to monitor physical activity patterns in the population. Data compiled by the Centers for Disease Control and Prevention and the National Center for Health Statistics are available online. Scientists can access the data to conduct additional analyses or research, professionals can access the data to provide updated statistics in presentations, and consumers can access the information to learn more about health issues. The national data from the Behavioral Risk Factor Surveillance system are posted separately for each state and tracked each year to allow users to graph important patterns and trends. Visit the "On the Web" resource for this concept to learn more (www.mhhe.com/phys_fit/web05 Click 05).

Activity levels in the most recent report (Table 1) are similar to those reported in *Healthy People 2010*. However, there was a modest decrease in the proportion of people performing no activity (–1.7 percent). The proportion of people doing muscle fitness exercise was higher than in previous reports because this survey asked only if muscle fitness exercise was performed and did not require a specific number of days, as was the case in other reports, such as *Healthy People 2010*.

The proportion of people meeting national health goals varies based on age. www.mhhe.com/phys_fit/web05 Click 06. Because it is difficult to measure physical activity among young children, the evidence concerning activity levels of children under age twelve is not as prevalent as for adolescents and adults. It is clear, however, that children are the most active group in Western society, though they are active in ways different from adults. Young children are not likely to perform activity continuously but, rather, do intermittent bouts of activity followed by short rests. Recent guidelines indicate that this type of activity is appropriate for children and attempts to get children to be active in ways similar to adults are inappropriate. For children, 60 minutes and up to several hours of physical activity is recommended per day.

During adolescence, activity levels tend to decrease. Lack of physical education in the upper grades, TV watching, and video game playing are thought to be reasons for the decline with age. Nevertheless, teens do considerably more vigorous activity than adults in their twenties. As indicated, physical activity of all types decreases from ages eighteen to seventy-five, with 50 percent or more of adults sixty-five and older performing no leisure activity at all (see Table 1).

Table 1 ▶ The Percentage of Adults Meeting Activity Goals

Characteristic	Moderate Activity	Vigorous Activity	Mod/Vig or Both	Muscle Fitness Exercise	Flexibility Exercises	No Leisure Activity
Sex						
Female	13.1%	18.9%	27.3%	22.9%	31.0%*	40.9%
Male	15.7%	26.1%	34.4%	27.2%	29.0%*	35.4%
All	14.3%	22.3%	30.6	18.7%	30.0%*	38.3%
Age						
18–24	16.5%	31.7%	38.9%	36.5%	36.0%*	30.4%
25–44	17.9%	26.5%	37.5%	27.3%	32.0%*	33.2%
45–64	14.2%	20.3%	28.1%	18.3%	28.0%*	39.5%
65–74	15.9%	12.6%	24.9%	11.7%	24.0%*	47.9%
75+	11.0%	5.6%	15.4%	8.2%	22.0%*	61.3%
Education						
Grades 9–11	10.0%	11.8%	18.4%	15.2%	16.0%*	60.1%
HS graduate	13.4%	17.6%	26.1%	17.3%	23.0%*	43.3%
Some college	16.8%	24.2%	33.7%	25.7%	36.0%*	32.2%
College graduate	16.1%	32.7%	40.8%	34.5%	No data	22.7%
Ethnicity						
Native/Indian Alaskan	13.0%*	19.0%*	No data	No data	26.0%*	No data
Asian or Pacific Islander	12.3%	17.7%	25.9%	27.6%	34.0%*	38.2%
Black/African American	9.9%	16.7%	23.1%	30.3%	26.0%*	50.2%
Hispanic/Latino	10.3%	15.5%	22.2%	21.0%	22.0%*	53.2%
White/non-Hispanic	15.6%	24.4%	33.2%	27.6%	31.0%*	34.5%
Income						
Below poverty	11.3%	12.9%	20.5%	17.6%	No data	56.9%
1 to 4× Poverty	13.9%	18.4%	26.9%	22.1%	No data	40.5%
Above 4× poverty	17.4%	31.1%	40.4%	36.4%	No data	24.3%
Disability Status						
With	12.0%*	13.0%*	No data	14.0%*	29.0%*	56.0%*
Without	16.0%*	25.0%*	No data	20.0%*	31.0%*	36.0%*

Source: Data from National Health Interview Survey and *Healthy People 2010.**

The proportion of adults meeting national health goals varies based on a variety of characteristics. Among the major characteristics associated with different levels of physical activity are age, education level, ethnicity, income, and disability status. Some statistics for various groups' characteristics are illustrated in Table 1.

The proportion of adults meeting national health goals varies by many demographic factors. Age, education level, ethnicity, income, and disability status have all been associated with physical activity. Statistics in Table 1 reveal the differences that are typically found for these demographic factors.

Economic status and level of education show similar trends and are likely related. People at the poverty level are more than twice as likely to be totally inactive during leisure time, compared with those with high income. High school dropouts are three times more likely to be inactive than college grads. Minority groups have high rates of inactivity, but this is likely associated with educa-

tional and economic factors. Adults identified as having one or more of a wide variety of physical disabilities have an especially high probability of being inactive. One of the two major goals of *Healthy People 2010* is to eliminate health disparities among different segments of the population. Education, in general, and educating the public about the value of physical activity and other health issues, in specific, are important if we are to achieve this goal.

Strategies for Action

A self-assessment of your current activity at each level of the pyramid can help you determine future activity goals. Lab 5A provides you with the opportunity to assess your physical activity at each level of the pyramid. Later you will develop a program of activity, and these assessments will provide a basis for program planning.

Study Resources

Check out additional online study resources for this concept in the Student Edition of the Online Learning Center at www.mhhe.com/corbin13e.

Web Resources

American College of Sports Medicine **www.acsm.org**
Centers for Disease Control and Prevention (CDC)
  www.cdc.gov
Health Canada **www.healthcanada.ca**
Healthy People 2010 **www.health.gov/healthypeople**
Morbidity and Mortality Weekly Reports **www.cdc.gov/mmwr**
Surgeon General's Report on Physical Activity and Health
  www.cdc.gov/nccdphp/sgr/sgr.htm

Suggested Readings

 Additional reference materials for Concept 5 are available at **www.mhhe.com/phys_fit/web05 Click 07**.

Ainsworth, B. E. 2003. The compendium of physical activities. *President's Council on Physical Fitness and Sports Research Digest* 4(2):1–8.

American College of Sports Medicine. 2004. *ACSM's Health-Related Physical Fitness Assessment Manual.* Philadelphia, PA: Lippincott, Williams, & Wilkins.

American College of Sports Medicine. 2000. *ACSM's Guidelines for Exercise Testing and Prescription.* 6th ed. Philadelphia: Lippincott, Williams and Wilkins.

Barnes, P. M., and C. A. Schoenhorn. 2003. Physical activity among adults. *Advance Data from Vital and Health Statistics* 333(May 14):1–23.

Bassuk, S. S., and Manson, J. E. 2003. Physical activity and cardiovascular disease prevention in women: How much is good enough? *Exercise and Sport Sciences Reviews* 31(4):176–181.

Blair, S. N. 2004. The evolution of physical activity recommendations: How much is enough? *American Journal of Clinical Nutrition* 79(5):913A–920S.

Corbin, C. B., G. L. Le Masurier, and B. D. Franks. 2002. Making sense of multiple physical activity recommendations. *President's Council on Physical Fitness and Sports Research Digest* 3(19):1–8.

Corbin, C. B., et al. 2004. Physical activity for children: Current patterns and guidelines. *President's Council on Physical Fitness and Sports Research Digest* 4(6):1–8.

Manson, J. E., et al. 2002. Walking compared with vigorous exercise for the prevention of cardiovascular events in women. *New England Journal of Medicine* 347(10):716–725.

National Association for Sports and Physical Education. 2004. *Physical Activity for Children: A Statement of Guidelines.* Reston, VA: National Association for Sports and Physical Education.

Rankinen, T., and C. Bouchard. 2002. Dose-response issues concerning the relations between regular physical activity and health. *President's Council on Physical Fitness and Sports Research Digest* 3(18):1–8.

Schoenborn, C. A., and P. M. Barnes. 2002. Leisure-time physical activity status among American adults. *Advance Data from Vital and Health Statistics* 325(April 7):1–24.

U.S. Department of Health and Human Services. 1996. *Physical Activity and Health: A Report of the Surgeon General.* Atlanta: U.S. Department of Health and Human Services.

Yu, S., et al. 2003. What level of physical activity protects against premature cardiovascular death? *Heart* 89(5):502–506.

 In the News

Physical Activity Guidelines for Youth

Public health experts have recognized the importance of promoting physical activity in youth. The National Association for Sports and Physical Education recently released updated guidelines that describe the appropriate levels of physical activity for youth. According to the new physical activity guidelines, children should

- Accumulate at least 60 minutes, and up to several hours, of age-appropriate physical activity on all if not most days of the week. This daily accumulation should include moderate and vigorous physical activity, with the majority of the time being spent in intermittent activity. (Continuous physical activity is not a condition for meeting these guidelines.)

- Participate in several bouts of physical activity lasting 15 minutes or more each day.
- Participate each day in a variety of age-appropriate physical activities designed to achieve optimal health, wellness, fitness, and performance benefits.
- Avoid extended periods of inactivity (periods of 2 or more hours), especially during the daytime hours.

While this book focuses on adults, it is important for readers to understand that children's activity guidelines are very different from the adult guidelines presented in this concept. Adults play a major role in shaping children's activity patterns. Helping children meet these guidelines may help reduce the prevalence of inactive and overweight adults in future years.

Lab 5A Self-Assessment of Physical Activity

Name	Section	Date

Purpose: To estimate your current levels of physical activity from each category of the physical activity pyramid

Procedures

1. Place an X over the circle that characterizes your participation in each category in the pyramid.
2. Determine if you met the national goal for each type of activity. Place an X over the "yes" circle if you met the goal in each area (see Results).

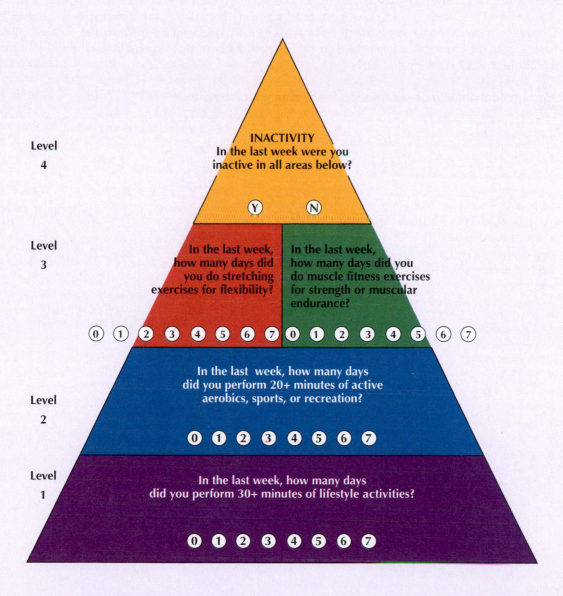

Level 4

INACTIVITY
In the last week were you inactive in all areas below?

Y   N

Level 3

In the last week, how many days did you do stretching exercises for flexibility?

In the last week, how many days did you do muscle fitness exercises for strength or muscular endurance?

0 1 2 3 4 5 6 7   0 1 2 3 4 5 6 7

Level 2

In the last week, how many days did you perform 20+ minutes of active aerobics, sports, or recreation?

0 1 2 3 4 5 6 7

Level 1

In the last week, how many days did you perform 30+ minutes of lifestyle activities?

0 1 2 3 4 5 6 7

Results

Activity Type	Level	National Goal	Did You Meet the National Health Goal?	
Lifestyle activity	1	5 days or more	Yes	No
Active aerobics/sports	2	3 days or more	Yes	No
Flexibility exercises	3	3 days or more	Yes	No
Muscle fitness	3	2 days or more	Yes	No
Inactivity	4	Avoid total inactivity	Yes	No

Conclusions and Implications: In the space below, write a brief paper describing your current physical activity patterns. Do you meet the national health goals in all areas? If not, in what types of activity from the pyramid do you need to improve? Are the answers you gave for the past week typical of your regular activity patterns? If you meet all national health goals, explain why you think this is so. Do you think that meeting the goals in the pyramid on the previous page indicates good activity patterns for you?

Write your physical activity assessment paper in the space below.

Learning Self-Planning Skills for Lifetime Physical Activity

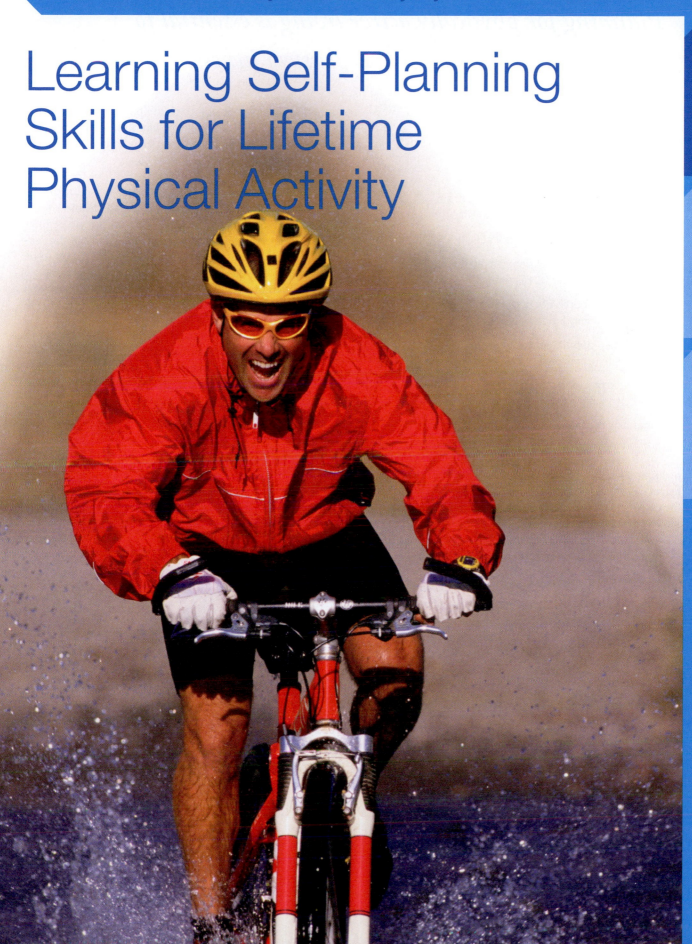

Planning for physically active living is essential to optimal health, wellness, and physical fitness.

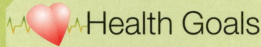

Health Goals

for the year 2010

- Improve health, fitness, and quality of life through regular, daily physical activity.
- Increase leisure-time physical activity.
- Increase proportion of people who do moderate daily activity for 30 minutes.
- Increase proportion of people who do vigorous physical activity 3 days a week.
- Increase proportion of people who do regular muscle fitness exercise.
- Increase proportion of people who do regular exercise for flexibility.
- Increase prevalence of a healthy weight.

In the first section of this book (Concepts 1 and 2), you learned some basic information about health, wellness, fitness, and healthy lifestyles. You also learned some of the self-management strategies that can be used to help you change a variety of lifestyles to promote health, wellness, and fitness. The second section of the book was devoted specifically to basic information about one healthy lifestyle: physically active living. In the third section of the book, you will learn more about planning for physically active living. First, you will learn about the six steps in personal programming (Concept 6). (See Table 1.) You will then learn to plan programs for each of the types of activities in the physical activity pyramid and the benefits associated with each type of activity (Concepts 7–11). Information about other healthy lifestyles is covered in later concepts. In the final concept of this book, you will have the opportunity to prepare a comprehensive lifetime program of physical activity, as well as to do planning for other healthy lifestyle changes.

Step 1: Clarifying Reasons

Clarifying your reasons for participating in physical activity is an important step in self-planning. As you continue your study in this book, you will be presented with a wide variety of physical activity choices. Your per-

sonal reasons for choosing to participate or not to participate should be clarified prior to planning your program. Over time, attitudes change, so periodic reassessment is recommended.

Knowing the most common reasons for inactivity can help you avoid sedentary living. Some of the common reasons given by those who do not do regular physical activity are outlined in Table 2. Many of the reasons for not being active are considered by experts to be barriers that can be overcome. Overcoming barriers is a self-management skill. Using the strategies for change in Table 2 helps inactive people to become more active.

 Knowing the reasons people give for being active can help you adopt positive attitudes. www.mhhe.com/phys_fit/web06 Click 01. Table 3 describes some of the major reasons why people choose to be active. It also offers strategies for changing behavior if you have more than one or two negative attitudes. Active people have more positive than negative attitudes. This is referred to by experts as a positive "balance of attitudes." The questionnaire in Lab 6A gives you the opportunity to

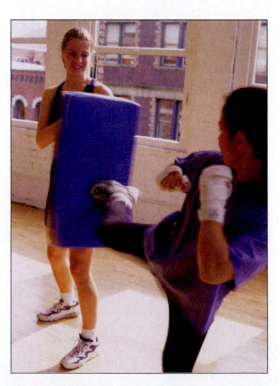

Active people have more positive than negative feelings about physical activity.

Table 1 ▶ Self-Planning Skills

Self-Planning	Description	Self-Management Skill
1. **Clarifying reasons**	Knowing the general reasons you might benefit helps you select activities that you will enjoy and adhere to for a lifetime.	Balancing attitudes: Sections of this concept and Lab 6A help you determine if you have more positive than negative attitudes and help clarify your reasons for doing physical activity.
2. **Identifying needs**	If you know your strengths and weaknesses, you can plan to build on your strengths and overcome weaknesses.	Self-assessment: In the concepts that follow, you will learn how to assess different health, wellness, and fitness characteristics. Learning these self-assessments will help you identify needs.
3. **Setting personal goals**	Goals are more specific than reasons (see #1). Establishing specific things that you want to accomplish can provide a basis for feedback that your program is working.	Goal setting: Guidelines in this concept will help you set goals. In subsequent concepts, you will establish goals for different types of activity from the pyramid.
4. **Selecting personal activities**	A personal plan should include activities that meet your needs and goals (see steps 1–3) and provide fun and enjoyment. Having skill improves enjoyment.	Performance skills: In subsequent concepts, you will learn how to enhance your performance skills. Self-assessments will also help you match your abilities to specific activities.
5. **Writing your plan**	Once you have determined which activities you will perform, you should put your plan in writing. This establishes your intentions and increases your chances of adherence.	Self-planning: This includes writing down the time of day, day of the week, and length of exercise session for each activity you will include in your plan.
6. **Evaluating progress**	Keeping records, including self-monitoring of activities performed and periodic self-assessment of fitness status, helps you adhere to your program.	Self-monitoring: This is used as the basis for keeping activity records (logs) and determining if activity goals are met. Self-assessment: This is used as a basis for determining if fitness goals are met.

assess your balance of attitudes. If you have a negative balance score, you can analyze your attitudes and determine how you can change them to view activity more favorably.

Step 2: Identifying Needs

Self-assessments are useful in establishing personal needs, planning your program, and evaluating your progress. You have already done some self-assessments of wellness, current activity levels, and current lifestyles. In the lab for this concept and others that follow, you will make additional assessments. The results of these assessments help you build a personal profile that can be used as the basis for program planning. With practice, self-assessments become more accurate. It is for this reason that it is important to repeat self-assessments and to pay careful attention to the procedures for performing them. If questions arise, get a professional opinion rather than making an error.

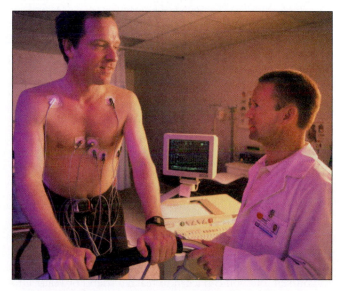

A fitness assessment by an expert can be useful.

Table 2 ▶ Common Reasons People Give for Not Being Active

Reason	Description	Strategy for Change
I don't have the time.	This is the number one reason people give for not exercising. Invariably, those who feel they don't have time know they should do more exercise. They say they plan to do more in the future when "things are less hectic." Young people say that they will have more time to exercise in the future. Older people say that they wish they had taken the time to be active when they were younger.	Planning a daily schedule can help you find the time for activity and avoid wasting time on things that are less important. Learning the facts in the concepts that follow will help you see the importance of activity and how you can include it in your schedule with a minimum of effort and with time efficiency.
It's too inconvenient.	Many who avoid physical activity do so because it is inconvenient. They are procrastinators. Specific reasons for procrastinating include "It makes me sweaty" and "It messes up my hair."	If you have to travel more than 10 minutes to do activity or if you do not have easy access to equipment, you will avoid activity. Locating facilities and finding a time when you can shower is important.
I just don't enjoy it.	Many do not find activity to be enjoyable or invigorating. These people may assume that all forms of activity have to be strenuous and fatiguing.	There are many activities to choose from. If you don't enjoy vigorous activity, try more moderate forms of activity such as walking.
I'm no good at physical activity.	"People might laugh at me," "Sports make me nervous," and "I am not good at physical activities" are reasons some people give for not being active. Some people lack confidence in their own abilities. This may be because of past experiences in physical education or sports.	With properly selected activities, even those who have never enjoyed exercise can get hooked. Building skills can help, as can changing your way of thinking. Avoiding comparisons with others can help you feel successful.
I am not fit, so I avoid activity.	Some people avoid exercise because of health reasons. Some who are unfit lack energy. Starting slowly can build fitness gradually and help you realize that you can do it.	There are good medical reasons for not doing activity, but many people with problems can benefit from exercise if it is properly designed. If necessary, get help adapting activity to meet your needs.
I have no place to be active, especially in bad weather.	Regular activity is more convenient if facilities are easy to reach and the weather is good. Opportunities have increased considerably in recent years. Some of the most popular activities require little equipment, can be done in or near home, and are inexpensive.	If you cannot find a place, if it is not safe, or if it is too expensive, consider using low-cost equipment at home, such as rubber bands or calisthenics. Lifestyle activity can be done by anyone at almost any time.
I am too old.	As people grow older, many begin to feel that activity is something they cannot do. For most people, this is simply not true! Properly planned exercise for older adults is not only safe but also has many health benefits—e.g., longer life, fewer illnesses, an improved sense of well-being, and optimal functioning.	Older people who are just beginning activity should start slowly. Lifestyle activities are a good choice. Setting realistic goals can help, as can learning to do resistance training and flexibility exercises.

Periodic self-assessments can aid in determining if a person is meeting health and fitness standards and is making progress toward personal goals. At some point, it is wise to have an expert test your fitness. This helps you get an accurate assessment of your current fitness level and helps you determine if your self-assessment results are accurate. Expert tests are often expensive and require time and effort on your part. When possible, you should learn to perform self-assessments, so that you can continue to assess your fitness for a lifetime without dependence on someone else. Tests such as skinfold measures are hard to administer to yourself, but you can learn to teach a friend or relative to assist you with the measurement.

For many components of physical fitness, multiple assessments are provided in this book. For example, four different cardiovascular fitness assessments are included for your selection. You are encouraged to try several assessments for each component of fitness and then decide which one best meets your personal needs.

Self-assessments have the advantage of consistent error rather than variable error. As noted previously, the best type of assessments are done by highly qualified experts using precise instruments. Eliminating error is always desirable. Following directions and practicing sound assessment techniques will reduce error significantly. Still,

Table 3 ▶ Common Reasons for Doing Regular Physical Activity

Reason	Description	Strategy for Change
I do activity for my health, wellness, and fitness.	Surveys show this is the number one reason for doing regular physical activity. Unfortunately, many adults say that a "doctor's order to exercise" would be the most likely reason to get them to begin a program. For some, however, waiting for a doctor's order may be too late.	Gaining information contained in this book will help you see the value of regular physical activity. Performing the self-assessments in the various concepts will help you determine the areas in which you need personal improvement.
I do activity to improve my appearance.	In our society, looking good is highly valued; thus, physical attractiveness is a major reason people participate in regular exercise. Regular activity can contribute to looking your best.	Some people have failed in past attempts to change their appearance through activity. Setting realistic goals and avoiding comparisons with others can help you to be more successful.
I do activity because I enjoy it.	A majority of adults say that enjoyment is of paramount importance in deciding to be active. Statements include experiencing the "peak experience," the "runner's high," or "spinning free." The sense of fun, well-being, and general enjoyment associated with physical activity are well documented.	Those people who do not enjoy activity often lack performance skills or feel that they are not competent in activity. Improving skills with practice, setting realistic goals, and adopting a new way of thinking can help you to be successful and to enjoy activities.
I do activity because it relaxes me.	Relaxation and release from tension rank high as reasons people do regular activity. It is known that activity in the form of sports and games provides a catharsis, or outlet, for the frustrations of daily activities. Regular exercise can help reduce depression and anxiety.	Activities, such as walking, jogging, or cycling, are ways of getting some quiet time away from the job or the stresses of daily living. In a later concept, you will learn about exercises that you can do to reduce stress.
I like the challenge and sense of personal accomplishment I get from physical activity.	A sense of personal accomplishment is frequently a reason for people doing activity. In some cases, it is learning a new skill, such as racquetball or tennis; in other cases, it is running a mile or doing a certain number of crunches. The challenge of doing something you have never done before is apparently a powerful experience.	Some people get little sense of accomplishment from activity. Taking lessons to learn skills or attempting activities new to you can provide the challenge that makes activity interesting. Also, adopting a new way of thinking allows you to focus on the task rather than competition with others.
I like the social involvement I get from physical activities.	"Why am I physically active?" "It is a good way to spend time with members of my family." "It is a good way to spend time with close friends." "Being part of the team is satisfying." Activity settings can also provide an opportunity for making new friends.	If you find activity to be socially unrewarding, you may have to find activities that you, friends, or family enjoy. Taking lessons together can help. Also, finding a friend with similar skills can help. Focus on the activity rather than the outcome.
Competition is the main reason I enjoy physical activity.	"The thrill of victory" and "sports competition" are two reasons given for being active. For many, the competitive experience is very satisfying.	Some people simply do not enjoy competing. If this is the case for you, select noncompetitive individual activities.
Physical activity helps me feel good about myself.	For many people, participation in physical activity is an important part of their identity. They feel better about themselves when they are regularly participating.	Physical activity is something that is self-determined and within your control. Participation can help you feel good about yourself, build your confidence, and increase your self-esteem.
Physical activity provides opportunities to get fresh air.	Being outside and experiencing nature are reasons that some people give for being physically active.	Many activities provide opportunities to be outside. If this is an important reason for you, seek out parks and outdoor settings for your activities.

errors will occur. One advantage of a self-assessment is that the person doing the assessment is always the same—you. Even if you make an error in a self-assessment, it is likely to be consistent over time, especially if you use the same equipment each time you make the assessment. For example, if you measure your own weight using a home scale and your measurement shows your weight to be 2 pounds higher than it really is, you have made a consistent error. You can determine if you are making improvement because you know the error exists. When different people using different instruments assess your fitness, the results may be inconsistent (variable error).

Results of fitness assessments are influenced by heredity. Many people get discouraged if improvements in fitness don't come as easily as expected or if other people achieve higher levels of fitness without being as active. Genetic factors influence many personal characteristics, including the rate and extent to which you can improve your fitness. Comparisons with others will almost always leave people feeling disappointed, so it is important to focus on personal goals and accomplishments. A hereditary predisposition may limit your potential for achieving exceptionally high levels of fitness (or becoming an elite athlete), but everyone can improve his or her personal level of fitness.

 Health-based criterion-referenced standards are recommended for rating your fitness. www.mhhe.com/phys_fit/web06 Click 02. Most experts now recommend **health-based criterion-referenced standards** to rate your current fitness. These standards are based on how much fitness is needed for good health. Other fitness standards may use norms or percentiles that compare a person's fitness against a reference population. Knowing how you compare with other people or population standards is not that important. In fact, such comparisons have been shown to be discouraging to many people. Determining if your fitness is adequate to enhance your health and wellness is much more relevant.

In this book, the health-related standard is referred to as the *Good Fitness Zone* (see Table 4). With reasonable amounts of physical activity, most people should be able to improve their fitness enough to make it into this range. For personal reasons, some may wish to aim for a higher level referred to as the *High Performance Zone*.

Attaining this level does not provide many additional health benefits but may be important for those interested in performance. The *Low Fit Zone* and *Marginal Zone* are levels of fitness that are not sufficient for optimal health benefits. If you score in these ranges, you should try to improve your levels of fitness.

 A comprehensive fitness profile can help you set program goals. www.mhhe.com/phys_fit/web06 Click 03. Compiling all of your self-assessments in one comprehensive profile can help you determine your strengths and weaknesses. The **fitness profile** will help you get a picture of the components of fitness in which you need improvement. A customized software program called the Interactive Personal Trainer is available for users of the book at the "On the Web" resource section.

⊙ Technology Update

Online Physical Activity Challenges

The President's Challenge is an online activity challenge program developed by the President's Council on Physical Fitness and Sports to encourage Americans to be more active. The Active Lifestyle Program is for adults who are beginning an exercise program or those who want to be more consistent in their activity patterns. The Presidential Champions Program is for people who are already active and want a special activity challenge. Both programs involve online tracking of activity and corresponding awards for those reaching their goal. There is also an option to set and monitor group exercise goals. For more information, visit the website (**www.presidentschallenge.org**).

Step 3: Setting Personal Goals

Learning to set realistic goals is useful as a basis for physical activity self-planning. If any lifestyle change is to be of value, it is important to determine—ahead of time—what you hope to accomplish. Goals are specific objectives you hope to accomplish as a result of a lifestyle change. To be effective, goals must be realistic—neither too hard nor too easy. If the goal is too hard, failure is likely. Failure is discouraging. By setting realistic and attainable goals, you have a greater chance of success.

Beginners are encouraged to focus on short-term goals. Focus on **short-term goals** first. Short-term goals are easier to accomplish than **long-term goals.**

Table 4 ▶ The Four Fitness Zones
High Performance Zone It is not necessary to reach this level to experience good health benefits. Achievement of high performance scores has more to do with performance than it does with good health. In some cases, extreme fitness scores can increase health risk—e.g., very low body fatness.
Good Fitness Zone If you reach the good fitness zone, you have enough of a specific fitness component to help reduce health risk. However, even reaching the good fitness zone may not result in optimal health benefits for inactive people.
Marginal Zone Marginal scores indicate that some improvement is in order, but you are nearing minimal health standards set by experts.
Low Fit Zone If you score low in fitness, you are probably less fit than you should be for your own good health and wellness.

Realistic short-term goals make you successful because one success leads to another. When you meet short-term goals, establish new ones. Long-term goals take a long time to accomplish and may be discouraging to beginners. After a series of short-term goals have been successfully accomplished, set long-term goals. In fact, setting and achieving a series of short-term goals is the best way to achieve long-term goals.

Short-term goals should be specific. Many individuals make the mistake of setting vague goals, such as "be more active" or "eat less." Although these may be your long-term objectives, goals should be more specific. Setting specific goals helps you commit to what you want to accomplish. It is also easier to assess whether you are making progress.

Short-term goals should be behavioral goals rather than outcome goals. A **behavioral goal** is associated with something you do. Performing physical activity for a specific period of time is something you do, so a **physical activity goal** is a type of behavioral goal. An example of a specific short-term behavioral goal is "to perform 30 minutes of brisk walking 6 days a week for the next 2 weeks." It is specific because you specify how long and how often you expect to do the exercise. It is short-term because you can accomplish it in a few weeks or less. The principal factor associated with success is your willingness to give effort. No matter who you are, you can accomplish this behavioral goal if you give a daily effort. In addition, behavioral goals are easy to self-monitor. Keeping an activity log of your weekly participation in brisk walking will reveal your compliance with the goal.

An **outcome goal** is associated with something you "can do." For example, **fitness goals** such as being able to do ten push-ups or to run a mile in 7 minutes are examples of outcome goals. Outcome and fitness goals are not recommended for beginners for three reasons:

- *Typically, it takes time (weeks or months) to reach fitness and other outcome goals.* For this reason short-term fitness goals are not recommended for beginners because they are often not achieved in the designated time, resulting in a perception of failure.
- *Outcome goals depend on many things other than your lifestyle behavior.* For example, your heredity affects your body fat and muscle development. Setting a goal of achieving a certain percentage of body fat or lifting a certain weight is influenced by heredity as well as your physical activity program. This makes it hard for beginners to set realistic fitness goals. Too often the tendency is to set the goal based on a comparative standard rather than on a standard that is possible for the individual to achieve in a short period of time. Those more experienced in physical activity learn to set more realistic outcome goals and learn that these goals often take time to achieve.
- *Different people progress at different rates.* People not only inherit a predisposition to fitness and body composition, but they also inherit a predisposition to benefit from training. In other words, if ten people do the exact same physical activities, there will be ten different results. One may improve performance by 60 percent, whereas another improves only 10 percent. Until you gain enough experience to see how you respond to physical activity, it is not wise to set fitness or outcome goals. You need experience to determine the areas of fitness in which you respond quickly and those areas in which your response to activity is slower. It is at this time that fitness and outcome goals become more appropriate.

Long-term goals can be either behavioral or outcome goals. Long-term goals can be of a behavioral nature similar to short-term goals. If you set as a goal participation in regular physical activity and meet the goal over a long period of time, fitness and other health

Health-Based Criterion-Referenced Standards The amount of a specific type of fitness necessary to gain a health or wellness benefit.

Fitness Profile A summary of the results of self-assessments of physical fitness.

Short-Term Goals Statements of intent to change a behavior or achieve an outcome in a period of days or weeks.

Long-Term Goals Statement of intent to change behavior or achieve a specific outcome in a period of months or years.

Behavioral Goal A statement of intent to perform a specific behavior (changing a lifestyle) for a specific period of time. An example is, "I will walk for 15 minutes each morning before work."

Physical Activity Goal A behavioral goal with exercise as the intended behavior.

Outcome Goal A statement of intent to achieve a specific test score (attainment of a specific standard) associated with good health, wellness, or fitness. An example is, "I will lower my body fat level by 3 percent."

Fitness Goals Outcome goals with a specific fitness score as the intended outcome.

benefits will occur to the extent that they are possible, given your genetics and body type. For this reason, behavioral, or physical activity, goals are appropriate. This type of goal is easy to monitor, and self-assessments of fitness will provide feedback of program success.

Outcome or fitness goals can also be useful to the person experienced in physical activity. If realistic, these goals will be met with appropriate physical activity and provide evidence of success. When establishing long-term fitness goals, be careful not to base them on what other people can do. You may be setting yourself up for failure. Be sure that the fitness outcomes you expect are based on health standards or scores slightly above what you can currently perform, rather than on the performance scores of other people.

It is appropriate to consider maintenance goals. There is a limit to the amount of fitness any person can achieve. You cannot improve forever. Limits on physical activity goals are appropriate. At some point, it is reasonable to set maintenance goals to help you to stay active and fit when improvement goals have already been met.

Set goals that you can maintain for a lifetime. Physical activity and fitness for a lifetime mean maintaining your program forever. If you set exercise or fitness goals that are excessive, you may burn out and quit exercising entirely. Consider the long term in setting your goals.

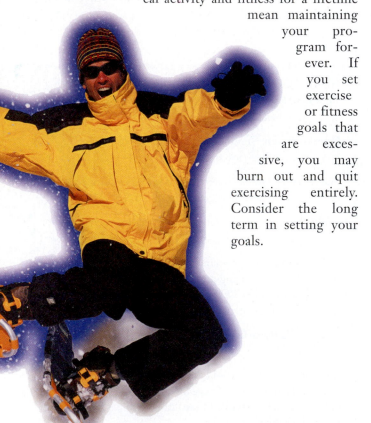

Select activities that help you meet personal goals.

Putting your goals in writing helps formalize them. Put your goals in writing. Otherwise, your goals will be easy to forget. Writing them helps establish a commitment to yourself and clearly establishes your goals. You can revise them if necessary. Written goals are not cast in concrete.

Step 4: Selecting Activities

🌍 **There are many activities from which you can choose to meet your goals.** www.mhhe.com/phys_fit/web06 Click 04. A good lifetime physical activity program will include a wide variety of activities. In the concepts that follow, you will learn more about activities from each level of the physical activity pyramid, including the benefits you can expect from each type of activity. The more you learn about each type of activity, the greater likelihood that you will select activities that meet your goals. Consider the following guidelines as you learn more about each type of activity:

- Choose activities you enjoy or find ways to make activity enjoyable.
- Choose activities that match your abilities.
- Practice to improve your performance skills or find activities that do not require a lot of skill.
- Choose activities that build all parts of fitness.

Step 5: Writing Your Plan

Preparing a written plan can improve your adherence to the plan. A written plan is a pledge, or a promise, to be active. Research shows that intentions to be active are more likely to be acted on when put in writing. In the concepts that follow, you will be given the opportunity to prepare written plans for all of the activities in the physical activity pyramid. This will be done one activity at a time. When you have developed a plan for each type of activity, you can then develop a comprehensive physical activity plan.

In Lab 21C, you will write a comprehensive lifetime activity plan. By then, you will have learned more about a variety of activities. You will also have learned more about a variety of self-management skills that will assist you.

Step 6: Evaluating Progress

🌍 **Self-monitoring of physical activity can help you evaluate progress.** www.mhhe.com/phys_fit/web06 Click 05. Once you have written a plan, it is important to assess your effectiveness in sticking with your plan. Keeping written records is one type of self-monitoring.

You can monitor your physical activity goals by keeping daily records of the activities you perform. Keeping records in the form of physical activity logs is the preferred method of self-monitoring for beginners. Activity logs help you comply with physical activity goals. In the concepts that follow, you will prepare a plan for different types of physical activity from the pyramid and keep activity logs to chart progress.

Advanced exercisers can evaluate progress by keeping records of fitness improvement. By the time you complete your studies associated with this book, you should have the experience necessary to establish and self-monitor fitness goals. You may already have the experience necessary, but you are encouraged to focus on physical activity recordkeeping as you perform the lab experiences presented early in this book.

Periodic self-assessments allow you to monitor progress toward fitness and other outcome goals. If fitness has improved, the results can be motivational. If done too frequently, monitoring improvements can be discouraging, since it takes time for fitness to improve. Also, changes that occur from day to day may not be representative of true changes in fitness. Fatigue, time of testing, and nutritional status are but a few of the factors that account for fitness differences from day to day. For example, strength test results may be low if done after a hard day's work, and your weight can vary from day to day or even hour to hour based on nutritional factors, such as water loss from physical activity.

Fitness recordkeeping is important. Periodic self-assessment of each of the different fitness dimensions is encouraged as long as it is not too often. Doing self-assessments under the same conditions, including the same time of the day, is important if self-monitoring is to be meaningful.

Strategies for Action

A self-assessment of your attitudes about physical activity is a good first step in planning for lifelong physical activity. The Physical Activity Attitude Questionnaire included in Lab 6A allows you the opportunity to consider your reasons for participating in physical activity. You will calculate a score for each of the nine attitudes described in Table 3. You will also calculate a balance of attitudes score, which will indicate whether you have more positive than negative attitudes about physical activity. If you have low scores for certain attitudes, you should consider the strategies for change outlined in Table 3. Efforts to change attitudes are especially important for people with a negative balance of attitudes (poor or very poor ratings).

Self-planning skills can be used for each of the different types of activity in the physical activity pyramid. In subsequent concepts, you will develop your own plans for each of the types of activity in the physical activity pyramid. As you develop those plans, it will be useful to refer to the self-planning skills outlined in this concept.

Study Resources

Check out additional online study resources for this concept in the Student Edition of the Online Learning Center at www.mhhe.com/corbin13e.

Web Resources

American College of Sports Medicine **www.acsm.org**
Centers for Disease Control and Prevention (CDC)
   www.cdc.gov
The Fitness Jumpsite **www.primusweb.com/fitnesspartner**
Health Canada-Physical Activity Guide **www.hc-sc.gc.ca/**
   hppb/paguide

Suggested Readings

Additional reference materials for Concept 6 are available at **www.mhhe.com/phys_fit/web06 Click 06**.

American College of Sports Medicine. 2000. *ACSM's Guidelines for Exercise Testing and Exercise Prescription.* 6th ed. Philadelphia: Lippincott, Williams and Wilkins.

American Journal of Preventive Medicine. 2002. Entire issue: Articles on how to become physically active. *American Journal of Preventive Medicine* 23(2)Supplement 1:1–108.

Blair, S. N., et al. 2001. *Active Living Every Day.* Champaign, IL: Human Kinetics.

Bray, S. A., and H. A. Born. 2004. Transition to university and vigorous physical activity: Implications for health and psychological well-being. *Journal of American College Health* 52(4):181–188.

Brehm, B. A. 2000. Maximizing the psychological benefits of physical activity. *ACSM's Health and Fitness Journal* 4(6):7–11.

Buckworth, J., and R. Dishman. 2002. *Exercise Psychology.* Champaign, IL: Human Kinetics.

Cardinal, B. J., and M. Kosma. 2004. Self-efficacy and the stages and processes of change associated with adopting and maintaining muscular fitness-promoting behaviors. *Research Quarterly for Exercise and Sport* 75(2):186–196.

Cox, R. H. 2002. *Sport Psychology: Concepts and Applications.* Chapter 6, Goal Setting in Sport. St. Louis: McGraw-Hill.

Kasch, F. 2001. Thirty-three years of aerobic activity adherence. *Quest* 53(3):362–365.

Locke, E. A. 2002. Setting goals for happiness. In C. R. Snyder and S. J. Lopez (eds.). *Handbook of Positive Psychology.* Oxford, UK: Oxford University Press.

Marcus, B., and L. A. Forsyth. 2003. *Motivating People to Be Physically Active.* Champaign, IL: Human Kinetics.

Porter, L., et al. 2003. *Motivation and Work Behavior.* Chapter 4, Role of Goals and Intentions in Motivation. St. Louis: McGraw-Hill.

Roitman, J. L. (ed.). 2001. *ACSM's Resource Manual for Guidelines for Exercise Testing and Prescription.* 4th ed. Philadelphia: Lippincott, Williams and Wilkins.

U.S. Department of Health and Human Services. 1996. *Physical Activity and Health: A Report of the Surgeon General.* Atlanta: U.S. Department of Health and Human Services.

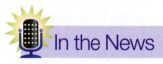 In the News

Essential Skills for Lifetime Activity

Are college students as active as they were in high school? According to a recent research study, college students are considerably less active in the first year of college than they were in high school. This is especially true for vigorous physical activity. During the last 2 months of high school, 66 percent of students were classified as vigorously active, but during the first few months of college only 44 percent of the students were vigorously active. The average frequency of vigorous physical activity dropped from 3.32 sessions per week during high school to 2.68 sessions per week during college. College students who were active reported higher levels of vigor and lower levels of tension and fatigue than inactive students.

Do college students need to use self-planning skills? The results cited earlier suggest that many college students need to use formal planning skills to maintain levels of physical activity. Do the steps in program planning really work? A study of people who have stayed active over a 33-year period of time suggest that they do. Of the fifteen people who were studied over the three decades of the study, all continued to adhere to their physical activity program; none dropped out. The steps in program planning described in this concept were among the most important factors related to the regular activity patterns over the years. These active people established their reasons and goals (steps 1 and 3) for participating, placing an emphasis on health and the reduction of hypokinetic disease risk. They performed regular oral and written evaluations (step 2) and kept records and progress reports (steps 5 and 6). In addition, they had the support of spouses and other regular exercisers.

Sometimes young people who are active feel that they do not have to do formal planning. Some say, "I am active, anyway. Why do I need to do all of that stuff?" Others, who are not active, say, "I don't have the time." Regular planning, including time management planning, can help inactive, busy people to become active and stay active. For those who are already active but who do not use more formal planning, learning the six steps in program planning can be important for staying active later in life. Evidence suggests that, as you grow older, your activities will change. The people in the study cited in this feature were able to stay active because of a commitment to personal goals and regular use of other self-management skills, such as self-assessment and self-monitoring. Even if you do not feel that you will use these skills now, learning about them and practicing them will help you use them in the future. Your long-term adherence to physical activity may depend on it.

Lab 6A Physical Activity Attitude Questionnaire

Name		Section		Date

Purpose: To evaluate your feelings concerning physical activity and to determine the specific reasons you do or do not participate in regular physical activity

The Physical Activity Attitude Questionnaire

Directions: The term *physical activity* in the following statements refers to all kinds of activities, including sports, formal exercises, and informal activities, such as jogging and cycling. Make an X over the circle that best represents your answer to each question.

	Strongly Disagree	Disagree	Undecided	Agree	Strongly Agree	Item Score		Attitude Score
1. I should do physical activity regularly for my health.	1	2	3	4	5			Health and Fitness Score
2. Doing regular physical activity is good for my fitness and wellness.	1	2	3	4	5	+	=	
3. Regular exercise helps me look my best.	1	2	3	4	5			Appearance Score
4. I feel more physically attractive when I do regular physical activity.	1	2	3	4	5	+	=	
5. One of the main reasons I do regular physical activity is because it is fun.	1	2	3	4	5			Enjoyment Score
6. The most enjoyable part of my day is when I am exercising or doing a sport.	1	2	3	4	5	+	=	
7. Taking part in physical activity helps me relax.	1	2	3	4	5			Relaxation Score
8. Physical activity helps me get away from the pressures of daily living.	1	2	3	4	5	+	=	
9. The challenge of physical training is one reason I do physical activity.	1	2	3	4	5			Challenge Score
10. I like to see if I can master sports and activities that are new to me.	1	2	3	4	5	+	=	
11. I like to do physical activity that involves other people.	1	2	3	4	5			Social Score
12. Exercise offers me the opportunity to meet other people.	1	2	3	4	5	+	=	
13. Competition is a good way to make physical activity fun.	1	2	3	4	5			Competition Score
14. I like to see how my physical abilities compare with those of others.	1	2	3	4	5	+	=	
15. When I do regular exercise, I feel better than when I don't.	1	2	3	4	5			Feeling Good Score
16. My ability to do physical activity is something that makes me proud.	1	2	3	4	5	+	=	
17. I like to do outdoor activities.	1	2	3	4	5			Outdoor Score
18. Experiencing nature is something I look forward to when exercising.	1	2	3	4	5	+	=	

Procedures

1. Read and answer each question in the questionnaire.
2. Write the number in the circle of your answer in the box labeled "Item Score."
3. Add scores for each pair of scores and record in the "Attitude Score" box.
4. Record each attitude score and a rating for each score (use Rating Chart) in the chart below.
5. Record the number of good and excellent scores in the box provided. Use the score in the box to determine your rating using the Balance of Feelings Rating Chart.

Results: Record your results as indicated in the Procedures section.

Physical Activity Attitude Questionnaire Results

Attitude	Score	Rating
Health and fitness		
Appearance		
Enjoyment		
Relaxation		
Challenge		
Social		
Competition		
Feeling good		
Outdoor		

Attitude Rating Chart

Rating Category	Attitude Score
Excellent	9–10
Good	7–8
Fair	5–6
Poor	3–4
Very poor	2

How many good or excellent scores do you have?

Balance of
Feeling Score

Having 5 or more in the box above indicates that you have a positive balance of feelings (more positive than negative attitudes).

Balance of Feelings Rating Chart

Excellent	6 to 9
Good	5
Fair	4
Poor	2–3
Very poor	0–1

In a few sentences, discuss your "balance of feelings" rating. Having more positive than negative scores (positive balance of feelings) increases the probability of being active. Include comments on whether you think your ratings suggest that you will be active or inactive and whether your ratings are really indicative of your feelings. Do you think that the scores on which you were rated poor or very poor might be reasons you would avoid physical activity? Explain.

Table 1 ▶ Classification of Physical Activity Intensities for a Person with Good Cardiovascular Fitness

Classification	Description	Examples
Maximum	Activities more than 12 times as intense as rest (12+ METs)	Running (10 mph, 6 min. mile)
Very hard	Activities more than 10 and up to 12 times as intense as rest (10 to 12 METs)	Running (8.5 mph, 7 min. mile), handball, full-court competitive basketball
Hard	Activities more than 7 and up to 10 times as intense as rest (7 to 10 METs)	Digging, level jogging (5 mph, 12 min. mile), cycling (13 mph), skiing, fencing
Moderate	Activity about 4 2/3 to 7 times as intense as rest (4.7 to 7 METs)	Brisk walking, lawn mowing, shoveling, social dancing
Light	Activity that is 2 1/2 to 4 2/3 times as intense as rest (2.5 to 4.7 METs)	Normal walking, walking downstairs, bowling, mopping
Very light	Activity about 2 to 2 1/2 times as intense as lying or sitting at rest (2 to 2.5 METs)	Washing your face, dressing yourself, typing, driving a car

selecting appropriate lifestyle physical activities. For example, activities considered very light to light for young fit people are equal to moderate activity for many people eighty and over. For many people over sixty-five, activities typically classified as light are equal to moderate activities.

🌐 **Because lifestyle activities are relatively easy to perform, they are popular among adults.** www.mhhe.com/phys_fit/web07 Click 03. Walking is the most popular of all leisure-time activities among adults eighteen years of age and over. Approximately 39 percent of all men and 48 percent of all women walk for exercise. Also, among the ten most popular activities among adults is gardening (including yard work), which is done by 34 percent of all male and 25 percent of all female adults. Approximately 10 percent of men and 12 percent of women report that they regularly use the stairs to increase their activity levels.

Interestingly, the number of people participating in lifestyle physical activities increases with age. For example, only 33 percent of men eighteen to twenty-nine walk regularly, but 50 percent of men over sixty-five walk for exercise. Among young women, 47 percent walk, while 50 percent over sixty-five are walkers. Nearly twice as many

🌐 **Activity classifications vary, depending on one's level of fitness.** www.mhhe.com/phys_fit/web07 Click 02. Normal walking is considered light activity for a person with good fitness (see Table 1), but for a person with low to marginal fitness the same activity is considered moderate. For a very low-fit person, brisk walking is considered to be hard. Table 2 helps you determine the type of lifestyle activity that would be considered moderate for you. Beginners with low fitness should start with normal rather than brisk walking, for example. Older people often have lower fitness levels than younger people and may find Table 2 useful in

Aerobic Physical Activities *Aerobic* means "in the presence of oxygen." Aerobic activities are activities or exercise for which the body is able to supply adequate oxygen to sustain performance for long periods of time; also called lifestyle activities.

MET One MET equals the amount of energy a person expends at rest. METs are multiples of resting activity (2 METS equals twice the resting energy expenditure).

Anaerobic Physical Activities *Anaerobic* means "in the absence of oxygen." Anaerobic activities are performed at an intensity so great that the body's demand for oxygen exceeds its ability to supply it.

Table 2 ▶ Classification of Lifestyle Physical Activities for People of Different Fitness Levels

Sample Lifestyle Activities	Activity Classification by Fitness Level			
	Low Fitness	Marginal Fitness	Good Fitness	High Performance
Washing your face, dressing, typing, driving a car	Light	Very light/light	Very light	Very light
Normal walking, walking downstairs, bowling, mopping	Moderate	Moderate	Light	Light
Brisk walking, lawn mowing, shoveling, social dancing	Hard	Moderate/hard	Moderate	Light/moderate

older men than young men do gardening, and the difference among women is almost as dramatic. As lifetime physical activity participation increases with age, involvement in sports dramatically decreases.

Lifestyle physical activities can easily be performed by most people, regardless of fitness level.

www.mhhe.com/phys_fit/web07 Click 04. Prior to the past two decades, the conventional wisdom concerning physical activity was that it had to be vigorous to provide health and fitness benefits. Long-term studies of large populations were conducted with a variety of groups, showing that moderate activity produced many benefits. For example, postal carriers who delivered mail showed benefits not present in the postal workers who sorted the mail, and bus drivers in England did not get the benefits found for conductors who climbed the stairs in double-deck buses many times during the day. More recently, a study in Finland showed that people who do gardening are much less likely to have health problems than sedentary people, and people who hunt and hike in the forest have even more dramatic reductions in health conditions. A recent study found that people who commuted to work by bicycle had fewer health problems and fewer early deaths than those who drove. These are only a few of the studies that show the benefits of lifestyle physical activity.

Because lifestyle activities are moderate, most people can easily perform them. This is one reason lifestyle physical activities are placed at the bottom of the pyramid (see Figure 1). They are basic and provide a foundation for other activities.

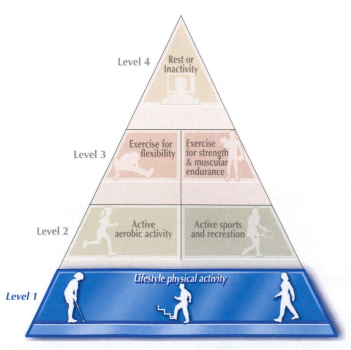

Figure 1 ▶ The physical activity pyramid level 1: lifestyle physical activity.

 Technology Update

Pedometers

Digital pedometers are popular self-monitoring tool used to track physical activity patterns. They are reasonably priced ($10–20) and provide an accurate indicator of the number of steps a person takes. Stride length and weight can be entered into some pedometers to provide estimates of distance traveled and/or calories burned. Many of the new pedometers also include walk timers. A built-in timer starts to count when you begin moving and continues to count until you stop moving. Pedometers can help you determine if you accumulate 30 minutes of walking per day. The most recent walk timers will also count the number of bouts of continuous movement of 10 minutes or more that you accumulate each day. Pedometers and walk timers are an excellent method of self-monitoring lifestyle physical activity. Pedometers vary greatly in quality, so this should be considered if purchasing one. Additional information on pedometers is available in the "On the Web" resource for this concept (www.mhhe.com/phys_fit/web07 Click 06).

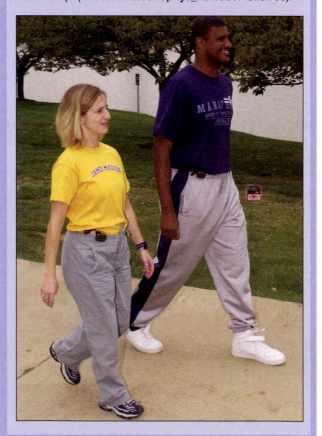

Moderate activity is more attractive than vigorous activity to many people. As the intensity of physical activity increases, it becomes less enjoyable to many people. Studies show that vigorous physical activity is a deterrent for more than a few people. This is another reason lifestyle physical activities are placed at the base of the physical activity pyramid. Not only does this type of activity provide many health benefits, but its intensity level makes it especially attractive to the people who most need to be active.

About 40 percent of all adult Americans do no leisure-time physical activity at all. They are totally sedentary. Statistics indicate that hundreds of thousands of premature deaths could be prevented if sedentary people would become active. Moderate physical activity is an alternative to vigorous activity that may be especially attractive to sedentary and/or less fit adults.

The Health Benefits of Lifestyle Physical Activity

Many health benefits can be achieved as a result of participation in lifestyle physical activities. Figure 2 illustrates that disease risk and early death decrease with moderate lifestyle physical activity. This figure, based on several large studies done worldwide, shows that a great proportion of the **health benefits** of physical activity described in this book result from participation in moderate lifestyle physical activities.

The first bar (red) in Figure 2 indicates that inactive or sedentary people have a high risk for hypokinetic diseases and early death. A modest increase in physical activity, such as the 30 minutes of daily moderate lifestyle activity recommended by the surgeon general, results in a substantial decrease in risk and early death (green bar). Additional activity (blue bar) has extra benefits, but the benefits are not as great as those that come from making the change from being inactive to doing some activity. As the final bar (black) indicates, very high levels of activity produce little additional health benefit.

Regular activity is important to achieving health benefits. For the benefits of activity, especially lifestyle physical activity, to be optimal it is important to exercise regularly. Daily, or nearly daily, lifestyle activity is recommended because each activity session has relatively short-term benefits that do not occur if the activity is not frequent enough. This is sometimes referred to as the **last bout effect.** Activity is most beneficial if you do the next bout before the effect of the previous bout has worn off. Some short-term benefits of activity last only a few hours, whereas others last longer. For this reason, the frequency of recommended activity depends on the type of activity and type of benefit expected.

The benefits of moderate or lifestyle physical activities are illustrated by the long arrow in Figure 2. The shorter arrow shows the additional benefits that result from more vigorous activity. The principle of diminishing returns applies. Even modest increases in physical activity are better than doing no activity at all. Clearly, the adage that "something is better than nothing" applies to physical activity.

Lifestyle activity builds some components of fitness more than others. Metabolic fitness has been previously defined as fitness of the systems that provide the energy for effective daily living. Indicators of good metabolic fitness include normal blood lipid levels, normal blood pressure, normal blood sugar levels, and healthy body fat levels. Though lifestyle physical activity does not promote high-level cardiovascular fitness, commonly referred to as a **performance benefit,** it effectively promotes metabolic fitness associated with health and wellness benefits. This type of activity can produce enough cardiovascular fitness to help unfit people escape from the low-fit category.

Lifestyle physical activity has wellness benefits. Reduction in disease risk and early death are important. But equally important is quality of life. Many of the wellness benefits previously described result from moderate lifestyle physical activity. For example, people who do moderate exercise have been shown to take less time to

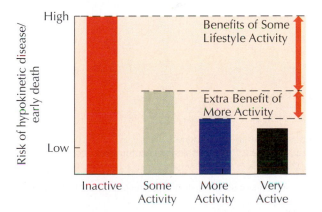

Figure 2 ▶ The health benefits from different levels of physical activity.

Health Benefits Reductions in hypokinetic disease risk, decreased risk of early death, and improved quality of life.

Last Bout Effect Some of the benefits of physical activity are short-term in nature. If the benefit of a bout of exercise lasts 24 hours, it is beneficial only if the last bout of activity was done before 24 hours elapsed.

Performance Benefit Improved ability to score well on physical fitness tests or to perform well in athletic or work activities requiring high-level performance.

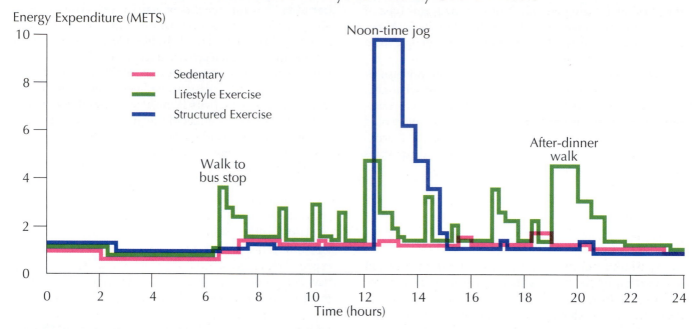

Figure 3 ▶ Comparison of structured exercise vs lifestyle activity.

go to sleep and sleep nearly an hour longer. A recent study shows that functional limitations are much lower in moderately active people than those who are sedentary. Lifestyle activity and its accompanying metabolic fitness benefits are also associated with enhanced self-esteem and less incidence of depression and anxiety.

How Much Lifestyle Physical Activity Is Enough?

There is a FIT formula for lifestyle physical activity. Perhaps the easiest way to keep track of lifestyle activity, especially for beginners, is counting minutes per day and minutes per week as recommended by the Surgeon Gen-

eral. However, there are other methods that can be used. For example you can use METS (see Table 1) or calories expended in activity. The threshold of training and target zones for these are presented in Table 3. Step counting can also be used to determine amounts of lifestyle activity but research has yet to clarify the exact number of steps necessary to achieve a health benefit. More sophisticated methods for monitoring physical activity levels include heart rate counting and ratings of perceived exertion (RPE). You will learn more about these methods in the concept on cardiovascular fitness that follows.

Keeping track of accumulated minutes per day and per week is an easy way to monitor physical activity. Brisk walking is used by the Surgeon General to indicate an intensity of activity necessary to be considered moderate

Table 3 ▶ The FIT Formula for Lifestyle Physical Activity		
	Threshold of Training	**Target Zone**
Frequency	Most days of the week	All, or most, days of the week
Intensity*	• Equal to brisk walking** • Approximately 150 calories accumulated per day • 3 to 5 METs**	• Equal to brisk to fast walking** • Approximately 150–300 calories accumulated per day • 3.0 to 7 METs**
Time (duration)	30 minutes or three 10-minute sessions per day	30–60 minutes accumulated in sessions of at least 10 minutes

*Heart rate and relative perceived exertion can also be used to determine intensity (see Concept 8).
**Depends on fitness level (see Table 2).

activity. Some people think that because walking was used as an example, that is the only lifestyle activity that is recommended. Any activity equal to brisk walking or at the appropriate MET level can be performed.

You can accumulate lifestyle physical activity to meet the recommendation. Previous recommendations suggested that physical activity had to be continuous to be effective. The evidence now indicates that all of the activity need not be done in one session to be effective. To achieve the health benefits, you can "accumulate activity" throughout the day. The diagram in Figure 3 demonstrates the different daily patterns of physical activity. The blue line reveals the pattern of a typical "exerciser" performing short bouts of vigorous activity, while the green line shows a lifestyle activity pattern. Note that both lines have a lot more daily activity than the low levels of activity for a sedentary individual. Although the bulk of the energy or calories expended should be in moderate activities, some light activity can also be beneficial. When some of the accumulated activity is in light activity, the duration of the activity must be increased (e.g., washing windows and floors, as seen in Table 4). Some lifestyle physical activities, such as shoveling snow and climbing stairs, are actually considered to be vigorous. These activities can be counted in the accumulation of daily activities. Performing some of these activities can offset the performance of light activity and make it possible to expend adequate calories in a 30-minute period.

Tracking energy expenditure from physical activity can help in monitoring lifestyle physical activity. www.mhhe.com/phys_fit/web07 Click 05. As shown in Table 3, an energy expenditure of between 150 to 300 kcal/day from physical activity is sufficient for meeting physical activity guidelines. While not as simple as tracking time, calories expended from physical activity can be estimated if the approximate MET value of the activity is known. The energy cost of resting energy expenditure (1 MET) is approximately 1 calorie per kilogram of body weight per hour (1 kcal/kg/hour). An activity such as walking (4 mph) requires an energy expenditure of about 4 METS, or 4 kcal/kg/hour. A 150 lb. person (~ 70 kg) walking for an hour would expend about 280 kcal (4 kcal/kg/hour × 70 kg × 1 hr.). Note that a 30-minute walk would burn approximately 150 calories and satisfy the guideline.

Energy expenditure estimates are often provided by many commercial pieces of fitness equipment. The workload MET level is determined by the pace or heart rate and the time is usually tracked internally. If body weight is recorded by the device during the start-up process, it can estimate energy expenditure using the same algorithm. To assist in using energy expenditure estimates, a listing of calories expended in many different activities is provided in Table 5. The table provides estimates for people of different weights performing exercise for an hour.

Pedometers are used by many individuals to monitor daily activity levels. www.mhhe.com/phys_fit/web07 Click 06. Pedometers can provide an accurate indicator of steps taken during the day and help remind people to be more active. The low cost and ease of use have led to widespread use of pedometers in schools, at worksites, and in community-based activity programs. The interest in and popularity of pedometers have been picked up by the media, and numerous reports have popularized a mythical standard of 10,000 steps per day for good health. This level was initially promoted in Japan, where pedometers were first developed, but research has demonstrated that this level may be too ambitious for sedentary individuals. A challenge in interpreting step counts is that people vary greatly in how many steps might occur in a day due to normal activities of daily living. Step count guidelines are therefore dependent on a variety of individual lifestyle factors, including age and occupation.

Most experts believe that wearing a digital pedometer to count steps can be motivating and an effective way of self-monitoring physical activity. The approach most frequently recommended for those who wish to use step counting is to wear the pedometer for 1 week to establish a baseline step count (average steps per day). Once this has been done, setting a goal of increasing steps per day by 1,000 to 3,000 steps per day is recommended. Keeping records of daily step counts will help you determine if you are meeting your goal. Setting a goal that you are likely to meet will help you find success. As you meet your goal, you can increase your step counts gradually.

Table 4 ▶ Examples of Lifestyle Physical Activities

Activity	Time (min.)	Less Intense More Time
Washing and waxing a car	45–60	
Washing windows or floors	45–60	
Gardening	30–45	
Wheeling self in wheelchair	30–40	
Social dancing	30	
Pushing a stroller (1 1/2 miles)	30	
Raking leaves	30	
Walking (2 miles)	30	
		More Intense Less Time

Adapted from the *Surgeon General's Report on Physical Activity and Health.*

Table 5 ▶ Calories Expended in Lifestyle Physical Activities

Activity Classification / Description	METs*	Calories Used per Hour for Different Body Weights				
		100 lb. (45 kg)	120 lb. (55 kg)	150 lb. (70 kg)	180 lb. (82 kg)	200 lb. (91 kg)
Gardening Activities						
Gardening (general)	5.0	227	273	341	409	455
Mowing lawn (hand mower)	6.0	273	327	409	491	545
Mowing lawn (power mower)	4.5	205	245	307	368	409
Raking leaves	4.0	182	218	273	327	364
Shoveling snow	6.0	273	327	409	491	545
Home Activities						
Child care	3.5	159	191	239	286	318
Cleaning, washing dishes	2.5	114	136	170	205	227
Cooking / food preparation	2.5	114	136	170	205	227
Home / auto repair	3.0	136	164	205	245	273
Painting	4.5	205	245	307	368	409
Strolling with child	2.5	114	136	170	205	227
Sweeping / vacuuming	2.5	114	136	170	205	227
Washing / waxing car	4.5	205	245	307	368	409
Leisure Activities						
Bocci ball / croquet	2.5	114	136	170	205	227
Bowling	3.0	136	164	205	245	273
Canoeing	5.0	227	273	341	409	455
Cross-country skiing (leisure)	7.0	318	382	477	573	636
Cycling (<10 mph)	4.0	182	218	273	327	364
Cycling (12–14 mph)	8.0	364	436	545	655	727
Dancing (social)	4.5	205	245	307	368	409
Fishing	4.0	182	218	273	327	364
Golf (riding)	3.5	159	191	239	286	318
Golf (walking)	5.5	250	300	375	450	500
Horseback riding	4.0	182	218	273	327	364
Swimming (leisure)	6.0	273	327	409	491	545
Table tennis	4.0	182	218	273	327	364
Walking (4 mph)	4.0	182	218	273	327	364
Walking (3 mph)	3.5	159	191	239	286	318
Occupational Activities						
Bricklaying / masonry	7.0	318	382	477	573	636
Carpentry	3.5	159	191	239	286	318
Construction	5.5	250	300	375	450	500
Electrical work / plumbing	3.5	159	191	239	286	318
Digging	7.0	318	382	477	573	636
Farming	5.5	250	300	375	450	500
Store clerk	3.5	159	191	239	286	318
Waiter / waitress	4.0	182	218	273	327	364

Note: MET values and caloric estimates are based on values listed in *The Compendium of Physical Activities* (see *Suggested Readings*).
*Based on values of those with "good fitness" ratings.

Pedometers do have some limitations as indicators of total physical activity. A person with longer legs will accumulate fewer steps over the same distance as someone with shorter strides (due to a longer stride length). A person running will also accumulate fewer steps over the same distance as a person who walks. Despite these limitations, pedometers can be helpful in monitoring your lifestyle activity levels. Table 6 includes some general guidelines for physical activity that may help provide motivation for your activity program. The basic suggestion is to first establish a personal baseline that represents your normal lifestyle steps (without activity). Depending on your starting point, try to progressively add activity into your routine to move into the *somewhat active*, *active*, or *very active* categories.

Table 6 ▶ Target Zones for Pedometer Step Counts in Healthy Adults

Category	Steps/Day
Sedentary	< 5000
Low active	5,000–7,500
Somewhat active	7,500–9,999
Active	10,000–12,500
Very active	> 12,500

Source: Based on values from Tudor-Locke, 2004.

Strategies for Action

A regular plan of lifestyle physical activity is a good place to start. Lifestyle physical activity is something that virtually anyone can do. In Lab 7A, you can set lifestyle physical activity goals and plan a 1-week lifestyle physical activity program. In the plan, you can indicate the lifestyle activities you plan to do on all, or most days, of the week. For some, this plan may be the main component of a lifetime plan. For others, it may be only a beginning that leads to the selection of activities from other levels of the physical activity pyramid. Even the most active people should consider regular lifestyle physical activity because it is a type of activity that can be done throughout life.

Self-monitoring lifestyle physical activity can help you stick with it. Self-monitoring is a self-management skill that can be valuable in encouraging long-term activity adherence. A self-monitoring chart is provided in Lab 7A to help you keep a log of the lifestyle activities (or step counts) you perform during a 1-week time period. This is a short-term record sheet. However, charts such as this can be copied to make a log book to allow long-term activity self-monitoring.

Because lifestyle physical activity is moderate, a specific warm-up may not be necessary. Lifestyle activities are similar to the cardiovascular portion of the warm-up described in the concept on preparing for physical activity. For this reason, it may not be necessary to perform a special warm-up prior to doing activities such as walking. It would be wise to perform the stretching activities after the walk as a cool-down.

Study Resources

Check out additional online study resources for this concept in the Student Edition of the Online Learning Center at www.mhhe.com/corbin13e.

Web Resources

American College of Sports Medicine **www.acsm.org**
ACSM's Health and Fitness Journal
    www.acsm-healthfitness.org
Centers for Disease Control and Prevention **www.cdc.gov**
National Center for Physical Activity and Disability
    www.ncpad.org

National Coalition for Promoting Physical Activity
    www.ncppa.org
Surgeon General's Report on Physical Activity and Health
    www.cdc.gov/nccdphp/sgr/sgr.htm

Suggested Readings

Additional reference materials for Concept 7 are available at **www.mhhe.com/phys_fit/web07 Click 7**.

Addy, C. L. et al. 2004. Associations of perceived social and physical environmental supports with physical activity and walking behavior. *American Journal of Public Health* 94(3):440–443.

Ainsworth, B. E. 2003. The compendium of physical activities. *President's Council on Physical Fitness and Sports Research Digest* 4(2):1–8.

American College of Sports Medicine. 2000. *ACSM's Guidelines for Exercise Testing and Prescription.* 6th ed. Philadelphia: Lippincott, Williams and Wilkins.

Blair, S. N., et al. 2001. *Active Living Every Day.* Champaign, IL: Human Kinetics.

Brown, D. W., et al. 2004. Associations between physical activity dose and health-related quality of life. *Medicine and Science in Sports and Exercise* 36(5): 890–896.

Ewing, R., et al. 2003. Relationship between urban sprawl and physical activity, obesity, and morbidity. *American Journal of Health Promotion* 18(1):47–57.

Eyler, A. A. 2004. The epidemiology of walking for physical activity in the United States. *Medicine and Science in Sports and Exercise* 35(9):1529–1536.

Franklin, B. A. 2001. Lifestyle activity: A new paradigm for exercise prescription. *ACSM's Health and Fitness Journal* 5(4):33–35.

Heath, G. W. 2003. Increasing physical activity in communities: What really works? *President's Council on Physical Fitness and Sports Research Digest* 4(4):1–8.

Lakka, T. A., et al. 2003. Sedentary lifestyle, poor cardiorespiratory fitness, and the metabolic syndrome. *Medicine and Science in Sports and Exercise* 35(8):1279–1286.

Le Masurier, G. C. 2004. Walk this way? *ACSM's Health and Fitness Journal* 8(1):7–10.

Manson, J. E., et al. 2002. Walking compared with vigorous exercise for the prevention of cardiovascular events in women. *New England Journal of Medicine* 347(10):716–725.

Meyer, M. 2004. Wiggle your toes, save your life. *AARP Bulletin* 45(6):18.

Public Health Service. 1996. *Surgeon General's Report on Physical Activity and Health.* Washington, DC: U.S. Government Printing Office.

Sidman, C. L. 2002. Count your steps to health and fitness. *ACSM's Health and Fitness Journal* 6(1):13–17.

Sidman, C. L., et al. 2004. Promoting physical activity among sedentary women using pedometers. *Research Quarterly for Exercise and Sport* 75(2):122–129.

Steiger, L. H., and J. L. Hesson. 2001. *Walking for Fitness.* 4th ed. St. Louis: McGraw-Hill.

Tudor-Locke, C. 2002. Taking steps toward increased physical activity: Using the pedometer to measure and motivate. *President's Council on Physical Fitness and Sports Research Digest* 3(17):1–8.

Tudor-Locke, C. 2004. How many steps/day are enough? Preliminary pedometer indices for public health. *Sports Medicine* 34(1):1–8.

Whelton, S. P., et al. 2002. Effects of aerobic exercise on blood pressure: A meta-analysis of randomized, controlled trials. *Annals of Internal Medicine* 136(7):493–503.

Wilde, B. E., C. L. Sidman, and C. B. Corbin. 2001. A 10,000 step count as a physical activity standard for sedentary women. *Research Quarterly for Exercise and Sport* 72(1):411–414.

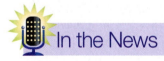 In the News

Walkable Communities

The continued reports of low levels of physical activity in the population have led researchers to attempt to identify factors that may cause people to be more or less active. Much recent attention has focused on aspects of our physical environment. Using GIS technology, researchers can accurately map cities and determine distances from residential areas to stores, parks, and greenspaces. Correlations are then made between these variables and measures of physical activity to study the effect of different environmental characteristics. One group of researchers demonstrated that the extent of urban sprawl is associated with population levels of physical activity and obesity. Counties with greater sprawl indices had lower amounts of activity and more obesity than counties with less sprawl. Researchers have also determined that certain characteristics of an environment can make it more or less "walkable." Sidewalks, safe neighborhoods, aesthetic surroundings, and good lighting are considered to be among the key factors that define walkable areas. A number of other similar findings have led to increased efforts by public health officials to promote more active environments in communities and cities. Increased coordination is also underway between public health officials and urban planners to plan and develop communities that are less dependent on automobiles and more conducive to active commuting and walking.

Lab 7A Planning and Self-Monitoring (Logging) Your Lifestyle Physical Activity

Name	Section	Date

Purpose: To self-monitor (log) physical activity and use it to plan a lifestyle physical activity program

Directions: Record the number of 5- or 10-minute activity blocks or steps taken each day (see back for procedures).

Chart 1 ▶ Lifestyle Activity Log

	5-Minute Blocks										10-Minute Blocks						Total Minutes or Steps
Day 1 Date: Activity: Activity: Activity: Activity:	1	2	3	4	5	6	7	8	9	10	1	2	3	4	5	6	Daily Total
Day 2 Date: Activity: Activity: Activity: Activity:	1	2	3	4	5	6	7	8	9	10	1	2	3	4	5	6	Daily Total
Day 3 Date: Activity: Activity: Activity: Activity:	1	2	3	4	5	6	7	8	9	10	1	2	3	4	5	6	Daily Total
Day 4 Date: Activity: Activity: Activity: Activity:	1	2	3	4	5	6	7	8	9	10	1	2	3	4	5	6	Daily Total
Day 5 Date: Activity: Activity: Activity: Activity:	1	2	3	4	5	6	7	8	9	10	1	2	3	4	5	6	Daily Total
Day 6 Date: Activity: Activity: Activity: Activity:	1	2	3	4	5	6	7	8	9	10	1	2	3	4	5	6	Daily Total
Day 7 Date: Activity: Activity: Activity: Activity:	1	2	3	4	5	6	7	8	9	10	1	2	3	4	5	6	Daily Total

Total Minutes or Steps for Week

101

Procedures

1. On Chart 1, record the time spent or steps taken per day in the various lifestyle activities.
2. If you record time spent in lifestyle activity, list all activities you perform each day. For each activity, record the number of minutes you were active using combinations of 5- or 10-minute blocks. For example, if you perform 15 minutes of brisk walking, place an X over one 5- and one 10-minute block for that activity. If you cannot keep the log with you during the day, complete it at the end of the day. Total the minutes of activity accumulated during the day and record it in the Daily Total box.
3. If you wear a pedometer to count daily activity, simply wear the pedometer from the time you get up until the time you go to bed. Record the number of steps taken in the Daily Total box.
4. Sum the total for each day to determine the total minutes or steps taken for the week.
5. Use the weekly log to help you develop a weekly plan. In Chart 2, record the number of minutes you plan to perform each activity in the coming week, or record the number of steps you plan to take. If you use minutes in your plan, try to reach 30 per day. If you use step counts in your plan, try to achieve 2,000–3,000 steps above your average daily count (if you averaged less than 10,000 steps a day in Chart 1), or at least 10,000 steps per day (if you averaged near or above 10,000 steps in Chart 1). Try to get your steps in blocks of time lasting at least 5 minutes.
6. Make a copy of Chart 1 and use it to self-monitor your activity for the week that you institute your plan.
7. Answer the questions in the Results and Conclusions and Interpretations sections.

Chart 2 ▶ Lifestyle Physical Activity Plan

Record the minutes or steps planned for each day. You may mix activities each day.

Activity	Day 1	Day 2	Day 3	Day 4	Day 5	Day 6	Day 7
Brisk walking							
Yard work/gardening							
Active housework							
Social dancing							
Occupational activity							
Wheeling self in wheelchair							
Bicycling							
Walking up and down stairs							
Other							
Other							
Other							
Daily Totals							

Results

Do you think you can consistently do 30 minutes of activity or meet your step goal each day?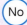

Conclusions and Interpretations

1. Do you feel that you will use lifestyle physical activity as a regular part of your lifetime physical activity plan, either now or in the future? Use several sentences to explain your answer.
2. Did the logging of your activity make you more aware of your daily activity patterns? Explain why or why not.

Cardiovascular Fitness

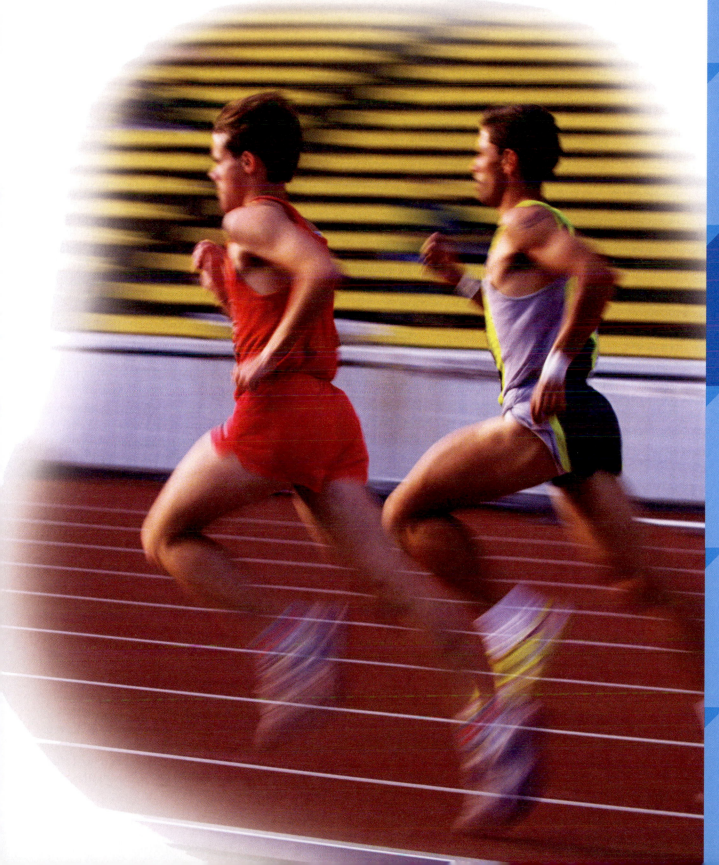

Cardiovascular fitness is probably the most important aspect of physical fitness because of its importance to good health and optimal physical performance.

Health Goals

for the year 2010

- Increase proportion of people who do vigorous physical activity that promotes cardiovascular fitness 3 or more days a week for 20 minutes per occasion.

- Decrease deaths from heart attack and stroke.

- Decrease incidence of heart attack, high blood pressure, stroke, and high blood lipids.

- Decrease heart disease among females.

- Increase public awareness of symptoms of heart disease.

Cardiovascular fitness is generally considered to be the most important aspect of physical fitness. Those who possess reasonable amounts of fitness have a decreased risk for heart disease, reduced risk for premature death, and improved quality of life. Regular cardiovascular exercise promotes fitness and provides additional health and wellness benefits that extend well beyond reducing risks for disease. This concept will describe the function of the cardiovascular system and explain how to determine the appropriate intensity of exercise needed to promote cardiovascular fitness.

Cardiovascular Fitness

Cardiovascular fitness is a term that has several synonyms. Cardiovascular fitness is sometimes referred to as *cardiovascular endurance* because a person who possesses this type of fitness can persist in physical activity for long periods of time without undue fatigue. It has been referred to as *cardiorespiratory fitness* because it requires delivery and utilization of oxygen, which is only possible if the circulatory and respiratory systems are capable of these functions.

The term *aerobic fitness* has also been used as a synonym for *cardiovascular fitness* because **aerobic capacity** is considered to be the best indicator of cardiovascular fitness, and aerobic physical activity is the preferred method for achieving it. Regardless of the words used to describe it, cardiovascular fitness is complex because it requires fitness of several body systems.

Good cardiovascular fitness requires a fit heart muscle. www.mhhe.com/phys_fit/web08 Click 01. The heart is a muscle; to become stronger, it must be exercised like any other muscle in the body. If the heart is exercised regularly, its strength increases; if not, it becomes weaker. Contrary to the belief that strenuous work harms the heart, research has found no evidence that regular, progressive exercise is bad for the normal heart. In fact, the heart muscle will increase in size and power when called upon to extend itself. The increase in size and power allows the heart to pump a greater volume of blood with fewer strokes per minute. For example, the average individual has a resting heart rate between 70 and 80 beats per minute (bpm), whereas a trained athlete's pulse is commonly in the low 50s or even in the 40s. A low resting heart rate (RHR) is not a perfect indicator of cardiovascular fitness, but decreases in your personal resting heart rate with training would indicate clear improvements in cardiovascular fitness.

The healthy heart is remarkably efficient in the work that it does. It can convert about half of its fuel into energy. An automobile engine in good running condition converts only one-fourth of its fuel into energy. By comparison, the heart is a more efficient engine. The heart of a normal individual beats reflexively about 40 million times a year. Over 4,000 gallons, or 10 tons, of blood are circulated each day. Every night the heart's workload is equivalent to a person carrying a 30-pound pack to the top of the 102-story Empire State building.

Good cardiovascular fitness requires a fit vascular system. As illustrated in Figure 1, blood containing a high concentration of oxygen is pumped by the left ventricle through the aorta (a major artery), where it is carried to the tissues. Blood flows through a sequence of arteries to capillaries and to veins. Veins carry the blood containing lesser amounts of oxygen back to the right side of the heart, first to the atrium and then to the ventricle. The right ventricle pumps the blood to the lungs. In the lungs, the blood picks up oxygen (O_2), and carbon dioxide (CO_2) is removed. From the lungs, the oxygenated blood travels back to the heart, first to the left atrium and then to the left ventricle. The process then repeats itself.

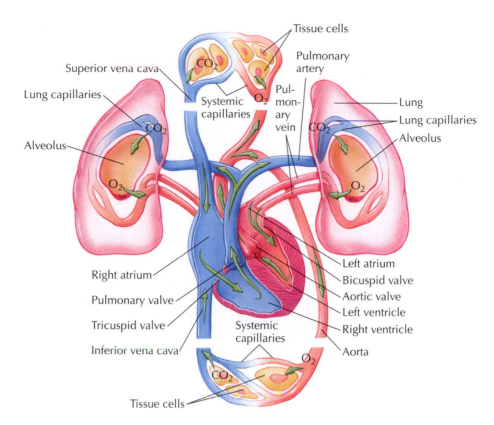

Figure 1 ▶ Cardiovascular system.

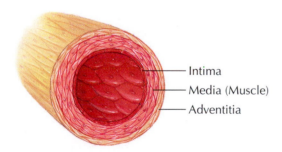

Figure 2 ▶ Healthy, elastic artery.

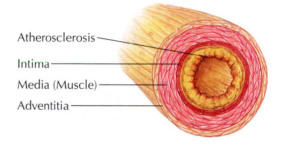

Figure 3 ▶ Unhealthy, rigid artery.

Healthy arteries are elastic, are free of obstruction, and expand to permit the flow of blood (see Figure 2). Muscle layers line the arteries and control the size of the arterial opening upon the impulse from nerve fibers. Unfit arteries (see Figure 3) may have a reduced internal diameter (atherosclerosis) because of deposits on the interior of their walls, or they may have hardened, nonelastic walls (arteriosclerosis).

Fit coronary arteries are especially important to good health. The blood in the four chambers of the heart does not directly nourish the heart. Rather, numerous small arteries within the heart muscle provide for coronary circulation. Poor coronary circulation precipitated by unhealthy arteries can be the cause of a heart attack.

Veins have thinner, less elastic walls than arteries, as shown in Figure 4. Also, veins contain small valves to prevent the backward flow of blood. Skeletal muscles assist the return of blood to the heart. The veins are intertwined in the muscle; therefore, when the muscle is contracted, the vein is squeezed, pushing the blood back to the heart. A malfunction of the valves results in a failure to remove used blood at the proper rate. As a result, venous blood pools, especially in the legs, causing a condition known as

Aerobic Capacity A measure of aerobic or cardiovascular fitness.

varicose veins. Regular physical activity helps reduce pooling of blood in the veins and helps keep the valves of the veins healthy.

Capillaries are the transfer stations where oxygen and fuel are released, and waste products, such as carbon diox-

ide, are removed from the tissues. The veins receive the blood from the capillaries for the return trip to the heart.

Good cardiovascular fitness requires a fit respiratory system and fit blood. The process of taking in oxygen (through the mouth and nose) and delivering it to the lungs, where it is picked up by the blood, is called external respiration (see Figure 5). External respiration requires fit lungs as well as blood with adequate **hemoglobin** in the red blood cells (erythrocytes). Insufficient oxygen-carrying capacity of the blood is called **anemia,** a condition caused by lack of hemoglobin.

Delivering oxygen to the tissues from the blood is called internal respiration. Internal respiration requires an adequate number of healthy capillaries. In addition to delivering oxygen to the tissues, these systems remove carbon dioxide. Good cardiovascular fitness requires fitness of both the external and internal respiratory systems.

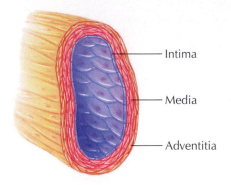

Figure 4 ▶ Healthy, nonelastic vein.

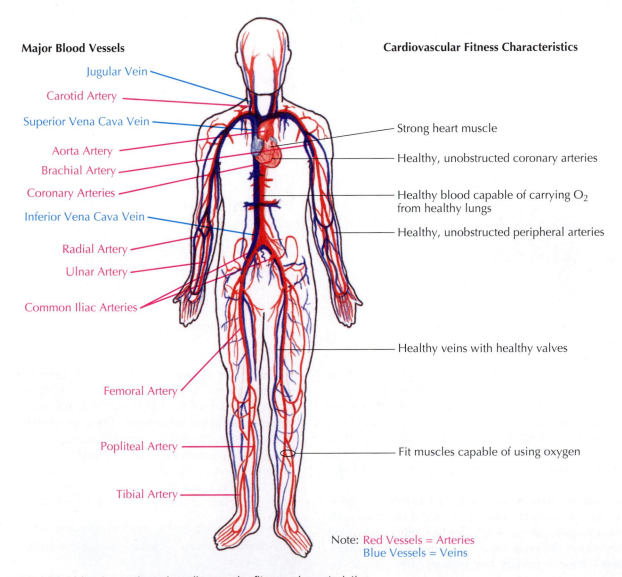

Figure 5 ▶ Major blood vessels and cardiovascular fitness characteristics.

Cardiovascular fitness requires fit muscle tissue capable of using oxygen. Once the oxygen is delivered, the muscle tissues must be able to use oxygen to sustain physical performance. Physical activity that promotes cardiovascular fitness stimulates changes in muscle fibers that make them more effective in using oxygen. Outstanding distance runners have high numbers of well-conditioned muscle fibers that can readily use oxygen to produce energy for sustained running. Training in other activities would elicit similar adaptations in the specific muscles used in those activities.

 Cardiovascular fitness is typically evaluated using an indicator known as maximum oxygen uptake, or $\dot{V}O_2$ max. www.mhhe.com/phys_fit/ web08 Click 02. A person's **maximum oxygen uptake ($\dot{V}O_2$ max),** commonly referred to as aerobic capacity, is determined in a laboratory by measuring how much oxygen a person can use in maximal exercise. The test is usually done on a treadmill using specialized gas analyzers to measure oxygen use. The treadmill speed and grade are gradually increased and, when the exercise becomes very hard, oxygen use reaches its maximum. The test is a good indicator of overall cardiovascular fitness because you cannot take in and use a lot of oxygen if you do not have good fitness throughout the cardiovascular system (heart, blood vessels, blood, respiratory system, and muscles).

Elite endurance athletes can extract 5 or 6 liters of oxygen per minute from the environment, and this high aerobic capacity is what allows them to maintain high speeds in both training and competition without becoming excessively tired. In comparison, an average person typically extracts about 2 to 3 liters per minute. $\dot{V}O_2$ max is typically adjusted to account for a person's body size

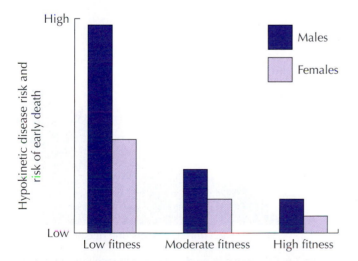

Figure 6 ▶ Risk reduction associated with cardiovascular fitness.

Adapted from Blair et al.

Table 1 ▶ Relative Risk of Major Risk Factors for Heart Disease and Early Death*

Risk Factor	Relative Risk for Heart Disease	Relative Risk for Early Death (All Causes)
Low cardiovascular fitness	2.69	2.03
Smoking	2.01	1.89
High systolic blood pressure	2.07	1.67
High cholesterol	1.86	1.45
Obesity (BMI)	1.70	1.33
Normal Risk	1.00	1.00

Based on Blair et al. (see *Suggested Readings*).
*Statistically adjusted to assure independence of risk factors.

because bigger people may have higher scores due to their larger size. Scores are reported in milliliters (mL) of oxygen (O_2) per kilogram (kg) of body weight (mL/kg/min.).

Cardiovascular Fitness and Health Benefits

Good cardiovascular fitness reduces risk of heart disease, other hypokinetic conditions, and early death. www.mhhe.com/phys_fit/web08 Click 03. One of the landmark studies documenting the importance of cardiovascular fitness is the Aerobics Center Longitudinal Study conducted at the Cooper Institute in Dallas, Texas. In this ongoing project, researchers have monitored fitness and health outcomes in a cohort of over 20,000 men and 10,000 women—over a span of 30 years. A major strength of this database is that maximal treadmill exercise tests were used to evaluate cardiovascular fitness on all participants. The data from this study (and many others) clearly demonstrate that cardiovascular fitness is associated with a reduced risk for heart disease and a

Hemoglobin Oxygen-carrying pigment of the red blood cells.

Anemia A condition in which hemoglobin and the blood's oxygen-carrying capacity is below normal.

Maximum Oxygen Uptake ($\dot{V}O_2$ max) A laboratory measure held to be the best measure of cardiovascular fitness. Commonly referred to as $\dot{V}O_2$ max or the volume ($\dot{V}$) of oxygen used when a person reaches his or her maximum (max) ability to supply it during exercise.

reduced risk for early death. A consistent finding in the study is that risks are highest for individuals with very low fitness (see Figure 6). In terms of longevity, one recent report from this study indicated that moderately fit individuals live approximately 5–6 years longer than low-fit individuals. Moving from the moderate fit to the high fit category provides additional benefits (and perhaps a few more years of life) but the key is to be out of the low fitness category.

The risk of low cardiovascular fitness is independent of other risk factors.

Good cardiovascular fitness has been shown to be independent of other risk factors in reducing heart disease risk and of reduction in early death from all causes. Table 1 shows the relative risk for heart disease in the first column and the relative risk for early death from all causes in the second column. People with low risk are assigned a relative risk of 1.0. A person with a relative risk of 2.0 would have two times the risk of a risk-free person. The highest relative risk for heart disease is among people low in cardiovascular fitness (2.69). Those with low cardiovascular fitness also have the highest relative risk for early death (2.03). All of the values in the table were adjusted statistically to exclude the influence of other risk factors. This illustrates that the benefits of good cardiovascular fitness are independent of other primary risk factors for heart disease and early death from all causes.

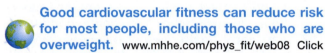 **Good cardiovascular fitness can reduce risk for most people, including those who are overweight.** www.mhhe.com/phys_fit/web08 Click 04. Some people think that they cannot be fit if they are overweight or overfat. It is now known that appropriate physical activity can build cardiovascular fitness in all types of people, including those with excess body fat. In fact, having good cardiovascular fitness greatly reduces risk for those who are overweight. Poor cardiovascular fitness, on the other hand, increases risk for both lean and overfat people. The greatest risk is among people who are unfit and overfat.

Good cardiovascular fitness enhances the ability to perform various tasks, improves the ability to function, and is associated with a feeling of well-being.

Moving out of the low fitness zone is of obvious importance to disease risk reduction. Achieving the good zone on tests further reduces disease and early death risk and promotes optimal wellness benefits, and a recent position statement by the American College of Sports Medicine shows an improved ability to function among older adults. Other wellness benefits include the ability to enjoy leisure activities and meet emergency situations, as well as the health and wellness benefits described earlier in this book. Cardiovascular fitness in the high performance zone enhances the ability to perform in cer-

tain athletic events and in occupations that require high performance level (e.g., firefighters). These benefits are commonly referred to as **performance benefits.**

Heredity influences your cardiovascular fitness.

It would be nice if all people who did appropriate physical activity achieved high levels of cardiovascular fitness. Genetic researchers have shown that the type of cardiovascular system you inherit has a good deal to do with your cardiovascular fitness. Further, we do not all respond similarly to physical activity because of our heredity. As illustrated in Figure 7, some people showed almost no improvement in fitness while others improved considerably even though they all performed the same amount of activity. This research led the researchers to draw the following conclusion: "Not only is it important to recognize that there are individual differences in the response to regular physical activity, but research indicates that there are non-responders in the population. Heredity may account for fitness differences as large as 3 to 10 fold when comparing low and high responders who have performed the same physical activity program" (Bouchard, see *Suggested Readings*). Those with low fitness in the beginning made more improvements than those who were already fit, but the researchers indicated that heredity was more of a factor than beginning fitness level.

You should not conclude from this information that achieving good cardiovascular fitness is impossible for some people. Rather, you should understand that it is harder for some people to get fit than others. No matter who you are, you can improve your cardiovascular fitness, but it takes longer for some than others. This study also points out the futility of comparing your own performance with that of others. Comparing yourself with fitness standards associated with good health is more reasonable.

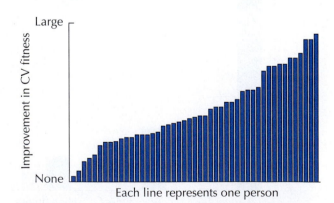

Figure 7 ▶ Difference in cardiovascular fitness improvement in forty-seven different people doing the same activity program for 15 to 20 weeks.

Adapted from Bouchard.

Threshold and Target Zones for Improving Cardiovascular Fitness

Aerobic physical activity that is more vigorous than lifestyle physical activities is necessary to produce optimal gains in cardiovascular fitness. Activities at the second level of the physical activity pyramid, including active aerobics and active sports and recreation, are recommended for promoting good cardiovascular fitness (Figure 8). The word *active* implies that these activities are more vigorous than lower-intensity activities from the lifestyle category. All physical activity can contribute to good health, but vigorous activity can also strengthen the cardiovascular system.

Cardiovascular fitness can be developed by exercising 3 to 6 days per week. Unlike less intense lifestyle physical activities, the types of activities that promote cardiovascular fitness may be done as few as 3 days a week. Additional benefits occur with added days of activity. However, because more vigorous physical activity has been shown to increase risk for orthopedic injury if done too frequently, most experts recommend at least 1 day a week off.

Various methods can be used to determine the appropriate intensity of aerobic activity. Like all dimensions of fitness, adaptations to cardiovascular fitness are based on the overload principle. When the body is regularly challenged, it essentially adapts to make the same amount of exercise easier on itself. Because individuals vary in their level of fitness, the appropriate intensity of exercise needed to maintain or improve fitness also varies. The relative intensity of a given bout of exercise can be directly determined if you have a measure of your **oxygen uptake reserve (VO$_2$R)** and the actual oxygen cost of a given activity. You would simply calculate what percentage of oxygen consumption the task requires, compared with your maximal capacity. Because these values cannot be calculated without special equipment, other indicators of relative intensity are more commonly used.

Heart rate provides a good indicator of the relative challenge presented by a given bout of exercise. Therefore, guidelines for the intensity of physical activity to build cardiovascular fitness are typically based on percentages of **heart rate reserve (HRR)** or maximal heart rate (max HR). Current guidelines from the ACSM indicate that exercise should be between 40 and 85 percent of your HRR or from 55 to 90 percent of your max HR to maintain or improve cardiovascular fitness. A fit individual will be able to work harder at a given heart rate, but the relative intensity of exercise will be equivalent for fit and unfit individuals using these types of ranges. Calculations of these ratings will be described in detail later.

Ratings of perceived exertion (RPE) have also been shown to be useful in assessing the intensity of aerobic physical activity. The RPE rating scale ranges from 6 (very very light) to 20 (very very hard), with 1 point increments in between (see Table 3). If the values are multiplied by 10, the RPE values loosely correspond to HR values (e.g., 60 = rest HR and 200 = max HR). The target zone for aerobic activity is from 12 to 16 (see Table 2).

The duration of physical activity for building cardiovascular fitness is 20 to 60 minutes. In the past, it was thought that the 20 to 60 minutes of active aerobic activity necessary to promote cardiovascular fitness should be done continuously in one session. Recent

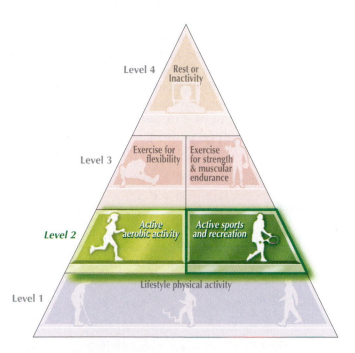

Figure 8 ▶ Select activities from level 2 of the pyramid for optimal cardiovascular fitness.

Performance Benefits In this concept, improved scores on a cardiovascular fitness test or in performance of activities requiring cardiovascular fitness.

Oxygen Uptake Reserve (VO$_2$R) The difference between your maximum oxygen uptake and your resting oxygen uptake. A percentage of this value is often used to determine appropriate intensities for physical activities.

Heart Rate Reserve (HRR) The difference between your maximum heart rate (highest heart rate in vigorous activity) and your resting heart rate (lowest heart rate at rest).

Ratings of Perceived Exertion (RPE) The assessment of the intensity of exercise based on how the participant feels; a subjective assessment of effort.

Table 2 ▶ Threshold of Training and Target Zones for Activities Designed to Promote Cardiovascular Fitness*

	Threshold of Training	Target Zone
Frequency	3 days a week	At least 3 days and no more than 6 days a week
Intensity		
Heart rate reserve (HRR)	40%*	40–85%
Maximal heart rate (maxHR)	55%*	55–90%
Relative perceived exertion (RPE)	12*	12–16
Time	20 minutes	20 to 60 minutes

*These values are for beginners—the threshold for fit individuals reaches higher into the target zone.

ACSM guidelines indicate that activity can be either intermittent or continuous if the total amount of exercise is the same and if the shorter sessions last at least 10 minutes. In other words, three 10-minute exercise sessions appear to give you the same benefit as one 30-minute session if the exercise is at the same intensity level.

There is a FIT formula for building cardiovascular fitness. Table 2 illustrates the threshold of training and target zones for performing physical activity designed to promote cardiovascular fitness.

Your current fitness status and activity patterns should influence the type and amount of activity you do to promote cardiovascular fitness. Making proper decisions about how much physical activity you should do is an art that is based on science. It is important that you listen to your body and not do too much too soon. Part of the art of making good decisions about

activity is using the principle of progression. The amount of activity performed by a beginner differs from that performed by a person who is more advanced.

Beginners with low fitness may choose to start with lifestyle physical activity of relatively moderate intensity. Performing this type of activity at about 40 percent of HRR or an RPE of 12 (rated as somewhat hard) for several weeks will allow the beginner to adapt gradually. Initial bouts of activity may be less than the recommended 20 minutes, but as fitness increases, at least 20 minutes a day should be accumulated. As fitness improves from the low to marginal range, the frequency, intensity, and time of activity can be increased (see Table 3). Cardiovascular fitness improvements for fit and active people are best when activity is at least 50 percent HRR, 65 percent max HR, and 13 RPE. Your current fitness and activity status will affect how quickly you progress. The type of activity you choose should be appropriate for the intensity of activity at each stage of the progression.

Learning to count heart rate can help you monitor the intensity of your physical activity. To determine the intensity of physical activity for building cardiovascular fitness, it is important to know how to count your pulse. Each time the heart beats, it pumps blood into the arteries. The surge of blood causes a pulse that can be felt by holding a finger against an artery. Major arteries that are easy to locate and are frequently used for pulse counts include the radial just below the base of the thumb on the wrist (see Figure 9) and the carotid on either side of the Adam's apple (see Figure 10). In Lab 8A, you will have the opportunity to practice counting your resting and postexercise heart rates.

To count the pulse rate, simply place the fingertips (index and middle finger) over the artery at the wrist or neck locations. Move the fingers around until a strong pulse can be felt. Press gently so as not to cut off the blood flow through the artery. Counting the pulse with the thumb is *not* recommended because the thumb has a relatively strong pulse of its own, and it could be confusing when counting another person's pulse.

Table 3 ▶ Progression of Activity Frequency, Intensity, and Time Based on Fitness Level

	Low Fitness	Marginal Fitness	Good Fitness
Frequency	3 days a week	3 to 5 days a week	3 to 6 days a week
Intensity			
Heart rate reserve (HRR)	40–50%	50–60%	60–85%
Maximum heart rate (maxHR)	55–65%	65–75%	75–90%
Relative perceived exertion (RPE)	12–13	13–14	14–16
Time	10–30	20–40	30–60

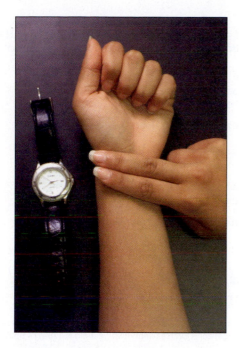

Figure 9 ▶ Counting your radial (wrist) pulse.

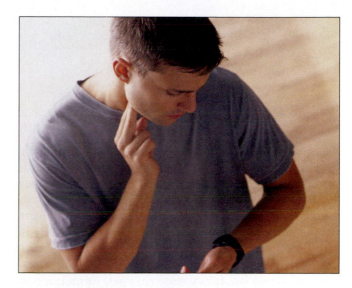

Figure 10 ▶ Counting your carotid (neck) pulse.

Counting the pulse at the carotid artery is the most popular procedure, probably because the carotid pulse is easy to locate. Some researchers suggest that caution should be used when taking carotid pulse counts because pressing on this artery can cause a reflex that slows the heart rate. This could result in incorrect heart rate counts. More recent research indicates that carotid palpation, when done properly, can be safely used to count heart rate for most people. Some have suggested that if the carotid pulse is taken on the right side of the neck, it should be taken with the right hand to avoid applying too much pressure to the artery. You may choose to use this procedure, though you can learn to be quite effective with either hand. The key is to press gently no matter which hand you use.

The radial pulse is a bit harder to find than the carotid pulse because of the many tendons near the wrist. Moving the fingers around to several locations on the wrist just above the thumb will help you locate this pulse. For older adults or those with known medical problems, the radial pulse is recommended. Though less popular, the pulse can also be counted at the brachial artery. This is located on the inside of the upper arm just below the armpit. Once the pulse is located, the heart rate can be determined in beats per minute. At rest, this is done simply by counting the number of beats in 1 minute.

Counting heart rates during exercise presents some additional challenges. To obtain accurate exercise heart rate values, it is best to count heart beats or pulses while moving; however, this is difficult during most activities.

The most practical method is to count the pulse immediately after exercise. During physical activity, the heart rate increases, but immediately after exercise, it begins to slow and return to normal. In fact, the heart rate has already slowed considerably within 1 minute after activity ceases. Therefore, it is important to locate the pulse quickly and to count the rate for a short period of time in order to obtain accurate results. For best results, keep moving while quickly locating the pulse, then stop and take a 15-second count. Multiply the number of pulses by 4 to convert heart rate to beats per minute.

You can also count the pulse for 10 seconds and multiply by 6, or count the pulse for 6 seconds and multiply by 10 to estimate a 1-minute heart rate. The latter method allows you to calculate heart rates easily by adding 0 to the 6-second count. However, short-duration pulse counts increase the chance of error because a miscount of one beat is multiplied by six or ten beats rather than by four beats.

The pulse rate should be counted after regular activity, not after a sudden burst. Some runners sprint the last few yards of their daily run and then count their pulse. Such a burst of exercise will elevate the heart rate considerably. This gives a false picture of the actual exercise heart rate. It would be wise for every person to learn to determine resting heart rate accurately and to estimate exercise heart rate by quickly and accurately making pulse counts after activity.

A person's maximal heart rate can be estimated reasonably with formulas. Calculations of threshold and target zone heart rates require an estimate of your maximal heart rate (maxHR). Your maxHR is the highest heart rate attained in maximal exercise. It could be

Table 4 ▶ Calculating Maximal Heart Rate (maxHR)		
	208.0	
	−15.4	.7 × 22 (age) = 15.4
	192.6	
maxHR = 193	(rounded up from 192.6)	

determined using an electrocardiogram while exercising to exhaustion; however, for most people it is easier to estimate by using a formula. Until recently a simple formula has been used (220 − age = maxHR). Although this formula gives a general estimate, recent research has found that it tends to overpredict for young people (twenty to forty) and underpredict for those over forty. Based on the extensive research involving a review of hundreds of past studies and new laboratory research, a new formula is now recommended. The formula is maxHR = 208 − (.7 × age). The formula has been shown to be useful for both sexes and for people of all activity levels. Table 4 illustrates the calculation of maxHR for a twenty-two-year-old using the new formula. The 193 (rounded up from 192.6) heart rate for the twenty-two-year-old example is five beats lower than if the old formula had been used.

The new formula is especially beneficial to older adults. Because the previous formula underpredicted maxHR, it also underestimated the true level of physical stress during a treadmill test and underestimated target heart rate values for older adults.

Two methods can be used to determine threshold and target zone heart rates. The procedures used in determining target heart rates vary in complexity and accuracy. The preferred method, known as the percent of heart rate reserve method (often referred to as the Karvonnen method), involves calculating a percentage of your HRR. This method is considered more accurate because it takes into account your individual resting heart rate (an indicator of fitness) in making the calculations. A simpler procedure, known as the percent of maximal heart rate method, is easier to calculate but less personalized. The two methods of determining threshold and target zone heart rates are described in the following sections. You can also use Chart 8 in the *Lab Resource Materials* to determine your threshold and target heart rates using your resting heart rate and your age.

Percent of Heart Rate Reserve (HRR) Method

To calculate your HRR, you must know your resting heart rate in addition to your maxHR. Resting heart rate is easily determined by counting the pulse for 1 minute while sitting or lying down. Ideally, this should be done early in the morning when you are rested, rather than late in the day when you have been involved in many activities.

Table 5 ▶ Calculating Threshold and Target Heart Rates Using the Percent of Heart Rate Reserve Method*	
Maximal heart rate	193 bpm
Minus resting heart rate	−68 bpm
Equals heart rate reserve (HRR)	125 bpm
Calculating Threshold Heart Rate	
HRR	125 bpm
× 40%	× .40
Equals	50 bpm
Plus resting heart rate	+68 bpm
Equals threshold heart rate	118 bpm
Calculating Upper Limit Heart Rate	
HRR	125 bpm
× 85%	× .85
Equals	106 bpm (106.25)
Plus resting heart rate	+68 bpm
Equals upper limit heart rate	174 bpm

*Example is for a twenty-two-year-old person with a resting heart rate of 68 bpm. The target zone for this twenty-two-year-old is 118–174 bpm.

HRR is determined by subtracting the resting heart rate from the maximal heart rate. The heart always works in the range between the resting (the lowest) and the maximal (the highest) rate of your pulse. The formula for calculating the working heart rate and an example for the twenty-two-year-old with a resting heart rate of 68 beats per minute are shown in Table 5.

The threshold of training, or minimum heart rate, for achieving health benefits is determined by calculating 40 percent of the working heart rate and then adding it to the resting heart rate. The upper limit of the target zone is 85 percent of the working heart rate added to the resting heart rate. The formula for determining threshold and the upper limit of the target heart rate zone and examples for a hypothetical exerciser are shown in Table 5. For best results, begin lower in the target zone and gradually increase exercise intensity.

It is important to note that activities that produce heart rates above 85 percent of heart rate reserve are considered to be **anaerobic activities** for most people. Physical activities of this high intensity may be needed for those in training for competition or for special physical tasks; however, it is not necessary for improving cardiovascular fitness associated with good health and wellness. Threshold and target zone values for anaerobic activities will be discussed in later concepts.

Percent of Maximal Heart Rate Method

To use this method, first estimate your maximal heart rate, just as you did for the previous method; then determine the threshold heart rate by calculating 55 percent of the maximal heart rate. The upper limit of the target zone

Table 6 ▶ Calculating Threshold and Target Heart Rates for Using Percent of Maximal Heart Rate*	
Calculating Threshold Heart Rate	
Maximal heart rate	193 bpm
× 55%	× .55
Equals threshold heart rate	106 bpm (106.15)
Calculating Upper Limit Heart Rate	
Maximal heart rate	193 bpm
× 85%	× .90
Equals upper limit heart rate	174 bpm (173.7)

*Example is of a twenty-two-year-old. The target zone for this twenty-two-year-old is 106–174 bpm.

is determined by calculating 90 percent of the maximal heart rate. Table 6 gives an example for a hypothetical twenty-two-year-old person. This procedure, using a percent of maximal heart rate, is deemed an acceptable alternative to the procedure using a percent of heart rate reserve because it provides target heart rates similar to those using 40–85 percent of the HRR method (see Table 6 for a worked example).

The ACSM recently increased the percentage of maxHR for calculating threshold heart rates because the percentage formerly used was underestimating these values. As the examples in Tables 5 and 6 indicate, the percent of maximal heart rate formula still underestimates threshold values but provides accurate values for the upper limit of the target zone.

Threshold and target zone heart rates should be used as general guidelines for cardiovascular exercise. You should learn to calculate your threshold and target zone heart rate values using one of the two methods described. Regardless of which method you use, the key is to bring your heart rate above threshold and into the target zone to get the health benefits from cardiovascular fitness. The ranges that result from these methods should be used as general guidelines because there are several possible sources of error that can influence the values.

First, the method of calculating maximal heart rate is an estimate based on typical values for typical people. Second, errors in counting heart rate are possible. Finally, it is possible that the count you make *after* exercise may not actually reflect your heart rate *during* the activity. For this reason, it is important that you make several estimates of your threshold and target heart rates, especially when you are first starting a cardiovascular fitness program.

The recent development of inexpensive watch-sized heart rate monitors has provided a reliable method of heart rate assessment for those who wish to use them

Technology Update

Heart Rate Monitors

Heart rate monitors have been used for years by competitive endurance athletes to monitor their training programs. Athletes learn what their heart rate is for certain paces and know how hard they can push to optimize their performance in a race. Technological advances have continued to enhance the utility of these devices, and the costs of the devices are now within the reach of many recreational exercisers.

A watch (receiver), typically worn on the wrist, receives a signal from a transmitter attached to a strap worn around the chest. Basic units display heart rate only, whereas more advanced models have alarms to indicate time spent in target zones and software that allows the heart rate signals to be downloaded and processed on a personal computer. The software can automatically track time spent in different target zones and allow users to see a graphical display of how hard they exercised. The immediate feedback on heart rate during exercise and the ability to log workouts over time may help some individuals maintain interest in their exercise program. See www.polarusa.com for more information.

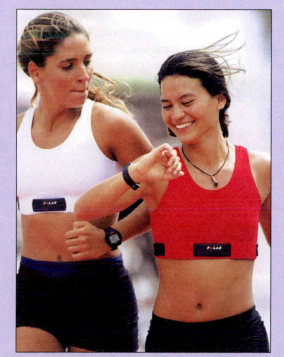

The heart rate monitor.

Anaerobic Activities Physical activities performed at an intensity that exceeds the body's capacity to supply oxygen.

Table 7 ▶ Ratings of Perceived Exertion (RPE)

Rating	Description
6	
7	Very, very light
8	
9	Very light
10	
11	Fairly light
12	
13	Somewhat hard
14	
15	Hard
16	
17	Very hard
18	
19	Very, very hard
20	

Data from Borg, 1982.

(see *Technology Update*). They give you a heart rate count *during* activity, allowing you to easily and quickly determine your heart rate at any time. Though these computerized monitors are helpful to some, they are not a requirement for accurate assessment of physical activity intensity.

Ratings of perceived exertion can be used as a method of monitoring the intensity of physical activity designed to promote cardiovascular fitness. The ACSM suggests that people experienced in physical activity can use RPE to determine if they are exercising in the target zone (see Table 7). Ratings of perceived exertion have been shown to correlate well with VO_2R and HRR. For this reason, RPE can be used to estimate exercise intensity among those who have learned to use the RPE rating categories. This avoids the need to stop and count heart rate during exercise. A rating of 12 is equal to threshold, and a rating of 16 is equal to the upper limit of the target zone. With practice, most people can recognize when they are in the target zone using ratings of perceived exertion.

Strategies for Action

An important step in taking action to develop and maintain cardiovascular fitness is assessing your current status. www.mhhe.com/phys_fit/web08 Click 05. For an activity program to be most effective, it should be based on personal needs. Some type of testing is necessary to determine your personal need for cardiovascular fitness. With proper instruction and practice, you can learn to self-assess your cardiovascular fitness.

Although a laboratory test of $\dot{V}O_2$ max is the ideal "gold standard" measure of cardiovascular fitness, a number of field tests are available that can be done with little or no equipment in or near your home. Commonly used tests are the step test, the swim test, the 12-minute run, the Astrand-Ryhming bicycle test, and the walking test. With proper instruction, you can learn to measure your own cardiovascular fitness using one of these methods (see *Lab Resource Materials*). These tests have been shown to estimate $\dot{V}O_2$ max with reasonable accuracy. Since these tests are not as accurate as laboratory tests of $\dot{V}O_2$ max, using more than one test is recommended to help you get a valid assessment of your cardiovascular fitness. www.mhhe.com/phys_fit/web08 Click 06. **The self-assessment you choose depends on your current fitness and activity levels, availability of equipment, and other factors.** The walking test is probably best for those at beginning levels because more vigorous forms of activity may cause discomfort and may discourage future participation. The step test is somewhat less vigorous than the running test and takes only a

few minutes to complete. The bicycle test is also submaximal or relatively moderate in intensity. It is quite accurate but requires more equipment than the other tests and requires more expertise. You may need help from a fitness expert to do this test properly. The swim test is especially useful to those with musculoskeletal problems and other disabilities. The running test is the most vigorous and for this reason may not be best for beginners. On the other hand, more advanced exercisers with high levels of motivation may prefer this test.

Results on the walking, running, and swimming tests are greatly influenced by the motivation of the test taker. If the test taker does not try hard, fitness results are underestimated. The bicycle and step tests are influenced less by motivation because one must exercise at a specified workload and at a regular pace. Because heart rate can be influenced by emotional factors, exercise prior to the test, and other factors, tests using heart rate can sometimes give incorrect results. It is important to do your self-assessments when you are relatively free from stress and are rested.

Prior to performing any of these, be sure that you are physically and medically ready. Prepare yourself by doing some regular physical activity for 3 to 6 weeks before actually taking the tests. If possible, take more than one test and use the summary of your test results to make a final assessment of your cardiovascular fitness. In Lab 8B, you will have the opportunity to self-assess your cardiovascular fitness using one or more tests.

Study Resources

Web Resources

American College of Sports Medicine **www.acsm.org**
American Heart Association **www.americanheart.org**
The Cooper Institute **www.cooperinst.org**

Suggested Readings

Additional reference materials for Concept 8 are available at **www.mhhe.com/phys_fit/web08 Click 07**.

Ainsworth, B. E. 2003. The compendium of physical activities. *President's Council on Physical Fitness and Sports Research Digest* 4(2):1–8.

American College of Sports Medicine. 2000. *ACSM's Guidelines for Exercise Testing and Exercise Prescription.* 6th ed. Philadelphia: Lippincott, Williams and Wilkins.

Bassuk, S. S., and J. E. Manson. 2004. Preventing cardiovascular disease in women: How much physical activity is good enough? *President's Council on Physical Fitness and Sports Research Digest* 5(3):1–8.

Blair, S. N., and A. S. Jackson. 2001. A guest editorial to accompany physical fitness and activity as separate heart disease risk factors: A meta-analysis. *Medicine and Science in Sports and Exercise* 33(5):762–764.

Blair, S. N., et al. 1996. Influence of cardiorespiratory fitness and other precursors on cardiovascular disease and all-cause mortality in men and women. *Journal of American Medical Association* 276(3):205–211.

Booth, F. W., and M. W. Chakravarthy. 2002. Cost and consequences of sedentary living: New battleground for an old enemy. *President's Council on Physical Fitness and Sports Research Digest* 3(16):1–8.

Borg, G. 1982. Psychological bases of perceived exertion. *Medicine and Science in Sports and Exercise* 14:377.

Bouchard, C. 1999. Heredity and health-related fitness. In C. B. Corbin and R. P. Pangrazi (eds.). *Toward a Better Understanding of Physical Fitness and Activity.* Scottsdale, AZ: Holcomb-Hathaway.

Carnethon, M. R., et al. 2003. Cardiorespiratory fitness of young adults and the development of cardiovascular disease risk factors. *Journal of the American Medical Association* 290(23):3092–3100.

Dziura, J., et al. 2004. Physical activity reduces Type 2 diabetes risk in aging independent of body weight change. *Journal of Physical Activity and Health* 1(1):19–28.

Farrell, S. W., et al. 2002. The relation of body mass index, cardiorespiratory fitness, and all-cause mortality in women. *Obesity Research* 10:417–423.

Franks, P. W., et al. 2004. Does the association of habitual physical activity with the metabolic syndrome differ by level of cardiorespiratory fitness? *Diabetes Care* 27(5):1187–1193.

Hootman, J. M., et al. 2001. Association among physical activity level, cardiorespiratory fitness, and risk of musculoskeletal injury. *American Journal of Epidemiology* 154(3):251–258.

Knuttgen, H. G. 2003. What is exercise? *The Physician and Sportsmedicine* 31(3):32–42.

Lakka, T. A. 2004. Sedentary lifestyle, poor cardiorespiratory fitness, and the metabolic syndrome. *Medicine and Science in Sports and Exercise* 35(8):1279–1286.

Lee, I., and R. S. Phaffenbarger. 2001. Preventing coronary heart disease: The role of physical activity. *The Physician and Sportsmedicine* 29(2):37–52.

Manson, J. E., et al. 2002. Walking compared with vigorous exercise for the prevention of cardiovascular events in women. *New England Journal of Medicine* 347(10):716–725.

Meyers, J., et al. 2002. Exercise capacity and mortality among men referred to for exercise testing. *New England Journal of Medicine* 346(11):793–801.

Schnirring, L. 2001. New formula estimates maximal heart rate. *The Physician and Sportsmedicine* 29(7):13–14.

Spain, C. G., and B. D. Franks. 2001. Healthy people 2010: Physical activity and fitness. *President's Council on Physical Fitness and Sports Research Digest* 3(13):1–16.

Tanaka H., K. D. Monahan, and D. R. Seals. 2001. Age-predicted maximal heart rate revisited. *Journal of the American College of Cardiology* 37(1):153–156.

U.S. Department of Health and Human Services. 1996. *Physical Activity and Health: A Report of the Surgeon General.* Atlanta: U.S. Department of Health and Human Services.

Williams, P. T. 2001. Physical fitness and activity as separate heart disease risk factors: A meta-analysis. *Medicine and Science in Sports and Exercise* 33(5):754–761.

Wilmore, J. H. 2003. Aerobic exercise and endurance. *The Physician and Sportsmedicine* 31(5):45–53.

Wong, S. L., et al. 2004. Cardiorespiratory fitness is associated with lower abdominal fat independent of body mass index. *Medicine and Science in Sports and Exercise* 36(2):286–291.

In the News

New Research on Cardiovascular Fitness

The evidence about the importance of aerobic fitness for good health continues to become stronger as researchers use more advanced designs and improved measurement techniques. In a recent report, people who were classified as unfit (bottom 20 percent of fitness distribution) were three to six times more likely to develop the symptoms of metabolic syndrome and were more likely to develop diabetes over a 15-year period. Another report revealed that the association between physical activity and metabolic syndrome was much stronger in the most unfit group. These studies clearly demonstrate the importance of having at least a base level of cardiovascular fitness (not in the lowest fitness category). The public health guidelines have emphasized the message that only small amounts of physical activity are needed to obtain important benefits, and these studies continue to support the merits of this approach.

Part of the benefit of aerobic activity appears to be its ability to promote the preferential loss of abdominal body fat. Several recent studies have demonstrated that higher levels of activity and/or higher cardiorespiratory fitness was associated with lower levels of abdominal body fatness independent of body mass index. In other words, individuals can be about the same size (similar weight for a given height) but individuals with lower activity levels (and lower fitness levels) will likely have higher levels of abdominal body fat. Abdominal body fat is considered to be more harmful than other forms of body fat. These studies provide a clear understanding of how fitness may protect against the health risks for obesity and improve overall health.

The importance of cardiovascular fitness for good health has led the Public Health Service to incorporate objective measures of aerobic fitness into a large-scale surveillance study known as NHANES (National Health and Nutrition Examination Survey). In this fourth (IV) version of the study, data collection teams travel around the country in mobile examination centers and complete comprehensive health and fitness assessments on a representative sample of adults. There have been many surveillance studies conducted using self-report measures of physical activity, but this is the first effort to systematically evaluate the fitness levels of the U.S. population. Results have not been released from this project, but the detailed measurements of fitness and other health parameters in a large sample of adults will surely add new information about the importance of cardiovascular fitness for good health. Visit the NHANES website at http://www.cdc.gov/nchs/nhanes.htm to take a virtual tour of the mobile testing center and to learn how this major public health study is being conducted.

Lab Resource Materials: Evaluating Cardiovascular Fitness

The Walking Test

- Warm up; then walk 1 mile as fast as you can without straining. Record your time to the nearest second.
- Immediately after the walk, count your heart rate for 15 seconds; then multiply by 4 to get a 1-minute heart rate. Record your heart rate.
- Use your walking time and your postexercise heart rate to determine your rating using Chart 1.

Chart 1 ▶ Walking Ratings for Males and Females

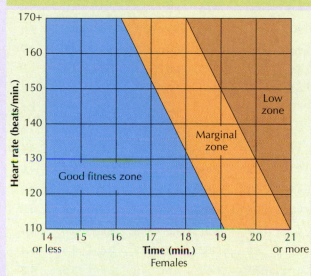

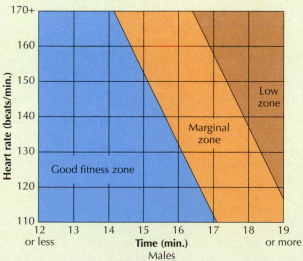

The ratings in Chart 1 are for ages twenty to twenty-nine. They provide reasonable ratings for people of all ages.

Note: The walking test is not a good indicator of high performance; the running and bicycle tests are recommended.

Source: James M. Rippe, M.D.

The Step Test

- Step up and down on a 12-inch bench for 3 minutes at a rate of twenty-four steps per minute. One step consists of four beats—that is, "up with the left foot, up with the right foot, down with the left foot, down with the right foot."
- Immediately after the exercise, sit down on the bench and relax. Don't talk.
- Locate your pulse or have someone locate it for you.
- Five seconds after the exercise ends, begin counting your pulse. Count the pulse for 60 seconds.
- Your score is your 60-second heart rate. Locate your score and your rating on Chart 2.

Chart 2 ▶ Step Test Rating Chart

Classification	60-Second Heart Rate
High-performance zone	84 or less
Good fitness zone	85–95
Marginal zone	96–119
Low zone	120 and above

As you grow older, you will want to continue to score well on this rating chart. Because your maximal heart rate decreases as you age, you should be able to score well if you exercise regularly.

Source: F. W. Kasch and J. L. Boyer.

The Astrand-Ryhming Bicycle Test

- Ride a stationary bicycle ergometer for 6 minutes at a rate of fifty pedal cycles per minute (one push with each foot per cycle). Cool down after the test.
- Set the bicycle at a workload between 300 and 1,200 kpm. For less fit or smaller people, a setting in the range of 300 to 600 is appropriate. Larger or fitter people will need to use a setting of 750 to 1,200. The workload should be enough to elevate the heart rate to at least 125 bpm but no more than 170 bpm during the ride. The ideal range is 140–150 bpm.
- During the sixth minute of the ride (if the heart rate is in the correct range—see previous step), count the heart rate for the entire sixth minute. The carotid or radial pulse may be used.
- Use Chart 3 (males) or 4 (females) to determine your predicted oxygen uptake score in liters per minute. Locate your heart rate for the sixth minute of the ride in the left column and the work rate in kp·m/min. across the top. The number in the chart where the heart rate and work rate intersect represents your predicted O_2 uptake in liters per minute. The bicycle you use must allow you to easily and accurately determine the work rate in kp·m/min.

- Ratings are typically assigned based on milliliters per kilogram of body weight per minute. To convert your score to milliliters per kilogram (mL/kg/min.) the first step is to multiply your score from Chart 3 or 4 by 1,000. This converts your score from liters to milliliters. Then divide your weight in pounds by 2.2. This converts your weight to kilograms. Then divide your score in milliliters by your weight in kilograms. This gives you your score in mL/kg/min.

- Example: An oxygen uptake score of 3.5 liters is equal to a 3,500-milliliter score ($3.5 \times 1,000$). If the person with this score weighed 150 pounds, his or her weight in kilograms would be 68.18 kilograms (150 divided by 2.2). The person's oxygen uptake would be 51.3 mL/kg/min. (3,500 divided by 68.18).
- Use your score in mL/kg/min. to determine your rating (Chart 5).

Chart 3 ▶ Determining Oxygen Uptake Using the Bicycle Test—Men (liters O$_2$/min.)

Heart Rate	450	600	900	1,200		Heart Rate	450	600	900	1,200	1,500		Heart Rate	450	600	900	1,200	1,500
123	3.3	3.4	4.6	6.0		139	2.5	2.6	3.6	4.8	6.0		155	2.0	2.2	3.0	4.0	5.0
124	3.3	3.3	4.5	6.0		140	2.5	2.6	3.6	4.8	6.0		156	1.9	2.2	2.9	4.0	5.0
125	3.2	3.2	4.4	5.9		141	2.4	2.6	3.5	4.7	5.9		157	1.9	2.1	2.9	3.9	4.9
126	3.1	3.2	4.4	5.8		142	2.4	2.5	3.5	4.6	5.8		158	1.8	2.1	2.9	3.9	4.9
127	3.0	3.1	4.3	5.7		143	2.4	2.5	3.4	4.6	5.7		159	1.8	2.1	2.8	3.8	4.8
128	3.0	3.1	4.2	5.6		144	2.3	2.5	3.4	4.5	5.7		160	1.8	2.1	2.8	3.8	4.8
129	2.9	3.0	4.2	5.6		145	2.3	2.4	3.4	4.5	5.6		161	1.7	2.0	2.8	3.7	4.7
130	2.9	3.0	4.1	5.5		146	2.3	2.4	3.3	4.4	5.6		162	1.7	2.0	2.8	3.7	4.6
131	2.8	2.9	4.0	5.4		147	2.3	2.4	3.3	4.4	5.5		163	1.7	2.0	2.8	3.7	4.6
132	2.8	2.9	4.0	5.3		148	2.2	2.4	3.2	4.3	5.4		164	1.6	2.0	2.7	3.6	4.5
133	2.7	2.8	3.9	5.3		149	2.2	2.3	3.2	4.3	5.4		165	1.6	1.9	2.7	3.6	4.5
134	2.7	2.8	3.9	5.2		150	2.2	2.3	3.2	4.2	5.3		166	1.6	1.9	2.7	3.6	4.5
135	2.7	2.8	3.8	5.1		151	2.2	2.3	3.1	4.2	5.2		167	1.5	1.9	2.6	3.5	4.4
136	2.6	2.7	3.8	5.0		152	2.1	2.3	3.1	4.1	5.2		168	1.5	1.9	2.6	3.5	4.4
137	2.6	2.7	3.7	5.0		153	2.1	2.2	3.0	4.1	5.1		169	1.5	1.9	2.6	3.5	4.3
138	2.5	2.7	3.7	4.9		154	2.0	2.2	3.0	4.0	5.1		170	1.4	1.8	2.6	3.4	4.3

Chart 4 ▶ Determining Oxygen Uptake Using the Bicycle Test—Women (liters O$_2$/min.)

Heart Rate	300	450	600	750	900		Heart Rate	300	450	600	750	900		Heart Rate	400	600	750	900
123	2.4	3.1	3.9	4.6	5.1		139	1.8	2.4	2.9	3.5	4.0		155	1.9	2.4	2.8	3.2
124	2.4	3.1	3.8	4.5	5.1		140	1.8	2.4	2.8	3.4	4.0		156	1.9	2.4	2.8	3.2
125	2.3	3.0	3.7	4.4	5.0		141	1.8	2.3	2.8	3.4	3.9		157	1.8	2.3	2.7	3.2
126	2.3	3.0	3.6	4.3	5.0		142	1.7	2.3	2.8	3.3	3.9		158	1.8	2.3	2.7	3.1
127	2.2	2.9	3.5	4.2	4.8		143	1.7	2.2	2.7	3.3	3.8		159	1.8	2.3	2.7	3.1
128	2.2	2.8	3.5	4.2	4.8		144	1.7	2.2	2.7	3.2	3.8		160	1.8	2.2	2.6	3.0
129	2.2	2.8	3.4	4.1	4.8		145	1.6	2.2	2.7	3.2	3.7		161	1.8	2.2	2.6	3.0
130	2.1	2.7	3.4	4.0	4.7		146	1.6	2.2	2.6	3.2	3.7		162	1.8	2.2	2.6	3.0
131	2.1	2.7	3.4	4.0	4.6		147	1.6	2.1	2.6	3.1	3.6		163	1.7	2.2	2.5	2.9
132	2.0	2.7	3.3	3.9	4.6		148	1.6	2.1	2.6	3.1	3.6		164	1.7	2.1	2.5	2.9
133	2.0	2.6	3.2	3.8	4.5		149	1.5	2.1	2.6	3.0	3.5		165	1.7	2.1	2.5	2.9
134	2.0	2.6	3.2	3.8	4.4		150	1.5	2.0	2.5	3.0	3.5		166	1.7	2.1	2.5	2.8
135	2.0	2.6	3.1	3.7	4.4		151	1.5	2.0	2.5	3.0	3.4		167	1.6	2.0	2.4	2.8
136	1.9	2.5	3.1	3.6	4.3		152	1.4	2.0	2.5	2.9	3.4		168	1.6	2.0	2.4	2.8
137	1.9	2.5	3.0	3.6	4.2		153	1.4	2.0	2.4	2.9	3.3		169	1.6	2.0	2.4	2.8
138	1.8	2.4	3.0	3.5	4.2		154	1.4	2.0	2.4	2.8	3.3		170	1.6	2.0	2.4	2.7

Chart 5 ▶ Bicycle Test Rating Scale (mL/O_2/kg/min.)

	Women				
Age	17–26	27–39	40–49	50–59	60–69
High-performance zone	46+	40+	38+	35+	32+
Good fitness zone	36–45	33–39	30–37	28–34	24–31
Marginal zone	30–35	28–32	24–29	21–27	18–23
Low zone	<30	<28	<24	<21	<18

	Men				
Age	17–26	27–39	40–49	50–59	60–69
High-performance zone	50+	46+	42+	39+	35+
Good fitness zone	43–49	35–45	32–41	29–38	26–34
Marginal zone	35–42	30–34	27–31	25–28	22–25
Low zone	<35	<30	<27	<25	<22

Source: Charts 4, 5, and 6 based on data from Astrand, P. O., and Rodahl, K.

The 12-Minute Run Test

- Locate an area where a specific distance is already marked, such as a school track or football field, or measure a specific distance using a bicycle or automobile odometer.
- Use a stopwatch or wristwatch to accurately time a 12-minute period.
- For best results, warm up prior to the test; then run at a steady pace for the entire 12 minutes (cool down after the tests).
- Determine the distance you can run in 12 minutes in fractions of a mile. Depending upon your age, locate your score and rating in Chart 6.

Chart 6 ▶ Twelve-Minute Run Test Rating Chart (Score in Miles)

	Men (Age)			
Classification	17–26	27–39	40–49	50+
High-performance zone	1.80+	1.60+	1.50+	1.40+
Good fitness zone	1.55–1.79	1.45–1.59	1.40–1.49	1.25–1.39
Marginal zone	1.35–1.54	1.30–1.44	1.25–1.39	1.10–1.24
Low zone	<1.35	<1.30	<1.25	<1.10

	Women (Age)			
Classification	17–26	27–39	40–49	50+
High-performance zone	1.45+	1.35+	1.25+	1.15+
Good fitness zone	1.25–1.44	1.20–1.34	1.15–1.24	1.05–1.14
Marginal zone	1.15–1.24	1.05–1.19	1.00–1.14	.95–1.04
Low zone	<1.15	<1.05	<1.00	<.94

For a metric version of this chart, see Appendix B.

Based on data from Cooper, K. H.

The 12-Minute Swim Test

- Locate a swimming area with premeasured distances, preferably 20 yards or longer.
- After a warm-up, swim as far as possible in 12 minutes using the stroke of your choice.

- For best results, have a partner keep track of your time and distance. A degree of swimming competence is a prerequisite for this test.
- Determine your score and rating using Chart 7.

Chart 7 ▶ Twelve-Minute Swim Rating Chart (Score in Yards)

Classification	Men (Age)			
	17–26	27–39	40–49	50+
High-performance zone	700+	650+	600+	550+
Good fitness zone	600–699	550–649	500–599	450–549
Marginal fitness zone	500–599	450–459	400–499	350–449
Low fitness zone	below 500	below 450	below 400	below 350

Classification	Women (Age)			
	17–26	27–39	40–49	50+
High-performance zone	600+	550+	500+	450+
Good fitness zone	500–599	450–549	400–499	450–549
Marginal fitness zone	400–499	350–359	300–399	250–349
Low fitness zone	below 400	below 350	below 300	below 250

For a metric version of this chart, see Appendix B.

Based on data from Cooper, K. H.

Directions:

To determine your threshold of training and target heart rates, locate your resting heart rate on the left and your age across the top. The values at the point where the lines intersect are your threshold and target heart rates.

Chart 8 ▶ Determining Threshold of Training* and Target Zone Heart Rates Using Resting Heart Rate and Age

Resting Heart Rate		Age									
		Less Than 25	25–29	30–34	35–39	40–44	45–49	50–54	55–59	60–64	Over 65
Below 50	Threshold	107	105	103	102	101	99	98	97	96	95
	target zone	107–170	105–167	103–164	102–161	101–159	99–155	98–151	97–148	96–146	95–139
50–54	Threshold	110	108	106	104	102	101	102	100	99	98
	target zone	110–170	108–167	106–164	104–162	102–160	101–156	102–153	100–150	99–147	98–140
55–59	Threshold	113	111	109	107	106	105	104	103	102	101
	target zone	113–171	111–168	109–163	107–162	106–160	105–157	104–154	103–150	102–146	101–140
60–64	Threshold	116	113	111	109	108	107	106	105	104	104
	target zone	116–171	113–169	111–166	109–163	108–161	107–159	106–155	105–151	104–147	104–141
65–69	Threshold	118	117	115	112	111	110	109	108	107	108
	target zone	118–172	117–170	115–166	112–163	111–161	110–159	109–155	108–152	107–148	108–142
70–74	Threshold	121	120	118	119	116	114	113	112	111	110
	target zone	121–173	120–171	118–167	119–164	116–162	114–160	113–156	112–153	111–149	110–143
75–79	Threshold	124	123	122	121	119	117	116	114	113	112
	target zone	124–173	123–172	122–168	121–164	119–163	117–160	116–157	114–155	113–151	112–143
80–85	Threshold	127	124	123	122	121	119	118	117	116	114
	target zone	127–174	124–172	123–169	122–165	121–164	119–161	118–158	117–156	116–152	114–144
86 and over	Threshold	130	125	126	125	124	123	121	119	117	117
	target zone	130–175	125–173	126–169	125–166	124–164	123–162	121–159	119–157	117–154	117–145

*Threshold for beginners. Mid target or above recommended after becoming a regular exerciser.

Lab 8A Counting Target Heart Rate and Ratings of Perceived Exertion

Name	Section	Date

Purpose: To learn to count heart rate accurately and to use heart rate and/or ratings of perceived exertion (RPE) to establish the threshold of training and target zones

Procedure

1. Practice counting the number of pulses felt for a given period of time at both the carotid and radial locations. Use a clock or watch to count for 15, 30, and 60 seconds. To establish your heart rate in beats per minute, multiply your 15-second pulse by 4, and your 30-second pulse by 2.
2. Practice locating your carotid and radial pulses quickly. This is important when trying to count your pulse after exercise.
3. Run a quarter-mile; then count your heart rate at the end of the run. Try to run at a rate you think will keep the rate of the heart above the threshold of training and in the target zone. Use 15-second pulse counts (choose either carotid or radial) and multiply by 4 to get heart rate in beats per minute (bpm). Record the bpm in the Results section.
4. Rate your perceived exertion (RPE) for the run (see RPE chart below). Record your results.
5. Repeat the run a second time. Try to run at a speed that gets you in the heart rate and RPE target zone. Record your heart rate and RPE results.

Results: Record your *resting* heart rates in the boxes below.

Carotid Pulse   **Heart Rate per Minute**   **Radial Pulse**   **Heart Rate per Minute**

[ ] 15 seconds × 4	[ ]	[ ] 15 seconds × 4	[ ]
[ ] 30 seconds × 2	[ ]	[ ] 30 seconds × 2	[ ]
[ ] 60 seconds × 1	[ ]	[ ] 60 seconds × 1	[ ]

Record your heart rate and rating of perceived exertion for run 1.

Pulse Count   **Heart Rate per Minute**

[ ] 15 seconds × 4   [ ]

Rating of Perceived Exertion [ ]

Record your heart rate and rating of perceived exertion for run 2.

Pulse Count   **Heart Rate per Minute**

[ ] 15 seconds × 4   [ ]

Rating of Perceived Exertion [ ]

Ratings of Perceived Exertion (RPE)	
Rating	**Description**
6	
7	Very, very light
8	
9	Very light
10	
11	Fairly light
12	
13	Somewhat hard
14	
15	Hard
16	
17	Very hard
18	
19	Very, very hard
20	

Source: Data from Borg, G.

Answer the following questions:

Which pulse-counting technique did you use after the runs?   Carotid ⬭   Radial ⬭

What is your heart rate target zone (calculate, see pages 112 and 113, or see Chart 8, page 120)? [＿＿＿＿] bpm

Was your heart rate for run 1 enough to get in the heart rate target zone?   Yes ⬭   No ⬭

Was your RPE for run 1 enough to get in the target zone (12–16)?   Yes ⬭   No ⬭

Was your heart rate for run 2 enough to get in the heart rate target zone?   Yes ⬭   No ⬭

Was your RPE for run 2 enough to get in the target zone (12–16)?   Yes ⬭   No ⬭

Conclusions and Implications: In several sentences, discuss your results, including which method you would use to count heart rate and why. Also discuss heart rate versus RPE (Rating of Perceived Exertion) for determining the target zone.

[blank response box]

Lab Supplement*: You may want to keep track of your exercise heart rate over a week's time or longer to see if you are reaching the target zone in your workouts. Shade your target zone with a highlight pen and plot your exercise heart rate for each day of the week (see sample).

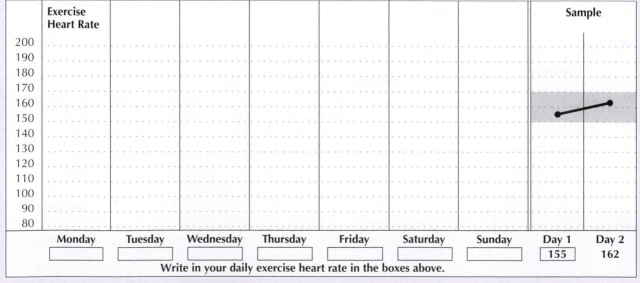

*Thanks to Ginnie Atkins for suggesting this lab supplement.

Lab 8B Evaluating Cardiovascular Fitness

Name	**Section** **Date**

Purpose: To acquaint you with several methods for evaluating cardiovascular fitness and to help you evaluate and rate your own cardiovascular fitness

Procedure: Perform one or more of the four cardiovascular fitness tests described in the *Lab Resource Materials*. Determine your ratings on the test(s) using the rating charts provided.

Results: Record the information obtained from taking the cardiovascular fitness test(s) (one or more) in the space provided.

Walking Test

Time _____ minutes

Heart rate _____ bpm

Rating _____ (see Chart 1, page 117)

Step Test

Heart rate _____ bpm

Rating _____ (see Chart 2, page 117)

Bicycle Test

Workload _____ kpm

Heart rate _____ bpm

Weight _____ pounds

Weight in kg* _____

mL/O_2/kg _____

Rating _____ (see Chart 5, page 119)

12-Minute Run

Distance _____ miles

Rating _____ (see Chart 6, page 119)

12-Minute Swim Test

Distance _____ yards

Rating _____ (see Chart 7, page 120)

*Weight in lb. ÷ 2.2.

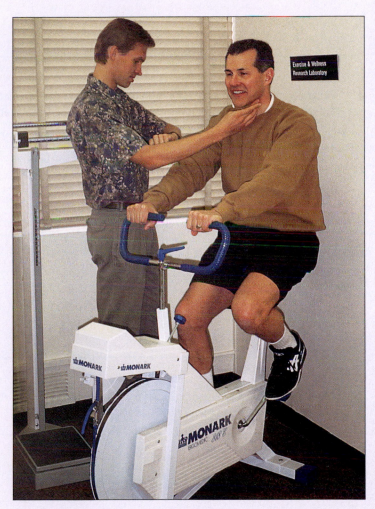

The bicycle test.

123

Conclusions and Implications

1. In several sentences, explain why you selected the test or tests you chose. If you selected only one test, explain why.

2. In several sentences, explain your results. Discuss your perception of the accuracy of the test results. Also, discuss whether you think you might have different results if you had taken another test and, if so, why.

3. In several sentences, discuss your current level of cardiovascular fitness and steps that you need to take to maintain or improve your cardiovascular fitness.

Active Aerobics, Sports, and Recreational Activities

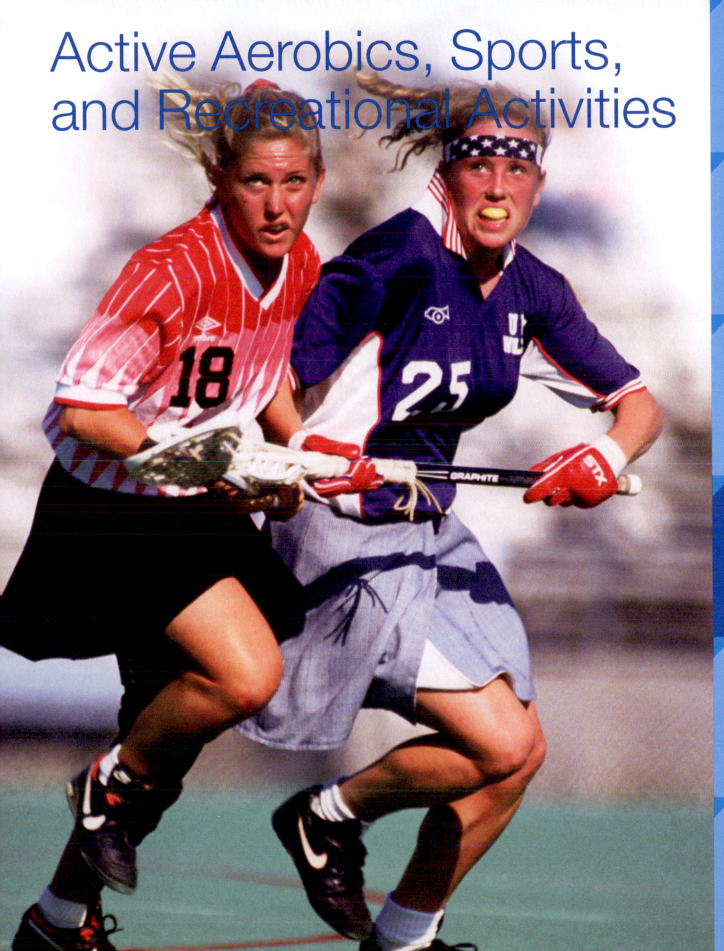

Active aerobics, sports, and recreational activities can promote health, develop fitness, and enhance performance.

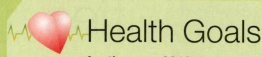

Health Goals

for the year 2010

- Increase proportion of people who do vigorous physical activity that promotes cardiovascular fitness 3 or more days a week for 20 minutes per occasion.

- Increase adoption and maintenance of daily physical activity.

- Increase leisure-time physical activity.

- Decrease incidence of and deaths from heart diseases.

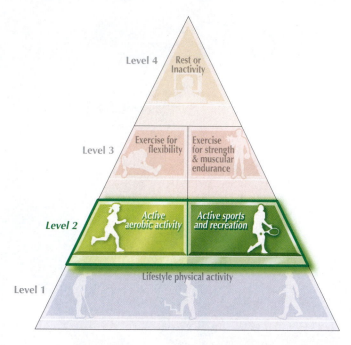

Figure 1 ▶ Active aerobics, sports, and recreational activities are included in the second level of the physical activity pyramid.

Aerobic physical activity provides the foundation for comprehensive fitness programs. Aerobic activity provides numerous health benefits, contributes to long-term weight control, and can be helpful in reducing stress. Improvements in cardiovascular fitness that result from aerobic activity also contribute to high quality of life and are essential for enhancing sports performance. Aerobic activity is generally defined as activity that is rhythmical, utilizes large muscle groups, and is performed in a continuous manner. However, aerobic activity does not have to be continuous to promote health or improve cardiovascular fitness.

This concept will review the two types of activity at the second level of the activity pyramid (active aerobic activity and active sports and recreation). These activities are more vigorous than those at the first level of the pyramid and are among the most popular types of activity.

Physical Activity Pyramid: Level 2

A variety of popular aerobic activities are included at level 2 of the pyramid. www.mhhe. com/phys_fit/web09 Click 01. While lifestyle activities at the bottom of the pyramid are considered to be "aerobic," the activities at the second level of the pyramid refer to those that are more vigorous (see Figure 1). **Active aerobics** are popular forms of activity among adults. Walking, swimming, exercising with machines, cycling, and jogging are consistently among the top fifteen participation activities

(see Table 1). These activities are often used by adults to obtain the regular aerobic activity needed for good health.

The word aerobic literally means "with oxygen," but the reference to *aerobic activity* was popularized by Dr. Kenneth Cooper in his pioneering book *Aerobics*, published in 1967. Dr. Cooper was an early advocate of and a leader in the fitness movement, and his book helped to increase awareness about the importance of regular physical activity. The Cooper Aerobic Points System emphasized that a variety of aerobic activities can contribute to cardiovascular health. Today, the concept of using various types of activities as part of an overall aerobic activity program is known as cross training.

Active recreation and sports are included at level 2 because they can provide the same benefits as structured aerobic activity. www.mhhe. com/phys_fit/web09 Click 02. Activities such as hiking, boating, fishing, horseback riding, and other outdoor activities are generally classified as recreation. Because many of these activities can be performed at intensities suitable for building cardiovascular fitness, some can be categorized as **active recreational activities.** Camping is a popular participation activity that may promote a variety of outdoor activities. It is equally popular (ranked

Table 1 ▶ Most Popular Participation Activities

Activity	Rank	Male	Female
Walking	1	2	1
Swimming	2	3	2
Camping	3	4	4
Fishing	4	1	10
Exercising with machines	5	8	3
Bowling	6	7	5
Cycling	7	5	7
Billiards/Pool	8	9	8
Basketball	9	10	14
Golf	10	6	*
Hiking	11	13	9
Running/jogging	12	14	11
Aerobics (dance)	13	*	6
Boating	14	15	12
Resistance training	15	12	15
Hunting	*	11	*
Rollerblading	*	*	13

Source: National Sporting Goods Association.

*Not in top fifteen.

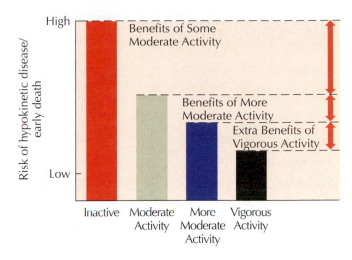

Figure 2 ▶ The extra benefits of vigorous physical activities.

Physical activities at level 2 of the pyramid produce improvements in cardiovascular fitness and health in addition to those produced by lifestyle physical activities. Participation in lifestyle activity provides important health benefits and additional vigorous aerobic activity results in additional health benefits. In fact, vigorous aerobic activity and active sports produce more benefits even if the total amount of activity (or energy expenditure) is the same. This difference can be seen in Figure 2. The green and blue bars show that a person's disease risk decreases as the amount of moderate activity increases. The black bar reveals the additional benefits provided by more vigorous activity. For each level of total activity, health risks are lower if a person performs more vigorous forms of physical activity. The Surgeon General's Report and other public health documents have encouraged Americans to meet at least the minimal activity threshold. The American College of Sports Medicine also emphasizes that "additional benefits can be gained through greater amounts of physical activity."

The activities included in the second level of the activity pyramid can be done less frequently than activities at level 1 of the pyramid. The lower the level in the pyramid, the more frequently an activity

fourth) among males and females. Other examples of popular active recreational activities are backpacking, kayaking, and canoeing. Recreational activities such as fishing and boating, also among the most popular activities, are done at less intensity and can be considered as lifestyle physical activities. Fishing and hunting are two activities that are much more popular among men than women.

Active **sports** can also be included in level 2 of the pyramid because they are vigorous. Basketball is the only active sport in the top fifteen activities. It is typically anaerobic and intermittent. Other aerobic sports include racquetball, tennis, soccer, and hockey. When done consistently with the FIT formula for cardiovascular fitness, these sports can provide benefits similar to those of active aerobics. Swimming and cycling are popular activities that can be considered sports. However, most people do these activities noncompetitively, so they are considered as active aerobics in this book.

Sports such as golf, bowling, and billiards/pool are aerobic but are light to moderate in intensity. For this reason, they are classified as lifestyle physical activities. Basketball and golf are much more popular among men than women. Basketball, football, and baseball are most popular among youth and young adults, whereas golf and bowling are much more popular among middle-aged and older adults.

Active Aerobics Physical activities of enough intensity to produce improvements in cardiovascular fitness. They are more intense than aerobic lifestyle physical activities.

Active Recreational Activities Activities done during leisure time that do not meet the characteristics of sports. Many types of active aerobics are recreational activities.

Sports Typically considered to be competitive physical activities that have an organized set of rules along with winners and losers.

Table 2 ▶ Risk for Injury in Exercise

Activity	Injury per 1,000 Hours of Activity
Skating (including rollerblading)	20
Basketball	18
Average competitive sports	16
Running/jogging	16
Racquetball	14
Average aerobic activity	10
Tennis	8
Cycling	6
High-impact dance aerobics	6
Step aerobics	5
Aerobic exercise machines	3
Walking	2
Low-impact dance aerobics	2

Source: Data from the Center for Sports Medicine at St. Francis Hospital, San Francisco, CA.

should be performed. Lifestyle physical activities need to be performed all, or most, days of the week. Active aerobics, sports, and recreation can be performed as few as 3 days a week (see FIT formula, Table 3 in Concept 8). They can be done less often because the activities are performed at a more vigorous level. This is important for young people who feel that their time is limited. Performing more vigorous activities provides health and fitness benefits with a relatively small time commitment.

Not all activities at level 2 of the pyramid are equally safe. Sports medicine experts indicate that certain types of physical activities are more likely to result in injury than others (see Table 2). Walking and low-impact dance aerobics are among the least risky activities. Skating, an aerobic activity, is the most risky, followed by basketball and competitive sports. Among the most popular aerobic activities, running has the greatest risk, with cycling, high-impact dance aerobics, and step aerobics having moderate risk for injury. Water activities were not considered in the study on which Table 2 was based, but other studies show that swimming and water aerobics are among those least likely to cause injuries because they do not involve impact, falling, or collision.

Injury rates vary among populations—for example, studies of high school and college athletes show that cheerleading and gymnastics are activities that result in the most injuries. A recent study of baby boomers, adults aged thirty-five to fifty-four, showed that bicycling, basketball, baseball/softball, running/jogging, and aerobic dance exercise were among the activities most likely to

result in emergency room treatment for that age group. No matter what the age group, activities that require high-volume training (aerobics and jogging), collision (football, basketball, and softball), falling (biking, skating, cheerleading, and gymnastics), the use of specialized equipment that can fail (biking), and repetitive movements that stress the joints (tennis and high-impact aerobics) increase risk for injury. These statistics point out the importance of using proper safety equipment, proper performance techniques, and proper training techniques.

Active Aerobic Activities

Many types of active aerobics can be done in group settings. Although most aerobic activities can be done individually, many people prefer the social interactions and challenge of group exercise classes. Group exercise classes are offered at many fitness centers and community recreation centers.

Active aerobics can be done either continuously or intermittently. We generally think of active aerobics as being continuous. Jogging, swimming, and cycling at a steady pace for long periods are classic examples. Experts have shown that aerobic exercise can be done intermittently as well as continuously. Both **continuous** and **intermittent aerobic activities** can build cardiovascular fitness. For example, recent studies have shown that three 10-minute exercise sessions in the target zone are as effective as one 30-minute exercise session. Still, experts recommend bouts of 20 to 60 minutes in length, with several 10 to 15 minute bouts being an acceptable alternative when longer sessions are not possible. The advantages and disadvantages of continuous and intermittent exercise are presented in Table 3.

There are many varieties of active aerobic activities to suit individual interests and needs. Active aerobic activities share some characteristics. They involve large muscle groups and are rhythmical. This allows these activities to be performed continuously. An advantage of active aerobic activities is that they provide a good cardiovascular workout in a short time and can often be done by oneself. A disadvantage (or barrier) for some people is that they are generally more vigorous and fast-paced than other forms of activity. The more vigorous nature is the most likely explanation for the age-related patterns that exist for participation in active aerobic activity. Young adults are far more likely to participate in active aerobic activity than oder adults. Most statistics report three- to five-fold differences in participation rates for young adults and older adults (forty to sixty). The declining interest in vigorous activity for older adults is only a concern to public health officials, if older adults fail to substitute moderate physical activity when they discontinue more vigorous activity.

Table 3 ▶ Continuous versus Intermittent Exercise: Advantages and Disadvantages

Continuous	Intermittent
• Done slowly and continuously, rather than in short, vigorous bursts; considered to be less demanding and more enjoyable	• When done in the target zone, has the same benefits as continuous
• Less intense with lower injury risk; may be best for beginners, older people, and those starting after a long layoff	• If done intensely, can increase risk of soreness and injury
• Provides health benefits associated with cardiovascular fitness	• Three 10-minute or two 15-minute sessions easier to schedule than one longer period
• May not provide optimal performance benefits for competitors	• May be more interesting to some people
	• If done at relatively high intensity with alternating rest periods, can produce superior improvements in fitness

Because there are so many choices of different activities, many beginning exercisers want to know which type of aerobic exercise is best. The best form of exercise is clearly whatever one you enjoy and will do regularly. Some of the more popular forms of active aerobic activities are described in this concept. Active sports and recreation provide additional alternatives, and these are described later. Some of these forms of active aerobic activity are described in the following sections. Additional information on each activity is available in the *On the Web* feature at the end of this concept.

Aerobic Exercise Machines

Weather, traffic, and darkness can limit the time available to perform outdoor activities. Aerobic exercise machines, such as treadmills, stair climbers, cross-country ski machines, rowing machines, stationary bicycles, and "elliptical trainers," are alternatives that make it easier to perform exercise indoors. The advantage of such machines is that they can be used in the home. Also, they do not require excessive amounts of skill. Use of these machines can be fun and interesting initially, but interest may decrease with repeated use. Ski machines seem to be most useful for people who ski on a regular basis, and stationary bicycles seem to be the best choice for regular cyclists, but many people enjoy using different machines to provide some degree of "cross training" and to have more variety in their program. Aerobic exercise machines can be useful in developing cardiovascular fitness as long as the intensity is sufficient to put the heart rate into the target zone. The key to the effectiveness of the machines is persistent use over long periods of time. Therefore, the type of device you choose should be based on your personal needs and interests.

Many features have been developed to enhance interest and ease of use. Most newer machines feature feedback systems that provide continuous readouts of total exercise time, distance traveled, target and goal intensity, and estimates of calories burned. Some models also include modes that provide built in warm-up and cool-down phases or a series of predetermined intervals with varying intensities. Models at some clubs have personalized key systems that automatically track personal preferences and settings and record time spent on each machine. This information can then be downloaded onto computers for automatic logging. Future developments likely will include interactive displays that allow you to compete against a virtual or real opponent. These features provide additional feedback that may enhance motivation or provide for a customized experience.

Bicycling

www.mhhe.com/phys_fit/web09 Click 03. Bicycling can be an excellent active aerobic activity, but it requires a properly fitted bike, as well as safety equipment, such as a helmet and light if done after dark. There are different types of bikes to fit the needs and interests of the rider. Road bikes are most common but mountain bikes are becoming increasingly popular. Many people appreciate having a versatile bike suitable for different conditions and select a "city bike," which still has upright handlebars but more durable wheels and tires for more rugged conditions.

Cycling is more efficient than running and some other aerobic activities because of the mechanical efficiency of the bicycle. Cycling on the level at 5 mph is about three times less intense than running the same speed. It would take a pace of 13 mph to expend a similar number of calories, compared with running at 5 mph. The speed of cycling will give you an indicator of intensity, but this can be influenced by hills and wind. A better indicator of intensity is heart rate or a rating of perceived exertion (RPE). Because biking may involve periods of coasting, it may need to be performed for longer periods of time than jogging to get the same benefit.

Cross-Country Skiing

www.mhhe.com/phys_fit/web09 Click 04. In most colder climates, cross-country skiing is one of the more popular forms of aerobic activity. Of course, this sport requires snow and some specialized equipment. Because it involves both the arms and legs in a coordinated movement, cross-country skiing is one of the most

Continuous Aerobic Activities Aerobic activities that are slow enough to be sustained for relatively long periods without frequent rest periods.

Intermittent Aerobic Activities Aerobic activities, relatively high in intensity, alternated with frequent rest periods.

effective types of cardiovascular fitness exercises. The downside is that it requires some degree of skill to be able to perform the movements correctly. There are two main types of cross-country skiing: classic, or diagonal stride, and skating. Each requires a different type of ski and technique.

Dance and Step Aerobics

This type of activity was first popularized by Jackie Sorensen in the 1970s as "aerobic dance." Since then, other versions of the activity have been promoted as rhythmic aerobics, Jazzercise, and Dancercize, to note just a few of the popular names. Dance aerobics is a choreographed series of dance steps and exercises done to music. Certified instructors may tailor dance routines to individuals, but many dance routines are preplanned (e.g., dance aerobic videos). Most of the early programs were considered to be high-impact because they included jumping, leaping, and hopping dance steps that resulted in stress on the feet and legs.

A variety of forms of aerobic dance are available for different interests and abilities. "Low-impact" aerobics were developed to reduce the risk for injury or soreness. In this form, one foot stays on the floor at all times. Low impact is an especially wise choice for beginners or older exercisers. Traditional "high impact" is still common in many settings. In this form, both feet leave the ground simultaneously for a good part of the routine. It is recommended only for advanced exercisers. Even for these people high-impact aerobics can increase risk for injuries. A hybrid aerobic dance format known as "hi-lo" is gaining in popularity. This form integrates the two types of impact to provide a more balanced routine. The use of alternating sequences moderates the risks associated with both types and is considered to reflect movements more typical of the activities of daily living.

Step aerobics, also known as bench stepping and step training, is an adaptation of dance aerobics. In this activity, the performer steps up and down on a bench when performing various dance steps. In most cases, step aerobics is considered to be low-impact but higher in intensity than many forms of dance aerobics. Step training has been used by professional athletic teams to promote cardiovascular fitness. A major benefit is the ability to change the height of the step to meet the needs of individual participants.

Dance and step aerobics, when planned appropriately for individual participants, can be very effective in building cardiovascular fitness for both men and women. However, one problem with dance aerobics is that it is often a preplanned exercise program; therefore, it requires all participants to do the same activity regardless of their fitness or activity levels. A vigorous routine can cause unfit people to overextend themselves, whereas an easy routine may not result in fitness gains for those who are already quite fit.

Also, some dance aerobic routines have been known to include dangerous exercises. Dance and step aerobics require skill, so instruction from a qualified instructor and practice are necessary for optimal enjoyment.

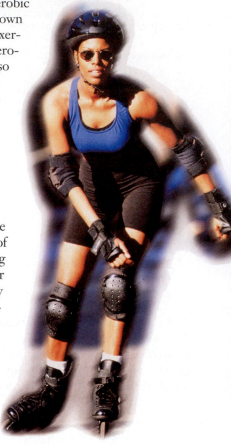

Inline skating is an effective and enjoyable type of aerobic exercise.

Inline Skating

 www.mhhe.com/ phys_fit/web09
Click 05. Because of the speed and freedom of movement, inline skating has become a popular form of aerobic activity and recreation. Technological advances in equipment have made it much safer, though injury rates are still high, compared with other aerobic activities (see Table 2). Because of the injury risk, precautions should be taken. Special equipment is recommended, including a helmet, knee and elbow pads, wrist supporters, and hand protectors. Some degree of skill is necessary to perform skating safely and effectively, so it is wise to practice a bit in a controlled environment before taking to the streets.

Jogging/Running

www.mhhe.com/phys_fit/web09 Click 06. A consistently popular form of active aerobics among both adult men and women is jogging or running. Though no official distinction exists between jogging and running, those who run more than a few miles per day, who participate in races, and who are concerned about improving the time in which they run a certain distance often prefer to be called "runners" rather than "joggers." Fifteen to 20 million American adults report that they jog or run on a regular basis.

The major advantage of jogging/running is that it requires only a good pair of running shoes, some inexpensive clothing, and little skill. With effort, almost anyone can benefit from the activity and even improve performance if that is the goal. There are some techniques that every jogger should be familiar with before starting a jogging program:

- *Foot placement.* The heel of the foot hits the ground first in jogging. Your heel should strike before the rest of your foot (but not hard); then you should rock forward and push off with the ball of your foot. Contrary to some opinions, you should *not* jog on your toes. (A flat-foot landing can be all right as long as you push off with the ball of your foot.) Your toes should point straight ahead. Your feet should stay under your knees and *not* swing out to the sides as you jog.
- *Length of stride.* For efficiency, you should have a relatively comfortable stride length. Your stride should be several inches longer than your walking stride. If necessary, you may have to reach to lengthen your stride. Most older people find it more efficient to run with a shorter stride.
- *Arm movement.* While you jog, you should swing your arms as well as your legs. The arms should be bent and should swing freely and alternately from front to back in the direction you are moving, not from side to side. Keep your arms and hands relaxed.
- *Body position.* While jogging, you should hold your upper body in a relatively erect position with your head and chest up. Don't lean forward, as you would with sprinting or fast running.

Martial Arts Exercise

A variety of martial arts have become popular active aerobic activities. In addition to traditional martial arts such as karate and tae kwon do, a number of other alternative formats have been developed, including kickboxing, aerobic boxing, cardio-karate, box-fitness, and tae-bo. These activities involve intermittent bouts of high-intensity movements and lower-intensity recovery phases. Because martial arts involve a lot of arm work, they can be effective in promoting good overall fitness. Some activities are more intense than others, so consider the alternatives to find the best fit for you. Good instruction is critical for this form of activity, so look for appropriate certifications and credentials before choosing a facility or setting. Many of the disciplines involve a number of contraindicated movements that may increase risk for injury, so it is important to be aware of the risks and minimize your use of bad movements (see Concept 12). If contact is involved, it is important to be matched with a person of similar size and ability.

Spinning

Spinning is a type of stationary cycling typically performed in a group. A group leader typically instructs participants on what pace, gear, and/or cadence to use. In most cases, the routines involve intermittent bursts of high-intensity

 ## Technology Update
Global Positioning Systems

Global positioning systems (GPS) use coded satellite signals that provide accurate coordinates to determine exact location. GPS were developed by the Federal Government primarily for use by the military, but they are now used for a variety of purposes. There are numerous examples of how GPS technology has become integrated into the sport and fitness industries. GPS can be helpful for hikers or backpackers who are out in the wilderness and may not have clear ideas of their location. Some golf courses now include GPS systems on their carts to allow golfers to know precisely where they are on the course and how far they have remaining to the pin. Fishermen can use GPS systems to navigate and plot coordinates on lakes and rivers more effectively.

The technology has also been incorporated into sports watches that are commonly used by runners and cyclists. The integration of GPS technology into the watches makes it possible to determine distance traveled and speed. The system includes a GPS receiver and a watch monitor, which are connected by a radio signal. The receiver (typically strapped to the upper arm) gets the signal from a satellite and sends it to the watch for immediate feedback. Because the system uses an atomic clock, it is quite accurate. For more information on this application of GPS, visit **www.timex.com**.

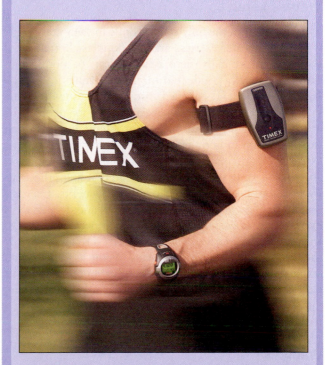

GPS system for runners.

intervals followed by spinning at lower resistance to recover. The instructor may help riders simulate hill climbing or extended sprints to simulate competitive biking conditions. Although the class relates most directly to cycling, the format has appealed to a broader set of fitness enthusiasts who just enjoy the challenge it provides.

Swimming

www.mhhe.com/phys_fit/web09 Click 07. Surveys typically rank swimming as one of the most popular forms of regular activity among adults. Data from the Surgeon General's report show that swimming for exercise ranks ninth among participation activities. The discrepancy is most likely because many people swim occasionally but fewer people swim as exercise on a regular basis. Because it requires considerable skill to move efficiently through the water, many individuals are not able to swim long enough to benefit. Even highly trained athletes can be exhausted after a few hundred yards if they do not have good skills. For those who do swim, it can be an excellent form of physical activity to promote cardiovascular fitness. Because of the water environment and the nonweight-bearing status, the heart rate response to swimming is typically lower for the same intensity of exercise. The heart rate does not increase as rapidly in response to swimming, so target heart rates should be set about five to ten beats lower than for other aerobic activities.

Water Exercise

Swimming is not the only activity done in the water. Water walking and water exercise are two popular alternatives to swimming. Although these activities can be done alone, they are typically conducted in group settings to provide access to pools and certified instructors trained in water safety. Water aerobics are especially good for people with arthritis or other musculoskeletal problems and for people relatively high in body fat. The body's buoyancy in water assists the participant and reduces injury risk. The resistance of the water provides an overload that helps the activity promote health and cardiovascular benefits. Exercises done in shallow water are low in impact, and deeper-water exercises are considered to be higher-impact activities. An advantage of water walking and water exercise is that neither requires the ability to swim. Many classes include activities designed to promote flexibility and muscle fitness development, as well as cardiovascular benefits. Many injured athletes use water activity as a way to rehabilitate from injuries without losing too much fitness.

Walking

www.mhhe.com/phys_fit/web09 Click 08. Walking is generally considered as a lifestyle physical activity and is effective in promoting metabolic fitness and overall health. If cardiovascular fitness is desired, walking must be done intensely enough to elevate the heart rate to target zone levels. For elderly and unfit individuals, walking often provides an intensity sufficient to maintain or improve cardiovascular fitness. For younger and more fit individuals, walking needs to be quite brisk to enhance cardiovascular fitness.

Crosstraining and Calisthenics

Some forms of cross training or calisthenics can provide aerobic exercise benefits. Many people combine a variety of exercises into routines that can provide both cardiovascular and muscular fitness benefits. The use of circuit resistance training, continuous calisthenics, and rope jumping are described in this context.

Circuit Resistance Training (CRT)

Originally, circuit training was a type of physical training involving movement from one exercise station to another. A different type of exercise was performed at each station. In order to complete the circuit, you had to complete all the exercises at all of the stations. The goal was to perform the circuit in progressively shorter time periods. Circuit resistance training (CRT) principally promotes muscle fitness development. However, when performed frequently enough and for enough time at the appropriate intensity, CRT can make a contribution to cardiovascular fitness. When aerobic exercise, such as riding on stationary bicycles and running on treadmills, is incorporated in the continuous exercise circuit, the contribution of this type of exercise to cardiovascular fitness increases.

If cardiovascular fitness is the goal, rest breaks should be minimized. Some clubs promote exercise circuits as a method of building both strength and cardiovascular fitness, yet exercise stations are often crowded, and it is next to impossible to perform the circuit without long waiting periods. You may want to add aerobic exercise to your circuit during periods of waiting.

Continuous Calisthenics

Survey results repeatedly show that calisthenics are among the most frequently performed participant activities. Calisthenic exercises, such as the crunch and push-ups, are designed to build flexibility, strength, or muscular endurance in specific muscle groups. Even though most calisthenics are aerobic, they are usually done intermittently. That is, calisthenic exercises are done a few at a time, followed by a rest period. They will do little for cardiovascular fitness or fat control unless they are done continuously.

Continuous calisthenics, or calisthenics that are done without stopping or with walking, jogging, rope jumping, or some other aerobic activity performed during the rest period, can develop almost all health-related aspects of physical fitness. Fitness pioneer Dr. Thomas Cureton long advocated the use of continuous calisthenics, or what he referred to as "continuous rhythmical endurance exercise."

Active Recreation Activities

Active recreation can provide important health benefits and contribute to high quality of life. Activities that you do in your free time for personal enjoyment or to "re-create" yourself are considered to be recreation activities. Recreation activities that exceed threshold intensity for cardiovascular fitness are considered to be "active" in nature. They are more vigorous than recreation activities such as fishing, bowling and golf that are typically classified as lifestyle or moderate level activities (level 1 in the pyramid).

Many of the active aerobic activities such as walking, jogging, and skiing could easily be classified in the active recreation as well as in the active aerobics section. Also many of the sports that are described in a later section of this concept can be considered as active recreation activities. The distinction somewhat depends on how the activities are viewed by the individual. Some people may view recreation as what they do for fun, but it can also contribute to a healthy lifestyle. Some common types of active recreation are described in the following sections.

Dance

There are many forms of dance that, when done continuously, can contribute significantly to cardiovascular fitness. Among the more popular are ballet, country, disco, folk, hip-hop, Latin (e.g., cha-cha, tango), modern, tap, square, and swing. There are many other forms as well. For dance to be considered active, it should be performed in the target zone for cardiovascular fitness. Less active dance (e.g., slow social dance) is equivalent to a lifestyle activity.

Hiking and Climbing

Like walking and jogging, hiking is a recreational activity that can promote cardiovascular fitness. Hiking has the advantage of an outdoors setting, often in a scenic environment. It requires some equipment, mainly good hiking shoes, but specialized skills are not needed. Backpacking is a form of hiking that usually covers longer distances and involves an overnight stay, often in the mountains. Rock climbing is another popular recreation

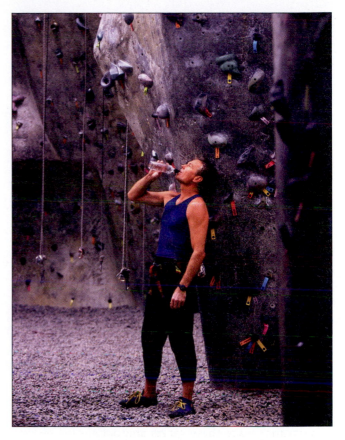

Indoor rock climbing walls are a popular exercise option.

activity that requires considerable strength, muscle endurance, and flexibility. Special skills are required for this activity, so a training course is recommended.

Skiing

Cross-country (Nordic skiing) was described in the active aerobics section. Cross-country and other forms of skiing can also be considered active recreation. For example, downhill (Alpine) skiing and snowboarding are active recreation activities that can be classified at the second level of the pyramid.

Rowing, Canoeing, and Kayaking

Rowing, canoeing, and kayaking are recreational activities that can be done at a leisurely pace or at a more vigorous pace. When done continuously for periods of 10 minutes or longer and with an intensity in the target zone, these activities are classified as a type of active recreation that produces benefits similar to those of active aerobics. When done at a leisurely pace with more floating than paddling or rowing, the activities are more appropriately considered to be similar to lifestyle physical activity.

Active Sport Activities

Some sports are more active than others. Some sports require more activity than others. Activities that involve muscles from different parts of the body are more active than those that involve fewer muscles. Some are of high intensity and others are less intense. When done vigorously, tennis and basketball involve many different muscle groups and are high in intensity. Soccer is an activity that involves many muscle groups and is high in intensity but does not emphasize the use of the arms. Golf, on the other hand, is less intense, and it relies more on skill and technique. The action in basketball, tennis, and soccer involves bursts of activity followed by rest but requires persistent vigorous activity over a relatively long period of time. Golf requires little vigorous activity. Sports that have characteristics similar to those of basketball, tennis, and soccer have similar benefits to active aerobic activities. Of course, any given sport can be more or less active, depending on how you perform the activity. Shooting baskets or even playing half-court basketball is not as vigorous as a full-court game.

The most popular sports share characteristics that contribute to their popularity. The most popular sports (see Table 1) are often considered to be lifetime sports because they can be done at any age. The characteristics that make these sports appropriate for lifelong participation probably contribute significantly to their popularity. Four of the top five are individual sports that do not require a large group of people to participate. Often the popular sports are adapted so people without exceptional skill can play them. For example, bowling uses a handicap system to allow people with a wide range of abilities to compete. Slow-pitch softball is much more popular than fast-pitch softball or baseball because it allows people of all abilities to play successfully.

One of the primary reasons sports participation is so popular is that sports provide a challenge. For the greatest enjoyment, the challenge of the activity should be balanced by the person's skill in the sport. If you choose to play against a person with lesser skill, you will not be challenged. On the other hand, if you lack skill or your opponent has considerably more skill, the activity will be frustrating. For optimal challenge and enjoyment, the skills of a given sport should be learned before competing. Likewise, choose an opponent who has a similar skill level.

There are benefits to watching and participating in sports. Active involvement in sports can have many physical, social, and personal benefits. Though watching sports will not build physical fitness, it does have other benefits. According to recent research, watching sports almost always makes people feel happy when their team wins and gives them a feeling of accomplishment and pride, even though they did not participate. On the downside, when the favorite team loses, feelings of depression and lack of accomplishment may occur. In extreme cases, displays of poor sportsmanship and even violence have occurred. Celebrations that have resulted in property destruction and violence after NCAA and NBA championship victories are examples.

Becoming skillful will help you enjoy sports. Improving your performance skill can increase the probability that you will perform sports for a lifetime. The following self-management guidelines can help you improve your sport performance:

- *When learning a new activity, concentrate on the general idea of the skill first; worry about details later.* For example, a diver who concentrates on pointing the toes and keeping the legs straight at the end of a flip may land flat on his or her back. To make it all the way over, the diver should concentrate on merely doing the flip. When the general idea is mastered, then concentrate on details.
- *The beginner should be careful not to emphasize too many details at one time.* After the general idea of the skill is acquired, the learner can begin to focus on the details, one or two at a time. Concentration on too many details at one time may result in **paralysis by analysis.** For example, a golfer who is told to keep the head down, the left arm straight, and the knees bent cannot possibly concentrate on all of these details at once. As a result, neither the details nor the general idea of the golf swing is performed properly.
- *Once the general idea of a skill is learned, a skill analysis of the performance may be helpful.* Be careful not to over-analyze; it may be helpful to have a knowledgeable

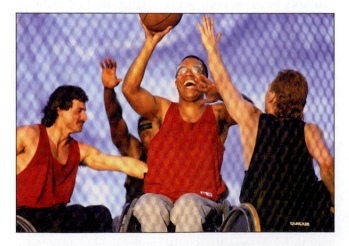

Sports can be effective in promoting fitness and health.

person help you locate strengths and weaknesses. Movies and videotapes of skilled performances can be helpful to learners.

- *In the early stages of learning a lifetime sport or physical activity, it is not wise to engage in competition.* Beginners who compete are likely to concentrate on beating their opponent rather than on learning a skill properly. For example, in bowling, the beginner may abandon the newly learned hook ball in favor of the sure thing straight ball. This may make the person more successful immediately, but is not likely to improve the person's bowling skills for the future.

- *To be performed well, sports skills must be overlearned.* Oftentimes, when you learn a new activity, you begin to play the game immediately. The best way to learn a skill is to overlearn it, or practice it until it becomes habit. Frequently, games do not allow you to overlearn skills. For example, during a tennis match is not a good time to learn how to serve because there may be only a few opportunities to do so. For the beginner, it is much more productive to hit many serves (overlearn) with a friend until the general idea of the serve is well learned. Further, the beginner *should not* sacrifice speed to concentrate on serving for accuracy. Accuracy will come with practice of a properly performed skill.

- *When unlearning an old (incorrect) skill and learning a new (correct) skill, a person's performance may get worse before it gets better.* For example, a golfer with a baseball swing may want to learn the correct golf swing. It is impor-

tant for the learner to understand that the score may worsen during the relearning stage. As the new skill is overlearned, skill will improve, as will the golf score.

- *Mental practice may aid skill learning.* Mental practice (imagining the performance of a skill) may benefit performance, especially if the performer has had previous experience in the skill. Mental practice can be especially useful in sports when the performer cannot participate regularly because of weather, business, or lack of time.

- *For beginners, practicing in front of other people may be detrimental to learning a skill.* An audience may inhibit the beginner's learning of a new sports skill. This is especially true if the learner feels that his or her performance is being evaluated by someone in the audience.

- *There is no substitute for good instruction.* Getting good instruction, especially at the beginning level, will help you learn skills faster and better. Instruction will help you apply these rules and use practice more effectively.

> **Paralysis by Analysis** An overanalysis of skill behavior. This occurs when more information is supplied than a performer can use or when concentration on too many details results in interference with performance.
>
> **Self-Promoting Activities** Activities that do not require a high level of skill to be successful.

Strategies for Action

You can take steps to become successful in physical activity. You can use self-management skills to help enjoy activities at the second level of the pyramid:

- *Improve your performance skills.* Consider taking lessons and practice the skills you want to learn. Using the guidelines listed earlier in this concept.

- *Select self-promoting activities.* **Self-promoting activities** require relatively little skill and can be done in a way that avoids comparison with other people. They allow you to set your own standards of success and can be done individually or in small groups that are suited to your personal needs. Examples include wheelchair distance events, jogging, resistance training, swimming, bicycling, and dance exercise.

- *Change your way of thinking.* Change your way of thinking to increase positive feelings about yourself. Avoid self-criticism and resist negative feelings if you do not

perform as well as others. The key is to reward yourself for being active—it's what you do that counts.

- *Develop a plan for performing level 2 activities.* All people are not equally good at all activities. Virtually all people can find something in which they can succeed. Lab 9A helps you try jogging. In Lab 9B, you can plan level two activities. You may do these activities instead of lifestyle physical activities or in addition to them.

- *Self-monitor your activity to help you stick with your plan.* Self-monitoring is a self-management skill that can be valuable in encouraging long-term activity adherence. A self-monitoring chart is provided in Lab 9B to help you log the activities you perform in a 1-week period. This is a short-term record sheet. However, it can be copied to make a log book to allow long-term self-monitoring. Consider using a heart rate monitor to help you determine self-monitor level 2 activities (see Concept 8).

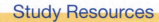

Web Resources

American Council on Exercise **www.acefitness.org**
American Running Association **www.americanrunning.org**
Disabled Sports USA **www.dsusa.org**
National Association for Sports and Physical Education
      www.aahperd.org/naspe/
Ordering information for GPS system **www.timex.com**
President's Council on Physical Fitness and Sports
      www.fitness.gov
Special Olympics International **www.specialolympics.org**
Sport Quest **www.sportQuest.com**
X Sports **www.expn.com**

Suggested Readings

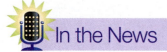 Additional reference materials for Concept 9 are available at **www.mhhe.com/phys_fit/web09 Click 09.**

Aggens, A., and C. Townsend. 2003. *Encyclopedia of Outdoor and Wilderness Skills.* Camden, ME: Ragged Mountain Press.

Brown, R. 2003. *Fitness Running.* 2nd ed. Champaign, IL: Human Kinetics.

Burke, E. 2003. *High-Tech Cycling.* 2nd ed. Champaign, IL: Human Kinetics.

Cochran, J., and J. Graden. 2001. *The Ultimate Martial Arts Question and Answer Book.* New York: McGraw-Hill.

Cooper, K. H. 1982. *The Aerobics Program for Total Well-Being.* New York: M. Evans.

Decker, J., and M. Mize. 2002. *Walking Games and Activities.* Champaign, IL: Human Kinetics.

Dinoffer, J. 2003. *Tennis Practice Games.* Champaign, IL: Human Kinetics.

Elling, R. 2002. *All-Mountain Skier.* New York: McGraw-Hill.

Kestenbaum, R. 2001. *The Ultralight Backpacker: The Complete Guide to Simplicity and Comfort on the Trail.* St. Louis: McGraw-Hill.

Lee, B. 2003. *Jump Rope Training.* Champaign, IL: Human Kinetics.

Magill, R. A. 2004. *Motor Learning: Concepts and Applications.* 7th ed. St. Louis: McGraw-Hill.

Maglischo, E. 2003. *Swimming Fastest.* Champaign, IL: Human Kinetics.

Miller, L. 2003. *Get Rolling: A Beginners Guide to In-Line Skating.* Camden, ME: Ragged Mountain Press.

Pryor, E. 2000. *Keep Moving: Fitness through Aerobics and Step.* 4th ed. St. Louis: McGraw-Hill.

U.S. Consumer Product Safety Commission. 2000. Baby boomer sports injuries. **www.cpsc.gov.**

Walker, J. 2003. *Self-Defense Techniques and Tactics.* Champaign, IL: Human Kinetics.

In the News

Aerobic Exercise Machines

The popularity of sports and recreation continues to grow in the United States. The Sporting Goods Manufacturing Association estimates that overall sales of U.S. recreational products is about $70 billion a year and the largest category of sports equipment is personal exercise machines ($3.8 billion). Treadmills account for over 25 percent of the total sales in this category, with the next largest contributions coming from home gyms and exercise cycles. The sale of elliptical trainers increased by 17 percent, indicating that this is becoming a more popular type of machine.

While some of the equipment is purchased for home use, the majority of purchases are probably by commercial or corporate fitness centers. These centers compete to keep people interested in their facilities and regularly upgrade their equipment to provide the latest technology to their clients. A trend in recent years has

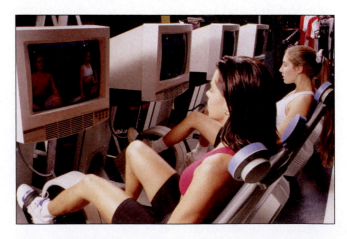

been the development of video-based exercise machines that allow pacing and even competition with other exercisers (see photo).

Lab 9A Jogging/Running

Name	**Section**	**Date**

Purpose: To give you an opportunity to experience one type of jogging program that can be used to develop and maintain cardiovascular fitness and to acquaint you with basic jogging techniques

Procedure

1. Work with a partner and evaluate each other on jogging techniques.
   a. Stand 20 yards in front of your partner while he or she jogs toward you; watch his/her arm and leg swing and foot placement.
   b. Jog along 10 yards behind your partner while he or she is jogging and watch for arm and leg swing and foot placement.
   c. Stand 10 yards to one side as your partner jogs past you; watch for body position and foot placement.
   d. Change places with your partner and repeat this procedure.
2. Check the appropriate Correct or Incorrect boxes in Chart 1.
3. Using proper jogging technique, jog for 15 minutes at your own cardiovascular threshold of training. You may use a heart rate monitor or count postexercise heart rate to determine jogging heart rate.

Results

Record your target zone heart rate here. _____ bpm

Record your heart rate after the jog. _____ bpm

Have your partner evaluate your jogging technique and then record your results in Chart 1.

Chart 1 ▶ Jogging Technique

Body Segment	Check Appropriate Circles		Technique
	Correct	Incorrect	
Foot placement	○	○	Heel hits ground first
	○	○	Rock forward, push off ball of foot
	○	○	Toes point straight ahead
	○	○	Feet under knees, do not swing side to side
Length of stride	○	○	Stride several inches longer than regular step
Arm movement	○	○	Elbows bent at 90 degrees
	○	○	Arms swing front to back, not side to side
	○	○	Arms and legs move in opposition
	○	○	Hands and arms are relaxed
Body position	○	○	Upper body nearly erect
	○	○	Head and chest are up

Conclusions and Implications

1. In several sentences, give an overall evaluation of your jogging technique.

2. In several sentences, indicate whether jogging is an appropriate activity for you. Indicate your reasons for your answer.

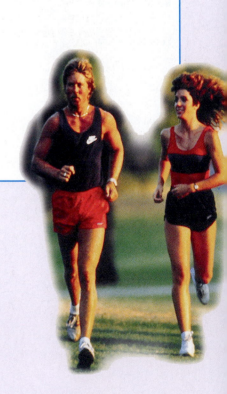

Lab 9B Planning and Logging Participation in Active Aerobics, Sports, and Recreation

Name		Section	Date

Purpose: To set 1-week lifestyle physical activity goals, to prepare a plan, and to self-monitor progress in your 1-week active aerobics, active sports, and active recreation plan

Procedures

1. Use the planning calendar (Chart 1) to schedule several aerobic exercise sessions for the week. Plan at least three sessions, but be realistic in your plan. Schedule activities that you enjoy and that you can perform conveniently. You may mix different activities each day for variety. Indicate the days you expect to do them, and the length of time you expect to do the activity.
2. Keep a 1-week log of your actual participation using Chart 2. If possible, keep the log with you during the day. Anytime you perform an activity for 10 minutes, check one of the boxes. If you perform more than 10 minutes of activity in one session, check additional 10-minute blocks. If you cannot keep the log with you, fill in the log at the end of the day. If you choose to keep a log for more than 1 week, use the extra log (Chart 3) or make copies of the extra log sheet.
3. Log only those activities for which you meet the target zone for cardiovascular fitness. Remember that 5 or 6, rather than 7, days a week of more vigorous activity is recommended. You can create a log book using several log sheets.
4. Sum the total number of minutes for each day by tallying the number of activity blocks.
5. Answer the questions in the Results section.

Chart 1 ▶ Planning Calendar

Write the number of minutes you plan to do each activity each day: You may mix activities each day.	Monday	Tuesday	Wednesday	Thursday	Friday	Saturday	Sunday
Aerobic exercise machines							
Cycling (including stationary)							
Circuit training or calisthenics							
Dance or step aerobics							
Hiking or backpacking							
Jogging or running (or walking)							
Skating/cross-country skiing							
Swimming							
Water activity							
Sport							
Other							
Other							
Daily totals							

Results

	Yes	No
Did you do 20 or more minutes at each session?	○	○
Did you do 20 or more minutes of activity on at least 3 days?	○	○

Conclusions and Interpretations

1. Do you feel that you will use active aerobics, active sports, or active recreation as a regular part of your lifetime physical activity plan, either now or in the future? Use several sentences to explain your answer.

2. Did the logging of your activity make you more aware of your daily activity patterns? In several sentences, explain why or why not.

Chart 2 ▶ Aerobic Activity Log

Record the type and length of each activity you performed.	10-Minute Blocks						Total Minutes	Comments*
Day 1 Date:	1	2	3	4	5	6		
Activity:								
Activity:								
Activity:								
Daily Total								
Day 2 Date:	1	2	3	4	5	6		
Activity:								
Activity:								
Activity:								
Daily Total								
Day 3 Date:	1	2	3	4	5	6		
Activity:								
Activity:								
Activity:								
Daily Total								
Day 4 Date:	1	2	3	4	5	6		
Activity:								
Activity:								
Activity:								
Daily Total								
Day 5 Date:	1	2	3	4	5	6		
Activity:								
Activity:								
Activity:								
Daily Total								
Day 6 Date:	1	2	3	4	5	6		
Activity:								
Activity:								
Activity:								
Daily Total								

*Optional: Record heart rate, pace, calories, or other details of your session.

Chart 3 ► Extra Aerobic Activity Log

Record the type and length of each activity you performed.

	10-Minute Blocks						Total Minutes	Comments*
Day 1 Date:	1	2	3	4	5	6		
Activity:								
Activity:								
Activity:								
Daily Total								
Day 2 Date:	1	2	3	4	5	6		
Activity:								
Activity:								
Activity:								
Daily Total								
Day 3 Date:	1	2	3	4	5	6		
Activity:								
Activity:								
Activity:								
Daily Total								
Day 4 Date:	1	2	3	4	5	6		
Activity:								
Activity:								
Activity:								
Daily Total								
Day 5 Date:	1	2	3	4	5	6		
Activity:								
Activity:								
Activity:								
Daily Total								
Day 6 Date:	1	2	3	4	5	6		
Activity:								
Activity:								
Activity:								
Daily Total								

*Optional: Record heart rate, pace, calories, or other details of your session.

Flexibility

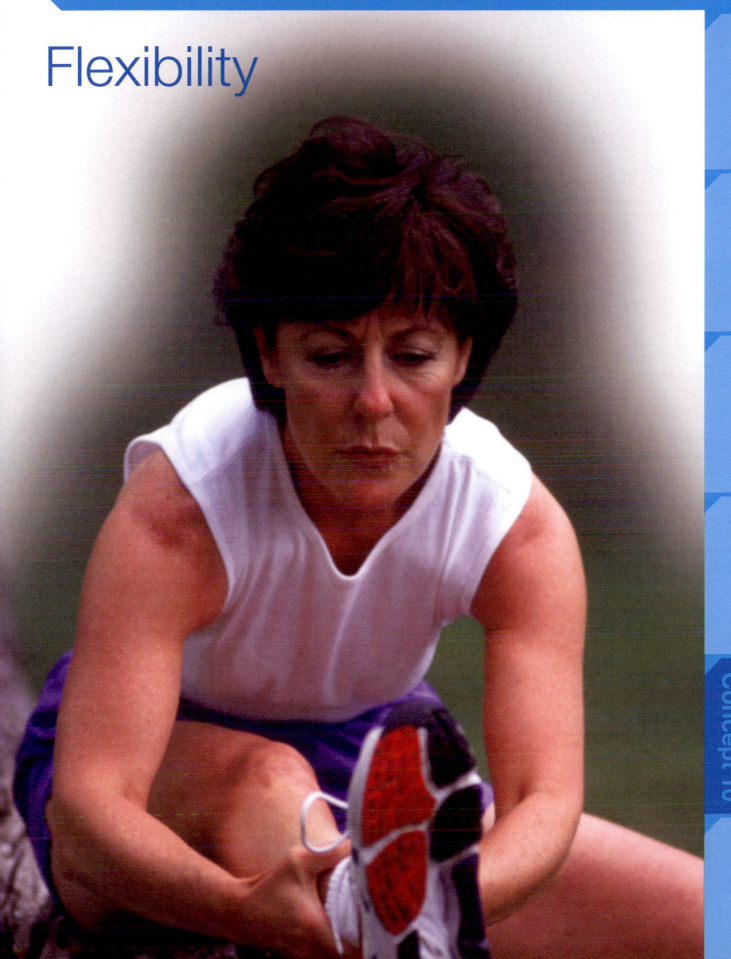

Regular stretching exercises promote flexibility—a component of fitness—that permits freedom of movement, contributes to ease and economy of muscular effort, allows for successful performance in certain activities, and provides less susceptibility to some types of injuries or musculoskeletal problems.

Health Goals

for the year 2010

- Increase proportion of people who regularly perform exercises for flexibility.

lexibility is a measure of the range of motion available at a joint or group of joints. It is determined by the shape of the bones and cartilage in the joint and by the length and extensibility of muscles, tendons, ligaments, and fascia that cross the joint. The range of movement at a joint may vary. In some cases, a joint has limited ability to bend or straighten and is said to be tight or stiff. The deformed hand of an arthritic is an example of this extreme. At the other end of the spectrum, a high degree of flexibility is referred to as loose jointedness, hypermobility, or erroneously as double-jointedness. An example of this extreme is the contortionist seen at the circus. Each person, depending upon his or her individual needs, must have a reasonable amount of flexibility to perform efficiently and effectively in daily life. The many types of stretching exercises designed to promote or maintain flexibility are described in this concept.

Flexibility is not the same thing as stretching. Flexibility is a component of health-related physical fitness. It is a state of being. Stretching is the primary technique used to improve the state of one's flexibility.

Each type of joint has a different range of motion. The **range of motion** in a joint is influenced most directly by the joint structure. A triaxial joint, such as the ball and socket joint in the hip (see Figure 1) and shoulder, allows for considerable range of motion. These joints can move to the side (adduction and abduction) and forward

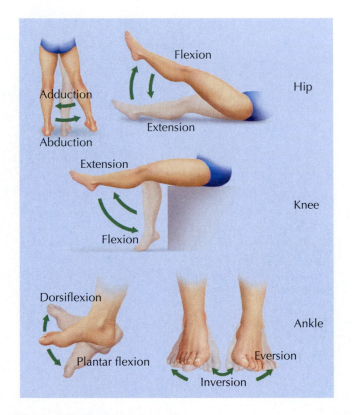

Figure 1 ▶ Ranges of joint motion.

and backward (flexion and extension). They also allow rotation such as moving your foot and leg in a circular motion (not pictured). Uniaxial joints, such as those in the knee (see Figure 1) and elbow, can move only forward and return to the original position (extension and flexion).

The ankle (see Figure 1) and wrist joints have many bones that can be moved in many directions. The ankle, for example, allows the foot to be pointed away from the body (plantar flexion) and to be flexed toward the shin (dorsiflexion). The ankle can also be turned so the sole of the foot faces toward the center of the body (inversion) or away from the body (eversion). A combination of these movements at this joint allows for rotation (not pictured).

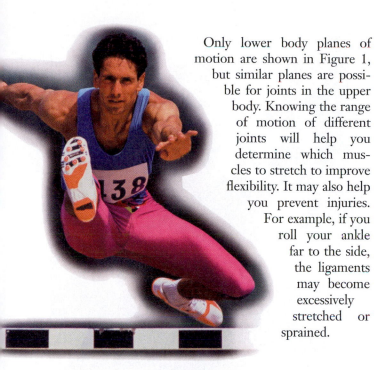

Only lower body planes of motion are shown in Figure 1, but similar planes are possible for joints in the upper body. Knowing the range of motion of different joints will help you determine which muscles to stretch to improve flexibility. It may also help you prevent injuries. For example, if you roll your ankle far to the side, the ligaments may become excessively stretched or sprained.

Flexibility aids athletic performance and may help reduce injury risk.

Factors Influencing Flexibility

Long muscle-tendon units (MTUs) are important to flexibility. Range of motion (ROM) in a joint is an indicator of one's flexibility. Joint ROM is influenced by the extensibility of **ligaments,** the surrounding muscles, and the **tendons** that connect the muscles to the bone. Having long muscles and tendons allows for greater range of motion and better flexibility. Together, the muscles and tendons are referred to as a **muscle-tendon unit (MTU).** Muscle fibers are more extensible and elastic than tendons but both are stretched together. However, for ease of understanding, the phrase "muscle stretching" rather than MTU stretching will be used.

Flexibility varies considerable across the life span. Flexibility is generally high in children but declines during adolescence because of the rapid changes in growth—essentially, the bones grow faster than the MTU. In early adulthood, the MTU catches up to the skeletal system, causing flexibility to peak in the mid- to late-twenties. With increasing age, range of motion tends to decline again. The reduced flexibility is due to a loss of elasticity in the MTU and cross-linkages within the collagen fibers of the tendons, ligaments, and joint capsules. Over the span of their working lives, adults typically lose 3 to 4 inches of lower back flexibility as measured by the common "sit and reach" test. In extreme old age, osteoarthritis can severely limit flexibility and make physical activity uncomfortable and even painful. Regular stretching can help people maintain good flexibility throughout life.

Gender differences exist in flexibility. Girls tend to be more flexible than boys at young ages, but the gender difference becomes smaller for adults. The greater flexibility of females is generally attributed to anatomical differences (e.g., wider hips) and hormonal influences. Preferred activity patterns may also explain some of the difference as females tend to be involved in sports and activities that require good flexibility and involve regular stretching (e.g., dance, gymnastics, swimming).

Genetic factors can explain some individual variability in flexibility. In some families, the trait for loose joints is passed from generation to generation. This **hypermobility** is sometimes referred to as joint looseness. Studies show that people with this trait may be more prone to joint dislocation. There is not much research evidence, but some experts believe that those with hypermobility, or **laxity** may also be more susceptible to athletic or dance injuries, especially to the knee, ankle, and shoulder, and may be more apt to develop premature osteoarthritis.

Lack of use or misuse can cause reductions in flexibility. The large declines in flexibility with age are not as evident in individuals who maintain regular patterns of physical activity. Planned stretching programs can also help to maintain flexibility with age.

Improper exercise that overdevelops one muscle group while neglecting the opposing group can lead to a shortening of muscles and ligaments. For example, bodybuilders who overdevelop their biceps in comparison to the triceps develop a *muscle-bound* look characterized by a restricted range of motion in the elbow joint. To avoid this, it is important to exercise muscles through the full range of motion and to provide sufficient exercise for the **antagonist muscles** involved in a specific movement.

Range of Motion (ROM) The full motion possible in a joint.

Ligaments Bands of tissue that connect bones. Unlike muscles and tendons, overstretching ligaments is not desirable.

Tendons Fibrous bands of tissue that connect muscles to bones and facilitate movement of a joint.

Muscle-Tendon Unit (MTU) The skeletal muscles and the tendons that connect them to bones. Stretching to improve flexibility is associated with increased length of the MTU.

Hypermobility Looseness or slackness in the joint and of the muscles and ligaments (soft tissue) surrounding the joint.

Laxity Motion in a joint outside the normal plane for that joint, due to loose ligaments.

Health Benefits of Flexibility and Stretching

No ideal standard for flexibility exists. We do not know how much flexibility any one person should have in a joint. Norms are available that list how hundreds of subjects of various ages, of both sexes, and in many walks of life have performed on different tests. But there is little scientific evidence to indicate that a person who can reach 2 inches past his or her toes on a sit-and-reach test is less fit than a person who can reach 8 inches past the toes. Too much flexibility could be as detrimental as too little. The standards presented in the *Lab Resource Materials* are based on the best available evidence.

Adequate flexibility is necessary for achieving and maintaining optimal posture. Short and tight muscles in certain body regions can result in poor posture. Shortness of muscles of the chest and back of the neck can result in "rounded shoulders" and a "forward head" position. Tightness of the hip flexor muscles can result in excessive lordosis, or arching, of the low back.

Extremes of inflexibility and hyperflexibility increase the likelihood of injury. Research linking stretching to the prevention of injury has been equivocal, with some studies showing benefits but others not. A recent critical review of this literature (see Thacker et al., 2004) reported that the problems lie in the extremes. Short, tight muscles and tendons are more likely to be involuntarily overstretched (strained) than long ones. However, excess flexibility can compromise the integrity of the joint capsule and increase tissue compliance to an extent that injuries are more likely. An appropriate amount of flexibility provides benefits without the risks. For individual bouts of activity, a good cardiovascular warm-up is definitely more important than a pre-exercise bout of stretching.

Adequate flexibility may help prevent muscle strain and such orthopedic problems as backache. Back pain is a leading medical complaint in Western culture. One common cause of backache is shortened lower back muscles and hip flexor muscles. Short hamstrings (muscles in the back of the leg) are also associated with lower back problems. Improving flexibility can decrease risk for back problems.

Good flexibility can improve performance, but stretching prior to competition is not recommended. Proper stretching can increase muscle length, reduce **stiffness,** and increase **stretch tolerance,** leading most experts to agree that regular stretching and improved flexibility can enhance athletic performance. For example, a diver must have flexibility to perform a

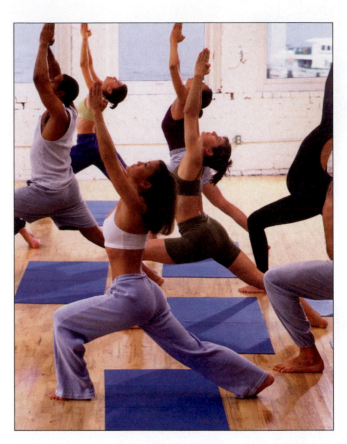

Yoga and other movement classes involving stretching are becoming increasingly popular.

pike dive and a hurdler must have good flexibility in the back, hip, and leg to perform well. The most recent evidence, however, suggests that under some circumstances stretching can actually impair performance. Excessive stretching during warm-ups has been shown to reduce strength performance, jumping height, and running economy. Similar to the literature on injuries, the consensus is that excessive flexibility and/or too much stretching prior to competition may negatively affect performance. A stretching warm-up is still recommended after a general warm-up, but the warm-up period is not the time to conduct an extensive flexibility program—especially for those preparing for high-level performance. Stretching to improve flexibility should be conducted at the end of training, when the muscles are warm and performance is not imminent.

Static muscle stretching is effective in relieving muscle spasms. A muscle spasm or cramp may result for various reasons, including overexertion, dehydration, and heat stress. Stretching a cramped (but not a strained) muscle will help relieve the cramp. Stretching should be done statically and can be done with active or passive assistance, though passive assistance should be applied carefully. For example, a person with a cramp or spasm in the calf muscle can pull the toe toward the shin using the shin muscles, or a partner can push the ball of the foot toward the shin to get the same benefit.

Trigger points may be prevented or inactivated by static or PNF stretching of the muscles involved. When body parts are held in static positions for long periods, or when muscles are chronically overloaded, fatigued, or chilled, **trigger points** may cause stiffness and local or referred pain. Often, the trigger point can be deactivated and the pain relieved by gentle but persistent stretching of the muscle, especially if heat or cold packs are applied.

Stretching exercises are useful in preventing and remediating some cases of dysmenorrhea in women. Painful menstruation (dysmenorrhea) of some types can be prevented or reduced by stretching the pelvic and hip joint fascia. Billig's exercise is an example of an effective exercise for this condition.

Static stretching is probably *ineffective* in preventing muscle soreness. In the past, it was suggested that stretching during a cool-down will *prevent* muscular soreness. In a controlled study, muscle soreness was deliberately induced in a group of subjects. When half of the group stretched immediately afterward and at intervals for 48 hours, they had as much soreness as the group who did not stretch.

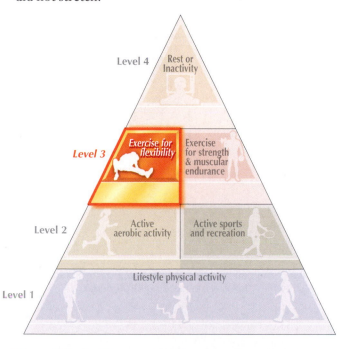

Figure 2 ▶ Flexibility or stretching exercises should be selected from level 3 of the physical activity pyramid.

Stretching Methods

To develop flexibility, do exercises from the flexibility exercise section of the physical activity pyramid. The activities in the first two levels of the physical activity pyramid (see Figure 2) do little to develop flexibility. To build this important part of fitness, stretching exercises from the third level of the pyramid are essential. Three commonly used types of stretching exercises are **static stretch, proprioceptive neuromuscular facilitation (PNF) exercise,** and **ballistic stretch.**

Static stretching is widely recommended because most experts believe it is less likely to cause injury. Static stretching is done slowly and held for a period of several seconds. With this type of stretch, the probability of tearing the soft tissue is low if performed properly. Static stretches can be performed with **active assistance** or with **passive assistance.**

When active assistance is used, you contract the opposing muscle group to produce a reflex relaxation **(reciprocal inhibition)** in the muscles you are stretching. This enables you to stretch the muscle more easily. For example, when doing a calf stretch exercise (see Figure 3A), the

Antagonist Muscles In this concept, *antagonist* refers to the muscle group on the opposite side of the limb from the muscle group being stretched (e.g., biceps is antagonist of triceps).

Stiffness Elasticity in the MTU; measured by force needed to stretch.

Stretch Tolerance Greater stretch for the same pain level.

Trigger Points Especially irritable spots, usually tight bands or knots in a muscle or fascia (a sheath of connective tissue that binds muscles and other tissues together). Trigger points often refers pain to another area of the body.

Static Stretch A muscle is slowly stretched, then held in that stretched position for several seconds.

Proprioceptive Neuromuscular Facilitation (PNF) Exercise A type of static stretch most commonly characterized by a precontraction of the muscle to be stretched and a contraction of the antagonist muscle during the stretch.

Ballistic Stretch Muscles are stretched by the force of momentum of a body part that is bounced, swung, or jerked.

Active Assistance An assist to stretch from an active contraction of the opposing (antagonist) muscle.

Passive Assistance Stretch imposed on a muscle with the assistance of a force other than the opposing muscle.

Reciprocal Inhibition Reflex relaxation in stretched muscle during contraction of the antagonist.

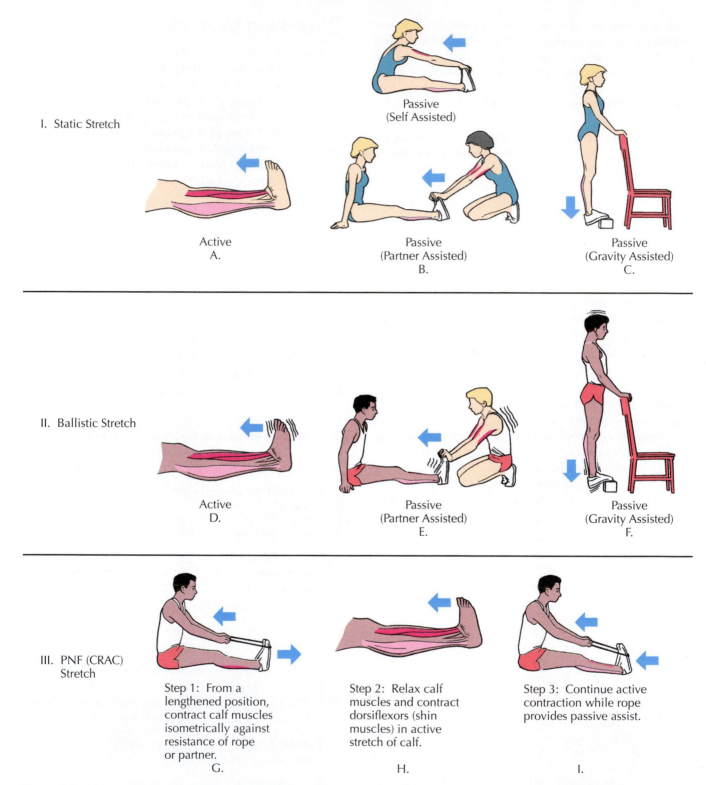

I. Static Stretch

Passive
(Self Assisted)

Active
A.

Passive
(Partner Assisted)
B.

Passive
(Gravity Assisted)
C.

II. Ballistic Stretch

Active
D.

Passive
(Partner Assisted)
E.

Passive
(Gravity Assisted)
F.

III. PNF (CRAC)
Stretch

Step 1: From a lengthened position, contract calf muscles isometrically against resistance of rope or partner.
G.

Step 2: Relax calf muscles and contract dorsiflexors (shin muscles) in active stretch of calf.
H.

Step 3: Continue active contraction while rope provides passive assist.
I.

Figure 3 ▶ Examples of static, ballistic, PNF, active, and passive stretches of the calf muscles (gastrocnemius and soleus). Muscles shown in dark pink are the muscles being contracted. Muscles shown in pink are those being stretched.

muscles on the front of the shin are contracted to assist in the stretch of the muscles of the calf. For this reason, many experts prefer static stretch with active assistance. However, active assistance to static stretching has one problem. It is almost impossible to produce adequate overload by simply contracting the opposing muscles.

When passive assistance (see Figures 3B, C) is used, an outside force, such as a partner, aids you in stretching. For example, in the calf stretch, passive assistance can be provided by another person (Figure 3B), another body part (Figure 3B), or gravity (Figure 3C). This type of stretch does not create the relaxation in the muscle associated with active assisted stretch. An unrelaxed muscle cannot be stretched as far, and injury may happen. Therefore, it is best to combine the active assistance with a passive assistance when performing a static stretch. This gives the advantage of a relaxed muscle and a sufficient force to provide an overload to stretch it.

A good way to begin static stretching exercises is to stretch until you begin to feel tension, back off slightly and hold the position several seconds, and then gradually stretch a little farther, back off, and hold. Decrease the stretch slowly after the hold.

PNF techniques have proven to be most effective at improving flexibility. www.mhhe.com/phys_fit/web10 Click 01. PNF has been popular for rehabilitation since the 1960s. It consists of dozens of techniques to stimulate muscles to contract more strongly or to relax more fully so that they can be stretched. Several PNF techniques have become popular in fitness programs to improve the flexibility of healthy people. The contract-relax-antagonist-contract (CRAC) technique is the most popular. CRAC PNF involves three steps: (1) move the limb so the muscle to be stretched is elongated initially; then contract it **(agonist muscle)** isometrically for several seconds (against an immovable object or the resistance of a partner); (2) relax the muscle; and (3) immediately statically stretch the muscle with the active assistance of the antagonist muscle and an assist from a partner, gravity, or another body part. Figures 3G, H, and I provide a detailed illustration of how this technique is applied to the calf stretch. Research shows that this and other types of PNF stretch are more effective than a simple static stretch.

Ballistic stretching is not recommended for most people. A ballistic stretch uses momentum to produce the stretch. Momentum is produced by vigorous motion, such as flinging a body part (bobbing) or rocking it back and forth to create a bouncing movement. As with static stretching, the ballistic movement can be provided either actively or passively. For example, in the calf stretch shown in Figures 3D, E, and F, the foot is actively bounced forward by the antagonist muscle force or passively by an assist from another person or gravity. The

forceful movement in ballistic stretching may increase risks for injury. Therefore, this form of stretching is not recommended for most people.

The inherent problem with most ballistic stretching is the lack of control over the force and range of movement. Experts have begun to characterize *dynamic stretching* as a safe derivative of ballistic stretching. This form of stretching uses gradual and controlled movement of body parts up to the limit of a joint's range of motion. Stretches may involve arm or leg swings of increasing reach or increasing speed. The key is to perform the movement in a controlled manner through the normal range of motion. This approach allows dynamic stretching to be a safe and efficient means to utilize active stretching techniques.

How Much Stretch Is Enough

Stretching exercises should be done regularly to achieve optimal benefits. Threshold and target zones for each type of stretching to improve and maintain flexibility are presented in Table 1. The values in this table illustrate how the principles of overload and progression are best applied to promote and maintain flexibility through regular stretching.

Note that stretching should be done at least three times a week and that daily stretching is preferable. Evidence suggests that even 1 week without stretching can lead to decreases in muscle length and increases in stiffness, so it is important to develop a regular routine of stretching. However, like other forms of activity, 1 day is clearly better than none.

To increase the length of a muscle, you must stretch it more than its normal length (overload) but not overstretch it. www.mhhe.com/phys_fit/web10 Click 02. The best evidence suggests that muscles should be stretched to about 10 percent beyond their normal length to bring about an improvement in flexibility. More practical indicators of the intensity of stretching are to stretch just to the point of tension or just before discomfort. Exercises that do not cause an overload will not increase flexibility. Once adequate flexibility has been achieved, **range of motion (ROM) exercises** that do not require stretch greater than normal can be performed to maintain flexibility and joint range of motion.

Agonist Muscle Muscle group being stretched.

Range of Motion (ROM) Exercises Exercises used to maintain existing joint mobility (to prevent loss of ROM).

Table 1 ▶ Flexibility Threshold of Training and Target Zones

	Threshold of Training			Target Zones		
	Static	Ballistic	PNF (CRAC)	Static	Ballistic	PNF (CRAC)
Frequency	• 3 days per week for all methods			• 3 to 7 days per week for all methods		
Intensity	• Stretch as far as you can without pain; with slow movement, hold at the end of the range of motion.	• Stretch muscle beyond normal length with gentle bounce or swing, but do not exceed 10 percent of active-static range of motion.	• Same as static except use a maximum isometric contraction of muscle prior to stretch	• Add assist. • Avoid overstretch and pain for all methods.	• Same as threshold	• Same as static • Add assist.
Time	• Hold 15 seconds. • 3 reps • Rest 30 seconds between reps.	• Continuous reps for 30 seconds (this is 1 set)	• Hold isometric contraction 3 seconds. • Hold stretch 15 seconds. • 3 reps • Rest 30 seconds between reps.	• Hold 15–60 seconds. • 3–5 reps • Rest 30 seconds between reps. • Rest 1 minute between sets.	• 1–3 sets • Rest 1 minute between sets.	• 3–5 reps of 3-second contraction and 15- to 60-second hold • Rest 30 seconds between reps. • 1–3 sets • Rest 1 minute between sets.

For flexibility to be increased, you must stretch and hold muscles beyond normal length for an adequate amount of time. When a muscle is stretched (lengthened), the stretch reflex acts to resist the stretch (see Figure 4). Sensory receptors (A) in the MTU (muscle tendon unit) send a signal to the sensory neurons (B) and these neurons signal the motor neurons (C) to contract (shorten) the muscles (D). This reflex restricts initial efforts at stretching; however, if the stretch is held and maintained over time, the stretch reflex subsides and allows the muscle to lengthen (this phase is called the

development phase because it is at this time that improvements occur). This reflex is important to understand because it explains why it is important to hold a stretch for an extended period of time. Attempts to stretch for shorter durations are limited by the opposing action of the stretch reflex (see Figure 4). In the past, stretches of 10 to 30 seconds were recommended. New studies, however, suggest that, to get the most benefit for the least effort, stretching for at least 15 seconds and up to 30 to 60 seconds for each repetition is recommended (see Figure 5).

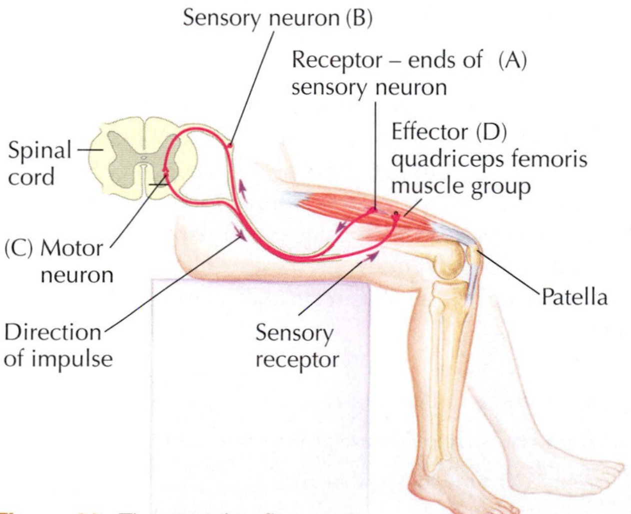

For flexibility to be increased, you must repeat stretching exercises an adequate number of times. Figure 5 provides a graphic representation of the typical responses to a stretched muscle during a series of stretches. Tension in a muscle decreases as the stretch is held. The majority of the decrease occurs in the first 15 seconds. The tension curves are lower with each successive repetition of stretching, which is why multiple sets of stretching are recommended. The ACSM recommends three or four repetitions because this number seems to give the most benefits for the amount of time spent in exercise. Recent evidence suggests that one or two repetitions are adequate for most healthy people not interested in high-level performance.

Performing warm-up exercises is not the same as doing a stretching workout for flexibility development. The warm-up typically includes stretching exercises to prepare you for the workout and to reduce the risk for injury. Modest static stretching exercises done after a general warm-up are recommended by most

Figure 4 ▶ The stretch reflex.
Source: Shier, D., Butler, J., and Lewis, R.

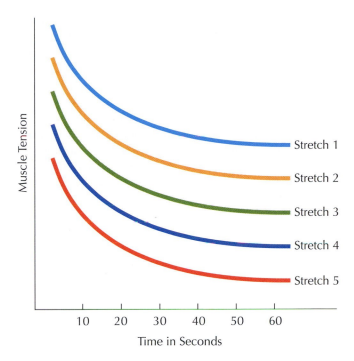

Figure 5 ▶ Typical responses to a stretched muscle during a series of stretches.

experts (see the concept on preparing for physical activity). Stretching exercises are typically done later in the workout to promote flexibility.

The best time for stretching is when the muscles are warm. Some studies have shown that increasing the temperature of the muscle through warm-up exercises or applying heat packs has resulted in improved ability to stretch the muscle. Other studies have failed to find a difference between the flexibility of subjects who warmed up and those who did not warm up. Some experts believe that cooling the muscle with ice packs in the final phases of stretching aids in lengthening the muscle, but a recent study has failed to confirm this. Until scientists reach a consensus, it seems wise to perform the stretching phase of your workout when the muscles are warm. This means that stretching can be done in the middle or near the end of the workout. Since some people do not want to interrupt their workout in the middle, they prefer to stretch at the end. Stretching at the end of the workout serves a dual purpose—building flexibility and cooling down. It is, however, appropriate to stretch at any time in the workout after the muscles have been active and are warm.

Guidelines for Safe and Effective Stretching

 There is a correct way to perform flexibility exercises. www.mhhe.com/phys_fit/web10 Click 03. Remember that stretching can *cause* muscle soreness, so "easy does it." Start at your threshold if you are unaccustomed to stretching a given muscle group, then increase within the target zone. The list in Table 2 will help you to gain the most benefit from your exercises.

Stretching is specific to each muscle or muscle group. No single exercise can produce total flexibility. For example, stretching tight hamstrings can increase the length of these muscles but will not lengthen the

Table 2 ▶ Do and Don't List for Stretching

Do	Don't
Do warm muscles before you attempt to stretch them.	Don't stretch to the point of pain. Remember, you want to stretch muscles, not joints!
Do stretch with care if you have osteoporosis or arthritis.	Don't use ballistic stretches if you have osteoporosis or arthritis.
Do use static or PNF stretching rather than ballistic stretching if you are a beginner.	Don't perform ballistic stretches with passive assistance unless you are under the supervision of an expert.
Do stretch weak or recently injured muscles with care.	Don't ballistically stretch weak or recently injured muscles.
Do use great care in applying passive assistance to a partner; go slowly and ask for feedback.	Don't stretch a muscle after it has been immobilized (such as in a sling or cast) for a long period.
Do perform stretching exercises for each muscle group and at each joint where flexibility is desired.	Don't bounce a muscle through excessive range of motion. Ballistic stretches should be gentle and should not involve excessive range of motion.
Do make certain the body is in good alignment when stretching.	Don't stretch swollen joints without professional supervision.
Do stretch muscles of small joints in the extremities first; then progress toward the trunk with muscles of larger joints.	Don't stretch several muscles all at one time until you have stretched individual muscles. For example, stretch muscles at the ankle, then the knee, then the ankle and knee simultaneously.
Do precede sport-specific ballistic stretch with static or PNF stretching.	

Technology Update

Stretching ropes

An advance in equipment technology for flexibility training is the development of "stretching ropes." These ropes have multiple loops which enable individuals to change the length of the rope and perform a variety of exercises. Because you can apply resistance through the elastic nature of the straps, it is even possible to perform PNF stretching without the assistance of a partner. A variety of stretching ropes are available on the market. One example is the Stretch Out strap available through Orthopedic Physical Therapy Products (OPTP—www.optp.com).

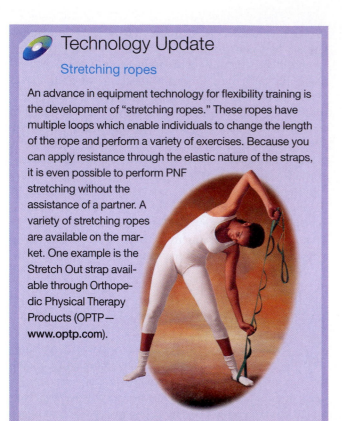

muscles in other areas of the body. For total flexibility, it is important to stretch each of the major muscle groups of the body and to use the major joints of the body through full range of normal motion.

Overstretching may make a person susceptible to injury or hamper performance. Muscles and tendons have the ability to lengthen (extensibility) and to return to their normal length after stretching (elasticity). Ligaments and the joint capsule are extensible but lack elasticity. When stretched, they remain in the lengthened state. If this occurs, the joint may lack stability and is susceptible to chronic dislocation or movement in an undesirable plane. This is particularly true of weight-bearing joints, such as the hip, knee, and ankle. Loose ligaments may allow the joint to twist abnormally, tearing the cartilage and other soft tissue.

Strategies for Action

An important step in taking action for developing and maintaining flexibility is assessing your current status. www.mhhe.com/phys_fit/web10 Click 04. An important early step in taking action to improve fitness is self-assessment. There are dozens of tests of flexibility. Four tests that assess range of motion in the major joints of the body, that require little equipment, and that can be easily administered are presented in the *Lab Resources Materials*. In Lab 10A, you will get an opportunity to try these self-assessments. It is recommended that you perform these assessments before you begin your regular stretching program and use these assessments to reevaluate your flexibility periodically.

Scores on flexibility tests may be influenced by several factors. Your range of motion at any one time may be influenced by your motivation to exert maximum effort, warm-up preparation, muscular soreness, tolerance for pain, room temperature, and ability to relax. Recent studies have found a relationship between leg or trunk length and the scores made on the sit-and-reach test. The sit-and-reach test used in this book is adapted to allow for differences in body build.

Select exercises that promote flexibility in all areas of the body. www.mhhe.com/phys_fit/web10 Click 05. The ACSM recommends that adults regularly perform eight to ten stretching exercises for the major muscle groups of the body. Table 3 provides eight exercises referred to as the Basic 8. These exercises are easy to perform and meet the ACSM guidelines. For most people, these are adequate for building flexibility for health and leisure-time recreational activities. Additional exercises are provided for people who may want alternatives to the Basic 8 or who want to do more than the basic exercises (see Table 4). The exercises presented in Tables 3 and 4 are static stretching exercises that can also be performed using PNF techniques. Ballistic stretching exercises are discussed in more detail in the concept on performance benefits of physical activity.

Keeping records of progress is important to adhering to a stretching program. An activity logging sheet is provided in Lab 10B to help you keep records of your progress as you regularly perform stretching exercises to build and maintain good flexibility.

Study Resources

Check out additional online study resources for this concept in the Student Edition of the Online Learning Center at www.mhhe.com/corbin13e.

Web Resources

Orthopedic Physical Therapy Products (source for stretching ropes) **www.optp.com**
The Physician and Sportsmedicine **www.physsportsmed.com**

Suggested Readings

Additional reference materials for Concept 10 are available at **www.mhhe.com/phys_fit/web10 Click 06.**

Alter, M. J. 1996. *Science of Stretch.* Champaign, IL: Human Kinetics.

Bracko, M. R. 2002. Can stretching prior to exercise and sports improve performance and prevent injury? *ACSM's Health and Fitness Journal* 6(5):17–22.

Chewning, B., T. M. A. Yu, and J. Johnson. 2000. Tai chi: Effects on health. *ACSM's Health and Fitness Journal* 4(3):17–19.

Greiner, S. G., C. Russell, and S. M. McGill. 2003. Relationships between lumbar flexibility, sit-and-reach test, and a previous history of low back pain in industrial workers. *Canadian Journal of Applied Physiology* 28(2):165–171.

Hootman, J. M., et al. 2002. Epidemiology of musculoskeletal injuries among sedentary and physically active adults. *Medicine and Science in Sports and Exercise* 34(5):838–844.

Knudsen, D. V. 2000. Stretching during warm-up: Do we have enough evidence? *Journal of Physical Education, Recreation and Dance* 70(2):271–277.

Knudsen, D. V., et al. 2000. Current issues in flexibility fitness. *President's Council on Physical Fitness and Sports Research Digest* 2(10):1–8.

Lemmink, K. A., et al. 2003. The validity of the sit-and-reach test and the modified sit-and-reach test in middle-aged to older men and women. *Research Quarterly for Exercise and Sport* 74(3):331–336.

Li, J. X., et al. 2001. Tai chi: Physiological characteristics and beneficial effects on health. *British Journal of Sports Medicine* 35(3):148–156.

McAtee, R. 1993. *Facilitated Stretching.* Champaign, IL: Human Kinetics.

Parks, K. A., et al. 2003. A comparison of lumbar range of motion and functional ability scores in patients with low back pain: Assessment for range of motion validity. *Spine* 28(4): 380–384.

Shier, D., J. Butler, and R. Lewis 2003. *Hole's Essentials of Anatomy and Physiology.* 8th ed. New York: McGraw-Hill.

Shrier, I., and K. Gossal. 2000. Myths and truths of stretching. *The Physician and Sportsmedicine* 28(8):57–63.

Thacker, S. B., et al. 2004. The impact of stretching on sports injury risk: A systematic review of the literature. *Medicine and Science in Sports and Exercise* 36(3):371–378.

In the News

Increasing Popularity of Tai Chi, Yoga, and Pilates

A major trend in recent years is the increasing popularity of more formalized stretching and movement disciplines. While participation in regular stretching in the overall population is quite low, the popularity of these offerings suggest that people may be more interested in flexibility when it is performed as part of a comprehensive movement or body awareness program. The following are brief descriptions of some of the most popular programs:

- *Tai chi* (often translated as Chinese shadow boxing) is considered a martial art but involves the slow, flowing movements called forms. Recent studies have demonstrated that participants in tai chi have improved balance and strength. These improvements have been shown to reduce the risk of falling in older populations.
- *Yoga* is an umbrella term that refers to a number of yoga traditions. The foundation for most yoga traditions is hatha yoga, which incorporates a variety of asanas (postures). Iyengar yoga is another popular variation. It uses similar asanas as hatha yoga but involves other props and cushions to enhance the movements. Emphasis is placed on balance through coordinated breathing and precise body alignment. A new version of yoga specific to the United States is power yoga, which incorporates elements of aerobics into the routines. Many yoga positions require movements that are contraindicated for good health, so it is important to be careful. The most extreme and/or challenging yoga positions may be impressive but, like any activity performed to extremes, there are increased risks for injury.
- *Pilates* is another increasingly popular class offered at many fitness clubs. It combines strength and flexibility movements. emphasis is on core stabilization movements and enhanced body awareness.

Table 3

Table 3 The Basic 8 for Stretching Exercises

1. Calf Stretch

This exercise stretches the calf muscles and Achilles tendon. Face a wall with your feet two or three feet away. Step forward on your left foot to allow both hands to touch the wall. Keep the heel of your right foot on the ground, toe turned in slightly, knee straight, and buttocks tucked in. Lean forward by bending your front knee and arms and allowing your head to move nearer the wall. Hold. Bend right knee, keeping heel on floor. Stretch and hold. Repeat with other leg.

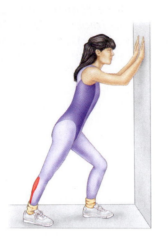

3. Sitting Stretch

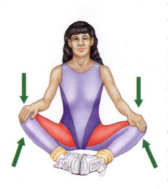

This exercise stretches the muscles on the inside of the thighs. Sit with soles of feet together; place hands on knees or ankles and lean forearms against knees; resist (contract) by attempting to raise knees. Hold. Relax and press the knees toward the floor as far as possible; hold. This exercise is useful for pregnant women and anyone whose thighs tend to rotate inward causing backache, knock-knees, and flat feet.

2. Hip and Thigh Stretch

This exercise stretches the hip (iliopsoas) and thigh muscles (quadriceps) and is useful for people with lordosis and back problems. Place right knee directly above right ankle and stretch left leg backward so knee touches floor. If necessary, place hands on floor for balance.

1. Tilt the pelvis backward by tucking in the abdomen and flattening the back.
2. Then shift the weight forward until a stretch is felt on the front of the thigh; hold. Repeat on opposite side. Caution: Do not bend front knee more than 90 degrees.

4. Hamstring Stretch

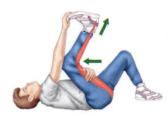

This exercise stretches the muscles on the back of the hip, thigh, knee, and ankle. Lie on your back with your knees bent. Bring right knee to chest and grasp toes with right hand. Place left hand on back of right thigh. Pull knee toward chest and push heel toward ceiling and pull toes toward shin. Attempt to straighten knee. Stretch and hold. Repeat on left side.

Table 3

5. Leg Hug

This exercise stretches the lower back and gluteals. Lie on your back with your knees bent in a hook-lying position. Contract gluteals and lumbar muscles. Lift hips. Hold for 3 seconds. Relax and pull knees to chest with arms as hard as possible; hold. Useful for people with backache and lordosis. Do not place the hands over the knees to apply stretch.

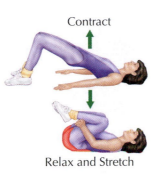

Contract

Relax and Stretch

7. Pectoral Stretch

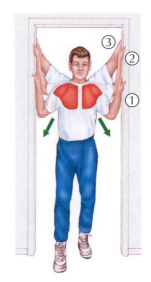

This exercise stretches the chest muscle (pectorals).

1. Stand erect in doorway with arms raised 45 degrees, elbows bent, and hands grasping door-jamb; feet in front-stride position. Press out on door frame, contracting the arms maximally for 3 seconds. Relax and shift weight forward on legs. Lean into doorway so muscles on front of shoulder joint and chest are stretched. Hold.
2. Repeat with arms raised 90 degrees.
3. Repeat with arms raised 135 degrees. Useful to prevent or correct round shoulders and sunken chest.

6. Trunk Twist

This exercise stretches the trunk muscles and muscles on the outside of hip. Sit with right leg extended, left leg bent and crossed over the right knee. Place right arm on the left side of the left leg and push against that leg while turning the trunk as far as possible to the left. Place left hand on floor behind buttocks. Stretch and hold. Reverse position and repeat on opposite side.

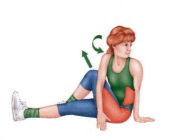

8. Arm Stretch

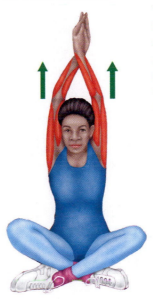

This exercise stretches the arm and chest muscles. Cross arms and turn palms of hands together. Raise arms overhead behind ears. Extend elbows. Stretch as high as possible. Hold.

Table 4

Table 4 Supplemental Stretching Exercises for Flexibility

1. Lower Leg Stretch

This exercise stretches the calf muscles and Achilles tendon. Stand with the toes on a stair step or thick book. Use hands to balance by holding a rail or wall. Keep toes pointed straight ahead or slightly inward. Rise up on toes (contract) as far as possible and hold for 3 seconds. Relax and lower heels to floor as far as possible; hold. Static stretch may alleviate spasms or cramps in calf muscles.

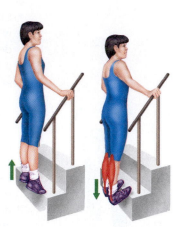

3. Lateral Thigh and Hip Stretch

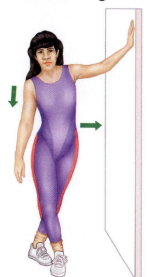

This exercise stretches the muscles and connective tissue on the outside of the legs (iliotibial band and tensor fascia lata). Stand with left side to wall, left arm extended and palm of hand flat on wall for support. Cross the left leg behind right and turn toes of both feet out slightly. Bend left knee slightly and shift pelvis toward wall (left) as trunk bends toward right. Adjust until tension is felt down outside of left hip and thigh. Stretch and hold. Repeat on other side.

2. Standing Thigh Stretch

This exercise stretches the hip flexor (iliopsoas) and thigh muscles (quadriceps). Stand near a wall so you can use one hand for balance. Place the top of one foot on a flat surface slightly higher than knee height (use a chair or table). Keep the knee of the elevated foot bent. Slide the leg backward until a stretch is felt on the front of the thigh. Keep the top of the pelvis tilted backward so the back does not arch. Repeat with the opposite leg.

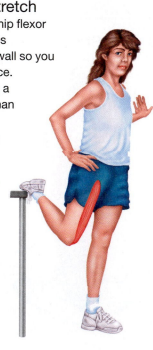

4. Back-Saver Hamstring Stretch

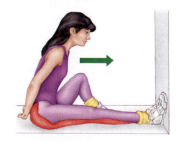

This exercise stretches the hamstrings and calf muscles and helps prevent or correct backache caused in part by short hamstrings. Sit on the floor with the feet against the wall or an immovable object. Bend left knee and bring foot close to buttocks. Clasp hands behind back. Contract the muscles of the back of the upper leg (hamstrings) by pressing the heel downward toward the floor; hold; relax. Bend forward from hips, keeping lower back as straight as possible. Let bent knee rotate outward so trunk can move forward. Lean forward keeping back flat; hold and repeat on each leg.

5. One-Leg Stretch

This exercise stretches the lower back and hamstring muscles. Stand with one foot on a bench, keeping both legs straight. Contract the hamstrings and gluteals by pressing down on bench with the heel for three seconds; then relax and bend the trunk forward, toward the knee. Hold for 10–15 seconds. Return to starting position 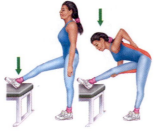 and repeat with opposite leg. As flexibility improves, the arms can be used to pull the chest toward the legs. Do not allow either knee to lock. This exercise is useful in relief of backache and correction of sway back.

7. Wand Exercise

This exercise stretches the front of the shoulders and chest. Sit with wand grasped at ends. Raise wand overhead. Be certain that the head does not slide forward. Keep the chin tucked and neck straight. Bring wand down behind shoulder blades. Keep spine erect. Hold. Press forward on the wand simulta- 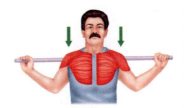 neously by pushing with the hands. Relax; then try to move the hands lower, sliding the wand down the back. Hold again. Hands may be moved closer together to increase stretch on chest muscles. If this is an easy exercise for you, try straightening the elbows and bringing the wand to waist level in back of you.

6. Lateral Trunk Stretch

This exercise stretches the trunk muscles. Sit on the floor. Stretch the left arm over head to right. Bend to the right at waist, reaching as far to right as possible with left arm and as far as possible to the left with right arm; hold. Do not let trunk rotate. Repeat on opposite side. For less stretch, overhead arm may be bent at elbow. This exercise can be done in the standing position but is less effective.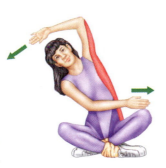

8. Arm Pretzel

This exercise stretches the shoulder muscles (lateral rotators). Stand or sit with elbows flexed at right angles, palms up. Cross right arm over left; grasp right thumb with left hand and pull gently downward, causing right arm to rotate laterally. Stretch and hold. Reverse arm position and repeat on left arm.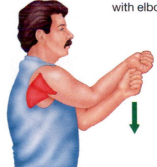

Table 4

Table 4 Supplemental Stretching Exercises for Flexibility

9. Shin Stretch

This exercise relieves shin muscle soreness by stretching muscles on front of shin. Kneel on knees, turn to right, and press down and stretch right ankle with right hand. Move pelvis forward. Hold. Repeat on opposite side. Except when they are sore, most people need to strengthen rather than stretch these muscles.

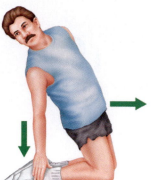

11. Billig's Exercise

This exercise stretches the pelvic fascia, hip flexors, and muscles of the inside thigh. Stand with side to a wall and place the elbow and forearm against the wall at shoulder height. Tilt the pelvis backward, tightening the gluteal and abdominal muscles. Place opposite hand on hip and push the hips toward the wall. Push forward and sideward (45 degrees) with the hips. Do not twist the hips. Hold. Repeat on opposite side. Useful for preventing some cases of dysmenorrhea (painful menstruation).

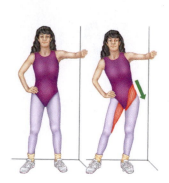

10. Spine Twist

This exercise stretches the trunk rotators and lateral rotators of the thighs. Start in hook-lying position, arms extended at shoulder level. Cross left knee over right. Push the right knee to the floor using pressure of the left knee and leg. Keep arms and shoulders on floor while touching knees to floor on left. Stretch and hold. Reverse leg position and lower knees to right.

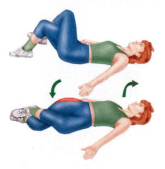

12. Two-Hand Ankle Wrap

This exercise is most useful for athletes or people interested in performance. It should not be done until after individual muscles have been stretched using other exercises. It stretches multiple muscle groups including the back, shoulders, and legs. Stand with heels together. Bend forward and place arms between knees; bend knees and wrap arms around legs, attempting to touch fingers in front of ankles. Hold.

Lab Resource Materials: Flexibility Tests

Directions: To test the flexibility of all joints is impractical. These tests are for joints used frequently. Follow the instructions carefully. Determine your flexibility using Chart 1.

Test

1. *Modified Sit-and-Reach* (Flexibility Test of Hamstrings)
   a. Remove shoes and sit on the floor. Place the sole of the foot of the extended leg flat against a box or bench, and place the head, back, and hips against a wall with a 90-degree angle at the hips.
   b. Place one hand over the other and slowly reach forward as far as you can with arms fully extended. Keep head and back in contact with the wall. A partner will slide the measuring stick on the bench until it touches the fingertips.
   c. With the measuring stick fixed in the new position, reach forward as far as possible, three times, holding the position on the third reach for at least 2 seconds while the partner reads the distance on the ruler. Keep the knee of the extended leg straight (see illustration).
   d. Repeat the test a second time and average the scores of the two trials.

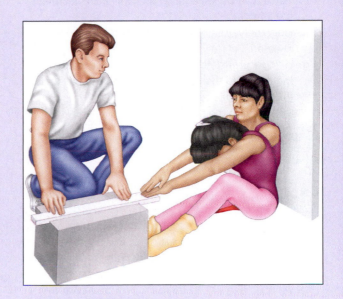

Test

2. *Shoulder Flexibility* ("Zipper" Test)
   a. Raise your arm, bend your elbow, and reach down across your back as far as possible.
   b. At the same time, extend your left arm down and behind your back, bend your elbow up across your back, and try to cross your fingers over those of your right hand as shown in the accompanying illustration.
   c. Measure the distance to the nearest half-inch. If your fingers overlap, score as a plus. If they fail to meet, score as a minus; use a zero if your fingertips just touch.
   d. Repeat with your arms crossed in the opposite direction (left arm up). Most people will find that they are more flexible on one side than the other.

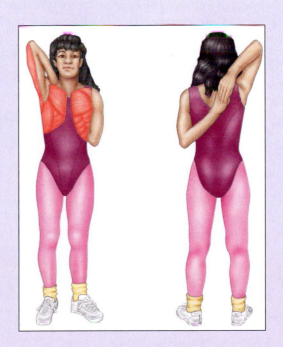

Test

3. *Hamstring and Hip Flexor Flexibility*
   a. Lie on your back on the floor beside a wall.
   b. Slowly lift one leg off the floor. Keep the other leg flat on the floor.
   c. Keep both legs straight.
   d. Continue to lift the leg until either leg begins to bend or the lower leg begins to lift off the floor.
   e. Place a yardstick against the wall and underneath the lifted leg.
   f. Hold the yardstick against the wall after the leg is lowered.
   g. Using a protractor, measure the angle created by the floor and the yardstick. The greater the angle, the better your score.
   h. Repeat with the other leg.*

*Note: For ease of testing, you may want to draw angles on a piece of posterboard as illustrated. If you have goniometers, you may be taught to use them instead.

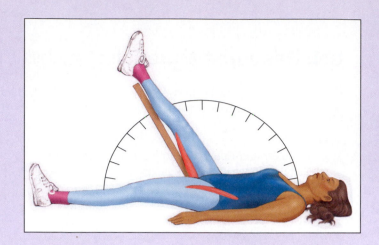

Test

4. *Trunk Rotation*
   a. Tape two yardsticks to the wall at shoulder height, one right side up and the other upside down.
   b. Stand with your left shoulder an arm's length (fist closed) from the wall. Toes should be on the line, which is perpendicular to the wall and even with the 15-inch mark on the yardstick.
   c. Drop the left arm and raise the right arm to the side, palm down, fist closed.
   d. Without moving your feet, rotate the trunk to the right as far as possible, reaching along the yardstick, and hold it 2 seconds. Do not move the feet or bend the trunk. Your knees may bend slightly.
   e. A partner will read the distance reached to the nearest half-inch. Record your score. Repeat two times and average your two scores.
   f. Next, perform the test facing the opposite direction. Rotate to the left. For this test you will use the second yardstick (upside down) so that the greater the rotation, the higher the score. If you have only one yardstick, turn it right side up for the first test and upside down for the second test.

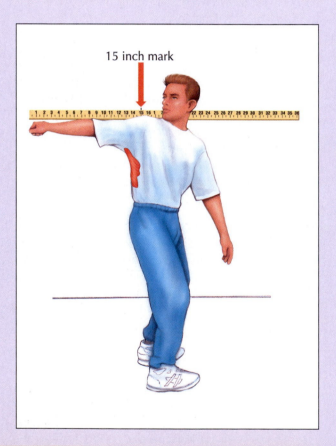

15 inch mark

Chart 1 ▶ Flexibility Rating Scale for Tests 1–4

Classification	Men					Women				
	Test 1	Test 2		Test 3	Test 4	Test 1	Test 2		Test 3	Test 4
		Right Up	Left Up				Right Up	Left Up		
High performance*	16+	5+	4+	111+	20+	17+	6+	5+	111+	20.5 or >
Good fitness zone	13–15	1–4	1–3	80–110	16–19.5	14–16	2–5	2–4	80–110	17–20
Marginal zone	10–12	0	0	60–79	13.5–15.5	11–13	1	1	60–79	14.5–16.5
Low zone	<9	<0	<0	<60	<13.5	<10	<1	<1	<60	<14.5

*Though performers need good flexibility, hypermobility may increase injury risk.

Lab 10A Evaluating Flexibility

Name	Section	Date

Purpose: To evaluate your flexibility in several joints

Procedures

1. Take the flexibility tests outlined in the *Lab Resource Materials*.
2. Record your scores in the Results section.
3. Use Chart 1 in *Lab Resource Materials* to determine your ratings on the self-assessments; then place an X over the circle for the appropriate rating.

Results

Flexibility Scores and Ratings

Record Scores			Record Ratings:			
			High Performance	Good Fitness	Marginal	Poor
Modified sit-and-reach						
Test 1	Left		◯	◯	◯	◯
	Right		◯	◯	◯	◯
Zipper						
Test 2	Left		◯	◯	◯	◯
	Right		◯	◯	◯	◯
Hamstring/hip flexor						
Test 3	Left		◯	◯	◯	◯
	Right		◯	◯	◯	◯
Trunk rotation						
Test 4	Left		◯	◯	◯	◯
	Right		◯	◯	◯	◯

Do any of these muscle groups need stretching? Check one circle for each muscle group.

	Yes	No
Back of the thighs and knees (hamstrings)	○	○
Calf muscles	○	○
Lower back (lumbar region)	○	○
Front of right shoulder	○	○
Back of right shoulder	○	○
Front of left shoulder	○	○
Back of left shoulder	○	○
Most of the body	○	○
Trunk muscles	○	○

Conclusions and Implications: In several sentences, discuss your current flexibility and your flexibility needs for the future. Include comments about your current state of flexibility, need for improvement in specific areas, and special flexibility needs for sports or other special activities.

Lab 10B Planning and Logging Stretching Exercises

Name	Section	Date

Purpose: To set 1-week lifestyle goals for stretching exercises, to prepare a stretching for flexibility plan, and to self-monitor progress in your 1-week plan

Procedures

1. On Chart 1, check the stretching exercises you plan to perform during the next week. Try to do at least eight exercises three times a week. The Basic 8 are listed. You may substitute other exercises by writing them in the "Other" blank. See Table 4 for additional exercises.
2. Keep a 1-week log of your actual participation using Chart 2. If possible, keep the log with you during the day. Place a check by each of the stretching exercises you perform each day, including ones that you didn't originally have planned. If you cannot keep the log with you, fill in the log at the end of the day. If you choose to keep a log for more than 1 week, make extra copies of the log before you begin.
3. Answer the questions in the Results section.

Chart 1 ▶ Stretching Exercise Plan

Place a check beside the stretching exercises you plan to do and under the days you plan to do them.	Day 1 Date:	Day 2 Date:	Day 3 Date:	Day 4 Date:	Day 5 Date:	Day 6 Date:	Day 7 Date:
1. Calf stretch							
2. Hip and thigh stretch							
3. Sitting stretch							
4. Hamstring stretch							
5. Back stretch (leg hug)							
6. Trunk twist							
7. Pectoral stretch							
8. Arm stretch							
Other:							
Other:							
Other:							
Other:							

Results

	Yes	No
Did you do eight exercises at least 3 days in the week?	◯	◯
Did you do eight exercises more than 3 days in the week?	◯	◯

Chart 2 ▶ Stretching Exercise Log

Place a check beside the stretching exercises you actually performed and the days on which you performed them.	Day 1 Date:	Day 2 Date:	Day 3 Date:	Day 4 Date:	Day 5 Date:	Day 6 Date:	Day 7 Date:
1. Calf stretch							
2. Hip and thigh stretch							
3. Sitting stretch							
4. Hamstring stretch							
5. Back stretch (leg hug)							
6. Trunk twist							
7. Pectoral stretch							
8. Arm stretch							
Other:							
Other:							
Other:							
Other:							

Conclusions and Interpretations

1. Do you feel that you will use stretching exercises as part of your regular lifetime physical activity plan, either now or in the future? Use several sentences to explain your answer.

2. Discuss the exercises you feel benefited you and the ones that did not. What exercises would you continue to do and which ones would you change? Use several sentences to explain your answer.

3. Did the logging of your stretching exercise help you to adhere to your program? In several sentences, explain why or why not.

Muscle Fitness

Progressive resistance exercise promotes muscle fitness that permits efficient and effective movement, contributes to ease and economy of muscular effort, promotes successful performance, and lowers susceptibility to some types of injuries, musculoskeletal problems, and some illnesses.

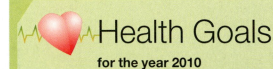

Health Goals

for the year 2010

- Increase proportion of people who regularly perform exercises for strength and muscular endurance.

- Reduce steroid use, especially among youth.

- Increase screening and reduce incidence of osteoporosis.

- Reduce activity limitations due to chronic back pain.

There are two components of muscle fitness: strength and muscular endurance. Strength is the amount of force you can produce with a single maximal effort of a muscle group. Muscular endurance is the capacity of the skeletal muscles or group of muscles to continue contracting over a long period of time. You need both strength and muscular endurance to increase work capacity; to decrease the chance of injury; to prevent low back pain, poor posture, and other hypokinetic conditions; to improve athletic performance; and perhaps to save a life or property in an emergency. Muscle fitness training increases the fitness of the bones, tendons, and ligaments, as well as the muscles. It has been found to be therapeutic for patients with chronic pain.

Progressive resistance training is the type of physical activity done with the intent of improving muscle fitness. The many types of progressive resistance exercises designed to promote or maintain muscle fitness are described in this concept.

Factors Influencing Strength and Muscular Endurance

There are three types of muscle tissue. www.mhhe.com/phys_fit/web11 Click 01. The three types of muscle tissue—smooth, cardiac, and skeletal—have different structures and functions. Smooth muscle tissue consists of long, spindle-shaped fibers with each fiber containing only one nucleus. The fibers are involuntary and are located in the walls of the esophagus, stomach, and intestines, where they move food and waste products through the digestive tract. Cardiac muscle tissue is also involuntary and, as its name implies, is found only in the heart. These fibers contract in response to demands on the cardiovascular system. The heart muscle contracts at a slow, steady rate at rest but contracts more frequently and forcefully during physical activity. Skeletal muscle tissues consist of long, cylindrical, multinucleated fibers. They provide the force needed to move the skeletal system and may be controlled voluntarily.

Leverage is an important mechanical principle that influences strength. The body uses a system of levers to produce movement. Muscles are connected to bones via tendons and some muscles (referred to as "primary movers") cross over a particular joint to produce movement. The movement occurs because when a muscle contracts it physically shortens and pulls the two bones connected by the joint together. Figure 1 shows the two heads of the biceps muscle inserting on the forearm. When the muscle contracts, the forearm is pulled up toward the upper arm (elbow flexion). A person with long arms and legs has a mechanical advantage in most movements, since the force that is exerted can act over a longer distance. Although it is not possible to change the length of your limbs, it is possible to learn to use your muscles more effectively. The ability of Tiger Woods to hit golf balls 350 yards is due to his ability to generate torque and power rather than to his actual strength.

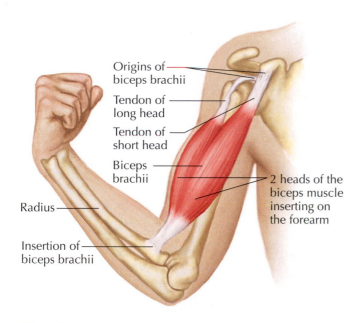

Origins of
biceps brachii

Tendon of
long head

Tendon of
short head

Biceps
brachii

2 heads of the
biceps muscle
inserting on
the forearm

Radius

Insertion of
biceps brachii

Figure 1 ▶ Muscle action on body levers.

Skeletal muscle tissue consists of different types of fibers that respond and adapt differently to training. www. mhhe.com/phys_fit/web11 Click 02. There are three distinct types of muscle fibers, slow-twitch (Type I), fast-twitch (Type IIb), and an intermediate fiber type (Type IIa). The slow-twitch fibers are generally red in color and are well suited to produce energy with aerobic metabolism. Slow-twitch fibers generate less tension but are more resistant to fatigue. Endurance training leads to adaptations in the slow-twitch fibers that allow them to produce energy more efficiently and better resist fatigue. Fast-twitch fibers are generally white in color and are well suited to produce energy with anaerobic processes. They generate greater tension than slow-twitch fibers, but they fatigue more quickly. These fibers are particularly well suited to fast, high-force activities, such as explosive weight-lifting movements, sprinting, and jumping. Progressive resistance exercise enhances strength primarily by increasing the size (muscle **hypertrophy**) of fast-twitch fibers, but cellular adaptations also take place to enhance various metabolic properties. Intermediate fibers have biochemical and physiological properties that are between those of the slow-twitch and fast-twitch fibers. A distinct property of these intermediate fibers is that they are highly adaptable, depending on the type of training that is performed.

An example of fast-twitch muscle fiber in animals is the white meat in the flying muscles of a chicken. The chicken is heavy and must exert a powerful force to fly a few feet up to a perch. A wild duck that flies for hundreds of miles has dark meat (slow-twitch fibers) in the flying muscles for better endurance.

People who want large muscles will use progressive resistance exercises designed to build strength (fast-twitch

fibers). People who want to be able to persist in activities for a long period of time without fatigue will want to use progressive resistance training programs designed to build muscular endurance (slow-twitch fibers).

Genetics, gender, and age affect muscle fitness performance. www.mhhe.com/phys_fit/web11 Click 03. Each person inherits a certain percentage of fast-twitch and slow-twitch muscle fibers. This allocation influences the potential a person has for muscle fitness activities. Individuals with a larger percentage of fast-twitch fibers will generally increase muscle size and strength more readily than individuals endowed with a larger percentage of slow-twitch fibers. People with a larger percentage of slow-twitch fibers have greater potential for muscular endurance performance. Regardless of genetics, all people can improve their strength and muscular endurance with proper training.

Women have smaller amounts of the anabolic hormone testosterone and, therefore, have less muscle mass than men. Because of this, women typically have 60 to 85 percent of the **absolute strength** of men. When expressed relative to lean body weight, women have **relative strength** similar to that of men. For example, a 150-pound female who lifts 150 pounds has relative strength equivalent to that of a 250-pound male who lifts 250 pounds, even though she has less absolute strength. **Absolute muscular endurance** is also greater for males, but the difference again is negated if **relative muscular endurance** is considered. Relative strength and endurance are better indicators of muscle fitness, since they take into account differences in size and muscle mass, but, for some activities, absolute strength and endurance are more important.

Hypertrophy Increase in the size of muscles as a result of strength training; increase in bulk.

Absolute Strength The maximum amount of force one can exert—e.g., maximum number of pounds or kilograms that can be lifted on one attempt.

Relative Strength Amount of force that one can exert in relation to one's body weight or per unit of muscle cross section.

Absolute Muscular Endurance Endurance measured by the maximum number of repetitions one can perform against a given resistance—e.g., the number of times you can bench press 50 pounds.

Relative Muscular Endurance Endurance measured by the maximum number of repetitions one can perform a given percent of your absolute strength—e.g., the number of times you can lift 50 percent of your absolute strength.

Maximum strength is usually reached in the twenties and typically declines with age. Though muscular endurance declines with age, it is not as dramatic as decreases in absolute strength. As people grow older, regardless of gender, strength and muscular endurance are better among people who train than people who do not. This suggests that progressive resistance training is one antidote to premature aging.

Some endurance tests penalize the weaker person. If you are tested on absolute endurance (the number of times you can move a designated number of pounds), a stronger person has an advantage. However, if you are tested on relative muscular endurance (the number of times you can move a designated percentage of your maximum strength), the stronger person does not have an advantage. For this reason, men and women can compete more evenly in relative muscular endurance activities. In fact, on some endurance tasks, women have done as well or better than men. For example, the women at the United States Military Academy do as well as the men on tests of abdominal muscular endurance.

Muscular endurance is related to cardiovascular endurance, but it is not the same thing. Cardiovascular endurance depends upon the efficiency of the heart muscle, circulatory system, and respiratory system. It is developed with activities that stress these systems, such as running, cycling, and swimming. Muscular endurance depends upon the efficiency of the local skeletal muscles and the nerves that control them. Most forms of cardiovascular exercise, such as running, require good cardiovascular and muscular endurance. For example, if your legs lack the muscular endurance to continue contracting for a sustained period of time, it will be difficult to perform well in running or other aerobic activities.

Health Benefits of Muscle Fitness and Resistance Exercise

Good muscle fitness is associated with reduced risk for injury. People with good muscle fitness are less likely to suffer joint injuries (e.g., neck, knee, ankle) than those with poor muscle fitness. Weak muscles are more likely to be involuntarily overstretched than are strong muscles.

Muscle balance is important in reducing the risk for injury. Resistance training should build both agonist and **antagonist muscles.** For example, if you do resistance exercise to build the quadriceps muscles (front of the thigh), you should also exercise the hamstring muscles (back of the thigh). In this instance, the quadriceps are the agonist (muscle being used), and the hamstrings are

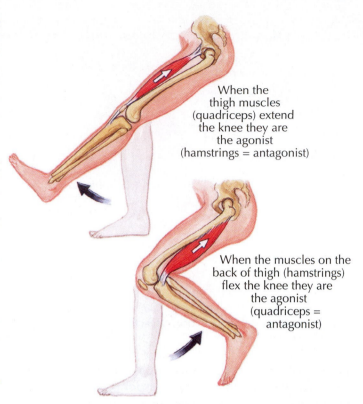

When the thigh muscles (quadriceps) extend the knee they are the agonist (hamstrings = antagonist)

When the muscles on the back of thigh (hamstrings) flex the knee they are the agonist (quadriceps = antagonist)

Figure 2 ▶ Agonist and antagonist muscles.

the antagonist. If the quadriceps become too strong relative to the antagonist hamstring muscles, the risk for injury increases (see Figure 2).

Good muscle fitness is associated with good posture and reduced risk of back problems. When muscles in specific body regions are weak or overdeveloped, poor posture can result. Lack of fitness of the abdominal and low back muscles is particularly related to poor posture and potential back problems. Excessively strong hip flexor muscles can lead to swayback. Poor balance in muscular development can also result in postural problems. For example, the muscles on the sides of the body must be balanced to maintain an erect posture.

Good muscle fitness can bring about improved athletic performance. Many sports depend on strength and muscular endurance. A football player must have good muscle strength to block and tackle effectively. A swimmer or a wrestler requires good muscular endurance to perform optimally. Also, people in jobs requiring high-level performance, such as law enforcement and fire safety, are likely to benefit from good muscle fitness.

Good muscle fitness is associated with wellness and quality of life. Wellness is reflected in quality of life and well-being. A person with muscle fitness is able to perform for long periods of time without undue fatigue. As a result, the person has energy to perform daily work efficiently and effectively and has reserve energy to enjoy leisure time. Among older people, maintenance of strength is associated with increased balance, less risk for falling, and greater ability to perform the tasks of daily living independently. Muscle fitness also contributes to looking one's best.

Resistance exercise is associated with reduced risk for osteoporosis.
Progressive resistance exercises (PRE) provide a positive stress on the bones. Together with good diet, including adequate calcium intake, this stress on the bones reduces the risk for osteoporosis. Evidence suggests that young people who do PRE develop a high bone density. As we grow older, bone mass decreases, so people who have a high bone density when they are young have a "bank account" from which to draw as they grow older. These people have bones that are less likely to fracture or be injured. Injuries to the bones, particularly the hip and back, are common among older adults. Regular PRE can reduce the risk for these conditions. Postmenopausal women are especially at risk for osteoporosis (see Concept 4).

PRE contributes to weight control and looking your best.
Regular PRE results in muscle mass increases. Muscle or lean body mass takes up less space than fat, contributing to attractive appearance. Further, muscle burns calories at rest, so extra muscle built through PRE can contribute to increased resting and basal metabolism. For each pound of muscle gained, a person can burn approximately 35 to 50 calories more per day. A typical strength training program performed at least three times a week can lead to 2 additional pounds of muscle after 8 weeks, so this can amount to an additional 100 calories a day, or 700 over a week. Conversely, muscle mass tends to decrease with age, and this can slow metabolism by a similar amount and contribute to gradual increases in body fatness. PRE can help people retain muscle mass as they grow older.

Types of Progressive Resistance Exercise

There are different types of PRE, and each has its advantages and disadvantages.
The main types of PRE are isotonic, isometric, and isokinetic. These terms refer to the way in which a load or stimulus is provided to the muscles. Each type of exercise has some advantages and disadvantages, which are described in the following sections. Table 1 compares the various types.

Isotonic exercise is the most common type of PRE.
www.mhhe.com/phys_fit/web11 Click 04. **Isotonic** exercise includes activities in which a resistance is raised and then lowered, as in weight training and calisthenics (also called dynamic exercise). When performing isotonic exercise, both **concentric** (shortening) and **eccentric** (lengthening) **contractions** should be used. For example, in an overhead press exercise, the muscles on the back of the arm (triceps) shorten

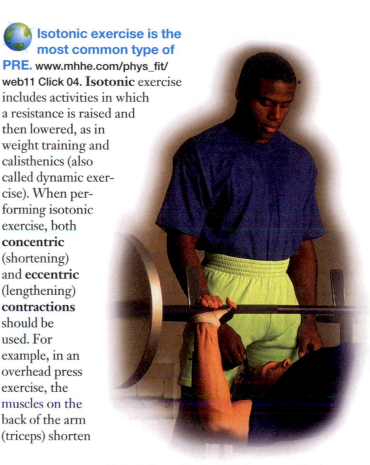

Progressive resistance exercises are methods of training designed to build muscle fitness.

Antagonist Muscles The muscles that have the opposite action from those that are contracting (agonists); normally, antagonists reflexively relax when agonists contract.

Progressive Resistance Exercises (PRE) Exercises done against a resistance; also referred to as progressive resistance training (PRT).

Isotonic Type of muscle contraction in which the muscle changes length, either shortening (concentrically) or lengthening (eccentrically).

Concentric Contractions Isotonic muscle contractions in which the muscle gets shorter as it contracts, such as when a joint is bent and two body parts move closer together.

Eccentric Contractions Isotonic muscle contractions in which the muscle gets longer as it contracts—that is, when a weight is gradually lowered and the contracting muscle gets longer as it gives up tension. Eccentric contractions are also called negative exercise.

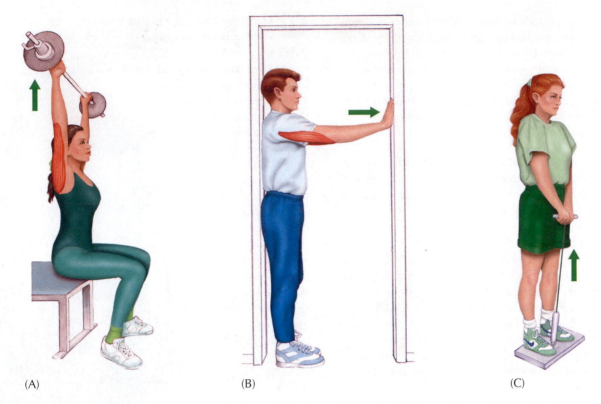

(A)   (B)   (C)

Figure 3 ▶ Examples of three types of muscle fitness exercises: (A) isotonic, (B) isometric, and (C) isokinetic.

(contract concentrically) to lift the weight overhead (see Figure 3A). When the weight is lowered, the muscles lengthen (contract eccentrically) if the weight is lowered slowly. Both concentric and eccentric contractions build the muscle. Eccentric contractions, sometimes called negative contractions, are more likely to cause delayed-onset muscle soreness than concentric contractions. Typically, the stress on the muscle in either concentric or eccentric exercises varies with speed, joint position, and muscle length. Thus, the muscle may work harder at the beginning of a lift than it does near the end of the range of motion.

🌎 Isometric exercise does not require special equipment. www.mhhe.com/phys_fit/web11 Click 05.

Isometric exercises are those in which no movement takes place while a force is exerted against an immovable object (see Figure 3B). They are effective for developing strength and muscular endurance but build **static strength** and **static muscular endurance,** as opposed to **dynamic strength** or **dynamic muscular endurance.** They work the muscle only at the angle of the joint used in the exercise and promote less hypertrophy and strength than isotonic resistance exercise. Thus, isometric exercises are probably less effective as an overall training method than isotonic exercises. On the other hand, isometrics have been found to be quite

useful for some athletes, such as wrestlers and gymnasts, and work especially well for people in the early stages of some rehabilitation programs. Research has shown that strength can be enhanced significantly by using isometric training at the **sticking points** of isotonic lifts.

🌎 Isokinetic exercises are often used for sports training and rehabilitation. www.mhhe.com/phys_fit/web11 Click 06.

Isokinetic exercises are isotonic-concentric muscle contractions performed on machines that keep the velocity of the movement constant through the full range of motion. This rate-limiting mechanism prevents the performer from moving faster, no matter how much force is exerted. Isokinetic devices essentially match the resistance to the effort of the performer, permitting maximal tension to be exerted throughout the range of motion (see Figure 3C). Thus, isokinetic devices overcome the basic weakness of isotonic exercise in which the muscle is only maximally challenged for a small part of the overall motion. A limitation is that these devices do not permit acceleration, so it is not possible to train specifically for sport skills, such as throwing or kicking, in which the limb is accelerated while applying maximum force. Another limitation is that some of these devices permit only concentric contractions. Isokinetic exercise has the advantage of being safer than most other forms of exercise and may

Table 1 ▶ Advantages and Disadvantages of Isotonic, Isometric, and Isokinetic Exercises

	Advantages	Disadvantages
Isotonic	• Can effectively mimic movements used in sport skills • Enhance dynamic coordination • Promote gains in strength	• Do not challenge muscles through the full range of motion • Require equipment or machines • May lead to soreness
Isometric	• Can be done anywhere • Low cost/little equipment needed • Can rehabilitate an immobilized joint	• Build strength at only one position • Less muscle hypertrophy • Poor link or transfer to sport skills
Isokinetic	• Build strength through a full range of motion • Beneficial for rehabilitation and evaluation • Safe and less likely to promote soreness	• Require specialized equipment • Cannot replicate natural acceleration found in sports • More complicated to use and cannot work all muscle groups

be better for developing power (see Concept 14). It is not better for developing pure strength, however. More research is needed to determine the best training regimen for isokinetic exercise.

Plyometrics is a form of isotonic exercise that promotes athletic performance. www.mhhe.com/phys_fit/web11 Click 07. **Plyometrics** is a form of isotonic exercise that is especially useful for athletes training for power development. High jumpers, long jumpers, and volleyball and basketball players often use this technique, which includes jumping from boxes, hopping on one foot, and engaging in similar types of activities. For most people interested primarily in the health benefits of physical activity, plyometrics are not a preferred type of exercise. In fact, they can increase risk for injury, especially among beginners. For more information on plyometrics, refer to the concept on the performance benefits of physical activity.

Resistance Training Equipment

There are advantages of both free weights and machine weights. www.mhhe.com/phys_fit/web11 Click 08. Free weights are weights that are not attached to a machine or an exercise device. Typically, they come in the form of a barbell or dumbbell that can be adjusted as necessary for different exercises to provide optimal resistance. Weight training with free weights is very popular because it can be done in the home with inexpensive equipment. Because free weights require balance and technique, they may be somewhat difficult for beginners to use. Competitive weight lifters generally prefer them because they can exercise muscle groups in a very specific way.

Resistance training machines can be effective in developing strength and muscular endurance if used properly. They can save time because, unlike free weights, the resistance can be changed easily and quickly. They may be safer because you are less likely to drop weights. A disadvantage is that the kinds of exercises that can be done on these machines are more limited than free weight exercises. They also may not promote optimal balance in muscular development, since a stronger muscle can often make up for a weaker muscle in the completion of a lift.

Some machines, such as Nautilus and Universal, offer what is called "variable" or "accommodating resistance." The Nautilus, for example, uses a cam to adapt the

Isometric Type of muscle contraction in which the muscle remains the same length. Also known as static contraction.

Static Strength A muscle's ability to exert a force without changing length; also called isometric strength.

Static Muscular Endurance A muscle's ability to remain contracted for a long period. This is usually measured by the length of time you can hold a body position.

Dynamic Strength A muscle's ability to exert force that results in movement. It is typically measured isotonically.

Dynamic Muscular Endurance A muscle's ability to contract and relax repeatedly. This is usually measured by the number of times (repetitions) you can perform a body movement in a given time period. It is also called isotonic endurance.

Sticking Points Points in the range of motion where the weight cannot be lifted any farther without extreme effort or assistance; the weakest points in the movement.

Isokinetic Isotonic-concentric exercises done with a machine that regulates movement velocity and resistance.

Plyometrics A training technique used to develop explosive power. It consists of isotonic-concentric muscle contractions performed after a prestretch or eccentric contraction of a muscle.

resistance as the performer moves through the range of motion. The Universal Trainer uses a rolling pivot to do the same thing. These adaptations attempt to compensate for an inherent weakness in isotonic constant-resistance exercises done with free weights and other machines. They are only partially successful, however, in adapting to the shapes, sizes, and torques of individual human bodies. There is no evidence that variable-resistance machines develop more strength or muscular endurance than other devices, although they may offer advantages in muscle fitness by allowing movement through an extended range of motion. Table 2 provides a comparison of free weights with weight machines. Common free weight exercises and machine exercises are shown in Tables 6 and 7, respectively.

Many resistance training exercises can be done with little or no equipment. www.mhhe.com/phys_fit/web11 Click 09. Calisthenics are among the most popular forms of muscle fitness exercise among adults. Calisthenics, such as curl-ups and push-ups, are suitable for people of different ability levels and can be used to improve both strength and muscular endurance. One disadvantage is that this type of exercise does little to increase strength unless resistance in addition to your body weight is added. For example, doing a push-up will build strength to a point. However, once you can do several, adding more repetitions will only build muscular endurance but not strength. To develop additional strength, you can add more weights to increase the resistance or change the body position so there is a greater

gravitational effect or more torque. For example, you can elevate your feet or wear a weighted vest while doing push-ups.

Other alternatives to expensive resistance training machines or commercially made free weights are homemade weights and elastic exercise bands. Homemade weights can be constructed from pieces of pipe or broom sticks and plastic milk jugs filled with water. Elastic tubes or bands available in varying strengths may be substituted for the weights and for the pulley device used in many resistance training machines to impart resistance.

Muscular endurance can be developed through activities such as running, swimming, circuit training, and aerobic dance if they are designed appropriately. Lifestyle activities such as gardening (e.g., raking, shoveling) or housework (lifting groceries) can also contribute to muscular endurance.

Progressive Resistance Exercise: How Much PRE Is Enough?

PRE is the best type of training for muscle fitness. PRE is the most common type of training for building muscle fitness and it is the most effective. It is sometimes referred to as progressive resistive training (PRT). The word *progressive* is used in both instances because the frequency, intensity, and length of time of muscle overload are gradually, or progressively, increased as muscle fitness increases. PREs are typically done in one to three sets, though more are used in some instances, such as for

Table 2 ▶ Advantages and Disadvantages of Free Weights and Weight Machines

		Free Weights		Machine Weights
Isolation of Major Muscle Groups	–/+	Movements require balance and coordination; more muscles are used for stabilization.	+/–	Other body parts are stabilized during lift, allowing isolation, but muscle imbalances can develop.
Applications to Real-Life Situations	+	Movements can be developed to be truer to real life.	–	Movements are determined by the paths allowed on the machine.
Risk for Injury	–	There is more possibility for injury because weights can fall or drop on toes.	+	They are safer because weights cannot fall on participants.
Needs for Assistance	–	Spotters are needed for safety with some lifts.	+	No spotters are required.
Time Requirement	–	More time is needed to change weights.	+	It is easy and quick to change weights or resistance.
Number of Available Exercises	+	Unlimited number of exercises is possible.	–	Exercise options are determined by the machine.
Cost	+	They are less expensive but good (durable) weights are still somewhat expensive.	–	They are expensive; often have to have access to a club, since usually need multiple machines.
Space Requirement	+/–	Equipment can be moved but loose weights may clutter areas.	–/+	Machines are stationary but take up large spaces.

high-performance benefits. A set is a group of repetitions (reps) done in succession, followed by a rest period. For most people, a set consists of three to twenty-five reps.

The stimulus for strength is different than for muscular endurance.

The stimulus for strength is maximal exertion. Strength training should, therefore, utilize high resistance overload with low repetitions. The stimulus for muscular endurance is repeated contractions with short rests. Muscular endurance exercises should be performed with a relatively high number of repetitions and lower resistance.

The graph in Figure 4 illustrates the relationship between strength and muscular endurance. Training that requires high resistance and low repetitions (top bar) results in the least gain in endurance but the greatest gain in strength. Training with moderate resistance and moderate repetitions (second bar) results in moderate gains in both strength and endurance. Training that requires a high number of repetitions and a relatively low resistance (third bar) results in small gains in strength but large increases in muscular endurance.

PRE is not the same thing as weight lifting, powerlifting, or bodybuilding.

PRE is a method of training to build muscle fitness that provides health and performance benefits. It should not be confused with the following three competitive activities. Weight lifting is a competitive sport that involves two lifts: the snatch and the clean and jerk. Powerlifting is also a competitive sport that includes three lifts: the bench press, the squat, and the dead lift. Bodybuilding is a competition in which participants are judged on the size and **definition** of their muscles. All three of these competitive events rely on progressive resistance exercise to improve performance. Weight training is a form of PRE and is a method of improving muscle fitness that is different from weight lifting—the competitive event.

Although strength training promotes strength, studies show that the person who is strength-trained will fatigue as much as four times faster than the person who is endurance-trained. However, there is a modest correlation between strength and endurance. A person who trains for strength will develop some endurance, and a person who trains for endurance will develop some strength.

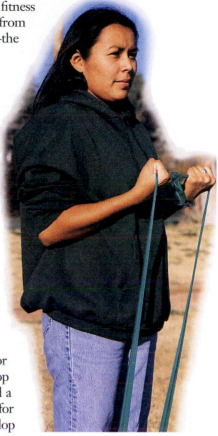
Elastic bands can provide resistance to build muscle fitness.

Muscular endurance and strength are part of the same continuum.

Though strength and muscular endurance are developed in different ways, strength and muscular endurance are part of the same continuum (Figure 5). This has led some writers to refer to muscular endurance as strength endurance. "Pure" strength is approached as one nears the end (right) of the continuum, where only one maximum contraction is made. As the number of repetitions increases and the force of the contractions decreases, one nears the other end (left) of the continuum and approaches "pure" endurance. In between the two extremes, varying degrees of strength and endurance are combined. The activities listed along the continuum are examples that might represent points along the scale. Most of the activities of daily living are at the middle of the continuum, indicating that they take a combination of strength and muscular endurance.

There are different thresholds and target zones for muscle fitness development.

The amount of resistance used in a PRE program is based on a percentage of

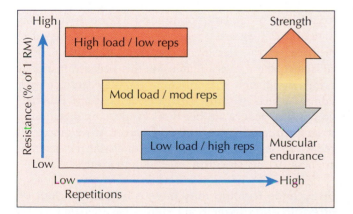

Figure 4 ▶ Comparison of muscular endurance with muscle strength developed by different repetitions and resistance.

Definition The detailed external appearance of a muscle.

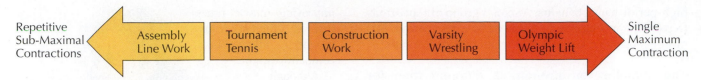

Repetitive Sub-Maximal Contractions ◀ | Assembly Line Work | Tournament Tennis | Construction Work | Varsity Wrestling | Olympic Weight Lift | ▶ Single Maximum Contraction

Figure 5 ▶ Muscle strength-endurance continuum.

your **1 repetition maximum (1RM)**—the maximum amount of resistance you can move (or weight you can lift) one time. The 1 RM value provides an indicator of your maximum strength, but desired levels of resistance are determined using percentages of the 1 RM value. The specific prescription depends on the program goals. For strength, the percentages typically vary 60 to 80 percent of the 1 RM value, whereas for endurance the percentages vary from 20 to 40 percent. Evidence suggests that very strong people interested in high-level performance can train at 80 percent and above. Individuals interested in a combination of strength and endurance should use values ranging from 40 to 60 percent.

A summary of the FIT formulas for muscular strength and muscular endurance are included in Table 3, along with guidelines for general muscle fitness. The guidelines are based on isotonic exercise, since this is the most common type of training equipment. The *On the Web* feature provides specific information on isotonic exercise (web11 Click04), isometric exercises (web11 Click05), and isokinetic exercises (web11 Click06).

A combined strength/muscle endurance program is the best choice for most individuals. Recent research has shown that for healthy adults most health benefits can be achieved using a combined strength/muscular endurance program. The American College of Sports Medicine guidelines indicate that young adults can achieve significant health benefits by performing one set of eight to twelve repetitions at least 2 days a week. For older adults (fifty and older), less intense exercises

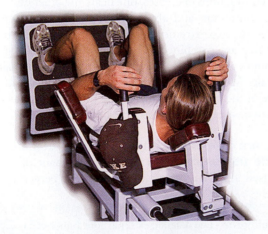

Resistance machines are safe and easy to use

performed ten to fifteen times appears to be sufficient. For both age groups, eight to ten basic exercises are recommended to promote good muscle fitness for the whole body. Individuals who want pure strength or high-level endurance for performance will benefit from extra sets and from more specific training protocols (see Kraemer & Ratamess, 2004).

Circuit resistance training (CRT) is an effective way to build muscular endurance and cardiovascular endurance. CRT consists of the performance of high repetitions of an exercise with low to moderate resistance, progressing from one station to another, performing a different exercise at each station. The stations are usually placed in a circle to facilitate movement. CRT typically employs about twenty to twenty-five reps against a resistance that is 30 to 40 percent of 1 RM for 45 seconds. Fifteen seconds of rest is provided while changing stations. Approximately ten exercise stations are used, and the participant repeats the circuit two to three times (sets). Because of the short rest periods, significant cardiovascular benefits have been reported in addition to muscular endurance gains.

CRT on weight or hydraulic machines has been found to be more effective than standard set weight training for caloric consumption during and after exercise and for improving cardiovascular endurance, although it is not as effective as aerobic exercises, such as cycling or bench stepping.

Programs intended to slim the figure/physique should be of the muscular endurance type. Many men and women are interested in exercises designed to decrease girth measurements. High-repetition, low-resistance exercise is suitable for this because it usually brings about some strengthening and may decrease body fatness, which in turn changes body contour. Exercises do not spot-reduce fat, but they do speed up metabolism so more calories are burned. However, if weight or fat reduction is desired, aerobic (cardiovascular) exercises are best. To increase girth, use strength exercises.

Endurance training may have a negative effect on strength and power. Some studies have shown that, for athletes who rely primarily on strength and power in their sport, too much endurance training can cause a loss of strength and power because of the modification of

Table 3 ▶ Threshold of Training and Fitness Target Zones for Muscular Fitness

		Threshold of Training	Fitness Target Zones
Muscular Strength			
	Frequency	2 days a week for each muscle group	2–3 days per week for each muscle group
	Intensity	60–65% of 1 RM for every repetition	60–80% of 1 RM for number of reps on every set
	Time	1 set of 3–8 reps	1–3 sets of 3–8 reps
General Muscular Fitness			
	Frequency	2–3 days a week	3 days a week
	Intensity	40–50% of 1 RM for young adults	40–60% of 1 RM for young adults
		30–50% for adults >50 years old	40–50% for adults >50 years old
	Time	1 set of 8–12 reps for young adults	1–3 sets of 8–12 reps for young adults
		1 set of 10–15 reps for adults >50 years old	1–3 sets of 10–15 reps for adults >50
Dynamic Muscular Endurance			
	Frequency	2 days per week	Every other day
	Intensity	Move 20–30% of the maximum resistance you can lift	Move 40%–60% of the maximum resistance you can lift
	Time	One set of 9 repetitions of each exercise	2–5 sets of 9–25 repetitions of each exercise
Static Muscular Endurance			
	Frequency	3 days per week	Every other day
	Intensity	Hold a resistance 50–100% of the weight you ultimately need to hold in your work or leisure activity	Hold a resistance 100%–150% of the weight you ultimately need to hold in your work or leisure activity
	Time	Hold for lengths of time 10–50% shorter than the time you plan to do the activity; repeat 10–20 times and rest 30 seconds between repetitions	Hold for lengths of time equal to and up to 20% greater than the time you plan to do the activity (for longer times use fewer repetitions); rest 30–60 seconds between repetitions

different muscle fibers. Strength and power athletes need some endurance training, but not too much, just as endurance athletes need some strength and power training, but not too much.

Training Principles for PRE

The overload principle provides the basis for PRE. For the body to adapt and improve, the muscles and systems of the body must be challenged. As noted earlier, the concept behind PRE is that the frequency, intensity, and duration of lifts are progressively increased to maintain an effective stimulus as the muscle fitness improves. It was in the area of muscle fitness development that the overload principle was first clearly outlined. Legend holds that centuries ago a Greek named Milo of Crotona became progressively stronger by repeatedly lifting his calf. As the calf grew into a bull, its weight increased, and

Milo's strength increased as well. We know now that for most people, PREs are necessary if muscle fitness is to be developed and maintained (see Figure 6). Activities from other levels of the physical activity pyramid do not provide an adequate stimulus, so specific resistance exercise is needed to improve this dimension of fitness.

🌐 **The muscle fitness workout should be based on the principle of progression.** www.mhhe.com/phys_fit/web11 Click 10. Many beginning resistance trainers experience soreness after the first few days of training.

1 Repetition Maximum (1RM) The maximum amount of resistance one can move a given number of times—for example, 1 RM = maximum weight lifted one time; 6 RM = maximum weight lifted six times.

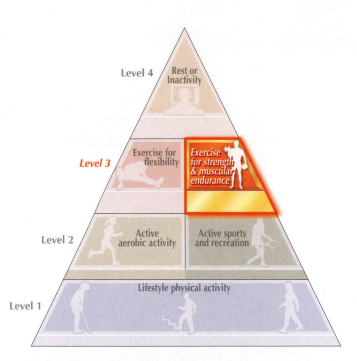

Figure 6 ▶ To build muscle fitness, activities should be selected from level 3 of the physical activity pyramid.

The reason for the soreness is that the principle of progression has been violated. Soreness can occur with even modest amounts of training if the volume of training is considerably more than normal. In the first few days or weeks of training, the primary adaptations in the muscle are due to motor learning factors rather than to muscle growth. Because these adaptations occur no matter how much weight is used, it is prudent to start your program slowly with light weights. After these adaptations occur and the rate of improvement slows down, it is necessary to follow the appropriate target zone to achieve proper overload.

The most common progression used in resistance training is the double progressive system, so-called because this system periodically adjusts both the resistance and the number of repetitions of the exercise performed. For example, if you are training for strength, you may begin with three repetitions in one set. As the repetitions become easy, additional repetitions are added. When you have progressed to eight repetitions, increase the resistance and decrease the repetitions in each set back to three and begin the progression again.

Other systems can be used within a training session to alter the training effect. Some recommend a "light to heavy" system (Delorme system), in which progressively heavier weights are lifted with each set. Others recommend the "heavy to light" system (Oxford system), in which the heaviest weight is used on the first set when the muscles are most rested. Still others advocate a preexhaust routine, in which small accessory muscle groups are fatigued before the exercises for major muscle groups are performed.

The principle of specificity applies to PRE. Depending on the specific muscle that you want to develop, you will use different types of resistance training programs. Factors that can be varied in your program are the type of muscle contraction (isometric or isotonic), the speed or cadence of the movement, and the amount of resistance being moved. For example, if you want strength in the elbow extensor muscles (e.g., triceps) so that you can more easily lift heavy boxes onto a shelf, you can train using isotonic contractions, at a relatively slow speed, with a relatively high resistance. If you want muscle fitness of the fingers to grip a heavy bowling ball, much of your training should be done isometrically using the fingers the same way you normally hold the ball. If you are training for a skill that requires explosive power, such as in throwing, striking, kicking, or jumping, your strength exercises should be done with less resistance and greater speed. If you are training for a skill that uses both concentric and eccentric contractions, you should perform exercises using these characteristics (e.g., plyometrics). More information on these techniques is included in the concept on the performance benefits of physical activity.

If you are not training for a specific task, but merely wish to develop muscle fitness for daily living, consider the advantages and disadvantages of isotonics, isometrics, and isokinetics, listed in Table 1. You may wish to use a variety of methods.

The principle of diminishing returns applies to resistance training. To get optimal strength gains from progressive resistance training, one or more sets of exercise repetitions are performed. Some high-level performers use as many as five sets of a particular exercise. Research indicates that most of the fitness and health benefits, however, are achieved in one set. Considerably more than 50 percent of the benefits may result in the first set, with each additional set producing less benefit. Because compliance with resistance training programs is less likely as the time needed to complete the program increases, the American College of Sports Medicine (ACSM) recommends single-set programs for most adults. It acknowledges that additional benefits are likely with more multiset routines but the ACSM believes that adults are more likely to participate if they can get most of the benefits in a relatively short amount of time. In sports or competition where small performance differences make a big difference, doing multiple sets is important.

The principle of rest and recovery especially applies to strength development. Progressive resistance training for strength development done every day of the week does not allow enough rest and time for recovery. Recent studies have shown that the greatest proportion of strength is accomplished in 2 days of training per week. Exercise done on a third day does result in additional increases, but the amount of gain is relatively small, compared with gains resulting from 2 days of training per week. For people interested in health benefits rather than performance benefits, 2 days a week saves time and may result in greater adherence to a strength-training program. For people interested in performance benefits, more frequent training may be warranted. Rotating exercises so that certain muscles are exercised on one day and other muscles are exercised the next allows for more frequent training.

The amount of exercise necessary to maintain strength is less than the amount needed to develop it. Recent evidence suggests that, once strength is developed, it can be maintained by performing fewer sets or exercising fewer days per week. For example, if you have performed three sets of an exercise 3 days a week to build strength, you may be able to maintain current levels of strength with one set a week. Also, you may be able to maintain strength by exercising 1 or 2 rather than 3 days per week. If schedules of fewer sets or days per week result in strength loss, frequency must be increased.

Some muscle groups seem to need training less often to maintain strength levels. For example, evidence suggests that muscle fitness of the back can be maintained using 1-day-a-week single-set exercises. Smaller muscles seem to need more frequent exercise.

Is There Strength in a Bottle?

Anabolic steroids are used by some athletes and a significant number of nonathletes to enhance performance and build muscular bodies. Anabolic steroids are a synthetic reproduction of the male hormone testosterone. Physicians prescribe them to treat such conditions as muscle diseases, breast cancer, severe burns, rare types of anemia, and kidney disease. Steroids have also been used to help people with AIDS and muscle-wasting diseases retain muscle mass. Because of their dangerous side effects, doctors prescribe minimal doses. At first, research showed steroids to be ineffective in promoting muscle gain. This was because the doses used in the studies were much smaller than those taken today for performance enhancement. Many athletes and people interested in muscle development have reportedly taken massive doses 20 to 100 times the normal therapeutic dose used for medical conditions. Studies now show that, when taken in large doses by people doing regular strength training, gains in muscle mass and strength can be considerable. Steroids act by increasing the rate of protein synthesis, and the effects have been shown to occur in a dose-response fashion.

Anabolic steroids are typically obtained on the black market or illegally from unethical physicians, coaches, trainers, bodybuilders, athletes, and other entrepreneurs. Whereas athletes use the drugs in an attempt to enhance performance, an increasing number of nonathletes use steroids to enhance their strength or improve their physique or appearance. Two million people are estimated to be using "roids." Steroid use has leveled off among males, but the levels among females has increased dramatically.

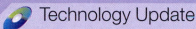 **Taking anabolic steroids is a dangerous way to build muscle fitness and is illegal.** www.mhhe. com/phys_fit/web11 Click 11. A number of significant side effects are associated with steroid use. In women, unlike men, some of these effects are irreversible (Figure 7). As can be seen in Figure 7, steroids (like all drugs) are dangerous. They can be addictive and produce

Technology Update
Resistance Training Equipment

Over the years, there have been major changes and developments in resistance training machines. Recent developments have allowed machines to overcome some of the well-known limitations. For example, many new machines allow movement to take place in multiple dimensions to allow for converging and diverging movements and independent arm function. Some examples include the Cybex VR2 line, the Paramount ART line, and the Arcuate Line by Pacific Fitness. These machines provide additional variety for strength training and a more natural motion. The Hammer Strength Line (Motion Technology Selectorized, or MTS) features independent arm function with dual-weight stacks to avoid one arm dominating the movement. Other companies have developed different "selectorized" technologies using cables and pulleys that allow exercisers to define their own path of motion. These machines allow the user to work multiple muscle groups and to target stabilizer muscles. Examples of this technology can be found in some of the new machines manufactured by Ground Zero, Vortex, Cybex, and Life Fitness.

Source: Fitness Management.

Anabolic Steroids Synthetic hormones similar to the male sex hormone testosterone. They function androgenically to stimulate male characteristics and anabolically to increase muscle mass, weight, bone maturation, and virility.

more than seventy serious side effects, some of which may be fatal. Many deaths have been attributed to their use. Twenty-five athletes from the former Soviet Union who competed in the 1980 Olympics died because of conditions attributed to steroid use, and the deaths of several American professional athletes, including former professional football player Lyle Alzado, have been attributed to steroid use. Former major league baseball player Ken Caminiti indicated in a *Sports Illustrated* interview that he used steroids and suggested that a high proportion of active players use them. His recent death at a very young age shocked the sports world, and although his death was directly attributable to a drug overdose, many have speculated that steriod use contributed to his early death. Studies show that most athletes who use anabolic steroids are familiar with the adverse effects but say, "I don't care and I will use them anyway." Most later say they regret this choice.

In addition to the physical effects, steroids have also been linked to other dangerous and unhealthy behaviors. Violent behavior, sometimes referred to as "roid rage," has been found to accompany steroid use. Recent research suggests that "roid rage" is most likely to result in people who are mentally unstable prior to use. Evidence indicates that steroid users are at greater risk of hepatitis or HIV/AIDS infections from shared needles.

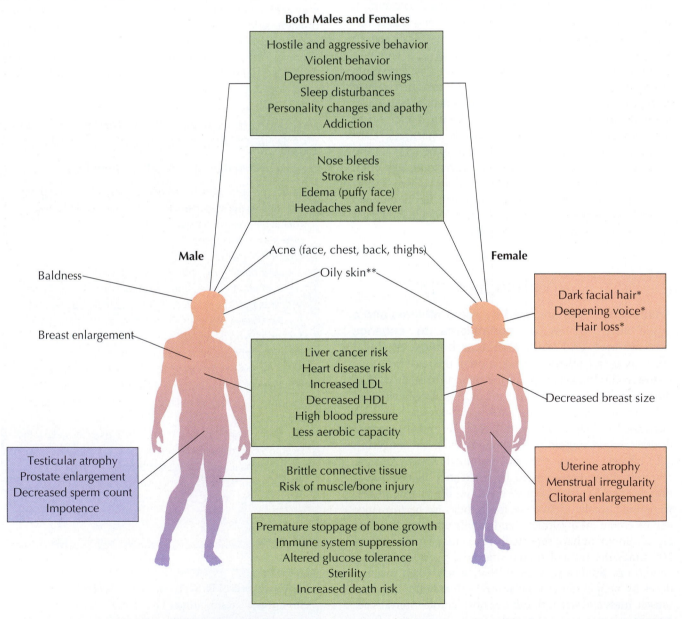

Both Males and Females

Hostile and aggressive behavior
Violent behavior
Depression/mood swings
Sleep disturbances
Personality changes and apathy
Addiction

Nose bleeds
Stroke risk
Edema (puffy face)
Headaches and fever

Male

Baldness

Breast enlargement

Acne (face, chest, back, thighs)
Oily skin**

Female

Dark facial hair*
Deepening voice*
Hair loss*

Liver cancer risk
Heart disease risk
Increased LDL
Decreased HDL
High blood pressure
Less aerobic capacity

Decreased breast size

Testicular atrophy
Prostate enlargement
Decreased sperm count
Impotence

Brittle connective tissue
Risk of muscle/bone injury

Uterine atrophy
Menstrual irregularity
Clitoral enlargement

Premature stoppage of bone growth
Immune system suppression
Altered glucose tolerance
Sterility
Increased death risk

*Among women, irreversible when use stops.
**Among women, partially reversible when use stops.

Figure 7 ▶ Adverse effects of anabolic steroids.

Injuries happen more easily and last longer in people who use steroids. Though steroids may make muscles stronger, tendons and ligaments do not proportionately increase in strength. Therefore, a strong muscle contraction can tear a tendon and/or a ligament. This is made more serious because steroids make the injury heal more slowly. When steroids increase muscle size, the extra muscle can grow around the bones and joints, causing them to break more easily. Many have attributed the increased muscle injuries in baseball players to steroids.

Androstenedione and THG are *not* safe alternatives to steroids. Androstenedione (andro) is a precursor of naturally occurring testosterone and estrogen. It became popular when baseball slugger Mark McGwire reported taking andro supplements during his assault on the season home run record. Early studies suggested that andro use did not lead to increases in testosterone levels, but recent evidence suggests that andro would probably have anabolic effects at the high doses most likely used by athletes. The side effects of andro use are similar to those of anabolic steroids, including disruption of normal sexual development, infertility, and increased risk for some forms of cancer. Use in children can lead to premature puberty and premature closure of the growth plates in bones. Andro has been banned by the International Olympic Committee, the NCAA, the NFL, and, most recently, major league baseball. The clear documentation of risks has also caused the FDA to require manufacturers to stop distributing products with androstenedione.

THG (tetrahydrogestrinone) is a chemically engineered steroid that, until recently, has been undetectable by standard drug tests. Many well-known athletes have recently tested positive for THG, and ongoing drug investigations will likely identify other THG users. The American College of Sports Medicine condemned THG as a threat to the health of athletes and the integrity of sports. The FDA declared that THG is a drug and not a "dietary supplement," as some purveyors or users of the product maintain. It is a purely synthetic steroid, which exhibits the same properties (and risks) of other anabolic steroids.

Recently, national legislation that was signed into law by the president prohibits the sale of steroid precursors and increases the penalties for their use. Eighteen substances, including andro and THG, were added to the list of illegal steroids and steroid alternatives.

Human growth hormone (HGH), taken to increase strength, may be even more dangerous than anabolic steroids. HGH is produced by the pituitary gland but is made synthetically. Some athletes are taking it in addition to anabolic steroids or in place of anabolic steroids because it is difficult to detect in urine tests. The effect of HGH is primarily on increasing bone size and not muscle size. Athletes often use growth hormone in combination with anabolic steroids so they can have gains in muscle mass along with the bone-strengthening effects of HGH. Athletes assume that this will protect them from some of the bone injuries that occur among steroid users. However, these athletes are further risking their health as the health risks of steroid use are compounded further with HGH use. Risks of HGH use include irreversible acromegaly (giantism) and growth deformities, cardiovascular disease, goiter, menstrual disorder, excessive sweating, lax muscles and ligaments, premature bone closure, decreased sexual desire, and impotence. In addition, the life span can be shortened by as much as 20 years. Like steroids, there are some medical uses for HGH, but HGH should be used only with physician recommendations and prescriptions.

Creatine use is becoming increasingly popular among people training for strength development. www.mhhe.com/phys_fit/web11 Click 12. Creatine is a nutrient involved in the production of energy during short-term, high-intensity exercise, such as resistance exercise. Creatine is produced naturally by the body from foods containing protein, but some athletes now take creatine supplements (usually a powder dissolved into a liquid) to increase the amounts available in the muscle. The concept behind supplementation is that additional creatine intake enhances energy production and therefore increases the body's ability to maintain force and delay fatigue. Some studies have shown improvements in athletic performance with creatine, but recent reviews indicate that the supplement may be effective only for athletes who are already well trained. Studies have been more consistent with regard to the ergogenic effects of creatine on muscle strength. It is important to recognize, though, that the benefits are due to the ability to work the muscles harder during an exercise session and not to the supplement itself. Increases in body weight may result, but this is likely due to water retention.

At present, creatine usage hasn't been linked to any major health problems but the long-term effects are unknown. The short-term side effects include stomach distress, cramping, and dehydration (see *In the News*, Concept 3). Additional side effects and complications may result if people take more than is recommended. The American College of Sports Medicine currently suggests that doses of 20 to 25 grams per day for 5 days followed by much smaller doses of 3 to 5 grams per day will result in maximal muscle saturation. Though not recommended for most people, if you are going to take creatine, it should not be taken in doses greater than those listed. Further, changes in the law in 1994 leave quality control issues up to the manufacturer rather than the government. For this reason, the quality of any food supplement (which creatine is considered) is only as good as the integrity of the supplier.

The safety and efficacy of many strength-related dietary supplements are not established. Many people use protein powders and various nutritional supplements in the hopes that they will help them make quick and easy gains in muscle mass. Claims for many of these products are often based on testimonials or articles in nonpeer-reviewed magazines. Studies using randomized, placebo-controlled designs that are published in high-quality journals have not demonstrated significant ergogenic benefits from protein supplementation. It is true that protein is needed for muscle synthesis, but the body does not store extra protein in the muscle, nor does extra protein increase muscle growth. Other dietary supplements such as chromium picolinate and DHEA have also been shown to be ineffective. Because of the unregulated nature of the dietary supplement industry, consumers should be wary about trying unproven products. (See "In the News" on page 184.)

Guidelines for Safe and Effective Resistance Training

 There are many fallacies, superstitions, and myths associated with resistance training. www. mhhe.com/phys_fit/web11 Click 13. Some common misconceptions about resistance training are described in Table 5.

There is a proper way to perform resistance training. Although resistance training offers considerable health benefits, there are also some risks if the exercises are not performed correctly or if safety procedures are not followed. A survey published in the *Physician and Sportsmedicine* estimated that there were over 1 million emergency room visits in the United States attributed to weight training during the 20-year period from 1978 to 1998. The leading predictor of injury identified in this survey was improper use of equipment. If you are unfamiliar with how to operate resistance training equipment, be sure to follow printed guidelines on the equipment and/or ask for general instruction. See Table 4 for specific safety tips.

Beginners should emphasize lighter weights and progress their program gradually. When beginning a resistance training program, start with weights that are too light, so that you can learn proper technique and avoid soreness and injury. As mentioned, most of the adaptations that occur in the first few months after beginning a program are due to improvements in the body's ability to recruit muscle fibers to contract effectively and efficiently. These neural adaptations occur in response to the movement itself and

are not due to how much weight is used. Therefore, beginning lifters can achieve significant benefits from lighter weights.

As experience and fitness levels improve, it is necessary to utilize heavier loads and more challenging sets to continually challenge the muscles. Information on how to determine appropriate workloads and how to balance more complex training programs is available in the article by Kraemer & Ratamess (2004).

Use good technique to reduce the risks for injury and to isolate the intended muscles. An important consideration in resistance exercise is to complete all lifts through the full range of motion using only the intended

Table 4 ▶ How to Prevent Injury (for the Beginner)
• Warm up 10 minutes before the workout and stay warm during the workout.
• Do not hold your breath while lifting. This may cause blackout or hernia.
• Avoid hyperventilation before lifting a weight.
• Avoid dangerous or high-risk exercises.
• Progress slowly.
• Use good shoes with good traction.
• Avoid arching your back. Keep the pelvis in normal alignment.
• Keep the weight close to the body.
• Do not lift from a stoop (bent over with back rounded).
• When lifting from the floor, do not let the hips come up before your upper body.
• For bent-over rowing, lay your head on a table and bend the knees, or use one-arm rowing and support the trunk with the free hand.
• Stay in a squat as short a time as possible and do not do a full squat.
• Be sure collars on free weights are tight.
• Use a moderately slow, continuous, controlled movement and hold the final position a few seconds.
• Overload but don't overwhelm! A program that is too intense can cause injuries.
• Do not pause between repetitions.
• Keep a steady rhythm.
• Do not allow the weights to drop or bang.
• Do not train without medical supervision if you have a hernia, high blood pressure, a fever, an infection, recent surgery, heart disease, or back problems.
• Use chalk or a towel to keep hands dry when handling weights.

muscle groups. A common cause of poor technique is using too heavy of a weight. If you have to jerk the weight up or use momentum to lift the weight, then it is too heavy. Using heavier weights will only provide a greater stimulus to your muscles if your muscles are actually doing the work. Therefore, it is best to use a weight that you can control safely. By lifting through the full range of motion, you will increase the effectiveness of the exercise and maintain good flexibility.

Perform lifts in a slow and controlled manner to enhance both effectiveness and safety. Lifting at a slow cadence will provide a greater stimulus to the muscles and increase strength gains. A common recommendation is to take 2 seconds on the lifting phase (concentric) and 4 seconds on the lowering (eccentric) phase. A recent study confirmed the effectiveness of this type of approach (see Westcott, 2003, *Suggested Readings*). In this study, novice exercisers were randomly assigned to perform a resistance training circuit at either a standard speed or a superslow speed. Following 8–10 weeks of training (two or three times per week), the gains in 10 RM and 5 RM lifts were significantly greater for the superslow group than for the normal-pace group.

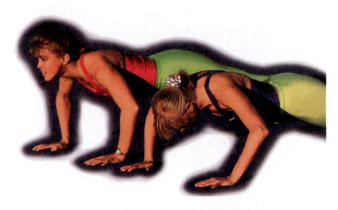

Well-planned resistance training helps you look your best.

Provide sufficient time to rest during and between workouts. The body needs time to rest in order to allow beneficial adaptations to occur. Choose an exercise sequence that alternates muscle groups so muscles have a chance to rest before another set. Lifting every other day or alternating muscle groups (if lifting more than 3 or 4 days per week) is also important in providing rest for the muscles.

Include all body parts and balance the strength of antagonistic muscle groups. A common mistake made by many beginning lifters is to perform only a few different exercises or to emphasize a few body parts.

Table 5 ▶ Facts and Fallacies about Resistance Training	
Myths and Fallacies	**Facts**
"Resistance training will make you muscle-bound and cause you to lose flexibility."	Normal resistance training will not reduce flexibility if exercises are done through the full range of motion and with proper technique. Powerlifters who do highly specific movements have been shown to have poorer flexibility than other weight lifters.
"Women will become masculine-looking if they gain strength."	Women will not become masculine-looking from resistance exercise. Women have less testosterone and do not bulk up from resistance training to the same extent as men. Women and men can make similar relative gains in strength and hypertrophy from a resistance training program, however. The greater percentage of fat in most women prevents the muscle definition possible in men and camouflages the increase in bulk.
"Strength training makes you move more slowly and look uncoordinated."	Strength training, if done properly, can enhance sport-specific strength and increase power. There are no effects on coordination from having high levels of muscular fitness.
"No pain, no gain."	It is not true that you have to get to the point of soreness to benefit from resistance exercise. It may be helpful to strive until you can't do a final repetition but you should definitely stop before it is painful. Slight tightness in the muscles is common 1 to 2 days following exercise but is not necessary for adaptations.
"Soreness occurs because lactic acid builds up in the muscles."	Lactic acid is produced during muscular work but is converted back into other substrates within 30 minutes after exercising. Soreness is due to microscopic tears or damage in the muscle fibers, but this damage is repaired as the body builds the muscle. Excessive soreness occurs if you violate the law of progression and do too much too soon.
"Strength training can build cardiovascular fitness and flexibility."	Resistance exercise can increase heart rate, but this is due primarily to a pressure overload rather than a volume overload on the heart that occurs from endurance (aerobic) exercise. Gains in muscle mass do cause an increase in resting metabolism that can aid in controlling body fatness.
"Strength training is beneficial only for young adults."	Studies have shown that people in their eighties and nineties can benefit from resistance exercise and improve their strength and endurance. Most experts would agree that resistance exercise increases in importance with age rather than decreases.

Training the biceps without working the triceps, for example, can lead to muscle imbalances that can compromise flexibility and increase risks for injury. In some cases, training must be increased in certain areas to compensate for stronger antagonist muscle groups. Many sprinters, for example, pull their hamstrings because the quadriceps are so overdeveloped that they overpower the hamstrings. The recommended ratio of quadriceps to hamstring strength is 60:40.

Customize your training program to fit your specific needs. Athletes should train muscles the way that they will be used in their skill, employing similar patterns, range of motion, and speed (the principle of specificity). If you wish to develop a particular group of muscles, remember that the muscle group can be worked harder when isolated than when worked in combination with other muscle groups.

Strategies for Action

An important step in taking action for developing and maintaining muscle fitness is assessing your current status. www.mhhe.com/phys_fit/ web11 Click 14. An important early step in taking action to improve fitness is self-assessment. A 1 RM test of isotonic strength is described in the *Lab Resource Materials*. This test allows you to determine absolute and relative strength for the arms and legs. In addition, the 1 RM values can be used to help you select the appropriate resistance for your muscle fitness training program. A grip strength test of isometric strength is also provided in the *Lab Resource Materials* for Lab 11A. In addition to descriptions of the 1 RM test, a body weight test for isotonic strength is provided in the "On the Web" feature for people who do not have the equipment to perform the 1 RM assessment.

Three tests of muscular endurance are described in the *Lab Resource Materials* for Lab 11B. It is recommended that you perform the assessments for both strength and muscular endurance before you begin your progressive resistance training program. Periodically reevaluate your muscle fitness using these assessments.

Many factors other than your own basic abilities affect muscle fitness test scores. If muscles are warmed up before lifting, more force can be exerted and heavier loads can be lifted. Muscle endurance performance may also be enhanced by a warm-up. Do not perform your self-assessments after vigorous exercise because that exercise can cause fatigue and result in suboptimal test results. It is appropriate to practice the techniques involved in the various tests on days preceding the

actual testing. People who have good technique achieve better scores and are less likely to be injured when performing tests than those without good technique. It is best to perform the strength and muscular endurance tests on different days.

Choose exercises that build muscle fitness in the major muscle groups of the body. The ACSM recommends eight to ten basic exercises for muscle fitness. Eight basic exercises, the Basic 8, for free weights (Table 6), resistance machines (Table 7), isometric exercises (Table 8), and calisthenics (Table 9) are presented to help you meet your muscle fitness needs. For most people the majority of the benefits associated with muscle fitness will result from performing the Basic 8 exercises using any of the four types of exercise. The Basic 8 for free weight and resistance machines would need to be supplemented with one or both of the abdominal exercises included in Table 10.

People interested in additional exercises that serve as alternates or that focus on improving fitness in other muscle groups are referred to the supplemental exercises in "On the Web" (web11 Click 09).

Keeping records of progress is important to adhering to a PRE program. Activity logging sheets are provided in Labs 11C and 11D to help you keep records of your progress as you regularly perform PRE to build and maintain good muscle fitness. A guide to the different muscles of the body is presented in Figure 8.

Study Resources

Check out additional online study resources for this concept in the Student Edition of the Online Learning Center at www.mhhe.com/corbin13e.

Web Resources

American College of Sports Medicine **www.acsm.org**
National Athletic Trainers Association **www.nata.org**
National Strength and Conditioning Association
   www.nsca-cc.org
The Physician and Sportsmedicine Online
   www.physsportsmed.com

Suggested Readings

 Additional reference materials for Concept 11 are available at www.mhhe.com/phys_fit/web11 Click 15.

American College of Sports Medicine. 2000. *ACSM's Guidelines for Exercise Testing and Prescription.* 6th ed. Philadelphia: Lippincott, Williams and Wilkins.

American College of Sports Medicine. "Creatine Supplementation: Current Content." (www.acsm.org).

Dohle, G., et al. 2003. Androgens and male fertility. *World Journal of Urology* 21:341–345.

Downing, J. H., and J. E. Lander. 2002. Performance errors in weight training and their correction. *Journal of Physical Education, Recreation and Dance* 73(9):44–52.

Earnest, C. P. 2001. Dietary androgen supplements. *The Physician and Sportsmedicine* 29(5):63–79.

Hartgens, F., et al. 2001. Androgenic-anabolic steroid-induced body changes in strength athletes. *The Physician and Sportsmedicine* 29(1):49–66.

Haykowsky, M. J., et al. 2003. Resistance exercise, the Valsalva maneuver, and cerebrovascular transmural pressure. *Medicine and Science in Sports and Exercise* 35(1):65–68.

Holt, S. July 2001. Mechanics of machines: Selecting the right piece of equipment. *Fitness Management* 56+.

Jones, C. S., C. Christenson, and M. Young. 2000. Weight training injury trends: A 20-year survey. *The Physician and Sportsmedicine* 28(7):61–72.

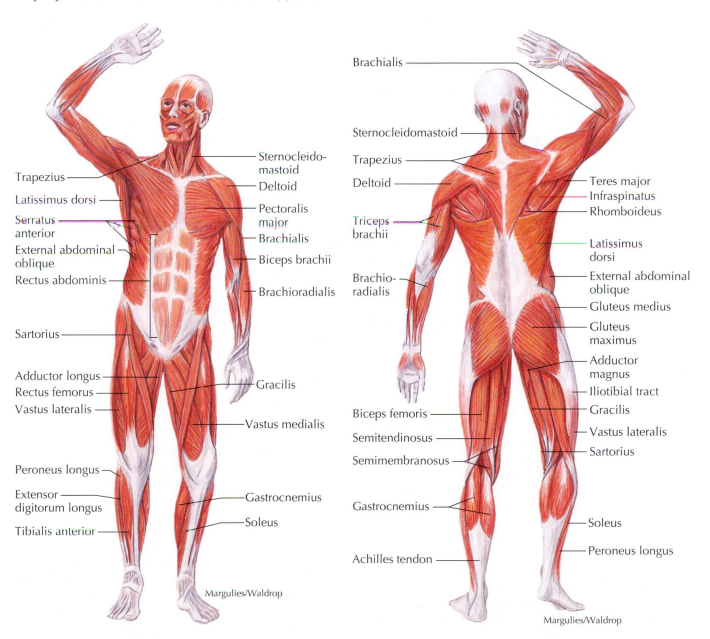

Figure 8 ▶ Muscles in the body.

Kraemer, W. J., and N. A. Ratamess. 2004. Fundamentals of resistance training: Progression and exercise prescription. *Medicine and Science in Sports and Exercise* 36(4):674–688.

Misic, M., and G. A. Kelley. 2002. The impact of creatine supplementation on anaerobic performance: A meta-analysis. *American Journal of Sportsmedicine* 4:116–124.

Nissen, S. L. and B. R. Sharp. 2003. Effects of dietary supplements on lean mass and strength gains with resistance exercise: A meta analysis. *Journal of Applied Physiology* 94(2):651–659.

Rhea, M. R., et al. 2003. A meta analysis to determine the dose response for strength development. *Medicine and Science in Sports and Exercise* 35(3): 456-464.

Rhea, M. R., et al. 2002. A comparison of linear and daily undulating periodized programs with equated volume and intensity for strength. *Journal of Strength and Conditioning Research* 16(2):250–255.

Sandler, D. 2003. *Weight Training Fundamentals.* Champaign, IL: Human Kinetics.

Urhausen, A., et al. 2004. Are the cardiac effects of anabolic steroids abuse in strength athletes reversible? *Heart* 90:496–501.

Volek, J. S. 2004. Influence of nutrition on responses to resistance training. *Medicine and Science in Sports and Exercise* 36(4):689–696.

Yesalis, C. E. and M. S. Bahrke. 2005. Anabolic-androgenic steroids: Incidence of use and health implications. *President's Council on Physical Fitness and Sports Research Digest* 6(1):1–8.

Wescott, W. 2003. *Building Strength and Stamina.* 2nd ed. Champaign, IL: Human Kinetics.

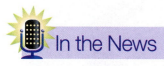 In the News

Guidelines to Improve the Safety of Dietary Supplements

Dietary supplements have continued to grow in popularity despite clear evidence that the overwhelming majority of the supplements are not effective. There are over 29,000 dietary supplements available to the American consumer and over 1,000 new products are released each year. Based on annual sales figures (over $16 billion last year), consumers seem willing to try almost any new product that hits the shelves and presumably believe that commercially available products are reasonably (or completely) safe. The now well-documented risks associated with ephedra clearly indicate that this is not the case, but consumers still seem to be willing to gamble by taking unproven supplements.

Under current guidelines from the Dietary Supplement Health and Education Act (DSHEA), manufacturers are not required to provide safety data on their products as drug companies are. Instead, dietary supplements are regulated as foods, meaning that they are considered safe unless proved otherwise, and they are not required to be clinically tested before they reach the market. The Food and Drug Administration (FDA) is responsible for determining whether a substance is harmful, but, with so many products, it is impossible for the FDA to keep up.

Concerns about the largely unregulated food supplement industry have led the Institute of Medicine (IOM) to recommend alternative procedures to help ensure the safety and efficacy of dietary supplements. The goal is to develop a system to identify supplement ingredients that may pose risks, prioritize them based on their level of potential risk, and then evaluate them for safety. The report also suggests that different kinds of data should be used to assess safety. Results from animal or laboratory tests, for example, may provide sufficient evidence to allow the FDA to cite that a product may pose an "unreasonable risk" to consumers and pull it from the market.

The IOM also recommended that manufacturers and distributors be required by the DSHEA to report adverse events to the FDA in a timely fashion to facilitate safety evaluations. Under the current rules, supplement manufacturers are not required to collect and report any health problems that they discover once the products are on the market. This loophole in the law hampers the FDA's ability to actively monitor supplement safety. According to recent estimates, the FDA receives reports on less than 0.5 percent of all adverse events associated with supplement use. A proposal to boost reporting is to include toll-free phone numbers on the product labels for consumers and health professionals to comment on products.

The biggest need cited in the report is for increased federal support for the FDA, so that it can carry out the consumer protection and education responsibilities mandated by the DSHEA. *Until changes are made in the law, consumers must use their own discretion and make their own decisions.* Students interested in more information should access the original IOM report (*Dietary Supplements: A Framework for Evaluating Safety*) from the National Academy Press (**www.nap.edu**).

1. Bench Press

This exercise develops the chest (pectoral) and triceps muscles. Lie supine on bench with knees bent and feet flat on bench or flat on floor in stride position. Grasp bar at shoulder level. Push bar up until arms are straight. Return and repeat. Do not arch lower back. Note: Feet may be placed on floor if lower back can be kept flattened. Do not put feet on the bench if it is unstable.

2. Overhead (Military Press)

This exercise develops the muscles of the shoulders and arms. Sit erect, bend elbows, palms facing forward at chest level with hands spread (slightly more than shoulder width). Have bar touching chest; spread feet (comfortable distance). Tighten your abdominal and back muscles. Move bar to overhead position (arms straight). Lower bar to chest position. Repeat. Caution: Keep arms perpendicular and do not allow weight to move backward or wrists to bend backward. Spotters are needed.

3. Biceps Curl

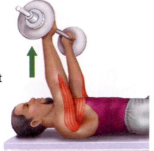

This exercise develops the muscles of the upper front part of the arms (biceps). Stand erect with back against a wall, palms forward, bar touching thighs. Spread feet in comfortable position. Tighten abdominals and back muscles. Do not lock knees. Move bar to chin, keeping body straight and elbows near the sides. Lower bar to original position. Do not allow back to arch. Repeat. Spotters are usually not needed. Variations: Use dumbbell and sit on end of bench with feet in stride position, work one arm at a time; or use dumbbell with the palm down or thumb up to emphasize other muscles.

4. Triceps Curl

This exercise develops the muscles on the back of the upper arms (triceps). Sit erect, elbows and palms facing up, bar resting behind neck on shoulders, hands near center of bar, feet spread. Tighten abdominal and back muscles. Keep upper arms stationary. Raise weight overhead, return bar to original position. Repeat. Spotters are needed. Variation: Substitute dumbbells (one in each hand, or one held in both hands, or one in one hand at a time).

Table 6 The Basic 8 for Free Weights

Table 6

5. Wrist Curl

This exercise develops the muscles of the fingers, wrist, and forearms. Sit astride a bench with the back of one forearm on the bench, wrist and hand hanging over the edge. Hold a dumbbell in the fingers of that hand with the palm facing forward. To develop the flexors, lift the weight by curling the fingers then the wrist through a full range of motion. Slowly lower and repeat. To strengthen the extensors, start with the palm down. Lift the weight by extending the wrist through a full range of motion. Slowly lower and repeat. Note: Both wrists may be exercised at the same time by substituting a barbell in place of the dumbbell.

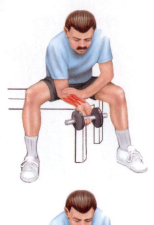
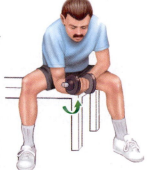

7. Half-Squat

This exercise develops the muscles of the thighs and buttocks. Stand erect, feet turned out 45 degrees. Rest bar behind neck on shoulders. Spread hands in a comfortable position. Squat slowly, keeping back straight, eyes ahead. Bend knees to approximately 90 degrees, and keep knees over feet. Pause; then stand. Repeat. Spotters are needed.

Variations: Substitute dumbbell in each hand at sides.

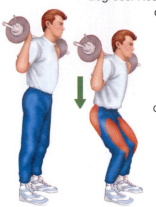

6. Dumbbell Rowing

This exercise develops the muscles of the upper back. It is best performed with the aid of a bench or chair for support. Grab a dumbbell with one hand and place opposite hand on the bench to support the trunk. Slowly lift the weight up until the elbow is parallel with the back. Lower the weight and repeat to complete the set. Switch hands and repeat with the opposite arm. The exercise can also be performed with one leg kneeling on the bench.

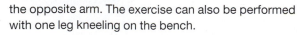

8. Lunge

This exercise develops the thigh and gluteal muscles. Place a barbell (with or without weight) behind your head and support with hands placed slightly wider than shoulder-width apart. In a slow and controlled motion, take a step forward and allow the leading leg to drop so that it is nearly parallel with the ground. The lower part of the leg should be near vertical and the back should be maintained in an upright posture. Take stride with opposite leg to return to standing posture. Repeat with other leg, remaining stationary or moving slowly in a straight line with alternating steps.

The Basic 8 for Resistance Machine Exercises Table 7

Table 7

1. Chest Press

This exercise develops the chest (pectoral) and tricep muscles. Position seat height so that arm handles are directly in front of chest. Position backrest so that hands are at a comfortable distance away from the chest. Push handles forward to full extension and return to starting position in a slow and controlled manner. Repeat. Note: Machine may have a foot lever to help position, raise, and lower the weight.

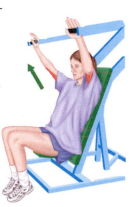

2. Seated Press

This exercise develops the muscles of the shoulders and arms. Position seat so that arm handles are slightly above shoulder height. Grasp handles with palms facing away and push lever up until arms are fully extended. Return to starting position and repeat. Note: Some machines may have an incline press.

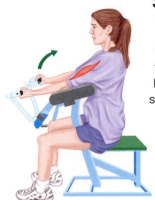

3. Bicep Curl

This exercise develops the elbow flexor muscles on the front of the arm, primarily the biceps. Adjust seat height so that arms are fully supported by pad when extended. Grasp handles palms up. While keeping the back straight, flex the elbow through the full range of motion.

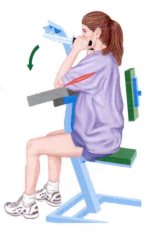

4. Tricep Press

This exercise develops the extensor muscles on the back of the arm, primarily the triceps. Adjust seat height so that arm handles are slightly above shoulder height. Grasp handles with thumbs toward body. While keeping the back straight, extend arms fully until wrist contacts the support pad (arms straight). Return to starting position and repeat.

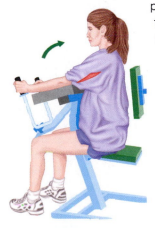

Table 7

Table 7 The Basic 8 for Resistance Machine Exercises

5. Lat Pull Down

This exercise primarily develops the latissmus dorsi, but the biceps, chest, and other back muscles may also be developed. Sit on the floor. Adjust seat height so that hands can just grasp bar when arms are fully extended. Grasp bar with palms facing away from you and hands shoulder-width (or wider) apart. Pull bar down to chest and return. Repeat.

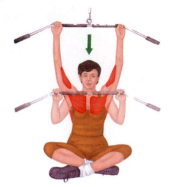

7. Knee Extension

This exercise develops the thigh (quadriceps) muscles. Sit on end of bench with ankles hooked under padded bar. Grasp edge of table. Extend knees. Return and repeat. Alternative: Leg press (similar to half-squat). Note: The knee extension exercise isolates the quadriceps but places greater stress on the structures of the knee than the leg press or half-squat.

6. Seated Rowing

This exercise develops the muscles of the back and shoulder. Adjust the machine so that arms are almost fully extended and parallel to the ground. Grasp handgrip with palms turned down and hands shoulder-width apart. While keeping the back straight, pull levers straight back to chest. Slowly return to starting position and repeat.

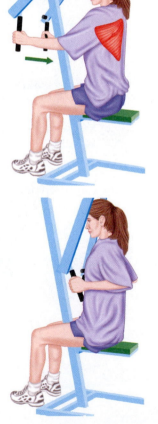

8. Hamstring Curl

This exercise develops the hamstrings (muscles on back of thigh) and other knee flexors. Lie prone on bench with ankles hooked under padded bar. Rest chin on hands or grasp bench. Flex knees as far as possible without allowing hips to raise. Return and repeat. Caution: Do not hyperextend the knees while assuming the starting position. If necessary, ask a partner to raise the pads while you place the heels under the bar.

Table 8

1. Arm Press in Doorway

This exercise develops the tricep and pectoral muscles. Stand in doorway, back flat on one side of doorway, hands placed on other side. Push with maximum force.

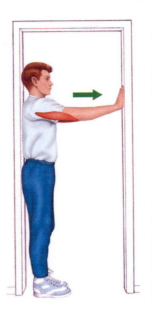

3. Curls

This exercise develops the muscles on the front of the arms. Place rope or towel loop behind thighs while standing in a half-squat position. Grasp loop, palms up, shoulder-width apart. Lift upward with maximum effort. Variation: Repeat, gripping with palms down.

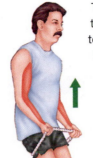

2. Overhead Press in Doorway

This exercise develops the muscles of the arms and shoulders. Stand in doorway, face straight ahead, hands shoulder-width apart, elbows bent. Tighten leg, hip, and back muscles. Push upward as hard as possible.

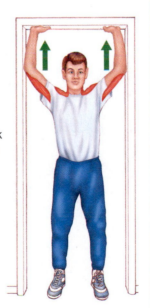

4. Triceps Press

This exercise develops the muscles on the back of the upper arm (triceps). Grasp towel or rope at both ends. Hold left hand at small of back, right hand over shoulder. Pull hands apart with maximum force. Repeat exercise, reversing position of hands.

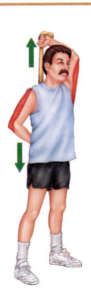

Table 8

Table 8 The Basic 8 for Isometric Exercises

5. Pelvic Tilt

This exercise develops the muscles of the abdomen and buttocks. Assume a supine position with the knees bent and slightly apart. Press the spine down on the floor and hold for several seconds. Keep abdominal and gluteal muscles tightened.

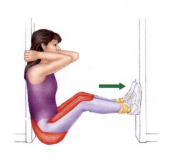

7. Wall Seat

This exercise develops the muscles of the legs and hips. Assume a half-sit position, back flat against wall, knees bent to 90 degrees. Push back against wall with maximum force and hold for several seconds.

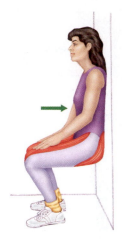

6. Leg Press in Doorway

This exercise develops the muscles of the legs and hips. Sit in doorway, facing side of door frame. Grasp molding behind head. Keep back flat on side of doorway, feet against other side. Push legs with maximum force and hold for several seconds.

8. Hamstring Curl

This exercise develops the muscles on back of legs. Stand on rope or towel loop with left foot. Place loop around right ankle. Flex knee until taut. Apply maximum force upward.

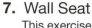

1. Bent Knee Push-Ups and Let-Down

This exercise develops the muscles of the arms, shoulders, and chest. Lie on the floor, face down with the hands under your shoulders. Keep your body straight from the knees to the top of the head. Push up until the arms are straight. Slowly lower chest (let-down) to floor. Repeat. Variation: full push-up and let-down performed the same way except body is straight from the toes to the top of head. Variation: Start from the up position and lower until the arm is bent at 90 degrees; then push up until arms are extended. Caution: Do not arch back.

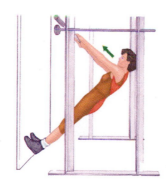

2. Modified Pull-Ups

This exercise develops the muscles of the arms and shoulders. Hang (palms forward and shoulder-width apart) from a low bar (may be placed across two chairs), heels on floor, with the body straight from feet to head. Bracing the feet against a partner or fixed object is helpful. Pull up, keeping the body straight, touch the chest to the bar, then lower to the starting position. Repeat. Note: This exercise becomes more difficult as the angle of the body approaches horizontal and easier as it approaches the vertical. Variation: Perform so that the feet do not touch the floor (full pull-up). Variation: Perform with palms turned up. When palms are turned away from the face, pull-ups tend to use all the elbow flexors. With palms facing the body, the biceps are emphasized more.

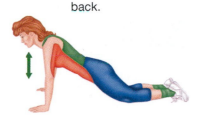

3. Dips

This exercise will develop the latissimus dorsi (on the back) and the tricep. Start in a fully extended position with hands grasping the bar (palms facing in). Slowly drop down until the upper part of the arm is horizontal or parallel with the floor. Extend the arms back up to the starting position and repeat. Note: Many gyms have a dip/pull-up machine with accommodating resistance that provides a variable amount of assistance to help you complete the exercise.

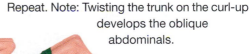

4. Crunch (Curl-Up)

This exercise develops the upper abdominal muscles. Lie on the floor with the knees bent and the arms extended or crossed with hands on shoulders or palms on ears. If desired, legs may rest on bench to increase difficulty. For less resistance, place hands at side of body (do not put hands behind head or neck). For more resistance, move hands higher. Curl up until shoulder blades leave floor; then roll down to the starting position. Repeat. Note: Twisting the trunk on the curl-up develops the oblique abdominals.

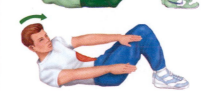

Table 9

Table 9 The Basic 8 for Calisthenics

5. (Trunk) Lift

This exercise develops the muscles of the upper back and corrects round shoulders. Lie face down with hands clasped behind the neck. Pull the shoulder blades together, raising the elbows off the floor. Slowly raise the head and chest off the floor by arching the upper back. Return to the starting position; repeat. For less resistance, hands may be placed under thighs. Caution: Do not arch the lower back. Lift only until the sternum (breastbone) clears the floor. Variations: arms down at sides (easiest), hands by head, arms extended (hardest).

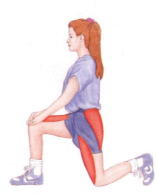

7. Lower Leg Lift

This exercise develops the muscles on the inside of thighs. Lie on the side with the upper leg (foot) supported on a bench. Note: If no bench is available, bend top leg and cross it in front of bottom leg for support. Raise the lower leg toward the ceiling. Repeat. Roll to opposite side and repeat. Keep knees pointed forward. Variation: An ankle weight may be added for greater resistance.

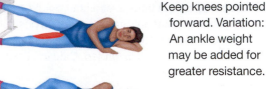
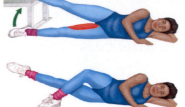

6. Side Leg Raises

This exercise develops the muscles on the outside of thighs. Lie on your side. Point knees forward. Raise the top leg 45 degrees; then return. Do the same number of repetitions with each leg. Caution: Keep knees and toes pointing forward. Variation: Ankle weights may be added for greater resistance.

8. Alternate Leg Kneel

This exercise develops the muscles of the legs and hips. Stand tall, feet together. Take a step forward with the right foot, touching the left knee to the floor. The knees should be bent only to a 90-degree angle. Return to the starting position and step out with the other foot. Repeat, alternating right and left.

Variation: Dumbbells may be held in the hands for greater resistance.

1. Crunch (Curl-Up)

This exercise develops the upper abdominal muscles. Lie on the floor with the knees bent and the arms extended or crossed with hands on shoulders or palms on ears. If desired, legs may rest on bench to increase difficulty. For less resistance, place hands at side of body (do not put hands behind neck). For more resistance, move hands higher. Curl up until shoulder blades leave floor, then roll down to the starting position. Repeat.

Note: Twisting the trunk on the curl-up develops the oblique abdominals.

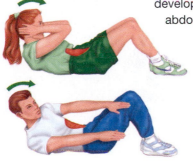

3. Crunch with Twist (on Bench)

This exercise strengthens the oblique abdominals and helps prevent or correct lumbar lordosis, abdominal ptosis, and backache. Lie on your back with your feet on a bench, knees bent at 90 degrees. Arms may be extended or on 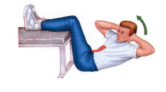 shoulders or hand on ears (the most difficult). Same as crunch except twist the upper trunk so the right shoulder is higher than the left. Reach toward the left knee with the right elbow. Hold. Return and repeat to the opposite side.

2. Reverse Curl

This exercise develops the lower abdominal muscles. Lie on the floor. Bend the knees, place the feet flat on the floor, and place arms at sides. Lift the knees to the chest, raising the hips off the floor. Do not let the knees go past the shoulders. Return to the starting position. Repeat.

4. Sitting Tucks

This exercise strengthens the lower abdominals, increases their endurance, improves posture, and prevents backache. (This is an advanced exercise and is not recommended for people 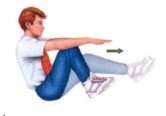 who have back pain.) Sit on floor with feet raised, arms extended for balance. Alternately bend and extend legs without letting back or feet touch floor.

Table 11

Table 11 Strength and Muscular Endurance Self-Assessments

1. Seated Press (Chest Press)

This test can be performed using a seated press (see below) or using a bench press machine. When using the seated press, position the seat height so that arm handles are directly in front of the chest. Position backrest so that hands are at comfortable distance away from the chest. Push handles forward to full extension and return to starting position in a slow and controlled manner. Repeat. Note: Machine may have a foot lever to help position, raise, and lower the weight.

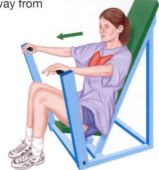

2. Leg Press

To perform this test, use a leg press machine. Typically, the beginning position is with the knees bent at right angles with the feet placed on the press machine pedals or a foot platform. Extend the legs and return to beginning position. Do not lock the knees when the legs are straightened. Typically, handles are provided. Grasp the handles with the hands when performing this test.

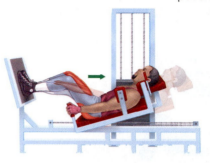

Lab Resource Materials: Muscle Fitness Tests

Evaluating Isotonic Strength: 1 RM

1. Use a weight machine for the leg press and seated arm press (or bench press) for the evaluation.
2. Estimate how much weight you can lift two or three times. Be conservative; it is better to start with too little weight than too much. If you lift the weight more than ten times, the procedure should be done again on another day when you are rested.
3. Using correct form, perform a leg press with the weight you have chosen. Perform as many times as you can up to ten.
4. Use Chart 1 to determine your 1 RM for the leg press. Find the weight used in the left-hand column and then find the number of repetitions you performed across the top of the chart.
5. Your 1 RM score is the value where the weight row and the repetitions column intersect.
6. Repeat this procedure for the seated arm press.
7. Record your 1 RM scores for the leg press and seated arm press in the Results section.
8. Next, divide your 1 RM scores by your body weight in pounds to get a "strength per pound of body weight" (str/lb./body wt.) score for each of the two exercises.
9. Finally, determine your strength rating for your upper body strength (arm press) and lower body (leg press) using Chart 2.

Chart 1 ▶ Predicted 1 RM Based on Reps-to-Fatigue

Wt.	1	2	3	4	5	6	7	8	9	10	Wt.	1	2	3	4	5	6	7	8	9	10
30	30	31	32	33	34	35	36	37	38	39	170	170	175	180	185	191	197	204	211	219	227
35	35	37	38	39	40	41	42	43	44	45	175	175	180	185	191	197	203	210	217	225	233
40	40	41	42	44	46	47	49	50	51	53	180	180	185	191	196	202	209	216	223	231	240
45	45	46	48	49	51	52	54	56	58	60	185	185	190	196	202	208	215	222	230	238	247
50	50	51	53	55	56	58	60	62	64	67	190	190	195	201	207	214	221	228	236	244	253
55	55	57	58	60	62	64	66	68	71	73	195	195	201	206	213	219	226	234	242	251	260
60	60	62	64	65	67	70	72	74	77	80	200	200	206	212	218	225	232	240	248	257	267
65	65	67	69	71	73	75	78	81	84	87	205	205	211	217	224	231	238	246	254	264	273
70	70	72	74	76	79	81	84	87	90	93	210	210	216	222	229	236	244	252	261	270	280
75	75	77	79	82	84	87	90	93	96	100	215	215	221	228	235	242	250	258	267	276	287
80	80	82	85	87	90	93	96	99	103	107	220	220	226	233	240	247	255	264	273	283	293
85	85	87	90	93	96	99	102	106	109	113	225	225	231	238	245	253	261	270	279	289	300
90	90	93	95	98	101	105	108	112	116	120	230	230	237	244	251	259	267	276	286	296	307
95	95	98	101	104	107	110	114	118	122	127	235	235	242	249	256	264	273	282	292	302	313
100	100	103	106	109	112	116	120	124	129	133	240	240	247	254	262	270	279	288	298	309	320
105	105	108	111	115	118	122	126	130	135	140	245	245	252	259	267	276	285	294	304	315	327
110	110	113	116	120	124	128	132	137	141	147	250	250	257	265	273	281	290	300	310	321	333
115	115	118	122	125	129	134	138	143	148	153	255	256	262	270	278	287	296	306	317	328	340
120	120	123	127	131	135	139	144	149	154	160	260	260	267	275	284	292	302	312	323	334	347
125	125	129	132	136	141	145	150	155	161	167	265	265	273	281	289	298	308	318	329	341	353
130	130	134	138	142	146	151	156	161	167	173	270	270	278	286	295	304	314	324	335	347	360
135	135	139	143	147	152	157	162	168	174	180	275	275	283	291	300	309	319	330	341	354	367
140	140	144	148	153	157	163	168	174	180	187	280	280	288	296	305	315	325	336	348	360	373
145	145	149	154	158	163	168	174	180	186	193	285	285	293	302	311	321	331	342	354	366	380
150	150	154	159	164	169	174	180	186	193	200	290	290	298	307	316	326	337	348	360	373	387
155	155	159	164	169	174	180	186	192	199	207	295	295	303	312	322	332	343	354	366	379	393
160	160	165	169	175	180	186	192	199	206	213	300	300	309	318	327	337	348	360	372	386	400
165	165	170	175	180	186	192	198	205	212	220	305	305	314	323	333	343	354	366	379	392	407

Source: JOPERD.

Evaluating Isometric Strength

Test: Grip Strength

Adjust a hand dynamometer to fit your hand size. Squeeze it as hard as possible. You may bend or straighten the arm, but do not touch the body with your hand, elbow, or arm. Perform with both right and left hands. *Note:* When not being tested, perform the Basic 8 isometric strength exercises, or squeeze and indent a new tennis ball (*after* completing the dynamometer test).

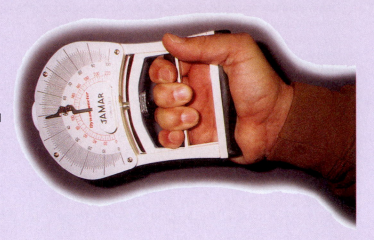

Evaluating Muscular Endurance

1. Curl-Up (Dynamic)

Sit on a mat or carpet with your legs bent more than 90 degrees so your feet remain flat on the floor (about halfway between 90 degrees and straight). Make two tape marks $4^{1}/_{2}$ inches apart or lay a $4^{1}/_{2}$-inch strip of paper or cardboard on the floor. Lie with your arms extended at your sides, palms down and the fingers extended so that your fingertips touch one tape mark (or one side of the paper or cardboard strip). Keeping your heels in contact with the floor, curl the head and shoulders forward until your fingers reach $4^{1}/_{2}$ inches (second piece of tape or other side of strip). Lower slowly to beginning position. Repeat one curl-up every 3 seconds. Continue until you are unable to keep the pace of one curl-up every 3 seconds.

Two partners may be helpful. One stands on the cardboard strip (to prevent movement) if one is used. The second assures that the head returns to the floor after each repetition.

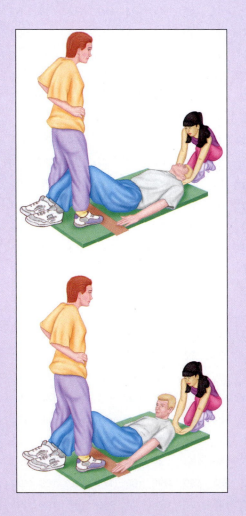

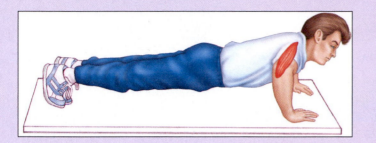

2. Ninety-Degree Push-Up (Dynamic)
Support the body in a push-up position from the toes. The hands should be just outside the shoulders, the back and legs straight, and the toes tucked under. Lower the body until the upper arm is parallel to the floor or the elbow is bent at 90 degrees. The rhythm should be approximately one push-up every 3 seconds. Repeat as many times as possible up to 35.

3. Flexed-Arm Support (Static)
Women: Support the body in a push-up position from the knees. The hands should be outside the shoulders, and the back and legs straight. Lower the body until the upper arm is parallel to the floor or the elbow is flexed at 90 degrees.
Men: Use the same procedure as for women except support the push-up position from the toes instead of the knees. (Same position as for 90-degree push-up.) Hold the 90-degree position as long as possible, up to 35 seconds.

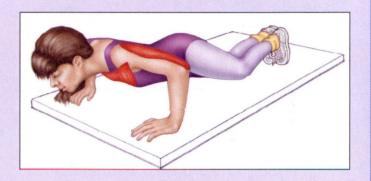

Chart 2 ▶ Strength per Pound of Body Weight Ratings						
Rating: Age: Men	Leg Press 30 or Less	31–50	51+	Arm Press 30 or Less	31–50	51+
High-performance zone	2.06+	1.81+	1.61+	1.26+	1.01+	.86+
Good fitness	1.96–2.05	1.66–1.80	1.51–1.60	1.11–1.25	.91–1.00	.76–0.85
Marginal	1.76–1.95	1.51–1.65	1.41–1.50	.96–1.10	.86–0.90	.66–0.75
Low fitness	1.75 or less	1.50 or less	1.40 or less	.96 or less	.80 or less	.65 or less
Women						
High-performance zone	1.61+	1.36+	1.16+	.75+	.61+	.51+
Good fitness	1.46\–1.60	1.21\–1.35	1.06–1.15	.65–0.75	.56–0.60	.46–0.50
Marginal	1.31–1.45	1.11–1.20	.96–1.05	.56–0.65	.51–0.55	.41–0.45
Low fitness	1.30 or less	1.10 or less	.95 or less	.55 or less	.50 or less	.40 or less

Chart 3 ▶ Isometric Strength Rating Scale (Pounds)

Classification	Left Grip	Right Grip	Total Score
Men			
High-performance zone	125+	135+	260+
Good fitness zone	100–124	110–134	210–259
Marginal zone	90–99	95–109	185–209
Low zone	less than 90	less than 95	less than 185
Women			
High-performance zone	75+	85+	160+
Good fitness zone	60–74	70–84	130–159
Marginal zone	45–59	50–69	95–129
Low zone	less than 45	less than 50	less than 95

Suitable for use by young adults between 18 and 30 years of age. After 30, an adjustment of 0.5 of 1 percent per year is appropriate because some loss of muscle tissue typically occurs as you grow older.

Chart 4 ▶ Rating Scale for Dynamic Muscular Endurance

Age:	17–26		27–39		40–49		50–59		60+	
Classification	Curl-Ups	Push-Ups	Curl-Ups	Push-Ups	Curl-Ups	Push-Ups	Curl-Ups	Push-Ups	Curl-Ups	Push-Ups
Men										
High-performance zone	35+	29+	34+	27+	33+	26+	32+	24+	31+	22+
Good fitness zone	24–34	20–28	23–33	18–26	22–32	17–25	21–31	15–23	20–30	13–21
Marginal zone	15–23	16–19	14–22	15–17	13–21	14–16	12–20	12–14	11–19	10–12
Low zone	<15	<16	<14	<15	<13	<14	<12	<12	<11	<10
Women										
High-performance zone	25+	17+	24+	16+	23+	15+	22+	14+	21+	13+
Good fitness zone	18–24	12–16	17–23	11–15	16–22	10–14	15–21	9–13	14–20	8–12
Marginal zone	10–17	8–11	9–16	7–10	8–15	6–9	7–14	5–8	6–13	4–7
Low zone	<10	<8	<9	<7	<8	<6	<7	<5	<6	<4

Chart 5 ▶ Rating Scale for Static Endurance (Flexed-Arm Support)

Classification	Score in Seconds
High-performance zone	30+
Good fitness zone	20–29
Marginal zone	10–19
Low zone	10

Lab 11A Evaluating Muscle Strength: 1 RM and Grip Strength

Name	Section	Date

Purpose: To evaluate your muscle strength using 1 RM and to determine the best amount of resistance to use for various strength exercises

Procedures: 1 RM is the maximum amount of resistance you can lift for a specific exercise. Testing yourself to determine how much you can lift only one time using traditional methods can be fatiguing and even dangerous. The procedure you will perform here allows you to estimate 1 RM based on the number of times you can lift a weight that is less than 1 RM.

Evaluating Strength Using Estimated 1 RM

1. Use a resistance machine for the leg press and arm or bench press for the evaluation part of this lab. (See page 200 or Table 11.)
2. Estimate how much weight you can lift two or three times. Be conservative; it is better to start with too little weight than too much. If you lift a weight more than ten times, the procedure should be done again on another day when you are rested.
3. Using correct form, perform a leg press with the weight you have chosen. Perform as many times as you can up to ten.
4. Use Chart 1 in *Lab Resource Materials* to determine your 1 RM for the leg press. Find the weight used in the left-hand column and then find the number of repetitions you performed across the top of the chart.
5. Your 1 RM score is the value where the weight row and the repetitions column intersect.
6. Repeat this procedure for the arm or bench press using the same technique.
7. Record your 1 RM scores for the leg press and bench press in the Results section.
8. Next divide your 1 RM scores by your body weight in pounds to get a "strength per pound of body weight" (str/lb./body wt.) score for each of the two exercises.
9. Determine your strength rating for your upper body strength (arm press) and lower body (leg press) using Chart 2 in *Lab Resource Materials*. Record in the Results section. If time allows, assess 1 RM for other exercises you choose to perform (see Lab 11C).
10. If a grip dynamometer is available, determine your right-hand and left-hand grip strength using the procedures in *Lab Resource Materials*. Use Chart 3 in *Lab Resource Materials* to rate your grip (isometric) strength.

Results:

Arm press (or bench press):	Wt. selected		Reps		Estimated 1 RM
					(Chart 1, *Lab Resource Materials*)
	Strength per lb. body weight (1 RM ÷ body weight)				Rating
					(Chart 2, *Lab Resource Materials*)
Leg press:	Wt. selected		Reps		Estimated 1 RM
					(Chart 1, *Lab Resource Materials*)
	Strength per lb. body weight (1 RM ÷ body weight)				Rating
					(Chart 2, *Lab Resource Materials*)
Grip strength:	Right grip score				Right grip rating
	Left grip score				Left grip rating
	Total score				Total rating

Seated Press (Chest Press)

This test can be performed using a seated press (see below) or using a bench press machine. When using the seated press position the seat height so that arm handles are directly in front of the chest. Position backrest so that hands are at a comfortable distance away from the chest. Push handles forward to full extension and return to starting position in a slow and controlled manner. Repeat. Note: machine may have a foot lever to help position, raise, and lower the weight.

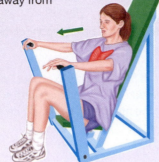

Leg Press

To perform this test use a leg press machine. Typically, the beginning position is with the knees bent at right angles with the feet placed on the press machine pedals or a foot platform. Extend the legs and return to beginning position. Do not lock the knees when the legs are straightened. Typically handles are provided. Grasp the handles with the hands when performing this test.

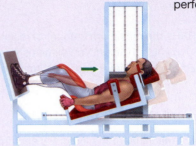

Conclusions and Implications: In several sentences, discuss your current strength, whether you believe it is adequate for good health, and whether you think that your "strength per pound of body weight" scores are really representative of your true strength.

Lab 11B Evaluating Muscular Endurance

Name	Section	Date

Purpose: To evaluate the dynamic muscular endurance of two muscle groups and the static endurance of the arms and trunk muscles

Procedures

1. Perform the curl-up, push-up, and flexed-arm support tests described in *Lab Resource Materials*.
2. In Chart 1, Record your test scores in the Results section. Determine and record your rating from Charts 4 and 5 in *Lab Resource Materials*.

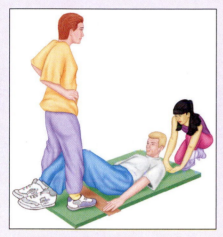

1. Curl-up (dynamic)

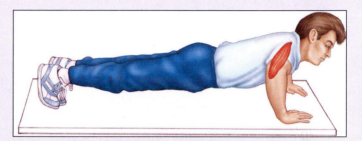

2. Ninety-degree push-up (dynamic)

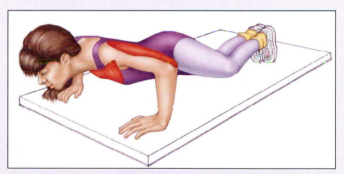

3. Flexed-arm support (static): women in knee position and men in full support position

Results

Record your scores below.

Curl-up [   ]   Push-up [   ]   Flexed-arm support (seconds) [   ]

Check your ratings in Chart 1.

Chart 1 ▶ Rating Scale for Static Endurance (Flexed-Arm Support)			
	Curl-up	**Push-up**	**Flexed-arm support**
High	○	○	○
Good	○	○	○
Marginal	○	○	○
Poor	○	○	○

On which of the tests of muscular endurance did you score the lowest?

Curl-up ◯   Push-up ◯   Flexed-arm support ◯

On which of the tests of muscular endurance did you score the best?

Curl-up ◯   Push-up ◯   Flexed-arm support ◯

Conclusions and Implications: In several sentences, discuss your current level of muscular endurance and whether this level is enough to meet your health, work, and leisure-time needs in the future.

Lab 11C Planning and Logging Muscle Fitness Exercises: Free Weights or Resistance Machines

Name		Section	Date

Purpose: To set lifestyle goals for muscle fitness exercise, to prepare a muscle fitness exercise plan, and to self-monitor progress for the 1-week plan

Procedures

1. The Basic 8 exercises are listed for free weights and resistance machines. Use Chart 1 to select eight exercises to represent your Basic 8 exercises. If you would like to add other exercises to your program, list them on the lines at the bottom of the chart. Descriptions of the exercises are provided in Tables 6 and 7.
2. In Chart 1, also indicate the days of the week that you plan on performing the exercises and the number of reps and the number of sets. Be sure to base your program on your goals (strength/endurance). If you are just starting out, it is best to start with one set of twelve to fifteen repetitions. Use the 1 RM procedure described in Lab 11A to help you determine the amount of weight or resistance to use. Plan to do at least eight exercises, two or three times a week. Note: All exercises do not have to be performed on the same day, but many people find this more convenient.
3. Though abdominal exercises are not typically done using free weights or resistance machines, an abdominal exercise is recommended as part of a resistance exercise program. Two abdominal exercises are provided in the "Other" category for you to consider (see Table 10).
4. In Chart 2, keep a 1-week log of your actual participation. For best results, keep the log with you during your workout session. Indicate the exercises you performed, including any that you didn't plan on performing when you developed your schedule. If you would like to keep a log for more than one week, make extra copies of the log before you begin.
5. Answer the question in the Results section.

Chart 1 ▶ Muscle Fitness Exercise Plan

What is your goal? Check one or more: Strength ❏   Endurance ❏   General Fitness ❏
Check boxes beside at least eight exercises; note days, reps, sets, and resistance to be used.

Primary Body Parts to Be Exercised	Free Weight Exercises (Basic 8)	Machine Weight Exercises (Basic 8)	Day 1 Date:	Day 2 Date:	Day 3 Date:	How Many Reps?	How Many Sets?	Weight or Setting
Chest	Bench press	Chest press						
Shoulder	Overhead press	Seated press						
Arm (bicep)	Bicep curl	Bicep curl						
Arm (tricep)	Tricep curl	Tricep press						
Arm (wrist)	Wrist curl	(No equivalent*)						
Back	Dumbbell rowing	Lat pull down						
Back (lower)	(No equivalent*)	Seated rowing						
Hip/leg (thigh)	Lunge	(No equivalent*)						
Leg (thigh)	Half squat	Knee extension						
Leg (hamstring)	(No equivalent*)	Hamstring curl						
Leg (calf)	Heel raise	(No equivalent*)						
Other exercises								
Abdominal	Crunch	Reverse curl						

*Note: Some free weight and machine exercises do not have equivalents.

Chart 2 ▶ Muscle Fitness Exercise Log

Check the exercises you performed and the days you performed them.

Primary Body Parts to Be Exercised	Free Weight Exercises (Basic 8)	Machine Weight Exercises (Basic 8)	Day 1 Date:	Day 2 Date:	Day 3 Date:
Chest	Bench press	Chest press			
Shoulder	Overhead press	Seated press			
Arm (bicep)	Bicep curl	Bicep curl			
Arm (tricep)	Tricep curl	Tricep press			
Arm (wrist)	Wrist curl	(No equivalent*)			
Back	Dumbbell rowing	Lat pull down			
Back (lower)	(No equivalent*)	Seated rowing			
Hip/leg (thigh)	Lunge	(No equivalent*)			
Leg (thigh)	Half squat	Knee extension			
Leg (hamstring)	(No equivalent*)	Hamstring curl			
Leg (calf)	Heel raise	(No equivalent*)			
Other exercises					
Abdominal	Crunch	Reverse curl			

*Note: Some free weight and machine exercises do not have equivalents.

Results

Were you able to do your Basic 8 exercises at least 2 days in the week?   Yes ◯   No ◯

Conclusions and Implications

1. Do you feel that you will use muscle fitness exercises as part of your regular lifetime physical activity plan, either now or in the future? Use several sentences to answer.

2. Discuss the exercises you feel benefited you and the ones that did not. What modifications would you make in your program for it to work better for you? Use several sentences to answer.

Lab 11D Planning and Logging Muscle Fitness Exercises: Calisthenics or Isometric Exercises

Name		Section	Date

Purpose: To set lifestyle goals for muscle fitness exercises that can easily be performed at home, to prepare a muscle fitness exercise plan, and to self-monitor progress for a 1-week plan

Procedures

1. The Basic 8 exercises are listed for calisthenics and isometric exercises. Use Chart 1 to select eight exercises to represent your Basic 8. If you would like to add other exercises to your program, then list them on the lines at the bottom of the chart. Descriptions of the exercises are provided in Tables 8 and 9.
2. In Chart 1, indicate the days of the week that you plan to perform the exercises and the number of reps and the number of sets. Plan to do at least eight exercises, two or three times a week. Note: All exercises do not have to be performed on the same day, but many people find this more convenient. Do what is best for your schedule.
3. In Chart 2, keep a 1-week log of your actual participation. For best results, keep the log with you during your workout session. Indicate the exercises you performed, including any that you did not plan on. If you would like to keep a log for more than 1 week, make extra copies of the log before you begin.
4. Answer the question in the Results section.

Chart 1 ▶ Muscle Fitness Exercise Log

What is your goal? Check one or more: Strength ☐   Endurance ☐   General Fitness ☐
Check boxes beside at least eight exercises; note days, reps, sets, and resistance to be used.

Primary Body Parts to Be Exercised	Calisthenic Exercises (Basic 8)	Isometric Exercises (Basic 8)	Day 1 Date:	Day 2 Date:	Day 3 Date:	How Many Reps?	How Many Sets?
Chest	Knee push-up	Arm press in door					
Shoulder	(No equivalent*)	Overhead press in door					
Arm (bicep)	Modified pull-up	Bicep curl					
Arm (tricep)	Dips	Tricep press					
Trunk/back	Trunk lift	(No equivalent*)					
Abdominals	Crunch	Pelvic tilt					
Leg (outer)	Side leg raise	(No equivalent*)					
Leg (inner)	Lower leg lift	(No equivalent*)					
Leg (thigh)	Leg kneel	Leg press					
Leg (thigh)	(No equivalent*)	Wall seat					
Leg (hamstring)	(No equivalent*)	Hamstring exercise					
Other							

*Note: Calisthenics and isometric exercises may not have exact equivalents.

Chart 2 ▶ Muscle Fitness Exercise Log

Check the exercises you performed and the days you performed them.

Primary Body Parts to Be Exercised	Calisthenic Exercises (Basic 8)		Isometric Exercises (Basic 8)		Day 1 Date	Day 2 Date	Day 3 Date
Chest	Knee push-up		Arm press in door				
Shoulder	(No equivalent*)		Overhead press in door				
Arm (bicep)	Modified pull-up		Bicep curl				
Arm (tricep)	Dips		Tricep press				
Trunk/back	Trunk lift		(No equivalent*)				
Abdominals	Crunch		Pelvic tilt				
Leg (outer)	Side leg raise		(No equivalent*)				
Leg (inner)	Lower leg lift		(No equivalent*)				
Leg (thigh)	Leg kneel		Leg press				
Leg (thigh)	(No equivalent*)		Wall seat				
Leg (hamstring)	(No equivalent*)		Hamstring exercise				
Other							

*Note: Calisthenics and isometric exercises may not have exact equivalents.

Results

Were you able to do your Basic 8 exercises at least 2 days in the week?   Yes ◯   No ◯

Conclusions and Implications

1. Do you feel that you will use these muscle fitness exercises as part of your regular lifetime physical activity plan, either now or in the future? Would the convenience of being able to do these exercises anywhere make it easier for you to stick with your program? Use several sentences to answer.

2. Discuss the exercises you feel benefited you and the ones that did not. What modifications would you make in your program for it to work better for you? Use several sentences to answer.

Safe Physical Activity and Exercises

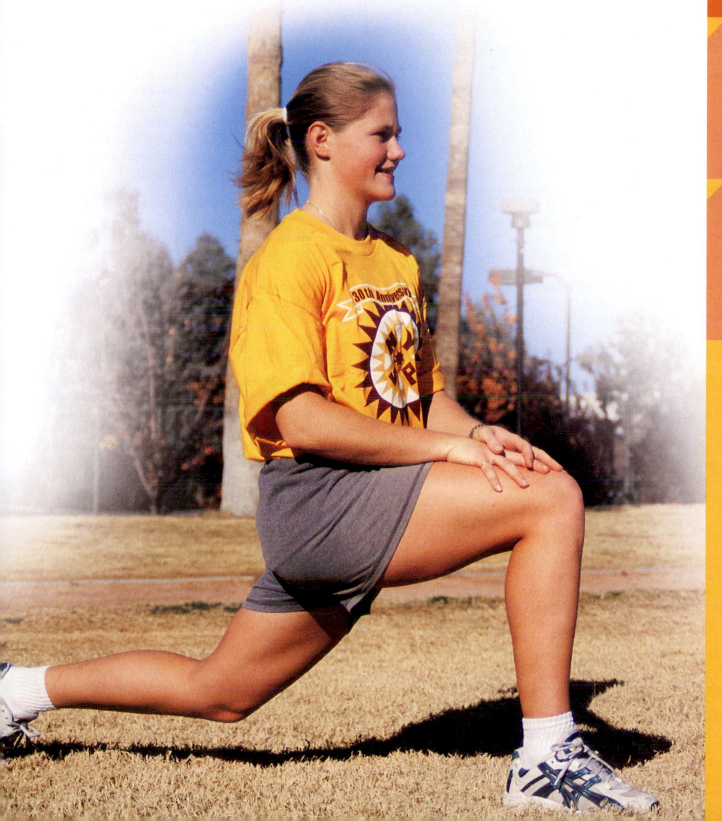

There are safe exercises that can be used as alternatives to questionable exercises that may cause more harm than good.

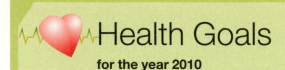

Health Goals

for the year 2010

- Increase incidence of people reporting "healthy days."
- Increase "active days" without pain.
- Reduce activity limitations.

Exercise need not be boring or mundane. Neither should it be harmful to the body. A wide variety of exercise programs exist today to suit the preferences, needs, and interests of most individuals. This array of choice, however, makes it difficult for many people to evaluate whether or not a particular exercise or exercise program is well suited to their personal needs. Recognizing that not all exercises are good for all people is important when choosing a safe exercise program.

"Safe" exercises are defined as those performed with normal body posture, mechanics, and movement in mind. They don't compromise the integrity or stability of one body part to the detriment of another. "Questionable" exercises, on the other hand, are exercises that may violate normal body mechanics and place the body at risk for injury. Certain questionable exercises can be regarded as poor choices for nearly everyone in the general population due to the reasonable risk for injury over time. Other questionable exercises may be poor choices for only certain segments of the general population because of a specific body type or health issue. Differentiating exercises as "safe" or "questionable" can be difficult—even experts in the field have different opinions on the subject.

With new knowledge comes change. What is regarded as "safe" today may be viewed differently over time as our understanding and knowledge base are shaped by new findings in the fields of anatomy, biomechanics, motor control, and kinesiology. For example, years ago it was acceptable to perform exercises such as a standing toe touch with the knees straight, neck circles, and leg stretches in a seated hurdler's position. These exercises are now regarded as hazardous due to the risks they impose on the normal structures of the body. It is important to keep abreast of changing views, so that your exercise program can be as safe and effective as possible.

When considering the merits and risks of different exercises, it may be necessary to consult with an expert. Professionals such as athletic trainers, biomechanists, physical educators, physical therapists, and certified strength and conditioning specialists are appropriate people to consult. These individuals typically have college degrees and four to eight years of study in such courses as anatomy, physiology, kinesiology, preventive and therapeutic exercise, and physiology of exercise. On-the-job training, a good physique or figure, and good athletic or dancing ability are not sufficient qualifications for teaching or advising about exercise. Most fitness centers prefer to hire instructors and personal trainers with appropriate certifications. Unfortunately, certification is not a requirement. When searching for advice on training or exercise, it is certainly appropriate to inquire about an individual's qualifications.

This concept will review the principles of safe physical activity and provide guidelines to reduce the risks from potentially harmful exercises. Examples of potentially hazardous exercises are provided at the end of this concept, with suggestions for safer alternative exercises.

Principles of Safe Physical Activity

Exercises that are prescribed for a particular individual differ from those that are good for everyone (mass prescription). In a clinical setting, a therapist works with one patient. A case history is taken and tests made to determine which muscles are weak or strong, short or long. Exercises are then prescribed for that person. For example, a tennis player with a recent history of shoulder dislocation would probably be prescribed specific shoulder-strengthening exercises to regain stability in the joint. Common shoulder stretching exercises would likely be **contraindicated** for this individual. In this case, the muscles and joint capsule on the front of the shoulder are already quite lax to have allowed dislocation to occur in the first place.

Exercises that are prescribed or performed as a group cannot typically take individual needs into account. For example, when a physical educator, an aerobics instructor, or a coach leads a group of people in exercise, there is little (if any) consideration for individual differences, except for some allowance made in the number of repetitions or in the amount of weight or resistance used. Some of the exercises performed in this type of group setting may not be appropriate for all individuals. Similarly, an exercise that is

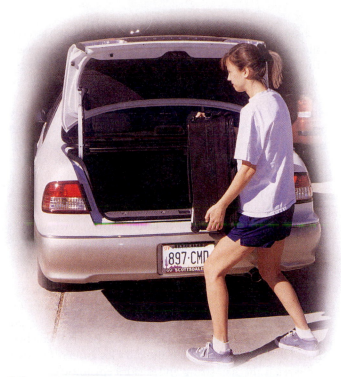

Safe exercise includes performing activities of daily living properly.

appropriate for a certain individual may not be appropriate for all members of a group. Since it is not always practical to prescribe individual exercise routines for everyone, it is often necessary to provide general recommendations that are appropriate for most individuals. The classification of exercises in this concept should be viewed in this context.

🌐 **Some exercises and movements can produce microtrauma, and some may cause acute injuries.** www. mhhe.com/phys_fit/web12 Click 01. **Microtrauma** is "a silent injury"—that is, an injury that results from repetitive motions such as those used in calisthenics or sports. These injuries also occur in occupations. Other terms that frequently appear in the scientific literature include *repetitive motion syndrome, repetitive strain injury (RSI), cumulative trauma disorder (CTD),* and *overuse syndrome.* They all refer to injury caused by repetitive movement. We may violate the integrity of our joints by performing, for example, forty backward arm circles with the palms down 3 days per week for 10 or 20 years. The wear and tear is not usually noticed by the participant until the friction over time causes microscopic changes in the joint, such as fibrosis of the synovial lining, abnormal thickening of the surrounding joint capsule, thinning and roughening of the articular cartilage cushioning joint surfaces, and calcifications in the rotator cuff tendon. Because these changes are unseen and often unfelt, the participant views the exercise as harmless. Later in life microtrauma becomes apparent, resulting in problems of tendonitis, bursitis, arthritis, or nerve compression. Chances are, when the injury reaches an acute

stage, the cause of the injury is never identified and is attributed to old age.

Acute injury is the more immediate onset of pain and abnormal tissue structure changes that occur within a few hours of performing an activity. For example, a basketball player who sprains an ankle will experience immediate onset of pain and swelling. This is an acute injury, caused by tearing of the ankle ligaments, and is referred to as an ankle sprain. As opposed to microtrauma, which is often "silent," the affects of an acute injury are almost always immediately obvious to the participant.

Decreasing Risks from Hazardous Activities and Exercises

Most hazardous exercises occur at the extreme ranges of motion. The human body is designed for motion. Nevertheless, there are certain movements that can put the joints and musculoskeletal system at risk and should therefore be avoided. With respect to care of the spine, many contraindicated movements involve the extremes of hyperflexion and hyperextension. Hyperflexion causes increased pressure in the disks, potentially leading to disk herniation. Hyperextension causes compressive wear and tear on the facet joints that join vertebral segments (see Figure 1). Hyperextension of the spine also causes narrowing of the intervertebral canal, potentially causing nerve impingement. With respect to the knee, hyperextension places excessive stress on the ligaments and joint capsule at the back of the knee, whereas hyperflexion increases compressive forces under the kneecap (patello-femoral joint).

🌐 **Maintaining a "neutral spine" is the cornerstone of core strengthening and dynamic stabilization exercises.** www.mhhe.com/phys_fit/web12 Click 02. When the body is aligned in "neutral," three normal curvatures of the spine are present (see Concept 13). These curves help balance forces on the body and minimize muscle tension. The degree of curvature is often influenced by the tilt of the pelvis. A forward pelvic tilt increases curvature in the neck and lower back, whereas a backward pelvic tilt tends to flatten the lower back. The most desirable position of the pelvis is one of "neutral tilt," in which the ideal amount of curvature of the spine occurs.

Contraindicated Not recommended because of the potential for harm.

Microtrauma Injury so small it is not detected at the time it occurs.

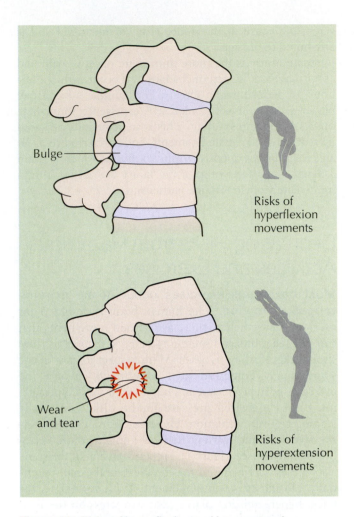

Bulge

Risks of hyperflexion movements

Wear and tear

Risks of hyperextension movements

Figure 1 ▶ Risks of hyperflexion and hyperextension.

Many fitness centers offer group classes in "core" strength to help promote back health and posture. Core strengthening focuses on using the abdominal, trunk extensor, and gluteal muscles to anchor the pelvis and spine in a neutral position. Dynamic stabilization exercises further challenge muscles to maintain neutral alignment. These exercises incorporate a variety of arm and leg movements to provide additional resistance. Programs often utilize stability balls and foam rollers (lightweight foam cylinders), but many exercises can also be done on mats.

The risks associated with a physical activity can be reduced by controlling the conditions under which the activity is performed. Variables that are under the direct control of the participant include exercise frequency, duration, intensity, speed, and quality. Some exercises may be reasonably safe for most people when performed only once but may induce microtrauma and become hazardous when done repetitively, incorrectly, too rapidly, or with little regard for smooth, controlled motion. For example, if hyperextension of the back during a prone press-up feels comfortable, then it is

probably safe when done once or twice as a static stretch following a series of abdominal-strengthening exercises. However, performing several dozen prone press-ups with a rapid, jerky style can be detrimental to the back.

High levels of physical fitness are especially important when the demands of a sport or an occupation include the repetitive use of questionable movements or postures. In baseball, the catcher has to assume and maintain a deep squat position for long periods of time. This causes microtrauma to the knee. Gymnasts frequently perform double-leg raises and movements resulting in hyperextension of the back. These movements cause microtrauma to the spine. Some workers (e.g., postal workers and construction workers) may also perform movements that produce microtrauma, even when adhering to guidelines for efficient and safe exercise. It is especially important that these people develop muscle fitness and flexibility in the regions of the body that are exposed to the dangerous movements. Baseball catchers should be sure to strengthen the muscles around the knee and stretch the hamstring and quadriceps muscles. Gymnasts should exercise to build strong abdominal and back muscles as well as stretch to lengthen the back, hamstring, and hip flexor muscles. Workers should similarly strengthen and lengthen the muscles associated with the movements commonly used in their jobs.

Some exercises performed in training for sports can predispose a person to injury. Many young athletes perform certain exercises because their coaches recommend them or their friends and teammates perform them in practice. Ballistic stretching or passive forms of resistance are often used in training programs, but these can lead to injury or instability in certain joints. Competitive swimmers, for example, often perform a variety of ballistic stretches or use passive forms of resistance to loosen up their shoulder muscles prior to swimming. One common exercise involves pulling the arms backward at shoulder level until they cross each other behind the back or pulling the bent elbows together, making them touch, while the hands are on the back of the head. Competitive swimmers sometimes begin such practices while they are in children's programs and continue them through their competitive years. Such overstretching has resulted in painful shoulders and disability.

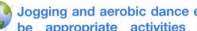 **Jogging and aerobic dance exercise may not be appropriate activities for all people.** www.mhhe.com/phys_fit/web12 Click 03. Jogging and aerobic dance exercises are excellent for cardiovascular conditioning, weight control, and improvement of a variety of conditions; however, reasonable caution should be observed. Jogging has been used successfully in rehabilitating cardiac patients and a variety of other health problems.

Like many other exercises, jogging should not be done without a physician's approval for people with arthritis, osteoporosis, and heart and circulatory diseases. The pounding from repeated strides can lead to shin splints, blisters, and a variety of foot, ankle, knee, and hip problems. Wearing the proper footwear and learning how to jog correctly will minimize these hazards. If you have poor leg or foot alignment, you would be wise to jog only 3 or 4 days per week because studies show that the risk for injury is greatest for those who jog every day. Or you should choose another activity, such as cycling or swimming.

Aerobic dance exercise has some of the same hazards as jogging; these include the overstress syndromes from too many hours of high-impact landings on the floor. The most common problems are shin splints, Achilles tendon injuries, arch strains, and pain under the knee cap. Most of these problems can be prevented by warming up and stretching properly before exercising, by using low-impact movements, and by avoiding hazardous exercises, such as those described in this concept. Some women may need to wear a sports bra as a comfort measure for either jogging or dance exercise.

 Movements and postures during daily activities can also put the body at risk. www.mhhe. com/phys_fit/web12 Click 04. Most people are aware that standing toe touches put a lot of strain on the lower back. The reason is that it causes hyperflexion in the lower back, which increases the pressure on the vertebral disks. Slouching in a chair can also put the back at risk (see Figure 2). Because we spend a large amount of time sitting, it is important to adopt good sitting postures to reduce damage to the lower back. (See Concept 13.)

Many lifestyle activities, such as raking leaves and shoveling snow, may be beneficial if done correctly but can put considerable strain on the back if done incorrectly. Ergonomically designed rakes and shovels may help main-

tain proper posture during these activities. Proper technique in these activities is important to reduce risks.

The valsalva maneuver should be avoided when exerting great force in weight lifting, calisthenics, and isometrics. Many people mistakenly hold their breath when lifting weights or exerting force. This action, known as a **valsalva maneuver** is potentially dangerous and should be avoided. A sharp increase in thoracic pressure and arterial blood pressure occurs when force is exerted in this way. The pressure decreases rapidly when the breath is released and can lead to a lag in blood flow to the heart. This can lead to dizziness, blackouts, and inguinal hernias. Do not hold your breath during exercises. **Hyperventilation** should also be avoided.

 ## Technology Update
Ergonomics

Ergonomics, also known as human factors engineering, is a discipline that helps to develop tools and workplace settings that put the least amount of strain on the body. Biomechanical principles are used to help identify movements and positions that may put individuals at greater risk for specific injuries or microtrauma. Many worksites take an active interest in ergonomic principles, since repetitive motion injuries and other musculoskeletal conditions are the leading cause of work-related ill health.

One application of ergonomics is the design of effective workstations for computer users. Properly fitting desks and chairs and effective positioning of the computer on the desk have been shown to minimize problems such as carpal tunnel syndrome (CTS), a painful and debilitating injury of the median nerve at the wrist. Risk for CTS increases if the fingers are forced to be above the wrists while typing, so care should be used to ensure proper desk and chair height. Wrist rests can also be used to provide support for the wrist. The Human Factors and Ergonomics Society has released a guidebook called *Human Factors Engineering of Computer Workstations* (for more information check **www.mhhe.com/phys_fit/web12 Click 04**).

Valsalva Maneuver Exerting force when holding your breath increases pressure in the chest cavity and raises arterial blood pressure. When breath is released, arterial pressure drops rapidly and blood vessels expand and are then filled, causing a lag in blood flow to the heart's left ventricle. When this occurs, the subject may become dizzy or feel faint. May be caused by holding the breath while exerting force.

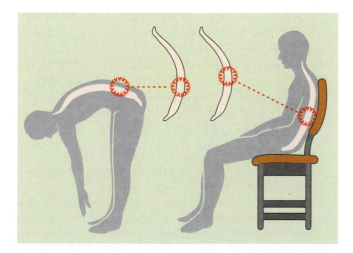

Figure 2 ▶ Poor sitting posture puts the back at risk.

Strategies for Action

Common exercises when misused or abused are potentially harmful. www.mhhe.com/phys_fit/ web12 Click 05. A number of commonly used exercises are considered by experts to be contraindicated for most individuals. These exercises typically put the body in a position that compromises the integrity of the joint or puts extra strain on the muscles and ligaments that support the body. No harm may be associated with doing the exercise once, but repeated use over time can lead to instability or more significant problems. In most cases, safer exercises target the same muscles or areas more effectively. Table 1 on the following pages shows a number of questionable exercises and safer alternatives.

Study Resources

Check out additional online study resources for this concept in the Student Edition of the Online Learning Center at www.mhhe.com/corbin13e.

Web Resources

American Academy of Orthopaedic Surgeons **www.aaos.org**
Human Factors and Ergonomics Society **www.hfes.org**

Suggested Readings

Additional reference materials for concept 12 are available at **www.mhhe.com/phys_fit/web12 Click 06.**

Bracko, M. R. 2004. Can we prevent back injuries? *ACSM's Health and Fitness Journal* 8(4):5–11.

Greiner, S. G., C. Russell, and S. M. McGill. 2003. Relationships between lumbar flexibility, sit-and-reach test, and a previous history of low back pain in industrial workers. *Canadian Journal of Applied Physiology* 28(2):165–171.

Hootman, J. M., et al. 2002. Epidemiology of musculoskeletal injuries among sedentary and physically active adults. *Medicine and Science in Sports and Exercise* 34(5):838–844.

Jones, C. S., C. Christenson, and M. Young. 2000. Weight-training injury trends: A 20-year survey. *The Physician and Sportsmedicine* 28(7):61–72.

Kraus, V. 2004. Joint flexibility may lessen wear and tear on joints. *Arthritis & Rheumatism* 50:2178–2183.

Liemohn, W., et al. 2004. Questionable exercises. In Corbin, C. B. et al. (eds.). *Toward an Understanding of Physical Fitness and Activity, Vol. II.* Scottsdale, AZ: Holcomb Hathaway Publishers.

McGibon, C. A. 2003. Toward a better understanding of gait changes with age and disablement. *Exercise and Sport Sciences Reviews* 31(2):102–108.

McGill, S. M. 2001. Low back stability: From formal description to issues for performance and rehabilitation. *Exercise and Sports Science Reviews* 29(1):26–31.

Neiman, D. C. 2000. Exercise soothes arthritis: Joint effects. *ACSM's Health and Fitness Journal* 4(3):20–27.

In the News

Treatment Options for Joint Conditions

The prevalence of many musculoskeletal conditions associated with both "old age" and microtrauma has been increasing in recent years. Examples are osteoarthritis (OA) and degenerative disk disease (DDD). A number of new treatment options are available to help people with these painful and debilitating conditions:

- Artificial lumbar disks have been approved by the FDA for use in replacing disks worn out from DDD. This new surgical procedure allows patients to have greater movement in their spine than treatments such as joint fusion. Increased mobility may enhance quality of life in people with this condition.
- A new class of medications, known as "viscosupplements," is available to help reduce pain associated with OA. Compounds such as Hyalgan, Supartz, and Synvisc are an artificial source of hyaluronic acid, the viscous substance that acts as a shock absorber in the joints. A single injection has been shown to reduce pain for up to 6 months in 70 percent of patients with OA.
- Two related neutraceuticals (glucosamine and chondroitin) have been developed to protect and stimulate cartilage (the protective lining of synovial joints) in joints. Both substances are produced naturally by the body in small quantities, but these "chondroprotective" supplements may provide additional benefits. Several recent studies have shown cartilage integrity and joint space to be better maintained and joint pain to be reduced in those taking supplements than in those taking a placebo.

Hyperventilation Overbreathing; forced, rapid, or deep breathing.

Questionable Exercise: The Swan

This exercise hyperextends the lower back and stretches the abdominals. These muscles are too long and weak in most people and should not be lengthened further. It can be harmful to the back, potentially causing muscle strain, nerve impingement, and facet joint compression. Other exercises in which this occurs include: cobras, back-bends, straight-leg lifts, straight-leg sit-ups, prone-back lifts, donkey kicks, fire hydrants, backward trunk circling, weight lifting with the back arched, and landing from a jump with the back arched.

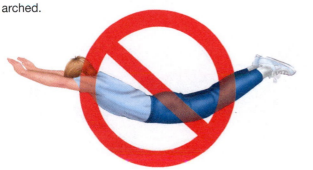

Safer Alternative Exercise: Back Extension

Lie prone over a roll of blankets or pillows and extend the back to a neutral or horizontal position.

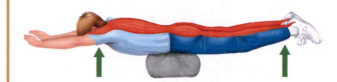

Questionable Exercise: Back-Arching Abdominal Stretch

This exercise can stretch the hip flexors, quadriceps, and shoulder flexors (such as the pectorals), but it also stretches the abdominals, which is not desired. Because of the armpull, it can potentially hyperflex the knee joint, and strain neck musculature.

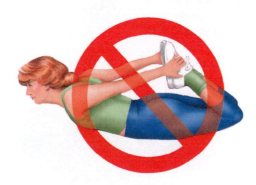

Note: All safer alternative exercises should be held 15 to 30 seconds unless otherwise indicated.

Safer Alternative Exercise: PNF Pectoral Stretch

Stand erect in the doorway with arms raised 45 degrees, elbows bent, and hands grasping door jambs, and feet in front stride position. Press forward on door frame, contracting the arms maximally for several seconds. Relax and shift weight on legs so muscles on front of shoulder joint and chest are stretched. Hold. Repeat with arms at 90 and 135 degrees. If your goal is stretching the hip flexors and quadriceps, substitute the hip and thigh stretch.

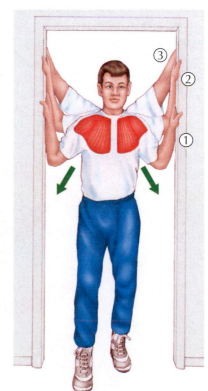

Table 1 Questionable Exercises and Safe Alternatives

Table 1

Questionable Exercise: Donkey Kick

This exercise may involve touching the nose with the knee followed by a ballistic backward kick, hyperextending the neck and the lower back when the leg is lifted above the horizontal.

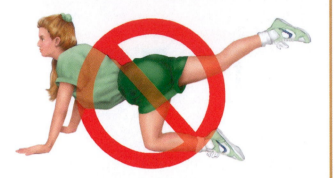

Safer Alternative Exercise: Knee-to-Nose

Kneel on all fours. Pull the knee up under the chest, then extend the leg backward, being sure not to raise the leg higher than the horizontal. Change legs. Avoid neck strain by looking down toward hands. Wrist and hand pain can be avoided by bearing weight on fists rather than an open hand.

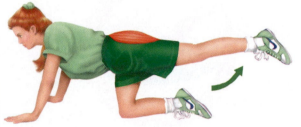

Questionable Exercise: Double-Leg Lift

This exercise is usually used with the intent of strengthening the abdominals, when in fact it is primarily a hip flexor (iliopsoas) strengthening exercise. Most people have overdeveloped the hip flexors and do not need to further strengthen those muscles because this may cause forward pelvic tilt. Even if the abdominals are strong enough to contract isometrically to prevent hyperextension of the lower back, the exercise produces excess stress on the discs.

Safer Alternative Exercise: Reverse Curl

This exercise strengthens the lower abdominals. Lie on your back on the floor and bring your knees in toward the chest. Place the arms at the sides for support. For movement, pull the knees toward the head, raising the hips off the floor. Do not let knees go past the shoulders. Return to starting position and repeat.

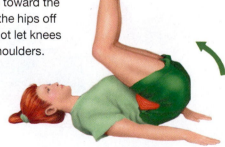

Questionable Exercises and Safe Alternatives Table 1

Table 1

Questionable Exercise: The Windmill

This exercise involves simultaneous rotation and flexion (or extension) of the lower back, which is contraindicated. Because of the orientation of the facet joints in the lumbar spine, these movements violate normal joint mechanics, placing tremendous torsional stress on the joint capsule and disks.

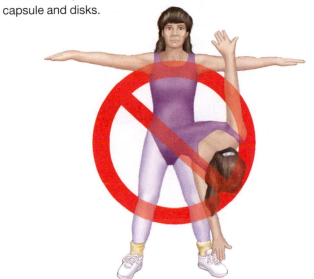

Safer Alternative Exercise: Back-Saver Hamstring Stretch

This exercise stretches the hamstring and lower back muscles. Sit with one leg extended and one knee bent, foot turned outward and close to the buttocks. Clasp hands behind back. Bend forward from the hips, keeping the low back as straight as possible. Allow bent knee to move laterally so trunk can move forward. Stretch and hold. Repeat with the other leg.

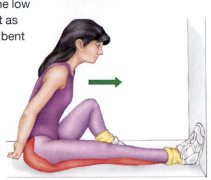

Questionable Exercise: Neck Circling

This exercise and other exercises that require neck hyperextension (e.g., neck bridging) can pinch arteries and nerves in the neck and at the base of the skull, cause wear and tear to small joints of the spine, and produce dizziness or myofascial trigger points. In people with degenerated discs, it can cause dizziness, numbness, or even precipitate strokes. It also aggravates arthritis and degenerated discs.

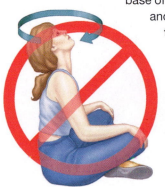

Safer Alternative Exercise: Head Clock

This exercise relaxes the muscle of the neck. Assume a good posture (seated with legs crossed or in a chair), and imagine that your neck is a clock face with the chin at the center. Flex the neck and point the chin at 6:00, hold, lift the chin; repeat pointing chin to 4:00, to 8:00, to 3:00 and finally to 9:00. Return to center position with chin up after each movement.

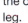

Table 1

Table 1 Questionable Exercises and Safe Alternatives

Questionable Exercise: Shoulder Stand Bicycle

This exercise and the yoga positions called the plough and the plough shear (not shown) force the neck and upper back to hyperflex. It has been estimated that 80 percent of the population has forward head and kyphosis (humpback) with accompanying weak muscles. This exercise is especially dangerous for these people. Neck hyperflexion results in excessive stretch on the ligaments and nerves. It can also aggravate preexisting arthritic conditions. If the purpose for these exercises is to reduce gravitational effects on the circulatory system or internal organs, lie on a tilt board with the feet elevated. If the purpose is to warm up the muscles in the legs, slow jog in place. If the purpose is to stretch the lower back, try the leg hug exercise.

Safer Alternative Exercise: Leg Hug

Lie on your back with the knees bent at about 90 degrees. Bring your knees to the chest and wrap the arms around the back of the thighs. Pull knees to chest and hold.

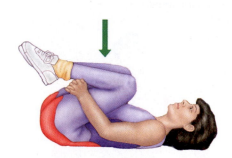

Questionable Exercise: Straight-Leg and Bent-Knee Sit-Ups

There are several valid criticisms of the sit-up exercise. Straight-leg sit-ups can displace the fifth lumbar vertebra causing back problems. A bent-knee sit-up creates less shearing force on the spine, but some recent studies have shown it produces greater compression on the lumbar discs than the straight-leg sit-up. Placing the hands behind the neck or head during the sit-up or during a crunch results in hyperflexion of the neck.

Safer Alternative Exercise: Crunch

Lie on your back with the knees bent more than 90 degrees. Curl up until the shoulder blades lift off the floor, then roll down to starting position and repeat. There are several safe arm positions. The easiest is with the arms extended straight in front of the body. Alternatives are with the arms crossed over the chest or the palms or fist held beside the ears.

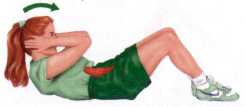

Questionable Exercise: Standing Toe Touches or Double-Leg Toe Touches

These exercises—especially when done ballistically—can produce degenerative changes at the vertebrae of the lower back. They also stretch the ligaments and joint capsule of the knee. Bending the back while the legs are straight may cause back strain, particularly if the movement is done ballistically. If performed only on rare occasions as a test, the chance of injury is less than if incorporated into a regular exercise program. Safer stretches of the lower back include the leg hug, the single knee-to-chest, the hamstring stretcher, and the back-saver toe touch.

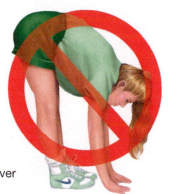

Safer Alternative Exercise: Back-Saver Toe Touch

Sit on the floor. Extend leg and bend the other knee, placing the foot flat on the floor. Bend at the hip and reach forward with both hands. Grasp one foot, ankle, or calf depending upon the distance you can reach. Pull forward with your arms and bend forward. Slight bend in the knee is acceptable. Hold. Repeat with the opposite leg.

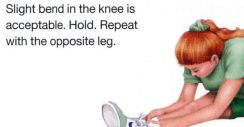

Questionable Exercise: Bar Stretch

This type of stretch may be harmful. Some experts have found that when the extended leg is raised 90 degrees or more and the trunk is bent over the leg, it may lead to **sciatica** and **pyriformis syndrome,** especially in the person who has limited flexibility.

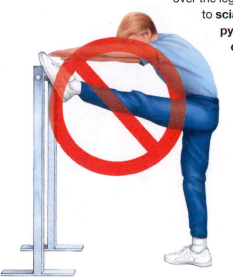

Safer Alternative Exercise: Hamstring Stretch

Lie on your back with the knees bent at about 90 degrees. Draw one knee to the chest by pulling on the thigh with the hands, then extend the knee and point the foot toward the ceiling. Hold. Pull to chest again and return to the starting position. Repeat with the other leg.

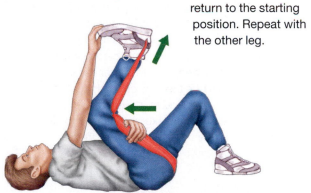

Sciatica Pain along the sciatic nerve in the buttock and leg.

Pyriformis Syndrome Muscle spasm and nerve entrapment in the pyriformis muscle of the buttocks region, causing pain in the buttock and referred pain down the leg (sciatica).

Table 1

Table 1 Questionable Exercises and Safe Alternatives

Questionable Exercise: Shin and Quadriceps Stretch

This exercise causes hyperflexion of the knee. When the knee is hyperflexed more than 120 degrees and/or rotated outward by an external **torque,** the ligaments and joint capsule are stretched and damage to the cartilage may occur. Note: One of the quadriceps, the rectus femoris, is not stretched if the trunk is allowed to bend forward because it crosses the hip as well as the knee joint. If the exercise is used to stretch the quadriceps, substitute the hip and thigh stretch. For most people it is not necessary to stretch the shin muscles, since they are often elongated and weak; however, if you need to stretch the shin muscles to relieve muscle soreness, try the shin stretch.

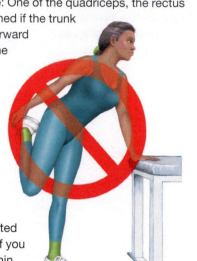

Safer Alternative Exercise: Hip and Thigh Stretch

Kneel so that the front leg is bent at 90 degrees (front knee directly above the front ankle). The knee of the back leg should touch the floor well behind the front foot. Press the pelvis forward and downward. Hold. Repeat with the opposite leg forward. Do not bend the front knee more than 90 degrees.

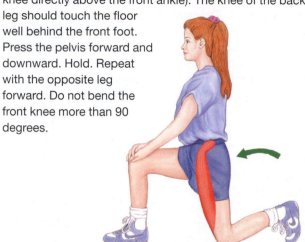

Questionable Exercise: The Hero

Like the shin and quadriceps stretch this exercise causes hyperflexion of the knee. It also causes torque on the hyperflexed knee. For these reasons the ligaments and joint capsule are stretched and the cartilage may be damaged. For most people it is not necessary to stretch the shin muscles since they are often elongated and weak; however, if you need to stretch the shin muscles use the shin stretch. If this exercise is used to stretch the quadricps substitute the hip and thigh stretch.

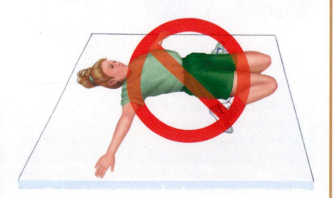

Safer Alternative Exercise: Shin Stretch

Kneel on your knees, turn to right and press down on right ankle with right hand. Hold. Keep hips thrust forward to avoid hyperflexing the knees. Do not sit on the heels. Repeat on the left side.

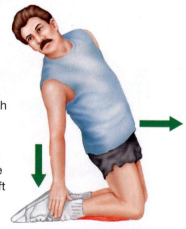

Torque A twisting or rotating force.

Questionable Exercise: Deep Squatting Exercises

This exercise, with or without weights, places the knee joint in hyperflexion, tends to "wedge it open," stretching the ligaments, irritating the synovial membrane, and possibly damaging the cartilage. The joint has even greater stress when the lower leg and foot are not in straight alignment with the knee. If you are performing squats to strengthen the knee and hip extensors, then try substituting the alternate leg kneel or half-squat with free weight or leg presses on a resistance machine.

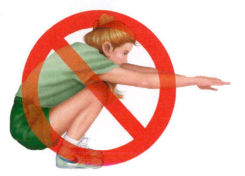

Safer Alternative Exercise: Alternate Leg Kneel

From a standing position, with or without a free weight, take a step forward with right foot, touching left knee to floor. The front knee should be bent only to a 90-degree angle. Return to start and lunge forward with other foot. Repeat, alternating right and left.

Questionable Exercise: Knee Pull-Down

This exercise can result in hyperflexion of the knee. The arms or hands placed on top of the shin places undue stress on the knee joint.

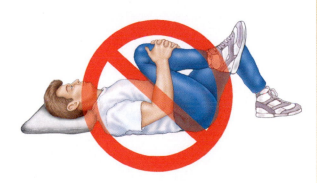

Safer Alternative Exercise: Single Knee-to-Chest

Lie down with both knees bent, draw one knee to the chest by pulling on the thigh with the hands, then extend the knee and point the foot toward the ceiling. Hold. Pull to chest again and return to starting position. Repeat with other leg.

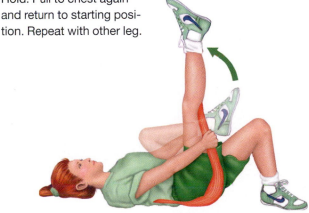

Table 1

Table 1 Questionable Exercises and Safe Alternatives

Questionable Exercise: Seated Forward Arm Circles with Palms Down

This exercise (arms straight out to the sides) may cause pinching of the rotator cuff and biceps tendons between the bony structures of the shoulder joint and/or irritate the **bursa** in the shoulder. The tendency is to emphasize the use of the stronger chest muscles (pectorals) to perform the motion rather than emphasizing the weaker upper back muscles.

Safer Alternative Exercise: Seated Backward Arm Circles with Palms Up

Sit, turn palms up, pull in chin, and contract abdominals. Circle arms backward.

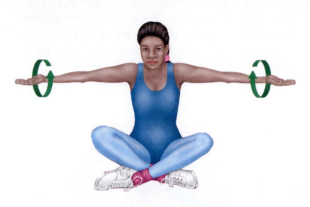

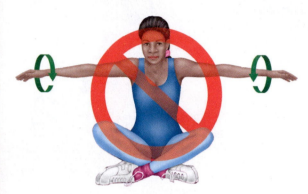

Bursa Small sacs filled with fluid and situated between muscles, or between muscles and bones, to prevent friction.

Lab 12A Safe Exercises

Name		Section	Date

Purpose: To perform safe exercises that are good alternatives to commonly performed questionable exercises and to self-monitor progress in your 1-week plan

Procedures

1. On Chart 1, check the questionable exercises you have performed.
2. Perform the safe exercises listed in the chart. Use the descriptions in this concept to help you perform them properly.
3. Place a check by the exercises you think you might consider using as part of your regular program.
4. Answer the question in the Results section.

Chart 1 ▶ Questionable Exercises and Safe Alternatives

Place a check beside the questionable exercises you have performed in the past.	Place a check beside the safe exercises you think you might include in your exercise program.
○ 1. Swan	○ 1. Back extension
○ 2. Back-arching abdominal stretch	○ 2. Pectoral stretch
○ 3. Donkey kick	○ 3. Knee-to-nose
○ 4. Double-leg lift	○ 4. Reverse curl
○ 5. Windmill	○ 5. Back-saver hamstring stretch
○ 6. Neck circling	○ 6. Head clock
○ 7. Shoulder stand bicycling, plough, or plough shear	○ 7. Leg hug
○ 8. Straight-leg or bent-knee sit-up	○ 8. Crunch
○ 9. Standing toe touch	○ 9. Back-saver toe touch
○ 10. Bar stretch	○ 10. Hamstring stretch
○ 11. Shin and quadriceps stretch	○ 11. Shin stretch
○ 12. Hero	○ 12. Hip and thigh stretch
○ 13. Deep squatting exercise	○ 13. Alternate leg kneel
○ 14. Knee pull-down	○ 14. Single knee-to-chest
○ 15. Forward arm circles (palms down)	○ 15. Backward seated arm circles (palms up)

Results: How many of the questionable exercises listed in Chart 1 have you performed?

Conclusions and Interpretations

1. In most cases, it takes a considerable amount of time for a questionable exercise and the microtrauma it causes to result in noticeable damage to the body. To what extent do you think that you might be affected by questionable exercises you have done in the past? Use several sentences to explain.

2. Will you change your way of exercising as a result of learning about questionable exercises and safe alternatives? Use several sentences to explain your answer.

Body Mechanics: Posture and Care of the Back and Neck

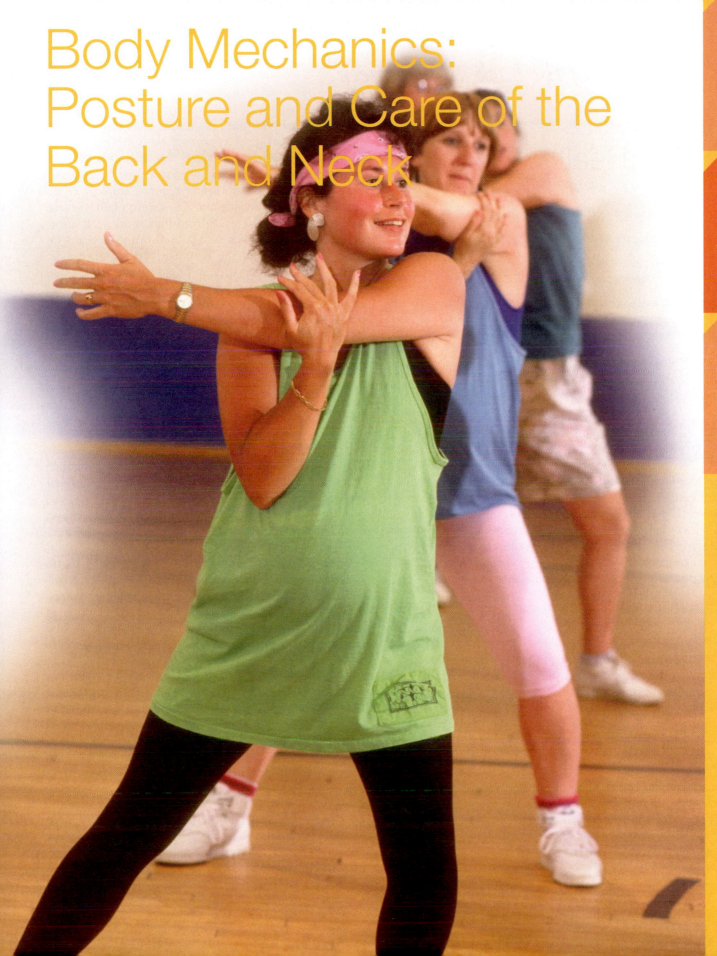

Proper body mechanics should be used for both static and dynamic postures to ensure the health, integrity, and function of the back and the neck.

Health Goals
for the year 2010

- Increase healthy and active days.

- Reduce days with pain and activity limitations.

- Increase assistance to those with pain and activity limitations.

- Increase proportion of people who regularly perform exercises for strength and muscular endurance.

- Increase proportion of people who regularly perform exercises for flexibility.

Neck and back pain are common in today's society. The potential consequences of chronic neck and back pain are far-reaching and include emotional and economic costs to individuals and society. This concept emphasizes the importance of healthy back and neck care. The role of good posture and body mechanics in maintaining a healthy spine are discussed, followed by descriptions of some common disorders of the spine. The concept concludes by focusing on exercises for improved postural alignment and trunk stability.

Facts about Backs

Most people (more than half) will see a physician about a backache during their lifetime. Back pain is second only to headache as a common medical complaint. An estimated 30 to 70 percent of Americans have recurring back problems, and 2 million of these people cannot hold jobs as a result. Back problems most often affect people between the ages of twenty-five and sixty, but one study indicated that up to 26 percent of teenagers report backaches. Athletes also have back problems, but the condition is more common in people who are not highly fit. Unfortunately, studies also indicate that back pain is the leading cause of inactivity among individuals under the age of forty-five. Therefore, taking preventive measures to reduce risk for back pain is important.

The prevention of back problems is an important goal in worksite health promotion programs. www.mhhe.com/phys_fit/web13 Click 01. Back pain is the most common reason for workers' compensations claims and for lost workdays among employed individuals. Statistics indicate that 27 percent of all workers' compensation claims result from musculoskeletal disorders of the neck and back. These disorders account for nearly 46 percent of the total workers' compensation costs. Given these statistics, it should come as no surprise that worksite health promotion programs place strong emphasis on measures to prevent or reduce back injury. These programs include structured exercise programs, the use of ergonomically designed workstations and equipment, and awareness education about proper lifting and carrying techniques.

Elements and Benefits of Good Posture

Good posture has aesthetic benefits. **Posture** is an important part of nonverbal communication. The first impression a person makes is usually a visual one, and good posture can help convey an impression of alertness, confidence, and attractiveness.

Proper posture allows the body segments to be balanced. The body is made in segments that are balanced in a vertical column by muscles and ligaments. Proper posture helps maintain an even distribution of force across the body, improve shock absorption, and minimize the degree of active muscle tension required to maintain the posture.

Awareness of good standing posture is important to a healthy spine. In the standing position, the head should be centered over the trunk; the shoulders should be down and back but relaxed, with the chest high and the abdomen flat. The spine should have gentle curves when viewed from the side but should be straight when seen from the back. There are three normal curvatures of the spine, including the **lordotic** (inward) **curve** of the neck and lower back and the **kyphotic** (outward) **curve** of the upper back. When the pelvis is tilted properly, the pubis falls directly underneath the lower tip of the sternum. The knees should be relaxed, with the kneecaps

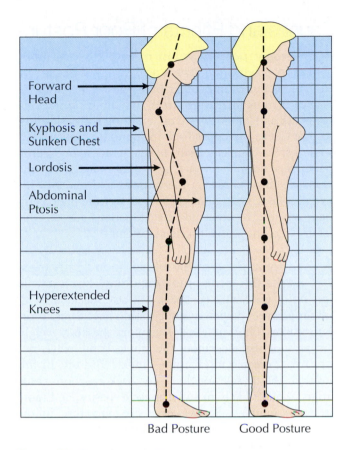

Figure 1 ▶ Comparison of bad and good posture.

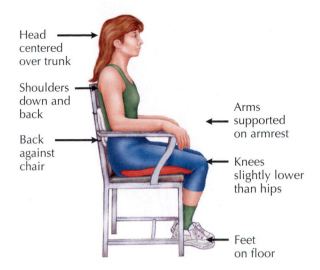

Figure 2 ▶ Good sitting posture.

pointed straight ahead. The feet should point straight ahead, and the weight should be borne over the heel, on the outside border of the sole, and across the ball of the foot and toes (see Figure 1).

🌐 **Awareness of good seated posture is important to a healthy spine.** www.mhhe.com/phys_fit/ web13 Click 02. A large percentage of our days are spent sitting as we attend class, commute to work, sit at a computer, dine out, or relax in front of the television. Good seated posture decreases pressure within the discs of the lower back and reduces fatigue of lower back muscles. In sitting, the head should be centered over the trunk, the shoulders down and back. If one is using a computer, the monitor should be at eye level with the screen 18–24 inches from the eyes. The seat of the chair should be at an angle that allows the knees to be positioned slightly lower than the hips. The back should firmly rest against the chair, with support to the lumbar spine. Feet should be supported on the floor and arms supported on armrests for ideal unloading of the spine (see Figure 2).

Maintaining proper alignment requires a balance of flexibility and strength in the muscles supporting the trunk. The muscles of the legs, trunk, and neck work in combination to maintain body alignment and posture (Figure 3). The abdominal muscles pull the bottom of the pelvis upward and keep the top of the pelvis tipped backward, eliminating excessive back curve. Strong hamstring muscles also help keep the pelvis tipped backward. If the hip flexor muscles are too strong, or not long enough, they have the opposite effect of strong abdominal muscles; that is, they tip the top of the pelvis forward, causing excessive low back curve (lordosis). (See Figure 4.) This is why it is important to have long, but not too strong, hip flexor muscles. As a general rule, flexibility exercises are needed to lengthen the hip flexor muscles, and strength and endurance exercises are recommended for the abdominal muscles. Sample exercises are provided later in this concept. Exercises to increase the strength of the hip flexor muscles are not recommended for people with back pain.

Posture The relationship among body parts, whether standing, lying, sitting, or moving. Good posture is the relationship among body parts that allows you to function most effectively, with the least expenditure of energy and with a minimal amount of stress and strain on muscles, tendons, ligaments, and joints.

Lordotic Curve The normal inward curvature of the cervical and lumbar spine that is necessary for good posture and body mechanics.

Kyphotic Curve The normal outward curvature of the thoracic spine that is necessary for good posture and body mechanics.

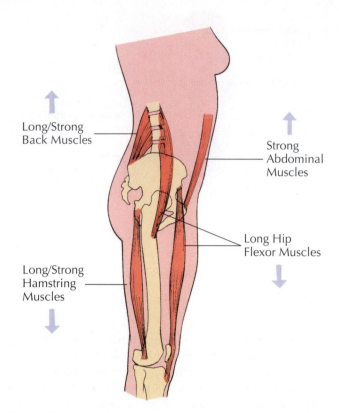

Figure 3 ▶ Balanced muscle strength and length permit good postural alignment.

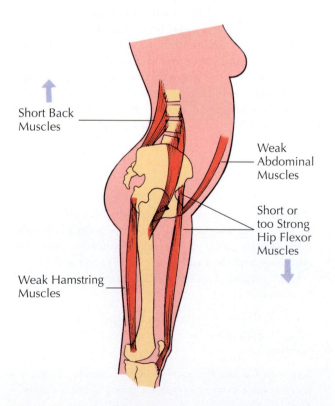

Figure 4 ▶ Unbalanced muscular development may cause poor posture or back problems.

Causes and Effects of Poor Posture

When proper posture is not maintained, the body begins to experience stress and strain. If one part of the body is out of line, other parts must compensate to balance it, thus increasing stress and strain on muscles, ligaments, and joints. For example, sitting with a slouched posture causes the upper back to round excessively. The cervical spine compensates by hyperextending in order to maintain a normal forward gaze. Excessive stress and strain are then placed on the muscles and joints of the posterior neck. Over time, chronic stress from poor alignment can lead to other postural deviations and possible deformity of the musculoskeletal system.

Chronic postural problems lead to a variety of health problems, including back strain and pain. www.mhhe.com/phys_fit/web13 Click 03. With proper posture, the lower spine should have a slight lordotic curve. This curve helps support the body weight and promote balance about the trunk. If the pelvis tips forward, it creates an excessive lumbar lordosis. In this position, the muscles of the lower back are more easily fatigued, more likely to suffer muscle spasms, and more prone to injury. Likewise, excessive curvature in the lower back can cause increased pressure on the small facet joints of the spine, narrowing of the canals where spinal nerves exit, and increased risk for pressure on nerve roots, thus contributing to **sciatica.** Due to these risks, some experts recommend that individuals with lordosis and weak abdominals eliminate exercises that hyperextend the spine.

Individuals who sit for long periods of time with the back flat and pelvis tilted backward can have the opposite postural problem of "flat back." The lower back curve in these individuals is absent or flattened. Regaining a normal lordotic curve would be beneficial in helping with shock absorption and decreasing pressure on the intervertebral bodies and discs. The use of lumbar support (rolls or pillows) placed behind the back during sitting may be helpful for this condition. Some examples of specific health problems that result from these and other postural problems are described in Table 1.

In addition to body alignment problems, hereditary, congenital, and disease conditions, as well as certain environmental factors, can cause poor posture. Some environmental factors that contribute to poor posture include ill-fitting clothing and shoes, chronic fatigue, improperly fitting furniture (including poor chairs, beds, and mattresses), emotional and personality problems, poor work habits, poor physical fitness due to inactivity, and lack of knowledge relating to good posture. Some posture problems, such as **scoliosis,** may be congenital, hereditary, or acquired, but may be corrected

Table 1 ▶ Health Problems Associated with Poor Posture

Posture Problem	Definition	Health Problem
Forward head	The head aligned in front of the center of gravity; also called poke neck	Headache, dizziness, and pain in the neck, shoulders, or arms
Kyphosis	Excessive curvature (flexion) in the upper back; also called humpback	Impaired respiration as a result of sunken chest and pain in the neck, shoulders, and arms
Lumbar lordosis	Excessive curvature (hyperextension) in the lower back (sway back), with a forward pelvic tilt	Back pain and/or injury, protruding abdomen, low back syndrome, and painful menstruation
Abdominal ptosis	Excessive protrusion of abdomen, also called protruding abdomen	Back pain and/or injury, lordosis, low back syndrome, and painful menstruation
Hyperextended knees	The knees bent backward excessively	Greater risk for knee injury and excessive pelvic tilt (lordosis)
Pronated feet	The longitudinal arch of the foot flattened with increased pressure on inner aspect of foot	Decreased shock absorption, leading to foot, knee, and lower back pain

with exercise, braces, and/or other medical procedures. Early detection is critical in treating scoliosis.

Back and Neck Pain

Often, back pain does not have a single isolated cause. Although back problems can result from an acute trauma (e.g., a diving accident or car accident), most are caused by a combination of lifestyle and behavioral factors. These factors include the avoidable effects of poor posture and body mechanics, the performance of questionable exercises (see the concept on safe physical activity), muscle imbalances, poor physical conditioning, overweight stature, and repetitive motion trauma from sports and worksite activities. Although there are also a number of potentially unavoidable causes of back pain, such as trauma, tumors, and congenital abnormalities, the overwhelming majority are avoidable. You will have the opportunity to assess your back and neck risk factors in the questionnaire in Lab 13A. Keep in mind that, with so many factors potentially influencing back health, it is often difficult to identify or diagnose a specific back problem. In fact, in 80 percent of cases, physicians are unable to pinpoint the exact cause of back and neck problems.

There is no such thing as a slipped disc. Disc problems are frequently misunderstood by the public. Between each vertebrae there are **intervertebral discs,** which act as shock absorbers for the spine. The disc has an outer fibrous ring (annulus fibrosus) and a gel-like center (nucleus pulposus). If the pulpy center of the disc protrudes through the fibrous ring, this is known as a **herniated,** or ruptured, **disc** (this is often referred to as a *slipped disc,* but this term is both outdated and technically incorrect). Once disc herniation occurs, the extruded material may begin to press on pain-sensitive structures within the intervertebral canal, such as spinal nerves, blood vessels, ligaments, and joint surfaces.

In addition to pain, unrelieved pressure on nerve roots can cause numbness and weakness in the arms or legs. It is important to note that not all herniated discs cause back pain. Contrary to popular literature and misleading statements by unethical "back doctors," studies show that only 5 to 10 percent of herniated discs are responsible for back pain. Similarly, there are individuals without back pain who still have radiographic evidence of a disc herniation.

Disc herniation is more common in young adults. Typically, herniation of the nucleus pulposus does not occur from a single incident. Instead, microtrauma to the back causes tears in the outer fibrous ring of the disc. This damage often goes unnoticed because only the outermost portion of the fibrous ring is supplied with sensory nerve fibers. Tears in the fibrous ring progress over time until enough damage is done to allow the inner disc material to protrude into the intervertebral space. Like the straw that broke the camel's back, it may take just one incident to progress a damaged disc to a herniated disc. Sudden twisting with flexion or extension movements,

Sciatica Pain radiating along the course of the sciatic nerve in the back of the hip and leg.

Scoliosis A lateral curvature with some rotation of the spine; the most serious and deforming of all postural deviations.

Intervertebral Discs Spinal discs; cushions of cartilage between the bodies of the vertebrae. Each disc consists of a fibrous outer ring (annulus fibrosus) and a pulpy center (nucleus pulposus).

Herniated Disc The soft nucleus of the spinal disc that protrudes through a small tear in the surrounding tissue; also called prolapse.

such as suddenly reaching for a ball in tennis or racquet-ball, may precipitate a disc herniation. Herniated discs are most common in the lumbar spine, as it is subjected to greater compressive forces and torque due to its location at the bottom of the spine. They are also more common in men than women and in people who do heavy manual labor. The risk for disc herniation is greatest for individuals in their thirties and forties and decreases with age as the disc degenerates and becomes less soft and pliable. (See Figure 5.)

Degenerative disc disease is a common part of aging. Many elderly people appear to get shorter as they age, often due to degenerative changes within the discs. One notable change is flattening of the discs as a result of lost water content. This in turn causes the vertebrae to sit closer together, increasing compressive forces on both the small facet joints and vertebral bodies, decreasing the size of the canal where the spinal nerves exit and increasing the likelihood of nerve impingement, bone spur formation, and arthritis. (See Figure 6.)

The neck is probably strained more frequently than the lower back. The neck is constructed with the same curve and has the same mechanical problems as the lower back. The postural fault of forward head places a chronic strain on the posterior neck muscles. Tension in these muscles can lead to **myofascial trigger points,** causing headache or **referred pain** in the face, scalp, shoulder, arm, and chest.

Kyphosis is a contributing factor in neck pain. The more the upper back is flexed, the greater the compensating curve **(cervical lordosis)** in the neck. The sharpest

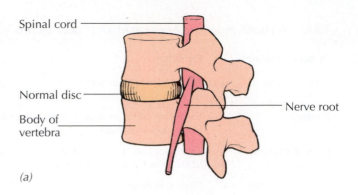

(a)

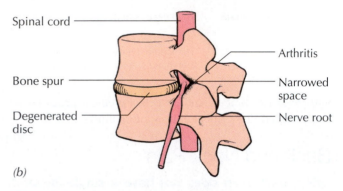

(b)

Figure 6 ▶ Normal disc (a) and degenerated disc with nerve impingement and arthritic changes (b).

angle is between the fourth and sixth cervical vertebrae, creating wear and tear (microtrauma) that accelerates disc degeneration and arthritic changes, which can ultimately result in nerve and artery impingement.

Because the exact causes of chronic neck pain are many and they vary from individual to individual, diagnosis is difficult. Some of the causes of chronic neck pain (and the often accompanying shoulder pain) include poor workplace design; poor posture, work habits, and physical fitness; and too much stress. Some examples of good body mechanics to prevent problems are shown in Figure 7.

Importance of Good Body Mechanics

Proper body mechanics can help prevent back and neck injury. Body mechanics is a discipline that applies mechanical laws and principles to study how the body can perform more efficiently and with less energy. Good body mechanics, as applied to back care, implies maintaining a "neutral spine" during activities of daily living. A neutral spine maintains the normal curvature of the spine, thus allowing an optimal balance of forces across the spine, reducing compressive forces and minimizing

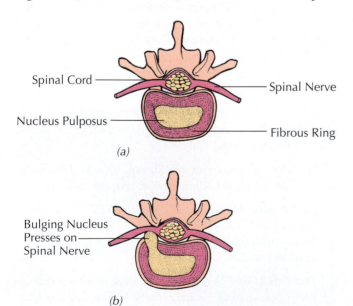

Figure 5 ▶ Normal disc (a) and herniated disc (b).

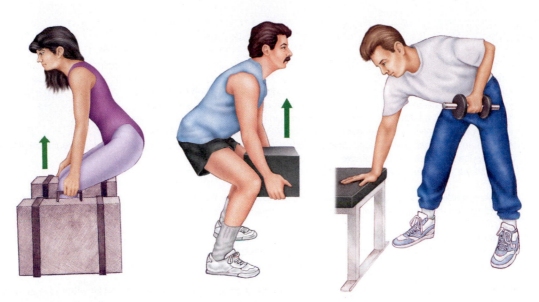

Figure 7 ▶ Good body mechanics can help prevent back and neck pain.

muscle tension. Table 2 provides specific recommendations and examples for good body mechanics in a variety of settings and positions.

Poor body mechanics can increase risks for back pain. A common cause of backache is muscle strain, frequently precipitated by poor body mechanics in daily activities, such as lifting or exercising. If lifting is done improperly, great pressure is exerted on the lumbar discs, and excessive stress and strain are placed on the lumbar muscles and ligaments. Many popular exercises also place too much strain on the back and should be avoided (see the concept on safe physical activity). Poor postures can also cause back strain. An example is sleeping flat on the back or abdomen on a soft mattress. By avoiding bad body mechanics you can reduce your risk of back pain.

Good lifting technique focuses on using the legs. Keep in mind that the muscles of the legs are relatively large and strong, compared with the back muscles. Likewise, the hip joint is well-designed for motion. It is less likely to suffer the same amount of wear and tear as the smaller joints of the spine. When lifting an object from the floor, an individual should strive to meet the following guidelines: straddle the object with a wide stance; squat down by hinging through the hips and bending the knees; maintain a slight arch to the lower back by sticking out the buttocks; test the load and get help if it is too heavy or awkward; rise by tightening the leg muscles, not the back; keep the load close to the waist; don't pivot or twist (see Figure 7).

Some additional general guidelines will help in preventing postural, back, and neck problems. In addition to the suggestions for improving body mechan-

ics noted in the previous sections, the following guidelines should be helpful:

- Do exercises to strengthen abdominal and hip extensors and to stretch the hip flexors and lumbar muscles if they are tight (see Tables 3–9).
- Avoid hazardous exercises (see the concept on safe physical activity).
- Do regular physical activity for the entire body, such as walking, jogging, swimming, and bicycling.
- Warm up before engaging in strenuous activity.
- Sleep on a moderately firm mattress or place a 3/4-inch-thick plywood board under the mattress.
- Avoid sudden, jerky back movements, especially twisting.
- Avoid obesity. The smaller the waistline, the less the strain on the lower back.
- Use appropriate back and seat supports when sitting for long periods.
- Maintain good posture when carrying heavy loads; do not lean forward, sideways, or backward.
- Adjust sports equipment to permit good posture; for example, adjust a bicycle seat and handle bars to permit good body alignment.
- Avoid long periods of sitting at a desk or driving; take frequent breaks and adjust the car seat and headrest for maximum support.

Myofascial Trigger Points A tender spot in the muscle or muscle fascia that refers pain to a location distant to the point.

Referred Pain Pain that appears to be located in one area, though it actually originates in another area.

Cervical Lordosis Excessive hyperextension in the neck region (swayback of the neck).

Table 2 ▶ Body Mechanics Guidelines for Posture and Back/Neck Care

Sitting	• Use a hard chair with a straight back and armrests, placing the spine against the back of the chair. A footrest reduces fatigue (see Figure 2). • Keep one or both knees lower than the hips and feet supported on the floor. • If your back flattens when you sit, place a lumbar roll behind your lower back. • When sitting at a table, keep the back and neck in good alignment. • Do not sit in front-row theater seats, which forces you to tip your head back. • When driving a car, pull the seat forward, so the legs are bent when operating the pedals. If your back flattens when you drive, use a lumbar support pillow. • Whenever possible, sit while working but stand occasionally.
Standing	• When standing for long periods of time, keep the lower back flat by propping a foot on a stool; alternate feet. • Avoid tilting the head backward (when shaving or washing your hair).
Lying	• Avoid lying on the abdomen. • When lying on the back, a pillow or lift should be placed under the knees. Do not use a thick head pillow. • When lying on your side, keep your knees and hips bent; place a pillow between the knees.
Lifting and Carrying	• When lifting, avoid bending at the waist. Keep the back straight, bend the knees, and lift with the legs. Assume a side-stride position with the object between the feet to allow you to get low and near the object (see Figure 7). • Perform one-hand lifting the same way as two-hand lifting; use the nonlifting hand (see Figure 7) for support. • When lifting, do not twist the spine. This can be more damaging from a sitting position than from a standing position. • When lifting, keep the object close to the body; do not reach to lift. Tighten the abdominal muscles before lifting. • If possible, avoid carrying objects above waist level. • When objects must be carried above the waist, carry them in the midline of the body, preferably on the back (use a backpack). Keep backpack weight low and use both straps for support. • Push or pull heavy objects, rather than lifting them. It takes thirty-four times more force to lift than to slide an object across the floor. Pushing is preferred over pulling. • Do not lift or carry loads too heavy for you. The most economical load for the average adult is about 35 percent of the body weight. Obviously, with strength training, you can lift a greater load, but heavy loads are a backache risk factor. • Divide the load if possible, carrying half in each hand/arm. If the load cannot be divided, alternate it from one side of the body to the other (see Figure 7). • When lifting and lowering an object from overhead, avoid hyperextending the neck and the back. Any lift above waist level is inefficient. • When objects must be carried in front of the body above the level of the waist, lean backward to balance the load, and avoid arching the back.
Working	• When working above head level, get on a stool or ladder to avoid tipping the head backward. • Work at eye level; for example, computer monitors should not be too high or low. • To avoid back and neck strain, climb a ladder or stand on a stool so you don't have to raise your arms over your head. • When working with the hands, the workbench or kitchen cabinet should be about 2 to 4 inches below the waist. The office desk should be about 29 to 30 inches high for the average man and about 27 to 29 inches high for the average woman. • Tools most often used should be the closest to reach. • Avoid constant arm extension, whether forward or sideward. • The arms should move either together or in opposite directions. When the conditions allow, use both hands in opposite and symmetrical motions while working. • Organize work to save energy. Vary the working position by changing from one task to another before feeling fatigued. When working at a desk, get up and stretch occasionally to relieve tension. • Use proper tools and equipment to reduce neck strain; for example, use a paint roller with an extension to reach overhead, thus reducing the need to hold the arms overhead and to hyperextend the neck. • Avoid stooping or unnatural positions that cause strain.

Exercises for Posture and Back/Neck Care

🌐 **Exercise is a frequently prescribed treatment for back or neck pain.** www.mhhe.com/phys_fit/ web13 Click 04. Treatments range from surgical removal of a disc or fusion to more conservative measures, such as injections, electrical stimulation, muscle relaxants, anti-inflammatory drugs, vapo-coolant spray, bracing, traction, bed rest, heat, cryotherapy, massage, and therapeutic exercise. Regardless of the treatment used, 70 to 85 percent of back patients recover spontaneously. Of those, 70 percent will have no symptoms at the end of 3 weeks, and 90 percent will recover in 2 months. The various treatment modalities may simply make patients more comfortable or may hasten the recovery.

Technology Update

MedX Back Machine

Although general resistance training may help to improve the strength and endurance of the back muscles, the exercises may not be specific enough to target the specific problems contributing to back pain. For years, physical therapists have used various rehabilitation devices to study muscle function in the back. Many of the equipment innovations used in clinical settings are becoming available to consumers. The inclusion of these machines in many clubs reflects the growing awareness in the population (and fitness professionals) of the importance of back care. One line of machines is made by a company called MedX. Similar to some clinical devices, these machines use a strain gauge and computer to evaluate isometric contractions at specific angular positions to determine the resistance profile supplied by the machine (this is similar to what clinical machines do). The machines include low minimal resistance levels and small increments in resistance to allow the machines to be used for individuals with different levels of back strength (see "On the Web" for more information).

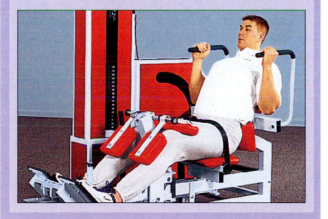

Exercise has been found to be helpful in treating all kinds of chronic pain. (Resistance exercises and aerobic exercises have been particularly helpful in pain clinics.) Aerobic exercise is also known to help nourish the spinal discs.

Exercise can prevent or correct some of the underlying causes of back and neck pain by strengthening weak muscles and stretching short ones. In the process of creating muscle balance, exercise improves postural alignment and body mechanics and relaxes muscle spasms. The dynamic nature of stability ball exercises make them well suited for correcting muscle imbalances. See Table 9 and the "On the Web" resource (Click 04).

Resistance exercise can often correct muscle imbalance, the underlying cause of many postural and back problems. www.mhhe.com/phys_fit/web13 Click 05. If the muscles on one side of a joint are stronger than the muscles on the opposite side, the body part is pulled in the direction of the stronger muscles. Corrective exercises are usually designed to strengthen the long, weak muscles and to stretch the short, strong ones in order to have equal pull in both directions. For example, people with lumbar lordosis may need to strengthen the abdominals and hamstrings and stretch the lower back and hip flexor muscles (see Figures 3 and 4).

Some people are unable to lift loads safely because tight and/or weak muscles prevent them from using proper body mechanics. Some people have backaches because they lift improperly. In many instances, the poor technique is caused by muscle imbalance. Examples include hamstrings or gluteals that are too tight to permit the lower back to retain its normal curve during lifting; calf muscles that are too tight to allow the heels to remain on the floor during squatting; and abdominal muscles that are too weak to support the back. Proper exercise can correct these problems.

Strategies for Action

An important step in taking action to assure good posture and good back and neck care is assessing your current status. www.mhhe.com/phys_fit/web13 Click 06. An important early step in taking action is self-assessment. The Healthy Back Tests consist of eight pass or fail items that will give you an idea of the areas in which you might need improvement. The Healthy Back Tests are described in *Lab Resource Materials*. You will take these tests in Lab 13A.

A posture test is included in Lab 13B to help you determine if you have any of the posture problems described in Table 1. Rating charts for both the back and posture tests are included in *Lab Resource Materials*.

Experts have identified behaviors associated with potential future back and neck problems. In addition to the back and posture tests, it may be useful to assess your risk factors. A questionnaire is provided in Lab 13A for assessing these risk factors.

Specific exercises are sometimes needed to prevent or help rehabilitate postural, neck, and back problems. www.mhhe.com/phys_fit/web13 Click 07. Exercises included in previous concepts were presented with health-related fitness in mind. The exercises included in this concept are not so different. They are either flexibility or strength/muscle endurance exercises for specific muscle groups; however, each is selected specifically to help correct a postural problem or to remove the cause of neck and back pain. To that extent, these exercises may be classified as therapeutic. The same exercises may be called preventive because they can be used to prevent postural or spine problems. Whether therapeutic or preventive, the exercises will not be effective unless they are done faithfully and with the FIT formula applied. People who have back and neck pain should seek the advice of a physician to make certain that it is safe for them to perform the exercises.

The exercises in Tables 3–9 are not necessarily intended for all people. Rather, you should choose exercises based on your own individual needs. Use your results on the Healthy Back Tests and the posture test to determine the exercises that are most appropriate for you.

To facilitate the use of these exercises for back or postural problems, the most effective exercises for various maladies are organized in Tables 3–9. Lab 13C is designed to help you choose specific exercises related to test items in Lab 13A.

Keeping records of progress is important to adhering to a back care program. An activity logging sheet is provided in Lab 13C to help you keep records of your progress as you regularly perform exercises to build and maintain good back and neck fitness.

Study Resources

Check out additional online study resources for this concept in the Student Edition of the Online Learning Center at www.mhhe.com/corbin13e.

Web Resources

American Back Care Company **www.americanback.com**
Back and Body Care **www.backandbodycare.com**
MedX **www.medxonline.com**
National Safety Council: **www.nsc.org**
National Osteoporosis Foundation: **www.nof.org**

Suggested Readings

Additional reference materials for Concept 13 are available at **www.mhhe.com/phys_fit/web13 Click 08.**

Bracko, M. R. 2004. Can we prevent back injuries? *ACSM's Health and Fitness Journal* 8(4):5–11.
Golderberg, L., and P. Twist, 2001. *Strength Ball Training: 69 Exercises Using Swiss Balls and Medicine Balls.* Champaign, IL: Human Kinetics.

Hamaoui, A., et al. 2004. Postural sway increase in low back pain subjects is not related to reduced spine range of motion. *Neuroscience Letters* 357(2):135–138.
Katzmarzyk, P. T., and L. C. Cora. 2002. Musculoskeletal fitness and risk of mortality. *Medicine and Science in Sports and Exercise* 34(5):740–744.
Liemohn, W., and G. Pariser. 2002. Core strength: Implications for fitness and low back pain. *ACSM's Health and Fitness Journal* 6(5):10–16.
McGill, S. M. 2001. Low back stability. *Exercise and Sport Science Reviews* 29(1):26–31.
Plowman, S. A. 1999. Physical fitness and healthy low back function. In C. B. Corbin and R. P. Pangrazi (eds.). *Towards a Better Understanding of Physical Fitness and Activity.* Scottsdale, AZ: Holcomb-Hathaway.
Rainville, J., et al. 2004. Exercise as a treatment for chronic low back pain. *Spine* 4(1):106–115.
Walters, P. H. 2000. Back to the basics: Strengthening the neglected lower back. *ACSM's Health and Fitness Journal* 4(4):19–25.
Worobey, S., et al. 2002. Strength training for posture. *Fitness Management* 6:46–49.

 In the News

Changes in Use of Hormone Replacement Therapies May Have Implications for Osteoporosis

Doctors have routinely prescribed hormone replacement therapy (HRT) for women to reduce risks for heart disease and osteoporosis following menopause. Over 6 million women were reported to be taking this type of regimen, but a major National Institutes of Health study reported increased risks for cardiovascular events and breast cancer in those taking HRT. The result caused the clinical trial on HRT to be halted and has caused doctors to recommend that women stop taking HRT. This change in medical practice could have major implications for other health risks in women, particularly for osteoporosis. The National Osteoporosis Foundation reports that over half of all women over the age of fifty will have an osteoporotic fracture sometime in their lifetime without supplemental estrogen to help preserve bone mass. Experts predict that the prevalence of osteoporosis to increase. Participation in regular weight-bearing exercise can help to maintain bone mass and prevent osteoporosis.

Stretching Exercises for the Hip Flexors and Hamstrings, and for Pelvic Stabilization Table 3

Table 3

When performed on a regular basis, these exercises will help maintain **neutral spine** posture and improve the flexibility of the hip flexor and hip extensor musculature. (Tightness of these muscles can, respectively, contribute to a forward or backward pelvic tilt due to their attachments to the pelvis.) Hold stretches for 15 to 30 seconds.

1. Back-Saver Hamstring Stretch

This exercise stretches the hamstrings and calf muscles. Sit on the floor with the feet against the wall or an immovable object. Bend left knee and bring foot close to buttocks. Clasp hands behind back. Bend forward from hips, keeping lower back as straight as possible. Let bent knee rotate outward so trunk can move forward keeping back flat. Hold and repeat on each leg.

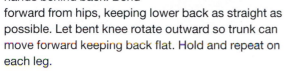

3. Hip and Low Back Stretch

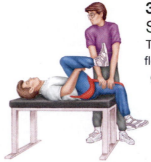

This exercise stretches the hip flexors of one leg and the gluteals and lumbar muscles of the opposite leg. Lie on your back. Draw one knee up to the chest and pull thigh down tightly with the hands, then slowly return to the original position. Repeat with other knee. Do not grasp knee—grasp thigh. If a partner or a weight stabilizes the extended leg, the hip flexor muscles on that leg will be stretched.

2. Single Knee-to-Chest

This exercise stretches the lower back, gluteals, and hamstring muscles. Lie on your back with knees bent. Use hands on back of thigh to draw one knee to the chest. Hold. Then extend the knee and point the foot toward the ceiling. Hold. Return to the starting position without arching your back. Repeat with other leg.

4. Hip and Thigh Stretch

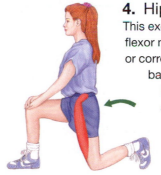

This exercise stretches the hip flexor muscles and helps prevent or correct forward pelvic tilt, lumbar lordosis, and backache. Place right knee directly above right ankle and stretch left leg backward so knee touches floor. If necessary, place hands on floor for balance. Press pelvis forward and downward. Hold. Repeat on opposite side. Caution: Do not bend front knee more than 90 degrees.

Neutral Spine Proper position of the spine to maintain a normal lordotic curve. The spine has neither too much nor too little lordotic curve.

Table 4 Pelvic Stabilization Exercises

These exercises help train the abdominal and buttock muscles to provide postural stability by maintaining the pelvis in a neutral position during activity. They help prevent or correct lumbar lordosis, abdominal ptosis (see Table 1, page 227), and backache. Hold stretches for 15 to 30 seconds.

Table 4

1. Pelvic Tilt

Lie on your back with knees bent. Tighten the abdominal muscles and tilt pelvis backwards slightly to "neutral." At the same time, tighten the hip and thigh muscles. Do not push with the legs. Hold, then relax. Breathe normally during the contraction; do not hold your breath.

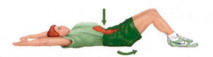

3. Wall Slide

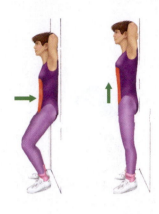

This exercise helps teach the feel of a neutral spine and pelvis. Stand with heels 4 to 6 inches from wall. Tighten abdominals and gently press lower back towards wall. Bend knees and slide down wall 8 to 10 inches maintaining pelvic tilt. Return to upright position. Repeat with hands behind neck.

2. Bridging

This exercise strengthens the hip extensors, especially the gluteal muscles. Lie on your back with knees bent and feet close to buttocks. Contract gluteals, lifting buttocks and lower back off floor. Hold, relax, and repeat. Do not arch low back. Variations: Alternately raise arms up and down while maintaining bridge and neutral spine. Repeat bridge while marching feet in place.

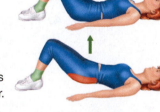

4. Pelvic Stabilizer

Lie on your back. Bend both knees up to chest. Place arms on floor for support. Tighten abdominals and hold neutral pelvic tilt while slowly extending one leg as far as possible without arching back. Return knee to chest. Alternate legs. Variation: Raise one arm overhead while extending opposite leg to floor.

Exercises for Muscle Fitness of the Abdominals 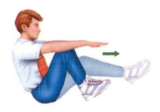**Table 5**

Table 5

These exercises are designed to increase the strength of the abdominal muscles. Strong abdominal muscles are important for maintaining a neutral pelvis, maintaining good posture, and preventing backache associated with lordosis. Hold stretches for 15 to 30 seconds.

1. Reverse Curl

Lie on your back. Bend the knees and bring knees in toward the chest. Place arms at sides for balance and support. Pull the knees toward the chest, raising the hips off the floor. Do not let the knees go past the shoulders. Return to the starting position. Repeat.

2. Crunch (Curl-Up)

Lie on your back with your knees bent and palms on ears. If desired, legs may rest on bench to increase difficulty. For less resistance, place hands at side of body. For more resistance, move hands higher. Curl up until shoulder blades leave floor, then roll down to the starting position. Repeat. Variation: extend the arms or cross the arms over your chest.

3. Crunch with Twist (on Bench)

Lie on your back with your feet on a bench, knees bent at 90 degrees. Arms may be extended or on shoulders or hands on ears (the most difficult). Same as crunch except twist the upper trunk so the right shoulder is higher than the left. Reach toward the left knee with the right elbow. Hold. Return and repeat to the opposite side. (This exercise is not recommended for people with lower back pain due to the combined motions of flexion and rotation.)

4. Sitting Tucks

Sit on floor with feet raised, arms extended for balance. Alternately bend and extend legs without letting your back or feet touch floor. (This is an advanced exercise and is not recommended for people who have back pain.)

235

Table 6

Table 6 Stretching and Strengthening Exercises for the Muscles of the Neck

These exercises are designed to increase strength in the neck muscles and to improve neck range of motion. They are helpful in preventing and resolving symptoms of neck pain and for relieving trigger points. Hold stretches for 15 to 30 seconds.

1. Neck Rotation Exercise

This PNF exercise strengthens and stretches the neck rotators. It should always be done with the head and neck in axial extension (good alignment). It is particularly useful for relieving trigger point pain and stiffness. Place palm of left hand against left cheek. Point fingers toward ear and point elbow forward. Turn head and neck to the left; contract while gently resisting with left hand. Contract neck muscle for 6 seconds. Relax and turn head to right as far as possible; hold stretch. Repeat four times; repeat on opposite side.

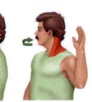

2. Isometric Neck Exercises

This exercise strengthens the neck muscles. Sit and place one or both hands on the head as shown. Assume good head and neck posture by tucking the chin, flattening the neck, and pushing the crown of the head up (axial extension). Apply resistance (a) sideward, (b) backward, and (c) forward. Contract the neck muscles to prevent the head and neck from moving. Hold contraction for 6 seconds. Repeat each exercise up to six times. Note: For neck muscles, it is probably best to use a little less than a maximal contraction, especially in the presence of arthritis, degenerated discs, or injury.

3. Chin Tuck

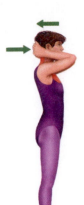

This exercise stretches the muscles at the base of the skull and reduces headache symptoms. Place hands together at the base of the head. Tuck in the chin and gently press head backward into your hands, while looking straight ahead. Hold.

4. Upper Trapezius Stretch

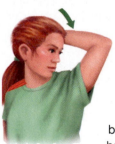

This exercise stretches the upper trapezius muscle and relieves neck pain and headache. To stretch the right upper trapezius, begin by placing right hand behind back and left hand on back of head. Gently turn head toward left underarm and tilt chin toward chest. Increase stretch by gently drawing head forward with left hand. Hold. Repeat to opposite side.

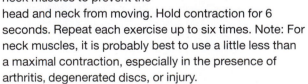

These exercises are designed to increase the strength and mobility of the muscles that move the trunk. They are especially helpful for people with chronic back pain. Hold stretches for 15 to 30 seconds.

1. Upper Trunk Lift

Lie on a table, bench, or a special-purpose bench designed for trunk lifts with the upper half of the body hanging over the edge. Have a partner stabilize the feet and legs while the trunk is raised parallel to the floor, then lower the trunk to the starting position. Lift smoothly, one segment of the back at a time. Place hands behind neck or on ears. Do not raise past the horizontal or arch the back or neck.

3. Side Bend

This exercise stretches the trunk lateral flexors. Stand with feet shoulder-width apart. Stretch left arm overhead to right. Bend to right at waist reaching as far to right as possible with left arm; reach as far as possible to the left with right arm. Hold. Do not let trunk rotate or lower back arch. Repeat on opposite side. Note: This exercise is made more effective if a weight is held down at the side in the hand opposite the side being stretched. More stretch will occur if the hip on the stretched side is dropped and most of the weight is borne by the opposite foot.

2. Trunk Lift

This exercise develops the muscles of the upper back and corrects round shoulders. Lie face down with hands clasped behind the neck. Pull the shoulder blades together, raising the elbows off the floor. Slowly raise the head and chest off the floor by arching the upper back. Return to the starting position. Repeat. For less resistance, hands may be placed under thighs. Caution: Do not arch the lower back or neck. Lift only until the sternum (breastbone) clears the floor. Variations: arms down at sides (easiest), hands by head, hands extended (hardest).

4. Supine Trunk Twist

This exercise increases the flexibility of the spine and stretches the rotator muscles. Lie on your back with your arms extended at shoulder level. Place left foot on right knee cap. Twist the lower body by lowering left knee to touch floor on right. Turn head to left. Keep shoulders and arms on floor. Hold.

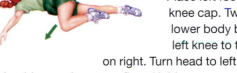

Table 7

Table 7 Exercise for the Trunk and Mobility

5. Lower Trunk Lift

This exercise develops low back and hip strength. Lie on your stomach on bench or table with legs hanging over the edge. Have a partner stabilize the upper back or grasp the edges of the table with hands. Raise the legs parallel to the floor and lower them. Do not raise past the horizontal or arch the back. Suggested progression: (1) begin by alternating legs; (2) when you can do 25 reps, add ankle weights; (3) when you can do 25 reps, lift both legs simultaneously (no weights).

6. Press-Up (McKenzie Extension Exercise)

This exercise increases flexibility of the lumbar spine, and restores normal lordotic curve, especially for people with a flat lumbar spine. Lie on your stomach with hands under the face. Slowly press up to a rest position on forearms. Keep pelvis on floor. Relax and hold 10 seconds. Repeat once. Do several times a day. Progress to gradually straightening the elbows while keeping the pubic bone on the floor. Caution: Do not perform if you have lordosis or if you feel any pain or discomfort in the back or legs. Note: A prone press-up will feel good as a stretch after doing abdominal strength or endurance exercises. This relaxed lordotic position can be performed while standing. Place the hands in the small of the back and gently arch the back and hold. This should feel good after sitting for a long period with the back flat.

Stretching and Strengthening Exercises for Round Shoulders Table 8

These exercises are designed to stretch the muscles of the chest and strengthen the muscles that keep the shoulders pulled back in good alignment (scapular adduction).

Table 8

1. Arm Lift

This exercise strengthens the scapular adductors. Lie on stomach with arms in reverse-T. Rest forehead on floor. Maintain the arm position and contract the muscles between the shoulder blades, lifting the arms as high as possible without raising head and trunk. Hold. Relax and repeat. Note: If the arms are first pressed against the floor before lifting, this becomes a PNF exercise and range of motion may be greater.
Variation: This more advanced exercise is performed in the same way except the arms are extended overhead.

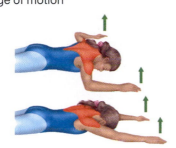

3. Wand Exercise

This exercise stretches the muscles on the front of the shoulder joint. Sit with wand grasped at ends. Raise wand overhead. Be certain that the head does not slide forward into a "poke neck" position. Keep the chin tucked and neck straight. Bring wand down behind shoulder blades. Keep spine erect; hold. Hands may be moved closer together to increase stretch on chest muscles.

2. Seated Rowing

This exercise strengthens the scapular adductors (rhomboid and trapezius). Sit facing pulley, feet braced and knees slightly bent. Grasp bar, palms down with hands shoulder-width apart. Pull bar to chest, keeping elbows high, and return.

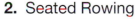
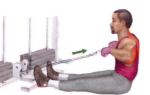

4. Pectoral Stretch

This exercise stretches the chest muscle (pectorals).

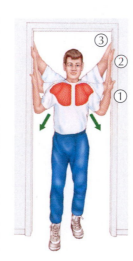

1. Stand erect in doorway with arms raised 45 degrees, elbows bent, and hands grasping door jambs; feet in front stride position. Press out on door frame, contracting the arms maximally for three seconds. Relax and shift weight forward on legs. Lean into doorway so muscles on front of shoulder joint and chest are stretched. Hold.
2. Repeat with arms raised 90 degrees.
3. Repeat with arms raised 135 degrees.

(This exercise is not recommended for people with shoulder instability. Discontinue if it causes numbness in the arms or hands.)

Table 9

Table 9 Lumbar Stabilization Exercises with Stability Balls

These exercises are designed to help improve the ability of the back to stabilize and support the trunk. The physioballs provide a useful way to learn to balance the body in these positions.

1. Balancing

Contract abdominal muscles. Straighten one knee and raise opposite arm over head. Alternate sides. To increase difficulty, position ball farther from your body.

Varriation: Slowly walk ball forward or backward with legs. Be careful not to arch back.

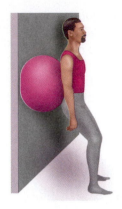

3. Wall Support

Stand against a wall with ball supporting low back. Contract abdominal muscles. Slowly bend knees 45 to 90 degrees and hold five seconds. Straighten knees and repeat. Raise both arms over head to increase difficulty.

2. Marching

Sit up straight with hips and knees bent 90 degrees. Contract abdominal muscles. Slowly raise one heel off the ground and opposite arm over head. Alternate sides. To increase difficulty, slowly raise one foot 2 inches from floor, alternating sides.

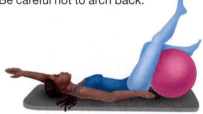

4. Stomach Roll

Lie prone over ball with abdominal region supported. Lower back and neck should be in neutral position with hands supported on floor directly under shoulders. Raise one leg off the floor while maintaining balance and a neutral spine. Alternate sides. To increase difficulty, raise one leg and opposite arm.

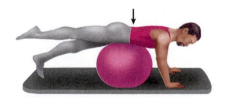

Lab Resource Materials: Healthy Back Tests

Chart 1 ► Healthy Back Tests

Physicians and therapists use these tests, among others, to make differential diagnoses of back problems. You and your partner can use them to determine if you have muscle tightness that may put you at risk for back problems. Discontinue any of these tests if they produce pain, numbness, or tingling sensations in the back, hips, or legs. Experiencing any of these sensations may be an indication that you have a low back problem that requires diagnosis by your physician. Partners should use *great caution* in applying force. Be gentle and listen to your partner's feedback.

Test 1-Back to Wall

Stand with your back against a wall with head, heels, shoulders, and calves of legs touching the wall as shown in the diagram. Flatten your neck and the hollow of your back by pressing your buttocks down against the wall. Your partner should just be able to place a hand in the space between the wall and the small of your back.

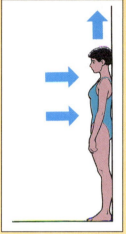

- If this space is greater than the thickness of his/her hand, you probably have lordosis with shortened lumbar and hip flexor muscles.

Test 2-Straight-Leg Lift

Lie on your back with hands behind your neck. The partner on your left should stabilize your right leg by placing his/her right hand on the knee. With the left hand, your partner should grasp the left ankle and raise your left leg as near to a right angle as possible. In this position (as shown in the diagram), your lower back should be in contact with the floor. Your right leg should remain straight and on the floor throughout the test.

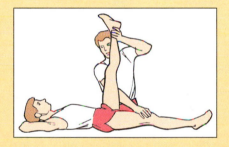

- If your left leg bends at the knee, short hamstring muscles are indicated. If your back arches and/or your right leg does not remain flat on the floor, short lumbar muscles or hip flexor muscles (or both) are indicated. Repeat the test on the opposite side. (Both sides must pass in order to pass the test.)

Test 3-Thomas Test

Lie on your back on a table or bench with your right leg extended beyond the edge of the table (approximately one-third of the thigh off the table). Bring your left knee to your chest and pull the thigh down tightly with your hands. Lower your right leg. Your lower back should remain flat against the table as shown in the diagram. Your right thigh should be at table level or lower.

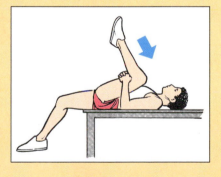

- If your right thigh lifts upward off the table while the left knee is hugged to the chest, a tight hip flexor (iliopsoas) on that side is indicated. Repeat on the opposite side. (Both sides must pass in order to pass the test.)

Test 4-Ely's Test*

Lie prone: flex right knee. Partner *gently* pushes right heel toward the buttocks. Stop when resistance is felt or when partner expresses discomfort.

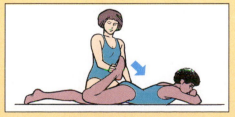

- If pelvis leaves the floor or hip flexes or knee fails to bend freely (135 degrees) or heel fails to touch buttocks, there is tightness in the quadriceps muscles. Repeat with left leg. (Both sides must pass in order to pass the test.)

*Ely's test is suitable as a diagnostic test when performed one time. This test item is not a good exercise for regular use. It is important to follow directions carefully. If pain or discomfort occurs stop the test.

Chart 1 ▶ Healthy Back Tests *(Continued)*

Test 5-Ober's Test

Lie on left side with left leg flexed 90 degrees at the hip and 90 degrees at the knee. Partner places right hip in neutral position (no flexion) and right knee in 90-degree flexion. Partner then allows the weight of the leg to lower it toward the floor.

- If there is no tightness in the iliotibial band (fascia and muscles on lateral side of leg), the knee touches the floor without pain and the test is passed. Repeat on the other side. (Both sides must pass in order to pass the test.)

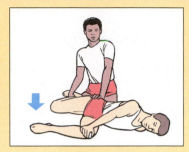

Test 6-Press-Up (Straight Arm)

Perform the press-up.

- If you can press to a straight-arm position, keeping your pubis in contact with the floor, and if your partner determines that the arch in your back is a continuous curve (not just a sharp angle at the lumbosacral joint), then there is adequate flexibility in spinal extension.

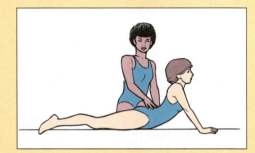

Test 7-Knee Roll

Lie supine with your knees and hips flexed 90 degrees, arms extended to the sides at shoulder level. Keep the knees and hips in that position and lower them to the floor on the right and then on the left.

- If you can accomplish this and still keep your shoulders in contact with the floor, then you have adequate rotation in the spine, especially at the lumbar and thoracic junction. (Both sides must pass in order to pass the test.)

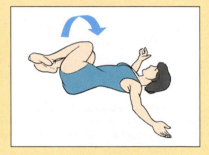

Test 8-Leg Drop Test*

Lie on your back on a table or on the floor with both legs extended overhead. Flatten the low back against the table or floor. Slowly lower legs while keeping the back flat.

- If your back arches before you reach a 45-degree angle, the abdominal muscles are too weak. A partner should be ready to support your legs if needed to prevent lower back arching or strain to the back muscles.

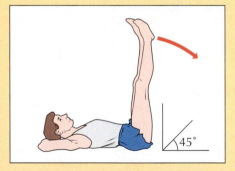

*The double leg-drop is suitable as a diagnostic test when performed one time. It is not a good exercise to be performed regularly by most people. If it causes pain, stop the test.

Chart 2 ▶ Healthy Back Test Ratings

Classification	Number of Tests Passed
Excellent	7–8
Very good	6
Good	5
Fair	4
Poor	1–3

Lab 13A The Healthy Back Tests and Back/Neck Questionnaire

Name	Section	Date

Purpose: To self-assess your potential for back problems using the Healthy Back Tests and the back/neck questionnaire

Procedures

1. Answer the questions in the back/neck questionnaire below. Count your points for nonmodifiable factors, modifiable factors, and total score and record these scores in the Results section. Use Chart 1 to determine your rating for all three scores and record them in the Results section.
2. With a partner, administer the Healthy Back Tests to each other (see *Lab Resource Materials*). Determine your rating using Chart 2. Record your score and rating in the Results section. If you did not pass a test, list the muscles you should develop to improve on that test.
3. Complete the Conclusions and Implications section.

Risk Factor Questionnaire for Back and Neck Problems

Directions: Place an X in the appropriate circle after each question. Add the scores for each of the circles you checked to determine your modifiable risk, nonmodifiable risk, and total risk scores.

Nonmodifiable

1. Do you have a family history of osteoporosis, arthritis, rheumatism, or other joint disease? ⓪ No   ① Yes

2. What is your age? ⓪ <40   ① 40–50   ② 51–60   ③ 61+

3. Did you participate extensively in these sports when you were young (gymnastics, football, weight lifting, skiing, ballet, javelin, or shot put)? ⓪ No   ① Some   ③ Extensive

4. How many previous back or neck problems have you had? ⓪ None   ① 1   ② 2   ⑤ 3+

Modifiable

5. Does your daily routine involve heavy lifting? ⓪ No   ① Some   ③ A lot

6. Does your daily routine require you to stand for long periods? ⓪ No   ① Some   ③ A lot

7. Do you have a high level of job-related stress? ⓪ No   ① Some   ③ A lot

8. Do you sit for long periods of time (computer operator, typist, or similar job)? ⓪ No   ① Some   ③ A lot

9. Does your daily routine require repetitive movements or holding objects for long periods of time (e.g., baby, briefcase, sales suitcase)? ⓪ No   ① Some   ③ A lot

10. Does your daily routine require you to stand or sit with poor posture (e.g., poor chair, reaching required while standing)? ⓪ No   ① Some   ③ A lot

11. What is your score on the Healthy Back Tests? ⓪ 6–7   ① 5   ③ 4   ⑤ 0–3

12. What is your score on the posture test in Lab 13B? ⓪ 0–2   ① 3–4   ③ 5–7   ④ 8+

Results

Tests	Pass	Fail	If you failed, what exercise should you do?
1. Back to wall	◯	◯	
2. Straight-leg lift	◯	◯	
3. Thomas test	◯	◯	
4. Ely's test	◯	◯	
5. Ober's test	◯	◯	
6. Press-up	◯	◯	
7. Knee roll	◯	◯	
8. Leg drop test	◯	◯	
Total	☐		

Chart 1 ▶ Back/Neck Questionnaire Ratings

Rating	Modifiable Score	Nonmodifiable Score	Total Score
Very high risk	7+	12+	19+
High risk	5–6	6–11	11–18
Average risk	3–4	4–6	7–10
Low risk	0–2	0–3	0–6

Chart 2 ▶ Healthy Back Tests Ratings

Classification	Number of Tests Passed
Excellent	7–8
Very good	6
Good	5
Fair	4
Poor	1–3

Back/Neck Questionnaire

Score [ ]   Rating [ ]

Back Tests

Score [ ]   Rating [ ]

Conclusions and Implications: In several sentences, discuss your need to do exercises for care of the back and neck. Include in your discussion whether you think your muscles are fit enough to prevent problems, the areas in which you are most likely to experience problems, and steps you might take to prevent future problems. Use your test results to answer.

Lab 13B Evaluating Posture

Name	**Section**	**Date**

Purpose: To learn to recognize postural deviations and thus become more posture conscious and to determine your postural limitations in order to institute a preventive or corrective program

Procedures

1. Wear as little clothing as possible (bathing suits are recommended) and remove shoes and socks.
2. Work in groups of two or three, with one person acting as the subject while partners serve as examiners; then alternate roles.
   a. Stand by a vertical plumb line.
   b. Using Chart 1 and Figure 1, check any deviations and indicate their severity (see points scale below).
   c. Total the score and determine your posture rating from the Posture Rating Scale (Chart 2).
3. If time permits, perform back and posture exercises (see Lab 13C).

Results

Record your posture score:

Record your posture rating from the Posture Rating Scale in Chart 2:

Chart 1 ▶ Posture Evaluation

Side View	Points	Back View	Points
Head forward	_____	Tilted head	_____
Sunken chest	_____	Protruding scapulae	_____
Round shoulders	_____	Symptoms of scoliosis	
		Shoulders uneven	_____
Kyphosis	_____	Hips uneven	_____
Lordosis	_____	Lateral curvature of	
		spine (Adam's position)	_____
Abdominal ptosis	_____	One side of back high	_____
		(Adam's position)	
Hyperextended			
knees	_____		
Body lean	_____		
		Total score	

Rate each using this point system:
- 0 = none
- 1 = slight
- 2 = moderate
- 3 = severe

Chart 2 ▶ Posture Rating Scale

Classification	Total Score
Excellent	0–2
Very good	3–4
Good	5–7
Fair	8–11
Poor	12 or more

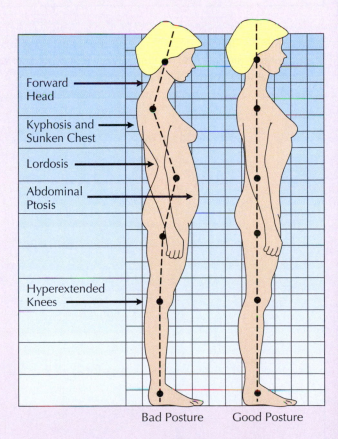

Forward Head

Kyphosis and Sunken Chest

Lordosis

Abdominal Ptosis

Hyperextended Knees

Bad Posture   Good Posture

Figure 1 ▶ Comparison of bad and good posture.

Conclusions and Implications

Were you aware of the deviations that were found?   Yes ⚪   No ⚪

1. List the deviations that were moderate or severe.

2. In several sentences, describe your current posture status. Include in this discussion your overall assessment of your current posture, whether you think you will need special exercises in the future, and the reasons your posture rating is good or not so good.

Lab 13C Planning and Logging Exercises: Care of the Back and Neck

Name _____   **Section** _____   **Date** _____

Purpose: To select several exercises for the back and neck that meet your personal needs and to self-monitor progress for one of these

Procedures

1. On Chart 1, check the tests from the Healthy Back Tests that you did *not* pass. Select at least one exercise from the group associated with those items. In addition, select several more exercises (a total of eight to ten) that you think will best meet your personal needs. If you passed all of the items, select eight to ten exercises that you think will best prevent future back and neck problems. Check the exercises you plan to perform in Chart 1.
2. Perform each of the exercises you select 3 days in 1 week.
3. Keep a 1-week log of your actual participation using the last three columns in Chart 1. If possible, keep the log with you during the day. Place a check by each of the exercises you perform for each day, including ones that you didn't originally have planned. If you cannot keep the log with you, fill in the log at the end of the day. If you choose to keep a log for more than 1 week, make extra copies of the log before you begin.
4. Answer the question in the Results section.

Chart 1 ▶ Back and Neck Exercise Plan

Check the tests you failed.	√	Place a check beside the exercises you plan to do. In the last 3 columns, check the exercises done and the days done.	√	Day 1 Date:	Day 2 Date:	Day 3 Date:
1. Back to wall		Pelvic tilt				
		Bridging				
		Wall slide				
		Pelvic stabilizer				
2. Straight-leg lift		Back-saver hamstring stretch				
		Calf stretch				
3. Thomas test		Hip and thigh stretch				
4. Ely's test		Single knee-to-chest				
5. Ober's test		Lateral hip and thigh stretch				
6. Press-up		Upper trunk lift				
		Trunk lift				
7. Knee roll		Side bend				
		Supine trunk twist				
8. Leg drop test		Reverse curl				
		Crunch				
Choose other exercises for the neck and shoulders.		Chin tuck				
		Neck rotation				
		Arm lift				
		Pectoral stretch				

Results

Did you do eight to ten exercises at least 3 days in the week?

Yes   No

◯   ◯

Conclusions and Interpretations

1. Do you feel that you will use back and neck exercises as part of your regular lifetime physical activity plan, either now or in the future? Use several sentences to explain your answer.

2. Discuss the exercises you did. What exercises would you continue to do and which ones would you change? Use several sentences to explain your answer.

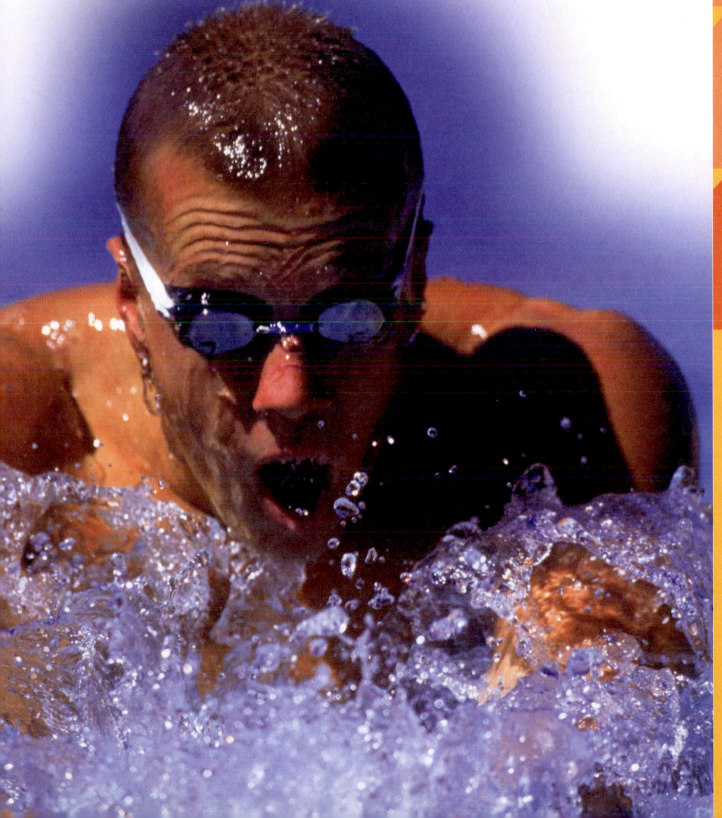

Performance Benefits of Physical Activity

Physical activity provides performance benefits above and beyond the benefits to health. These performance benefits can promote quality of life for the typical person and enhance the abilities of athletes and people in jobs requiring high levels of performance.

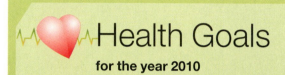

Health Goals

for the year 2010

- Increase leisure-time physical activity.

- Increase adoption and maintenance of regular daily physical activity.

- Increase proportion of people who participate in employee-sponsored activity programs.

- Reduce steroid use, especially among young people.

S ports and competitive athletics provide opportunities for individuals to explore the limits of their ability and to challenge themselves in competition. Some individuals enjoy challenges associated with competitive aerobic activities, such as running, cycling, swimming, and triathlons. Others enjoy the challenges associated with competitive resistance training activities, such as powerlifting and bodybuilding. High-level performance is also a requirement for some types of work. Examples are fire safety, military service, and police work. The heroic efforts of firefighters, law enforcement, and Port Authority officials following the events of September 11, 2001, are clear examples of how important high-level performance is in these careers.

In this concept, specific attention is devoted to the methods used to train for high-level performance. Several types of training will be discussed, including aerobic training, anaerobic training, special forms of resistance training (including plyometrics), and advanced techniques for flexibility. Methods for maximizing skill-related fitness and skill will also be presented.

High-Level Performance and Training Characteristics

Improving performance requires more specific training than the type needed to improve health. High levels of performance require good genetics, high levels of motivation, and a commitment to regular training. The effort and training required to excel in sports, competitive athletics, or work requiring high-level performance are greater than the amount required for good health and wellness. Because adaptations to exercise are specific to the type of activity that is performed, training should be matched to the specific needs of a given activity.

High-level performance requires health-related, skill-related fitness and the specific motor skills necessary for the performance. People who possess good fitness levels for each of the five health-related fitness components have enhanced health and wellness, as well as reduced risk for disease. To succeed in sports and certain jobs, high performance levels of health-related physical fitness are necessary, over and above what the normal person needs to enhance health. This is illustrated in Figure 1. **Training** (regular physical activity) builds health-related fitness to enhance health and high-level performance. This is why arrows in Figure 1 extend from health-related fitness to both health and high-level performance. To some extent, it can be said that high-level health-related fitness is much like skill-related fitness. High performance levels are not necessary for all people, only those who need exceptional performances. A distance runner needs exceptional cardiovascular fitness and muscular endurance, a lineman in football needs exceptional strength, a volleyball player needs power for jumping, and a gymnast needs exceptional flexibility.

Exceptional performance also requires high-level skill-related physical fitness. Skill-related physical fitness is especially affected by heredity. For example, speed is influenced greatly by the number of fast-twitch fibers you inherit, and reaction time is associated with the innate

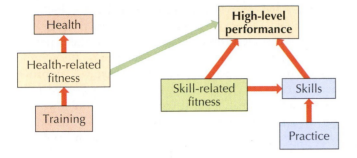

Figure 1 ▶ Factors influencing high-level performance.

characteristics of your nervous system. With specific training, you can make modest modifications in your skill-related fitness, but most experts believe that it is more important to do regular practice to enhance performance skills associated with the specific tasks of your sport or job. It is important to understand that skill-related fitness and skills are not the same thing.

Skill-related fitness components are abilities that help you learn skills faster and better, thus the arrow in Figure 1 from skill-related fitness to skills. Skills, on the other hand, are things such as throwing, kicking, catching, and hitting a ball. Practice enhances skills. Therefore, practicing the specific skills of a sport or a job is more productive to performance enhancement than more general drills associated with changing skill-related fitness. The most successful performers are those who inherit good potential for health and skill-related fitness, who train to improve their health-related fitness, and who do extensive practice to improve the skills associated with the specific activity in which they hope to excel.

High-level performers need high-performance levels of fitness.

Training for Endurance and Speed

🌐 **Success in endurance sports requires a high aerobic capacity.** www.mhhe.com/phys_fit/web14 Click 01. Regardless of the type of activity you perform, you derive energy from high-energy fuel that must be available to the muscle fibers. The breakdown of this high-energy fuel in the muscle cells allows you to perform all types of exercise. To continue exercising, the body must replenish these energy stores on a continual basis.

For some performers, success depends on the ability to sustain activity for long periods of time without stopping. Distance runners and swimmers are good examples. These types of performers are in special need of high levels of cardiovascular fitness, or aerobic capacity. In aerobic exercise, adequate oxygen is available to use the carbohydrates and fats available in the body to rebuild the high-energy fuel the muscles need to sustain performance. Aerobic exercise increases aerobic capacity (cardiovascular fitness) by enhancing the body's ability to supply oxygen to the muscles as well as their ability to use it. Slow-twitch muscle fibers appear to benefit most from aerobic exercise. Any performance that involves sustained performance places special demands on the slow-twitch fibers and requires a high level of aerobic capacity (cardiovascular fitness). The best measure of cardiovascular fitness is $\dot{V}O_2$ max (see cardiovascular fitness concept).

🌐 **Many types of high-level performance require anaerobic capacity.** www.mhhe.com/phys_fit/web14 Click 02. If adequate oxygen is supplied, activity can be sustained for long periods. Unfortunately, the energy resulting from the breakdown of the body's high-energy fuel is used in a matter of seconds if adequate oxygen is not supplied. Carbohydrates stored in the cells can be broken down to replenish the high-energy fuel supply to allow performance to continue for an additional time (30 to 40 seconds for most people). Short-term, vigorous exercise performed in the absence of an adequate oxygen supply is called **anaerobic exercise.** Anaerobic exercise

Training The type of physical activity performed by people interested in high-level performance—e.g., athletes, people in specialized jobs.

Anaerobic Exercise *Anaerobic* means "in the absence of oxygen." Anaerobic exercise is performed at an intensity so great that the body's demand for oxygen exceeds its ability to supply it.

results in **lactic acid** build-up in the process of energy production. Muscle fatigue occurs when anaerobic energy supplies are depleted, and lactic acid build-up occurs. Regular anaerobic exercise seems to allow the muscle to tolerate higher lactic acid levels before fatigue occurs. Also, anaerobic exercise improves anaerobic energy production capabilities, primarily in the fast-twitch fibers. These fibers appear to benefit most from anaerobic exercise.

Anaerobic capacity, or the ability to perform vigorous, short-term bouts of exercise and repeat them after relatively short rest periods, is necessary for success in many sports and jobs that require high-level performance. Anaerobic capacity is often measured in the laboratory using the Wingate test, an all-out, 30-second stationary bicycle ride at high resistance.

Training for activities requiring high levels of aerobic capacity can be achieved using a variety of techniques. The ability to perform sustained aerobic performance can be enhanced using a variety of techniques. The most common procedure is to perform the activity in which you plan to participate. For example, people who plan to run a marathon or a 10K race will commonly perform regular distance running at speeds similar to those required for their specific event. This type of training is also supplemented with aerobic interval training and long-slow distance training. Some training to enhance anaerobic capacity is also performed by most people interested in aerobic activities. Performers in other activities, such as swimming and cycling, use similar schedules of training.

Improved anaerobic capacity can contribute to performance in activities considered to be aerobic. Many physical activities commonly considered to be aerobic—such as tennis, basketball, and racquetball—have an anaerobic component. These activities require periodic vigorous bursts of exercise. Regular anaerobic training will help you resist fatigue in these activities. Even participants in activities such as long-distance running can benefit from anaerobic training, especially if performance times or winning races is important. A fast start may be anaerobic, a sprint past an opponent may be anaerobic, and a kick at the end will no doubt be anaerobic. Anaerobic training can help prepare a person for these circumstances.

🌐 **Interval training can be effective in building both aerobic and anaerobic capacity.** www. mhhe.com/phys_fit/web14 Click 03. High-level performance requires high-level training. **Interval training** is a commonly used technique used by many competitive athletes. The premise behind interval training is that by providing periodic rest you can increase the overall intensity of the exercise session and provide a greater stimulus to the body. Interval training can be performed in different ways to achieve different training goals.

In aerobic interval training, the goal is to challenge the aerobic system to work near maximal levels for extended periods of time. Research suggests that a period of 4 to 6 minutes of activity is needed to cause the aerobic system to elicit maximal adaptations that will improve aerobic capacity ($\dot{V}O_2$ max). The use of repeated mile runs at a faster than normal training pace would provide this type of challenge to the aerobic system. Alternately, shorter exercise bouts can be performed with brief rest periods to achieve the same goal. For example, a series of quarter-mile repeats with short rests is suitable as long as the total time at a high intensity is similar. In this case, the rest intervals must be short enough to only allow partial recovery between intervals.

Aerobic intervals are typically conducted at paces slower than the pace an individual would use in a race. An example of a schedule of aerobic interval training for a 10-km runner is illustrated in Table 1. To use the schedule, locate your typical 10-km time in the left-hand column. Perform 400-meter runs at the time specified in the "pace" column. Repeat twenty times with intervals of 10 to 15 seconds between runs. Similar schedules can be developed with other activities, such as swimming and cycling.

In anaerobic interval training, the goal is to challenge the anaerobic energy systems. This is typically accomplished with repeated high-intensity bouts of activity. In response to this training, the body improves its ability to

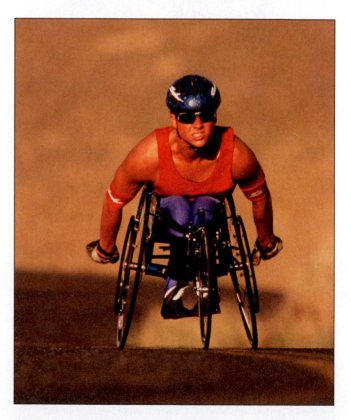

Interval training can be adapted for performers in a variety of activities.

Table 1 ▶ Aerobic Interval Training Schedules for a 10-Kilometer Runner

Best 10-km Times (Min:Sec)	Reps	Distance (Meters)	Rest (Sec)	Pace (Min:Sec)
46:00	20	400	10–15	2:00
43:00	20	400	10–15	1:52
40:00	20	400	10–15	1:45
37:00	20	400	10–15	1:37
34:00	20	400	10–15	1:30

Source: Wilmore, J. H. and D. L. Costill.

Table 2 ▶ Sample Anaerobic Interval Training Program (Moderate Intensity)

Short Intervals	Long Intervals
1. Do a flexibility and cardiovascular warm-up.	1. Do a flexibility and cardiovascular warm-up.
2. Run at 100% speed for 10 seconds (approximately 70–100 yards).	2. Run at 90% speed for 1 minute (approximately 300–500 yards).
3. Rest for 10 seconds by walking slowly.	3. Rest for 4 minutes by walking slowly.
4. Alternately repeat steps 2 and 3 until twenty runs have been completed.	4. Alternately repeat steps 2 and 3 until five runs have been completed.

produce energy anaerobically and improves its ability to tolerate and remove lactic acid from the blood.

Anaerobic interval training can be performed with either short or long intervals. Short-interval workouts should use maximum speed with rest intervals lasting from 10 seconds to 2 minutes. These should be repeated eight to thirty times. Long-interval training should use 90 to 100 percent speed, with rest intervals lasting from 3 to 15 minutes. These should be repeated four to fifteen times. A sample short anaerobic interval program and a sample long interval running program are presented in Table 2. These plans can be modified for use with other types of activities.

Principles of interval training can be adapted for different activities. The principles of interval training can be integrated into workouts in less structured ways. Runners sometimes use *fartlek* training to break up their workouts. A fartlek training run incorporates bursts of higher-intensity running followed by recovery periods of lower intensity. The difference from interval training is that the intermittent bursts in fartlek training are dictated by the nature of the terrain or the feelings of the moment. The term is from a Swedish word meaning "speed play," because the unstructured nature is more relaxed than structured interval training.

Many competitive sports involve alternating bursts of high-intensity activity followed by periods of recovery. Basketball, for example, involves intermittent sprints and jumps interspersed with periods of short recovery. Similarly, tennis involves bursts of activity separated by short recovery periods between points. To prepare for success in sports, it is important for athletes to incorporate intermittent interval-type training into their conditioning. Simulated games that require repeated sprints up and down the basketball court are a form of interval training specific to basketball players. Tennis players can incorporate a variety of forward and lateral movements into a high-intensity agility drill to improve conditioning for tennis.

Long-slow distance training is important for enhancing performances requiring aerobic capacity. The training techniques described in previous sections are necessary to achieve high-level aerobic performance. However, there is evidence that **long-slow distance (LSD) training** is also needed to promote high-level aerobic performances (such as long-distance running, cycling, or swimming). The reason for this is that there are specific adaptations that take place within the muscles when used for long periods of time. These adaptations improve the muscles' ability to take up and use the oxygen in the bloodstream. Adaptations within the muscle cell also improve the body's ability to produce energy from fat stores. Long-slow distance training involves performances longer than the event for which you are performing but at a slower pace. For example, a mile runner will regularly perform 6- to 7-mile runs (at 50 to 60 percent of racing pace) to improve aerobic conditioning, even though the event is much shorter. A marathoner may perform runs of 20 miles or more to achieve even higher levels of endurance. Although this 20-mile distance is shorter than the marathon race distance, research suggests that ample adaptations occur from this volume of exercise. Excess mileage in this case

Lactic Acid Substance that results from the process of supplying energy during anaerobic exercise; a cause of muscle fatigue.

Interval Training A training technique often used for high-level aerobic and anaerobic training; uses repeated bouts of activity followed by rest to maximize the quality of the workout.

Long-Slow Distance (LSD) Training Training technique that emphasizes long, slow distance. It is used by marathon runners and other endurance performers.

may just wear the body down. Long-slow distance training should be performed once every 1 to 2 weeks, and a rest day is recommended on the subsequent day to allow the body to recover fully.

Too much strength and flexibility training may impair endurance performance. The principle of specificity dictates that adaptations are specific to the type of training that is performed. While athletes should strive for a good balance of strength and flexibility, studies show that too much training in these areas can actually cause decreases in performance. Additional muscle mass from resistance training can reduce efficiency and impair performance. The use of weighted wristlets, anklets, or belts is also not recommended, as they may alter running mechanics and stride efficiency.

Flexibility has always been thought to be important for minimizing risks for injury, but recent studies have shown that running economy (the energy cost required to run a specific speed) is not as good in people with high flexibility as those who have poorer flexibility. Because running economy is an advantage for distance running performance, this suggests that extra flexibility may actually reduce performance. The theory behind these findings is that stiffer muscle-tendon structures may help to facilitate elastic energy return during running movements. This result shouldn't discourage you from stretching, but it does illustrate the complexities of high-level training. Regular stretching is still of value for most runners and endurance athletes.

Training for Strength and Muscular Endurance

Specific progressive resistance training programs are needed to achieve high-level muscular performance. A basic progressive resistance program for overall good health might involve performing a single exercise for each major muscle group two or three times a week. This level of training provides a regular stimulus to maintain healthy levels of muscular strength and endurance. However, many people enjoy challenging themselves to achieve higher levels of muscular performance. Olympic weight lifting competitors use free weights and compete in two exercises: the snatch and the clean and jerk. Powerlifting competitors use free weights and compete in three lifts: the bench press, squat, and dead lift. Bodybuilding competitors use several forms of resistance training and are judged on muscular hypertrophy (large muscles) and **definition of muscle.** Performers in these activities and athletes in strength-related sports need to use more advanced training methods to reach their full potential. The essential goal in high-level training is to provide the optimal stimulus, so that the muscles adapt in the desired way.

Because the goals are clearly different for athletes interested in strength/power, muscular hypertrophy, or muscular endurance, it is important to follow appropriate programs. The essential aspects of these different training programs are described in the sections that follow. The basic concepts are summarized in Figure 2.

Performers training for high-level strength should use multiple sets with heavier weights. www.mhhe.com/phys_fit/web14 Click 04. The best stimulus for strength gains is repeated lifts with very heavy loads. Guidelines for intermediate lifters call for multiple sets of six to twelve reps performed using 70 to 80 percent of 1 RM values. The load and intensity guidelines are higher for advanced lifters (one to twelve reps performed using 70 to 100 percent 1 RM) because they may need to use a higher overload to get continued improvements. Rest intervals must be long (2 to 3 minutes) for high-intensity strength training to allow full recovery of the muscles between sets.

Multiple joint exercises, such as the bench press, have been found to be more effective in strength enhancement, since they allow a greater load to be lifted. The sequencing of exercises within a workout is also an important consideration for strength development. When training all major muscle groups in a workout, large muscle groups should be done before small muscle groups, and multiple-joint exercises should be done before single-joint ones.

Performers training for muscular endurance should emphasize many repetitions with lighter weights. Completing multiple sets of ten to twenty-five

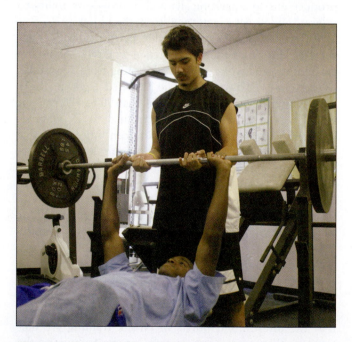

Strength training for high-level performance differs from strength training for health.

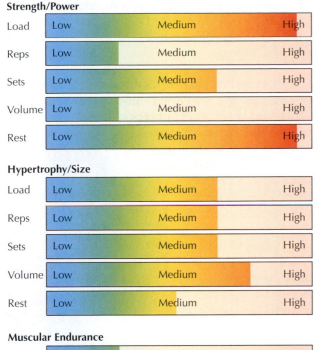

Strength/Power

Hypertrophy/Size

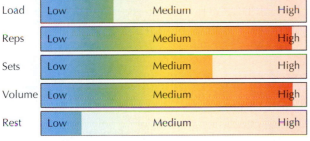

Muscular Endurance

Figure 2 ▶ Differences in training stimulus for different resistance training programs.

repetitions is required to build endurance. Short rest periods of 1 to 2 minutes are recommended for high-repetition sets and periods of less than 1 minute should be used for lower-repetition sets. This challenges the muscles to perform repeatedly and with little or no rest. Variation in the order in which exercises are performed is also recommended to vary the stimulus. Intermediate lifters should aim for two to four times per week, but advanced lifters may perform up to six sessions per week if appropriate variation in muscle groups is used between workouts.

Performers training for bulk and definition often use extra reps and/or sets. www.mhhe.com/phys_fit/web14 Click 05. Bodybuilders are more interested in definition and hypertrophy than in absolute strength. Gaining both size and definition requires a balance between strength and muscle endurance training. Most bodybuilders use three to seven sets of ten to fifteen repetitions, rather than the

three sets of three to eight repetitions recommended for most weight lifters. Sometimes definition is difficult to obtain because it is obscured by fat. It should be noted that people with the largest-looking muscles are not always the strongest.

Training for cardiovascular fitness along with strength training can limit adaptations. The body adapts to the type of training that is performed. If too much endurance training is performed, the body tries to adapt to the needs of aerobic activity, and this makes it more difficult to gain muscle mass or achieve maximal increases in strength. The effect would only be an issue for competitive strength or power athletes and should not detract people from getting the important health benefits associated with moderate amounts of aerobic activity. Regular aerobic activity is considered essential for bodybuilders to assist in reducing unwanted body fat.

Training for Power

Power is a combination of strength and speed, and it is both health-related and skill-related. Most experts classify power as a skill-related component of fitness because it is partially dependent on speed. On the other hand, power is also dependent on strength and can be classified as a health-related component to the extent that strength is involved. Thus, power falls somewhere between the two distinct groups of fitness attributes.

Some experts consider power to be the most functional mode in which all human motion occurs. Power is exceptionally important in sport activities such as hitting a baseball, blocking in football, putting the shot, or throwing the discus. Power is also essential for good vertical jumping—a movement critical for basketball and many other sports. A typical progressive resistance exercise program will build sufficient power for normal activities of daily living; however, people interested in high-level performance should consider using additional exercises that specifically develop power.

The stronger person is not necessarily the more powerful. Power is the amount of work per unit of time. To increase power, you must do more work in the same time or the same work in less time. If you extend your knee and move a 100-pound weight through a 90-degree arc in 1 second, you have twice as much power as

Definition of Muscle The detailed external appearance of a muscle.

a person who needs 2 seconds to complete the same movement. Power requires both strength and speed. Increasing one without the other limits power. Some power athletes (for example, football players) might benefit more by achieving less strength and more speed.

The principle of specificity applies to power development. If you need power for an activity in which you are required to move heavy weights, then you need to develop *strength-related power* by working against heavy resistance at slower speeds. If you need to move light objects at great speed, such as in throwing a ball, you need to develop *speed-related power* by training at high speeds with relatively low resistance. There must be trade-offs between speed and power because, the heavier the resistance, the slower the movement. Training adaptations are also specific to the type of training performed. Power exercises done at high speeds will help to enhance muscular endurance, whereas power exercises that use heavy resistance at lower speeds will increase strength.

Performers who need explosive power to perform their events should use training that closely resembles the event. Jumpers, for example, should jump as a part of their training programs in order to learn correct timing at the same time they are developing power. This also applies to Olympic weight lifters, shot putters, jumpers, ballet dancers, and others. These athletes need both strength and endurance; however, studies show that too much of either can have a negative effect on performance. If they use machines, it is better to use the leg press than a knee extension machine because the press more nearly resembles the leg action of the jump.

The performer's program should use similar speed, force, angle, and range of motion as the activity. However, if a performer is unable to do the specific skill because of weather or injury or is seeking variety, then plyometrics, isokinetics, and weight training (especially with free weights or pulleys if simulating a sport skill) are effective means of developing power.

Power training can be done with weight equipment, but care is needed to ensure safety and efficacy. Resistance training can be performed to optimize power development, but these movements are not recommended for beginning lifters. Studies have shown that heavy resistance training can actually decrease power unless training also includes some explosive movements. Current guidelines from the ACSM recommend heavy loading (85 to 100 percent of 1 RM) to increase the force component of the power equation and light to moderate loading (30 to 60 percent of 1 RM) performed at an explosive velocity to enhance the speed component of power. The guidelines recommend that a multiple set power program (three to six sets) be integrated within an overall strength training program. Exercises for power are most effectively done

with free weights or pulleys to simulate sport-related movements more effectively. Isokinetic devices, such as isokinetic swim benches, may also be useful for enhancing sport-specific power.

 Plyometrics may be useful in training for tasks or events requiring power. www.mhhe.com/ phys_fit/web14 Click 06. **Plyometrics** is an advanced training technique used by many athletes. It takes advantage of a quick pre-stretch prior to a movement to increase power. By repeatedly doing these movements in training, athletes can provide a greater stimulus to their muscles and improve their body's ability to perform power movements. Track and field athletes may do a hopping drill for 30 to 100 meters or alternate jumping from a box to the floor and back to the box (called depth jumping, drop jumping, or bounce loading). As the body lands, some of the major leg muscles lengthen in an eccentric contraction, then follow immediately with a strong concentric contraction as the legs push off for the next jump or stride. The prestretch of the muscle during landing adds an elastic recoil that provides extra force to the push-off (see Table 3).

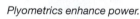
Plyometrics enhance power.

Plyometrics are used to apply the specificity principle to training for certain skills. Because eccentric exercise tends to result in more muscular soreness, it would be wise to proceed slowly with this type of training. It would also be important to have good flexibility before beginning a plyometrics program. Some safety guidelines for plyometrics are listed in Table 4.

Training for Flexibility

Stretching for performance may differ from stretching for good health. Guidelines for building flexibility using a variety of stretching exercises are presented in the concept on flexibility. It was noted in that concept that static stretching techniques are recommended for the warm-up, even for high-level performers. Ballistic stretching is appropriate for high-level performers because many of the motions of the activities in which they perform require ballistic movements. Nevertheless,

Table 3 ▶ Plyometric Exercise is a Technique for Developing Power

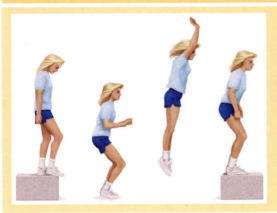

In this plyometric exercise called the "depth jump," the athlete jumps off a box and then quickly bounds upward to land on another box. The first phase of the exercise involves an eccentric contraction (shortening of muscle fibers to slow the body during the landing phase. This is followed immediately by a concentric (lengthening) of muscle fibers to leap onto the next box. The recoiling of the fibers increases the force that can be applied to the muscles. Several repeats of this type of exercise should be performed followed by brief rests. Because of the eccentric contractions, plyometric exercises can promote greater amounts of muscle soreness, so it is important to work up to this gradually.

Table 4 ▶ Safety Guidelines for Plyometrics

- Plyometrics for growing teens should begin moderately and progress slowly, compared with plyometrics for adults.
- Progression should be gradual to avoid extreme muscle soreness.
- Adequate strength should be developed prior to plyometric training. (As a general rule, you should be able to do a half-squat with one-and-a-half times your body weight.)
- Get a physician's approval prior to doing plyometrics if you have a history of injuries or if you are recovering from injury to the body part being trained.
- The landing surface should be semiresilient, dry, and unobstructed.
- Shoes should have good lateral stability, be cushioned with an arch support, and have a nonslip sole.
- Obstacles used for jumping-over should be padded.
- The training should be preceded by a general and specific warm-up.
- The training sequence should
  - Precede all other workouts (while you are fresh)
  - Include at least one spotter
  - Be done no more than twice per week, with 48 hours rest between bouts
  - Last no more than 30 minutes
  - (For beginners) include 3 or 4 drills, with 2 or 3 sets per drill, 10–15 reps per set and 1–2 minutes rest between sets

Source: G. Brittenham.

it is recommended that ballistic stretching be performed after initiating the workout with static or PNF stretching.

The ballistic stretching phase should use stretches that closely approximate the performance activity. Examples of ballistic stretching exercises for specific performances are presented in Table 5.

Training for High-Level Performance: Skill-Related Fitness and Skill

Good skill-related fitness is needed for success in many sports. As described in a previous concept, there are six primary components of skill-related fitness (agility, coordination, balance, reaction time, speed, and power). Possessing these attributes can make it easier to learn the skills that are important for many competitive sports. Balance and reaction time may be especially critical for hitting a baseball, considered by many to be the toughest skill in sports. Similarly, agility and coordination may help one master advanced dribbling skills for sports such as basketball or soccer. Because skill-related fitness can enhance performance in sports, it is often called **motor fitness** or **sports fitness.** Table 6 summarizes the general skill-related fitness requirements of forty-four different sport activities. In Lab 14A, you will evaluate your skill-related fitness and learn what activities you may be most suited for.

There are subcomponents of each component of skill-related physical fitness. Most of the six parts of skill-related physical fitness have subcomponents. For example, coordination includes foot-eye coordination

Plyometrics A training technique used to develop explosive power. Referred to as "speed-strength training" in Eastern Europe and the former Soviet Union, where it originated, it consists of concentric-isotonic contractions performed after a prestretch or an eccentric contraction of a muscle.

Motor Fitness A term commonly used for skill-related physical fitness.

Sports Fitness A term commonly used for skill-related fitness.

Table 5 ▶ Examples of Ballistic Stretch to Enhance Performance

Ballistic Stretch for Throwing and Striking

This exercise can improve flexibility to aid one-handed throwing and striking skills (for example, racket sports forehand, backhand, and serve; baseball throw, or discus and shot put) and/or two-handed throwing or striking skills (for example, batting a softball or executing a golf drive or hammer throw). Assume a position at the end of the backswing for any skill listed above. Partner grasps hand(s) and resists movement while the performer turns the trunk away from the partner, making a series of gentle bouncing movements, attempting to rotate the trunk as if performing the skill. Alternate roles with the partner. Note: Avoid overstretching by too vigorous bouncing. If no partner is available, use a door frame for resistance, or these sports actions can be practiced using elastic bands or inner tubes (attached to fixed objects) as resistance.

Ballistic Stretch for Golf Swing

This exercise is to improve flexibility for the golf swing. A similar exercise can be performed using one-handed throwing and striking skills (for example, racket sports forehand, backhand, and serve; baseball throw, or discus and shot put) and/or two-handed throwing or striking skills (for example, batting a softball or hammer throw). Stand and swing the club with or without a weight on the implement or on the wrist. Start by swinging backward and forward rhythmically and continuously. Gradually increase the speed and vigor of the swing to finally resemble the actual skill.

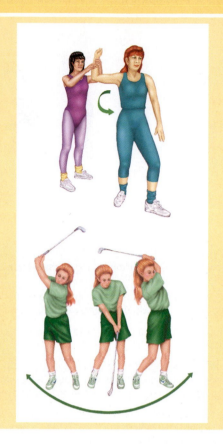

and hand-eye coordination, which are measured quite differently. Other abilities also contribute to performing skills. For example, many experts consider various perceptual abilities, such as depth and distance perception (ability to judge depth and distances accurately) and visual tracking (ability to visually follow a moving object), to be skill-related parts of physical fitness.

An individual might possess ability in one area and not in another. For this reason, general motor ability probably does not really exist, and individuals do not have one general capacity for performing. Rather, the ability to play games or sports is determined by combined abilities in each of the separate skill-related components. However, some performers will probably be above average in many areas.

Exceptional performers tend to be outstanding in more than one component of skill-related fitness. Though people possess skill-related fitness in varying degrees, great athletes are likely to be above average in most, if not all, aspects. Indeed, exceptional athletes must be exceptional in many areas of skill-related fitness.

Excellence in one skill-related fitness component may compensate for a lack in another. Each individual possesses a specific level of each skill-related fitness aspect. The performer should learn his or her other strengths and weaknesses in order to produce optimal performances. For example, a tennis player may use good coordination to compensate for lack of speed.

Excellence in skill-related fitness may compensate for a lack of health-related fitness when playing sports and games. As you grow older, health-related fitness potential declines more rapidly than many components of skill-related fitness. You may use superior skill-related fitness to compensate. For example, a baseball pitcher who lacks the power to dominate hitters may rely on a pitch such as a knuckle ball, which is more dependent on coordination than on power.

Practice can help skill-related fitness but is probably not as effective as practice to improve the specific skills of the activity you expect to perform. As noted in a previous section, power is the component of fitness especially likely to be changed with training. Drills for

Table 6 ▶ Skill-Related Requirements of Sports and Other Activities

Activity	Balance	Coordination	Reaction Time	Agility	Power	Speed
Archery	***	****	*	*	*	*
Backpacking	**	**	*	**	**	*
Badminton	**	****	***	***	**	***
Baseball/softball	***	****	****	***	****	***
Basketball	***	****	****	****	****	***
Bicycling	****	**	**	*	**	**
Bowling	***	****	*	**	**	**
Canoeing	***	***	**	*	***	*
Circuit training	**	**	*	**	***	**
Dance, aerobic	**	****	**	***	*	*
Dance, ballet	****	****	**	****	***	*
Dance, disco	**	***	**	****	*	**
Dance, modern	****	****	**	****	***	*
Dance, social	**	***	**	***	*	**
Fencing	***	****	****	***	***	****
Fitness calisthenics	**	**	*	***	**	*
Football	***	***	****	****	****	****
Golf (walking)	**	****	*	**	***	*
Gymnastics	****	****	***	****	****	**
Handball	**	****	***	****	***	***
Hiking	**	**	*	**	**	*
Horseback riding	***	***	**	***	*	*
Interval training	**	**	*	*	*	**
Jogging	**	**	*	*	*	*
Judo	***	****	****	****	****	****
Karate	***	****	****	****	****	****
Mountain climbing	****	****	**	***	***	*
Pool; billiards	**	***	*	**	**	*
Racquetball	**	****	***	****	**	***
Rope jumping	**	***	**	***	**	*
Rowing, crew	**	****	*	***	****	**
Sailing	***	***	***	***	**	*
Skating	****	***	**	***	**	***
Skiing, cross-country	**	****	*	***	****	**
Skiing, downhill	****	****	***	****	***	*
Soccer	**	****	***	****	***	***
Surfing	****	****	***	****	***	*
Swimming (laps)	**	***	*	***	**	*
Table tennis	**	***	***	**	**	**
Tennis	**	****	***	***	***	***
Volleyball	**	****	***	***	**	**
Walking	**	**	*	*	*	*
Waterskiing	***	***	*	***	**	*
Weight training	**	**	*	*	**	*

* = minimal needed; **** = a lot needed.

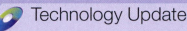

Technology Update

Illegal Drugs

An unfortunate application of technology in sports is the continued evolution and refinement of performance-enhancing drugs. Whereas safe and effective ergogenic aids (see page 261) have their place in sports, substances that give one athlete an unfair advantage are a major problem. The use of these illegal drugs puts many athletes at risk for health problems and damages the integrity of the sport. Reports of drug use in pro sports (particularly baseball in recent years) has led to discussions about whether to conduct random drug tests in professional sports. Because athletes typically use blocking agents and other supplements to mask illegal drug use, an issue of considerable importance is whether there is sufficient capability to detect illegal drugs. The technology of drug testing always seems to be a few steps behind the technology of drug use.

Steroids are certainly not the only drug that is abused by athletes. Among endurance athletes, the most commonly abused drug is erythropoietin, or EPO. The use of EPO is part of a practice called blood doping, which provides endurance athletes with additional red blood cells. This allows the blood to carry more oxygen. With a greater oxygen-carrying capacity, athletes can maintain aerobic activity at a higher intensity and perform better. The Tour de France was rocked a few years ago when athletes were found to be using illegal supplements. More than a few Olympic, NFL, and NBA athletes have failed drug tests but many others go undetected. The technology has improved but is less than perfect.

enhancing other aspects of skill-related physical fitness can help improve these abilities. For example, agility drills can improve scores on the specific agility drill that is practiced. Speed in running can be improved by increasing strength. However, experts generally agree that heredity highly influences skill-related fitness.

As illustrated in Figure 1, learning specific skills (not skill-related fitness) through regular practice is the preferred method of improving performance. To achieve high-level performance, regular and systematic practice is essential.

Guidelines for High-Performance Training

Overtraining is a common problem among athletes. Most Americans suffer from hypokinetic conditions resulting from too little activity. Athletes, on the other hand, often push themselves too hard in their pursuit of high-level performance and are susceptible to a variety of **hyperkinetic conditions.** Athletes who train too hard and do not allow adequate time for rest are susceptible to a hyperkinetic condition known as "overload syndrome." This condition is characterized by fatigue, irritability, and sleep problems, as well as an increased risk for injuries. Performance is known to decline sharply in an overtrained status, and this can cause athletes to train even harder and become even more overtrained. Athletes should pay close attention to possible symptoms of overtraining and back off their training if they notice increased fatigue, lethargy, or unexpected decreases in their performance. Lab 14B will allow you to identify some of the symptoms of overtraining.

A useful physical indicator of overtraining is a slightly elevated morning heart rate (four or five beats more than normal values). Essentially, an elevated morning heart rate reveals that the body has had to work too hard to recover from the exercise and wasn't in its normal resting mode. To use this indicator, you should regularly monitor your resting heart rate prior to getting out of bed in the morning. Another indicator that is increasingly used by elite endurance athletes is compressed or reduced "heart rate variability." A lower beat to beat variability indicates fatigue or overtraining, since it reflects sympathetic dominance over the normally dominant parasympathetic system that exists during more rested states. Newer heart rate monitors provide an indicator of heart rate variability.

A history of regular exercise and periodic rest are important to reduce the risk for overuse injuries.
The most common overuse injuries are joint injuries to the foot, ankle, and knee; stress fractures in the lower extremities; and muscle/connective tissue injuries, such as shin splints, strained hamstring muscles, and calf pain. These injuries are apparent among exercisers who train too hard or fail to get sufficient rest. Runners who train 7 days a week have more muscle and joint injuries than runners who take off at least 1 day a week or reduce training levels several days a week. Many aerobic dance instructors suffer from overuse injuries because they teach multiple sessions of aerobics every day for an extended period of time. Periodic rest is essential to allow the body to recover from the stress of continuous and vigorous training.

Considerable research on overuse injuries is conducted by the U.S. military to better prepare soldiers for battle. In one recent study, approximately 8.5 percent of new recruits suffered stress fractures during the grueling 8-week basic training regimen that they undergo upon enlistment. A variety of factors were found to influence risk. The study reported that a history of regular exercise was protective against stress fracture, and a longer history of exercise further decreased the relative risk for fracture. This suggests that regular progressive exercise can build up the strength and integrity of bones and joints and possibly reduce the risk for injury. In other words, experienced athletes can perform higher levels of training without injury because they have built up a greater tolerance.

 Periodization of training may help prevent overtraining. www.mhhe.com/phys_fit/web14 Click 07. When a person trains for a single performance or perhaps several competitive events such as games or matches during a sport season, it requires careful planning to reach peak performance at the right time and to avoid overtraining and injuries. Periodization is a modern concept of manipulating repetition, resistance, and exercise selection so there are periodic peaks and valleys during the training program. The peaks are needed to challenge the body, and the valleys are needed to allow the body to recover and adapt fully. Over the course of the season, there should be a gradual progression that allows the person to peak at just the right time. To accomplish this, training begins with an emphasis on base training in which the volume of training is gradually increased (increasing reps or performing large numbers of sets). As the season progresses, the focus shifts to an emphasis on the intensity of training (going faster or lifting heavier weights). Because higher-intensity exercise requires more time for recovery, the volume of training should be reduced at these times. A key concept in periodization is to provide opportunities for the body to fully adapt and recover prior to competition. Thus, the phase immediately prior to competition **(tapering)** is characterized by a reduced volume and intensity of training. By applying periodization to their training, athletes are able to optimize performance and minimize the risks of overtraining (see Figure 3).

Athletes should be aware of various psychological disorders related to overtraining.
Compulsive physical activity, often referred to as activity neurosis or exercise addiction, can be considered a hyperkinetic condition. People with activity neurosis become irrationally concerned about their exercise regimen. They may exercise more than

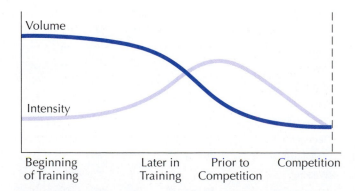

Figure 3 ▶ Volume and intensity of training during periodization.

once a day, rarely take a day off, or feel the need to exercise even when ill or injured. One condition related to body neurosis is an obsessive concern for having an attractive body. Among females, it is usually associated with an extreme desire to be thin, whereas among males it is more often associated with an extreme desire to be muscular. The excessive desire to be fit or thin can negatively affect other aspects of life, threaten personal relationships, and contribute high amounts of stress. Anorexia nervosa, an eating disorder associated with an excessive drive to be thin, has frequently been associated with compulsive exercise. Recent data suggest that at least 25 percent of people with anorexia nervosa do compulsive exercise (see Concept 15 for more information).

Ergogenic Aids

Many athletes look to ergogenic aids as an additional way to improve performance. Athletes are always looking for a competitive edge. In addition to pursuing rigorous training programs, many athletes look for alternative ways to improve their performance. Substances, strategies, and treatments that are designed to improve physical performance beyond the effects of normal training are collectively referred to as **ergogenic aids.** People interested in improving their appearance (including those with body neurosis) also abuse products they think will enhance their appearance. Ergogenic aids can be classified as mechanical, psychological, and physiological. Each category will be discussed in the subsequent sections.

Mechanical ergogenics (technology or equipment) may improve efficiency and performance. www.mhhe.com/phys_fit/web14 Click 08. Most competitive activities require equipment or special clothing. In many cases, technological innovations can greatly improve performance. In the 2002 winter Olympics in Salt Lake City, speed skaters used a new type of skate called klap skates (named for the sound it makes) to set a number of new speed records in their sport. The skates have a spring-loaded front hinge that allows the skater to raise the heel off the blade while skating to generate more force than with conventional skates. Swimmers now wear "skinsuits," which have less resistance than normal skin when gliding through the water. Wearing these suits provided a considerable advantage in many swimming events and essentially replaces the traditional practice of "shaving" to reduce resistance in the water. There are countless other examples of how improvements in technology have changed many sporting activities. Oversized tennis racquets revolutionized tennis, and refinements in golf club technology and balls have also helped golfers increase distance and improve accuracy. In general, mechanical ergogenics such as these will be of use only for individuals who already possess high levels of fitness or skill. For example, Andre Agassi could still beat most people with an old tennis racquet and Tiger Woods would still be a great golfer with old golf clubs. Still, it is useful to stay abreast of changing technology in sport equipment and clothing that can make activity more enjoyable. An example is running and cycling clothing featuring microfiber or Cool Max technology that helps keep you cool and dry in hot conditions.

Psychological ergogenics improve concentration and focus during competitive activities. Many competitive activities require extreme levels of concentration and focus. Athletes who are able to maintain this mental edge during an event are at a clear advantage over athletes who cannot. Psychological ergogenics are strategies such as mental imagery and hypnosis, which have been shown to help athletes achieve peak performance. Athletes are encouraged to use these psychological aids but to be wary of untested or unproven techniques, since quackery is prominent in this area.

Physiological ergogenics are designed to improve performance by enhancing biochemical and physiological processes in the body. www.mhhe.com/phys_fit/web14 Click 09. Physiological ergogenics primarily are nutritional supplements that are thought to have a positive effect on various metabolic processes. An example is fluid-replacement drinks that athletes consume during endurance exercise. Consumption of these drinks has been shown to maintain blood sugar levels and delay fatigue in exercise lasting over 1 hour. Whereas the ergogenic benefit of fluid-replacement beverages is clearly established, the safety and effectiveness of most other supplements are questionable. Because the supplement industry is largely unregulated, many products are developed and marketed with little or no research to document their effects. These products prey on an athlete's lack of knowledge and concern over performance. Products with little or no evidence of benefits also have questionable safety, so consumers should be cautious. Table 7 summarizes the potential effectiveness and safety issues of many commercially available supplements.

Hyperkinetic Conditions Condition caused by too much physical activity and/or insufficient rest.

Tapering A reduction in training volume and intensity that is used prior to competition to elicit peak performance.

Ergogenic Aids Substances, strategies, and treatments that are intended to improve performance in sports or competitive athletics.

Table 7 ▶ Effectiveness and Safety of Various Physiological Ergogenic Aids

ERGOGENIC AIDS WITH STRONG EVIDENCE FOR A PERFORMANCE BENEFIT		
Name of Supplement	**Proposed Effect (Claims)**	**Safe?**
Alkaline salts (e.g., sodium bicarbonate, sodium citrate)	Buffer metabolic acidosis produced from lactic acid buildup	Yes
Caffeine	Increases rate of fat metabolism and sparing glycogen depletion	Yes, in moderation, can dehydrate
Carbohydrates (e.g., glucose, fructose)	Maintain blood glucose levels and delay glycogen depletion	Yes
Creatine	Muscular strength	Some side effects; long-term safety unknown
Water	Minimizes dehydration during endurance exercise in the heat	Yes

ERGOGENIC AIDS WITH SOME EVIDENCE FOR A PERFORMANCE BENEFIT		
Name of Supplement	**Proposed Effect (Claims)**	**Safe?**
Aspartate salts (e.g., potassium, magnesium aspartate)	Mitigate the accumulation of ammonia during exercise	Probably safe
Carbohydrate metabolites (e.g., DHAP, pyruvate)	Maintain blood glucose levels and delay glycogen depletion	Probably safe
Glycerol	Promotes hyperhydration and improves thermoregulation during exercise in the heat	Probably safe
Hydroxy beta-methylbutyrate (HMB)	Thought to improve cellular repair of muscle and improve strength adaptations	Probably safe
Phosphates	Phosphates are a component of 2,3-DPG, which is essential for the release of oxygen from hemoglobin	Not clear

ERGOGENIC AIDS WITH LITTLE OR NO EVIDENCE FOR A PERFORMANCE BENEFIT		
Name of Supplement	**Proposed Effect (Claims)**	**Safe?**
Amino acids (general)	Alleged increase in muscle mass, prevents protein catabolism	Probably safe, unless consumed in extremely high doses
Amino acids (e.g., arginine, ornithine)	Alleged increase in strength by increasing levels of human growth hormone and insulin	Probably safe; however, extreme protein consumption is harmful
Androstenedione + dehydroepiandrosterone	Alleged hormone precursor to testosterone	Not safe
L-carnitine	Allegedly facilitates the transport of fatty acids, and oxidation of amino acids and pyruvate, which delays glycogen depletion	Not established
Choline	Allegedly maintains acetylcholine levels during exercise; acetylcholine is thought to be related to onset of fatigue	Not established
Coenzyme Q10 (Ubiquinone)	Allegedly improves oxygen uptake in the mitochondria to increase energy production	Not established
Inosine	A nucleic acid in DNA purported to increase energy production	Not established
Lipid metabolites (medium chain triglycerides)	Allegedly increases fat metabolism by increasing the availability of dietary fats in the circulation	Yes, if consumed as a part of diet
Protein metabolites (branched chain amino acids)	Alter the formation of serotonin, a neurotransmitter alleged to influence central nervous system fatigue	Yes, if consumed as a part of diet

Source: Williams, M. H.

Strategies for Action

Select activities that match your abilities. People differ in many factors, including skills and abilities that influence sports and athletic performance. You may be well suited to some sports but not to others. Behavioral scientists have also determined that perceptions of competence are important predictors of long-term exercise adherence. To give yourself the best chance of being successful in sports (and exercise involvement), it is important to choose activities that are well matched to your abilities. Lab 14A provides an assessment that will allow you to evaluate your levels of skill-related physical fitness. By referring to Table 6, you can determine the sports and activities that best match your individual abilities.

It should be noted that the assessments provided in Lab 14A are but a few of the many tests that can be done for each of the skill-related fitness parts. You may want to try other tests if you want more information about your abilities. If you have a personal desire to train for a specific sport or activity, but do not have a fitness profile that predicts success, you should not be deterred. Lab 14A will help you find an activity that you will enjoy and in which you have a good chance of success. People with good motivation, who persist in training, can often excel over others with greater ability.

Take time to plan and record your training sessions. Success in sports and competitive athletics requires careful planning and a lot of effort. To maximize your potential, it is important to take time to plan your training program. Coaches handle these tasks for many competitive athletes, but recreational athletes typically have to plan their own program. While you can contract with personal trainers to help with this task, adequate planning can be done by applying the principles described in this book. The key is to write out a workout plan and keep careful records of your progress. This will allow you to monitor how your training program is progressing.

Get adequate rest and listen to your body. Because high-performance training can be quite intense, it is important to get adequate rest. Many athletes make the mistake of training too hard. An essential part of a good training program is rest. Without rest, the body does not have sufficient time to make the needed adaptations and overtraining syndrome can result. Lab 14B provides an assessment of overtraining to help you learn how to monitor for signs of overtraining.

Study Resources

Check out additional online study resources for this concept in the Student Edition of the Online Learning Center at www.mhhe.com/corbin13e.

Web Resources

Gatorade Sports Science Institute **www.gssiweb.com**
National Athletic Trainers Association **www.nata.org**
National Collegiate Athletic Association **www.ncaa.org**
National Strength and Conditioning Association
    www.nsca-cc.org
Special Olympics International **www.specialolympics.org**
United States Olympic Committee **www.usoc.org**
Women's Sports Foundation
    www.womenssportsfoundation.org

Suggested Readings

Additional reference materials for Concept 14 are available at **www.mhhe.com/phys_fit/web14 Click 10.**

ACSM. 1997. Position stand on the female athlete triad. *Medicine and Science in Sports and Exercise* 29(5):i.

Albert, C. M., et al. 2000. Triggering of sudden death from cardiac causes by vigorous exertion. *New England Journal of Medicine* 243(19):1355–1361.

Bracko, M. R. 2002. Can stretching prior to exercise and sports improve performance and prevent injury? *ACSM's Health and Fitness Journal* 6(5):17–22.

Burke, E. 2003. *High-Tech Cycling.* 2nd ed. Champaign, IL: Human Kinetics.

Cobb, K. L. 2003. Disordered eating, menstrual irregularity and bone density in female runners. *Medicine and Science in Sports and Exercise* 35(5):711–719.

Delavier, F. 2001. *Strength Training Anatomy.* Champaign, IL: Human Kinetics.

Dufek, J. S. 2002. Exercise variability: A prescription for overuse injury prevention. *ACSM's Health and Fitness Journal* 6(4):18–23.

Hootman, J. M., et al. 2001. Association among physical activity level, cardiorespiratory fitness, and risk of musculoskeletal injury. *American Journal of Epidemiology* 154(3):251–258.

Jones, A. M. 2002 Running economy is negatively related to sit and reach test performance in international-standard distance runners. *International Journal of Sports Medicine* 23(1):40–43.

Kraemer, W. J., and N. A. Ratamess. 2004. Fundamentals of resistance training: Progression and exercise prescription. *Medicine and Science in Sports Exercise* 36(4):674–688.

Kraus, D. 2000. *Mastering Your Inner Game.* Champaign, IL: Human Kinetics.

Landry, G., and D. Bernhardt. 2003. *Essentials of Primary Care Sports Medicine.* Champaign, IL: Human Kinetics.

Manore, M., and J. Thompson. 2000. *Sport Nutrition for Health and Performance.* Champaign, IL: Human Kinetics.

Radcliffe, J. and R. Farebtinos. 2001. *High-Powered Plyometrics.* Champaign, IL: Human Kinetics.

Uusitalo, A. L. 2001. Overtraining. *The Physician and Sportsmedicine* 29(5):35–50.

Volek, J. S. 2004. Influence of nutrition on responses to resistance training. *Medicine and Science in Sports and Exercise* 36(4):689–696.

Weinberg, R., and D. Gould. 2003. *Foundations of Sport and Exercise Psychology.* 3rd ed. Champaign, IL: Human Kinetics.

Wescott, W. 2003. *Building Strength and Stamina.* 2nd ed. Champaign, IL: Human Kinetics.

Wilmore, J. H., and D. Costill. 2004. *Physiology of Sport and Exercise.* 3rd ed. Champaign, IL: Human Kinetics.

Wilmore, J. H. 2003. Aerobic exercise and endurance. *The Physician and Sportsmedicine* 31(5):45–53.

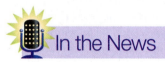 In the News

The 2004 Olympics

As this book went into final production, the 2004 Olympics were just being complete. Over 11,000 athletes from 202 countries participated in 301 different events. An estimated 4 billion people watched the Olympics making it perhaps the most visable worldwide event ever.

A particularly intriguing aspect of this year's Olympics was that it was held in Athens, Greece—site of the first modern Olympic Games back in 1896. This inaugural event 108 years earlier included a much smaller contingent of athletes (245 athletes from 13 countries) but many of the 43 original events are still being contested today. The Olympic spirit has always challenged athletes to try to go farther, high or faster and that same spirit drives modern Olympic athletes as well. Records keep dropping as athletes learn better ways to train or better ways to perform. The chart below compares performances in some of the events that were held in 1896 and 2004. An interesting observation from this comparison is that the improvements were fairly consistent (17–42%)

across different types and distances of events. Advances in training, technology and competition will continue to help athletes push for even faster records. The limits of human performance have always been intriguing. Will long jump records ever reach 10m or will someone ever run a sub 2 hour marathon? Only time will tell. Stay tuned.

Comparison of Olympic Performances (1896–2004)				
Sport	**Event**	**1896**	**2004**	**% imp**
Swimming	100m (s)	82	48	41.5%
Track	100m (s)	12	9.85	17.9%
	400m (s)	54.2	44	18.8%
	800m (m:s)	2:11	1:45	19.8%
	1500 (m:s)	4:33	3:34	21.65
	Marathon (h:s)	2:59	2:10	26.8%
Field	High Jump (m)	1.81	2.36	30.4%
	Long Jump (m)	6.35	8.59	35.3%

Lab Resource Materials: Skill-Related Physical Fitness

Important Note: Because skill-related physical fitness does not relate to good health, the rating charts used in this section differ from those used for health-related fitness. The rating charts that follow can be used to compare your scores to those of other people. You *do not* need exceptional scores on skill-related fitness to be able to enjoy sports and other types of physical activity; however, it is necessary for high-level performance. After the age of thirty, you should adjust ratings by 1 percent per year.

Evaluating Skill-Related Physical Fitness

I. Evaluating agility: The Illinois agility run

An agility course using four chairs 10 feet apart and a 30-foot running area will be set up as depicted in this illustration. The test is performed as follows:

1. Lie prone with your hands by your shoulders and your head at the starting line. On the signal to begin, get on your feet and run the course as fast as possible.
2. Your score is the time required to complete the course.

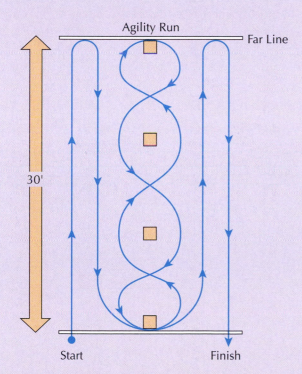

Agility Run

Far Line

30'

Start   Finish

II. Evaluating balance: The Bass test of dynamic balance

Eleven circles (9 1/2 inch) are drawn on the floor as shown in the illustration. The test is performed as follows:

1. Stand on the right foot in circle X. *Leap* forward to circle 1, then circle 2 through 10, alternating feet with each leap.
2. The feet must leave the floor on each leap and the heel may not touch. Only the ball of the foot and toes may land on the floor.
3. Remain in each circle for 5 seconds before leaping to the next circle. (A count of 5 will be made for you aloud.)
4. Practice trials are allowed.
5. The score is 50, plus the number of seconds taken to complete the test, minus the number of errors.
6. For every error, deduct 3 points each. Errors include touching the heel, moving the supporting foot, touching outside a circle, and touching any body part to the floor other than the supporting foot.

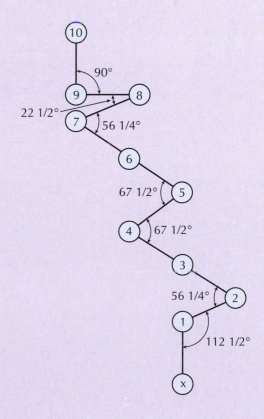

Chart 1 ▶ Agility Rating Scale

Classification	Men	Women
Excellent	15.8 or faster	17.4 or faster
Very good	16.7–15.9	18.6–17.5
Good	18.6–16.8	22.3–18.7
Fair	18.8–18.7	23.4–22.4
Poor	18.9 or slower	23.5 or slower

Source: Adams et al.

Chart 2 ▶ Balance Test Rating Scale

Rating	Score
Excellent	90–100
Very good	80–89
Good	60–79
Fair	30–59
Poor	0–29

Chart 3 ▶ Coordination Rating Scale

Classification	Men	Women
Excellent	14–15	13–15
Very good	11–13	10–12
Good	5–10	4–9
Fair	3–4	2–3
Poor	0–2	0–1

III. Evaluating coordination: The stick test of coordination

The stick test of coordination requires you to juggle three wooden sticks. The sticks are used to perform a one-half flip and a full flip, as shown in the illustrations.

1. *One-half flip*—Hold two 24-inch (1/2 inch in diameter) dowel rods, one in each hand. Support a third rod of the same size across the other two. Toss the supported rod in the air so that it makes a half turn. Catch the thrown rod with the two held rods.
2. *Full flip*—Perform the preceding task, letting the supported rod turn a full flip.

The test is performed as follows:
1. Practice the half-flip and full flip several times before taking the test.
2. When you are ready, attempt a half-flip five times. Score 1 point for each successful attempt.
3. When you are ready, attempt the full flip five times. Score 2 points for each successful attempt.

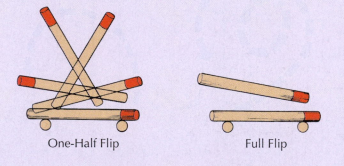

One-Half Flip   Full Flip

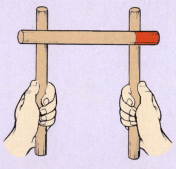

Hand Position

IV. Evaluating power: The vertical jump test

The test is performed as follows:

1. Hold a piece of chalk so its end is even with your fingertips.
2. Stand with both feet on the floor and your side to the wall and reach and mark as high as possible.
3. Jump upward with both feet as high as possible. Swing arms upward and make a chalk mark on a 5′ × 1′ wall chart marked off in half-inch horizontal lines placed 6 feet from the floor.
4. Measure the distance between the reaching height and the jumping height.
5. Your score is the best of three jumps.

Chart 4 ▶ Power Rating Scale

Classification	Men	Women
Excellent	25 1/2″ or more	23 1/2″ or more
Very good	21″–25″	19″–23″
Good	16 1/2″–20 1/2″	14 1/2″–18 1/2″
Fair	12 1/2″–16″	10 1/2″–14″
Poor	12″ or less	10″ or less

Metric conversions for this chart appear in Appendix B.

V. Evaluating reaction time: The stick drop test

To perform the stick drop test of reaction time, you will need a yardstick, a table, a chair, and a partner to help with the test. To perform the test, follow this procedure:

1. Sit in the chair next to the table so that your elbow and lower arm rest on the table comfortably. The heel of your hand should rest on the table so that only your fingers and thumb extend beyond the edge of the table.
2. Your partner holds a yardstick at the top, allowing it to dangle between your thumb and fingers.
3. The yardstick should be held so that the 24-inch-mark is even with your thumb and index finger. No part of your hand should touch the yardstick.
4. Without warning, your partner will drop the stick, and you will catch it with your thumb and index finger.
5. Your score is the number of inches read on the yardstick just above the thumb and index finger after you catch the yardstick.
6. Try the test three times. Your partner should be careful not to drop the stick at predictable time intervals so that you cannot guess when it will be dropped. It is important that you react only to the dropping of the stick.
7. Use the middle of your three scores (for example: if your scores are 21, 18, and 19, your middle score is 19). The higher your score, the faster your reaction time.

Chart 5 ▶ Reaction Time Rating Scale

Classification	Score
Excellent	More than 21″
Very good	19″–21″
Good	16″–18 3/4″
Fair	13″–15 3/4″
Poor	Below 13″

Metric conversions for this chart appear in Appendix B.

VI. Evaluating speed: 3-sec run

To perform the running test of speed, it will be necessary to have a specially marked running course, a stopwatch, a whistle, and a partner to help you with the test. To perform the test, follow this procedure:

1. Mark a running course on a hard surface so that there is a starting line and a series of nine additional lines, each 2 yards apart, the first marked at a distance 10 yards from the starting line.

2. From a distance 1 or 2 yards behind the starting line, begin to run as fast as you can. As you cross the starting line, your partner starts a stopwatch.

3. Run as fast as you can until you hear the whistle that your partner will blow exactly 3 seconds after the stopwatch is started. Your partner marks your location at the time when the whistle was blown.

4. Your score is the distance you were able to cover in 3 seconds. You may practice the test and take more than one trial if time allows. Use the better of your distances on the last two trials as your score.

Chart 6 ▶ Speed Rating Scale

Classification	Men	Women
Excellent	24–26 yards	22–26 yards
Very good	22–23 yards	20–21 yards
Good	18–21 yards	16–19 yards
Fair	16–17 yards	14–15 yards
Poor	Less than 16 yards	Less than 14 yards

Metric conversions for this chart appear in Appendix B.

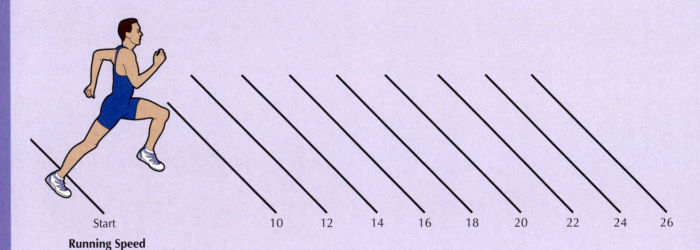

Start 10 12 14 16 18 20 22 24 26

Running Speed

Lab 14A Evaluating Skill-Related Physical Fitness

Name	Section	Date

Purpose: To help you evaluate your own skill-related fitness, including agility, balance, coordination, power, speed, and reaction time. This information may be of value in helping you decide which sports match your skill-related fitness abilities.

Procedures

1. Read the direction for each of the skill-related fitness tests presented in *Lab Resource Materials*.
2. Take as many of the tests as possible, given the time and equipment available.
3. Be sure to warm up before and to cool down after the tests.
4. It is all right to practice the tests before trying them. However, you should decide ahead of time which trial you will use to test your skill-related fitness.
5. After completing the tests, write your scores in the appropriate places in the Results section.
6. Determine your rating for each of the tests from the rating charts in *Lab Resource Materials*.

Results

Place a check in the circle for each of the tests you completed.

Agility (Illinois run)   ◯

Balance (Bass test)   ◯

Coordination (stick test)   ◯

Power (vertical jump)   ◯

Reaction time (stick drop test)   ◯

Speed (3-second run)   ◯

Record your score and rating in the following spaces.

	Score		Rating	
Agility				(Chart 1)
Balance				(Chart 2)
Coordination				(Chart 3)
Power				(Chart 4)
Reaction time				(Chart 5)
Speed				(Chart 6)

Conclusions and Implications: In two or three paragraphs, discuss the results of your skill-related fitness tests. Comment on the areas in which you did well or did not do well, the meaning of these findings, and the implications of the results with specific reference to the activities you will perform in the future.

Lab 14B Identifying Symptoms of Overtraining

| Name | Section | Date |

Purpose: To help you identify symptoms associated with overtraining

Procedures

1. Answer the questions concerning overtraining syndrome in the Results section. If you are in training, rate yourself; if not, evaluate a person you know who is in training. As an alternative, you may evaluate a person you know who was formerly in training (and who experienced symptoms) or evaluate yourself when you were in training (if you trained for performance in the past).
2. Use Chart 1 (below) to rate the person (yourself or another person) who is (or was) in training.
3. Use Chart 2 (page 272) to identify some steps that you might take to treat or prevent overtraining syndrome.
4. Answer the questions in the Conclusions and Implications section.

Results

Answer "Yes" (place a check in the circle) to any of the questions relating to overtraining symptoms you (or the person you are evaluating) experienced.

  ○ 1. Has performance decreased dramatically in the last week or two?

  ○ 2. Is there evidence of depression?

  ○ 3. Is there evidence of atypical anger?

  ○ 4. Is there evidence of atypical anxiety?

  ○ 5. Is there evidence of general fatigue that is not typical?

  ○ 6. Is there general lack of vigor or loss of energy?

  ○ 7. Have sleeping patterns changed (inability to sleep well)?

  ○ 8. Is there evidence of heaviness of the arms and/or legs?

  ○ 9. Is there evidence of loss of appetite?

  ○ 10. Is there a lack of interest in training?

Chart 1 ▶ Ratings for Overtraining Syndrome

Number of Yes Answers	Rating
9–10	Overtraining syndrome is very likely present. Seek help.
6–8	Person is at risk for overtraining syndrome if it is not already present. Seek help to prevent additional symptoms.
3–5	Some signs of overtraining syndrome are present. Consider methods of preventing further symptoms.
0–2	Overtraining syndrome is not present, but attention should be paid to the few symptoms that do exist.

Conclusions and Implications

Chart 2 lists some of the steps that may be taken to help eliminate or prevent overtraining syndrome. Check the steps that you think would be (or would have been) most useful to the person you evaluated.

Chart 2 ▶ Steps for Treating or Preventing Overtraining Syndrome
◯ 1. Consider a break from training.
◯ 2. Taper the program to help reduce symptoms.
◯ 3. Seek help to redesign the training program.
◯ 4. Alter your diet.
◯ 5. Evaluate other stressors that may be producing symptoms.
◯ 6. Reset performance goals.
◯ 7. Talk to someone about problems.
◯ 8. Have a medical checkup to be sure there is no medical problem.
◯ 9. If you have a coach, consider a talk with him or her.
◯ 10. Add fluids to help prevent performance problems from dehydration.

Discuss overtraining syndrome in general. Elaborate on one or two of the steps in Chart 2 that you think would be (or would have been) most effective in treating or preventing overtraining syndrome for the person you evaluated.

Body Composition

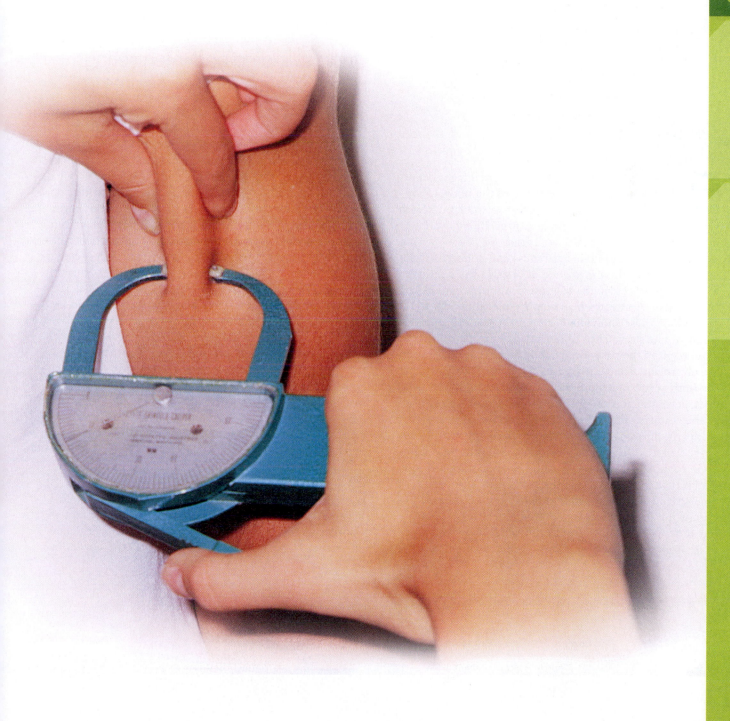

Possessing an optimal amount of body fat contributes to health and wellness.

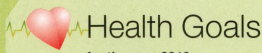

Health Goals
for the year 2010

- Increase proportion of adults who are at a healthy weight.

- Reduce proportion of adults who are obese.

- Reduce proportion of children and adolescents who are overweight or obese.

Body composition is the relative percentage of muscle, fat, bone, and other tissue of the body. Of primary concern, because of its association with various health problems, is body fatness. Being overfat or underfat can result in health concerns.

Despite general public awareness and concerns about weight control, the prevalence of obesity has continued to rise. Current estimates suggest that more than 60 percent of Americans are overweight, and about 20 to 25 percent of these individuals also meet the criterion for obesity. The prevalence of obesity has increased by over 50 percent in the past decade, indicating that this is a relatively recent trend. Increases in obesity were evident for both sexes and the trends were consistent across all ages, across socioeconomic classes, and across all regions of the country. The fact that similar trends are occurring in nearly all industrialized countries in the world suggests that the "epidemic of obesity" should be considered pandemic. The World Health Organization (WHO) recently concluded that "obesity's impact is so diverse and extreme that it should now be regarded as one of the greatest neglected public health problems of our time with an impact on health which may well prove to be as great as that of smoking." Since eating disorders, such as anorexia nervosa and bulimia, are also a significant health concern, especially among teens, the national goal is to keep the percentage of overfat teens from increasing while reducing the incidence of those who have too little fat associated with eating disorders.

Understanding and Interpreting Body Composition Measures

Standards have been established to determine how much body fat an individual should possess. www.com/phys_fit/web15 Click 01. Every person should possess at least a minimal amount of fat **(percent body fat)** for good health. This fat is called **essential fat** and is necessary for temperature regulation, shock absorption, and regulation of essential body nutrients, including vitamins A, D, E, and K. The exact amount of fat considered essential to normal body functioning has been debated, but most experts agree that males should possess no less than 5 percent and females no less than 10 percent. For females, an exceptionally low body fat percentage **(underfat)** is especially of concern. **Amenorrhea** may occur among women at fat levels as high as 16%. Some people feel that amenorrhea, when associated with low body fat levels, is a reversible condition that is merely the body's method of preventing pregnancy. However, low body fat levels, accompanied by amenorrhea, places a woman at risk for bone loss (osteoporosis). A body fat level below 10 percent is one of the criteria often used by clinicians for diagnosing eating disorders, such as anorexia nervosa.

In Table 1, standards for body fatness (percent body fat) are presented. Those classified as too low in body fat are below the essential body fat levels listed in Table 1. Because individuals differ in their response to low fatness, a borderline range is provided. No particular health benefits appear to be associated with being in the borderline

	Too Low	Borderline	Good Fitness (Healthy)	Marginal	Overfat
	Below Essential Fat Levels	Unhealthy for Many People	Optimal for Good Health	Associated with Some Health Problems	Unhealthy
Males	no less than 5%	6–9%	10–20%	21–25%	>25
Females	no less than 10%	11–16%	17–28%	29–35%	>35

Table 1 ▶ Standards for Body Fatness (Percent Body Fat)

range, and for some people there are health risks. Even though low body fat levels (borderline range) are not generally recommended, some individuals are interested in high-level performance and seek low body fatness in an attempt to enhance performance. Standards for high-level performers are typically lower than for normally active people primarily interested in good health. Performance levels considered to be in the borderline area for nonperformers can be acceptable if the performer eats well, avoids overtraining, and practices a healthy lifestyle. If symptoms such as amenorrhea, bone loss, and frequent injury occur, then levels of body fatness should be reconsidered, as should training techniques and eating patterns. For many people in training, maintaining performance levels of body fatness is temporary; thus, the risk of long-term health problems is diminished.

Nonessential fat is fat above essential fat levels that accumulates when you take in more calories than you expend. When nonessential fat accumulates in excessive amounts, **overfatness** or even **obesity** can occur. Just as the percent body fat should not drop too low, it should not get too high, either. A desirable range of fatness is associated with good metabolic fitness, good health, and wellness. It is referred to as the good fitness or healthy fatness range. People with more than healthy fat levels but who are not considered obese have scores in the marginal zone. Although reaching the healthy fitness zone is desirable, it is harder to reach for some people. Most experts agree that fat levels in the marginal zone are healthier than those in the overfat zone. Those who are overfat are at risk for the health problems described in this concept.

Body composition is considered a component of health-related fitness but can also be considered a component of metabolic fitness. Body composition is generally considered to be a health-related component of physical fitness. Most national fitness tests include either a skinfold test or the **body mass index (BMI)** as an indicator of this component. Like the other parts of health-related physical fitness, body composition is related to good health. However, body composition is unlike the other parts of health-related physical fitness in that it is not a performance measure. Cardiovascular fitness, strength, muscular endurance, and flexibility can be assessed using some type of movement or performance such as running, lifting, or stretching. Body composition requires no movement or performance. This is one reason some experts prefer to consider body composition as a component of metabolic fitness.

Metabolic fitness includes other nonperformance measures associated with increased risk for health problems, such as high blood fat, high blood pressure, and high blood sugar levels. Some experts have hypothesized that metabolic fitness is really one syndrome characterized by body composition (body fat) and the other highly related nonperformance measures described earlier. Whether you consider body composition to be a part of health-related or metabolic fitness, it is an important health-related factor.

Assessing body weight too frequently can result in making false assumptions about body composition changes. Taking body weight measurements too frequently can provide incorrect information and lead to false assumptions. For example, people vary in body weight from day to day and even hour to hour, based solely on their level of hydration. Short-term changes in weight are often due to water loss or gain, yet many people attribute the weight changes to their diet, a pill they have taken, or the exercise they are doing. In fact, short-term weight changes are more likely water changes than real body composition changes. We know this to be true because it takes a relatively long period of time for diet or exercise to affect weight changes. Monitoring your weight less frequently, once a week for example, is more useful than daily or multiple daily measures because it is more likely to represent real changes in body composition. Weighing at the same time of day, preferably early in the morning, is best because it reduces the chances that your weight variation will be a result of body water changes. Of course, it is best to use body composition assessments in addition to those based on body weight if accurate evaluations are expected.

Decisions about body composition should be based on more than one measurement. In Labs 15A and 15B, you will do several measurements of body composition. Using only one of the methods may result in

---

Percent Body Fat The percentage of total body weight that is composed of fat.

Essential Fat The minimum amount of fat in the body necessary to maintain healthful living.

Underfat Too little of the body weight composed of fat (see Table 1).

Amenorrhea Absence of, or infrequent, menstruation.

Nonessential Fat Extra fat or fat reserves stored in the body.

Overfatness Too much of the body weight comprised of fat (see Table 1).

Obesity Extreme overfatness.

Body Mass Index (BMI) A measure of body composition using a height-weight formula. High BMI values have been related to increased disease risk.

misinformation and unrealistic goals, which is why it is wise to use several techniques when making decisions about personal body composition goals. As you read about the various ways to assess body composition, consider the strengths and weaknesses of each technique and learn to use the techniques that provide the most information to you personally.

Being overfat is more important than overweight in making decisions about health and wellness. Many of the measures described in the following sections of this concept are indicators of the amount of body fat a person possesses. Others focus primarily on body weight. People who do regular physical activity and possess a large muscle mass can be high in body weight without being too fat. This is one of the limitations of measures based primarily on weight. Also, weight measures vary greatly based on your state of hydration or dehydration. You can lose weight merely by losing body water (becoming dehydrated) or gain weight by gaining body water (becoming hydrated). For this reason, measures that use weight as the primary indicator of body composition should be viewed with caution.

Methods Used to Assess Body Composition

Methods of body composition vary by accuracy and practicality. www.mhhe.com/phys_fit/web15 Click 02. Underwater weighing, also referred to as hydrostatic weighing, is a laboratory procedure for assessing body composition. In this procedure, a person is weighed underwater and out of the water. Corrections are made for the amount of air in the lungs when the underwater weight is measured. Using Archimedes' principle, the body's density can be determined. Because the density of various body tissues is known, the amount of the total body fat can be determined. Body fatness is usually expressed in

terms of a percentage of the total body weight. In the past, underwater weighing was considered the best method, but dual-energy X-ray absorptiometry (DXA) has now become the accepted "gold standard" for body composition measurements. This technique is available only in research laboratories or medical centers, but it may lead to changes in the accuracy with which other measures can estimate body fatness.

Other, more commonly used methods for measuring body fatness include skinfold measurements, bioelectric impedance, body circumferences, near-infrared interactance, and BMI. Table 2 provides a summary of the effectiveness of these methods. The procedures vary in terms of practicality and accuracy, so it is important to under-

Technology Update

DXA

Dual-energy X-ray absorptiometry (DXA) has emerged as the most accepted criterion measure of body composition. The technique utilizes the attenuation of two energy sources in order to estimate the density of the body. A specific advantage of DXA is that it can provide whole body measurements of body fatness as well as amounts stored in different parts of the body. For the procedure, the person lies on a table and the machine scans up along the body. Although some radiation exposure is necessary with the procedure, it is quite minimal, compared with X-ray and other diagnostic scans. Because the machine is quite expensive, this procedure is found only in medical centers and well-equipped research laboratories. Still, the use of this procedure as a gold standard can indirectly improve the accuracy of other measures, such as skinfold or bioelectric impedence, since these measures rely on comparisons with a criterion measure in order to provide estimates of body fatness.

Table 2 ▶ Ratings of the Validity and Objectivity of Body Composition Methods

Method	Precise	Objective	Accurate	Valid Equations	Overall Rating
Skinfold measurement	4.0	3.5	3.5	3.5	3.5
Bioelectric impedance	4.0	4.0	3.5	3.5	3.5
Circumferences	4.0	4.0	3.0	3.0	3.0
Body mass index (BMI)	5.0	5.0	1.5	1.5	2.0

Adapted from Lohman, T. G., L. H. Houtkooper, and S. B. Going.

Precise: Can the same person get the same results time after time?

Accurate: Do values compare favorably to underwater weighing?

5 = excellent; 4 = very good; 3 = good; 2 = fair; 1 = unacceptable.

Objective: Can two different people get the same results consistently?

Valid: Is the formula accurate for predicting fat from measurements?

stand the limitations of each method. It should be noted that even established techniques such as underwater weighing have potential for error.

A variety of other technologies have been developed to assess body composition. Different types of X rays and magnetic resonance machines (including DXA) have been used to assess body fatness in specific regions of the body for clinical research. Another relatively new device, called the Bod Pod, uses air displacement (rather than water displacement, as in underwater weighing) to assess body composition. Evidence suggests that it provides an acceptable alternative to underwater weighing and is particularly useful for special populations (the obese, older people, and the physically challenged).

 Skinfold measurements are a preferred, practical method of assessing body fatness. www.mhhe.com/phys_fit/web15 Click 03. Body fat is distributed throughout the body. About one-half of the body's fat is located around the various body organs and in the muscles. The other half of the body's fat is located just under the skin, or in skinfolds (Figure 1). A skinfold is two thicknesses of skin and the amount of fat that lies just under the skin. By measuring skinfold thicknesses of various sites around the body, it is possible to estimate total body fatness (Figure 2). Skinfold measurements are often used because they are relatively easy to do. They are not nearly as costly as underwater weighing and other methods that require expensive equipment. Research-quality skinfold calipers cost several hundred dollars, but consumer-models are available for less than ten dollars (see On the Web).

In general, the more skinfolds measured, the more accurate the fatness estimate. However, measurements with two or three skinfolds have been shown to be reasonably accurate and can be done in a relatively short period. Two skinfold techniques are used in Lab 15A. You are encouraged to try both. With adequate training, most people can learn to use calipers to get a good estimate of fatness. When performed by a trained person, skinfold techniques are rated favorably by experts (see Table 2), but it is a skill that takes practice. Measurements made by an untrained person can be inaccurate.

Body circumference measures can be used to assess body fatness. Body circumference, or girth, measurements can be used to estimate body fatness using various weight, height, waist, thigh, hip, and other girth measurements. They are not rated as favorably as skinfold measurements (see Table 2), but they are easy to do. One weakness of circumference measures is they may misclassify people who have a large muscle mass. For this reason, they are not as useful as skinfold measures for active people who have a relatively large muscle mass, compared with inactive people. As the sole measure of fatness, they should be used with caution. They can provide a useful second or third source of information about body fatness, however, and can be useful in monitoring change or improvement. Another technique that uses body circumferences—the waist-to-hip ratio—is described in *Lab Resource Materials*.

 Bioelectric impedance analysis has become a practical alternative for body fatness assessment. www.mhhe.com/phys_fit/web15 Click 04. Bioelectric impedance analysis ranks quite favorably for accuracy and has overall rankings similar to those of skinfold measurement techniques. The test can be performed quickly and is more effective for people high in body

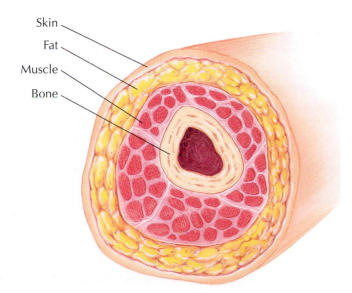

Figure 1 ▶ Location of body fat.

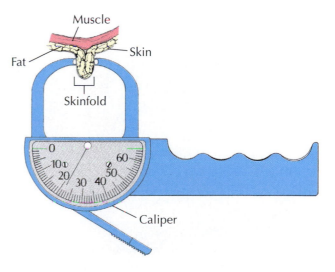

Figure 2 ▶ Measuring skinfold thickness with calipers.

fatness (a limitation of skinfolds). The technique is based on measuring resistance to current flow. Electrodes are placed on the body and low doses of current are passed through the skin. Because muscle has greater water content than fat, it is a better conductor and has less resistance to current. The overall amount of resistance and body size are used to predict body fatness. Dehydration can bias the result and it is critical to not have measures taken within 3 to 4 hours after a meal. Accurate measures require the use of high-quality equipment, but some commercially available "scales" provide estimates of body fatness that are based on the same principles. Instead of electrodes, you simply stand on metal plates that measure the current flow.

Infrared sensors are sometimes used to assess body fatness. Near-infrared interactance machines use the absorption of light to estimate body fatness. The technique was originally developed to measure the fat content of meats. Commercially available units for humans have not been shown to be effective for estimating body fat, and at least one company has faced sanctions from the government for selling an unapproved product. For this reason, this type of device is not included in Table 2.

BMI is considered to be a better measure than height and weight charts, but it has its limitations. www.mhhe.com/phys_fit/web15 Click 05. Individuals who are interested in controlling their weight often consult height and weight tables to determine their "desirable" weight. Being 20 percent or more above the recommended table weight is one commonly used indicator of obesity. New tables adopted by the federal government are based on relative risk for health problems rather than normative comparisons with other people. A limitation of height and weight tables is that they do not take into account a person's degree of body fatness. A person who has a large muscle mass as a result of regular physical activity can appear to be **overweight** using a height and weight table and still not be too fat. A more accurate way to use height and weight is with the body mass index. BMI is calculated using a formula and has a higher correlation with true body fatness than weights determined from height-weight tables. Nevertheless, the BMI may misclassify active people who have a large muscle mass. You can calculate your BMI using the procedures described in *Lab Resource Materials.* After much debate, there has been some consensus regarding standards of overweight and obesity based on BMI values. The accepted international standards used by the United States and the WHO is a BMI > 25 for overweight and a BMI > 30 for obesity.

Consensus regarding the definition of these body composition categories now makes it easier to examine trends within the United States or to compare body composition levels and research results across countries. For example, BMI is the measure that public health officials have used to determine that over half of the U.S. population is either overweight or obese and to document increases in the past 10 years. Nearly all other developed countries are observing similar trends in the prevalence of obesity.

Although the BMI is a useful indicator for large-scale research applications or to examine differences in groups, it is less valuable for making measurements for a specific individual at a particular point in time. Because the BMI is widely cited in news reports, it is important for all people to know how to calculate it and how to use it properly. Plotting changes in BMI over time can be useful in tracking personal changes. Together with other techniques, BMI can provide useful information, but the risk of misclassification is high among active people with a high amount of muscle if BMI is used by itself.

Health Risks Associated with Overfatness

Obesity has been elevated from a secondary to a primary risk factor for heart disease. Prior to 1998, obesity was considered to be a secondary risk factor for heart disease. The reason for this was that the effects of obesity were thought to be mediated by other risk factors, such as high blood pressure and blood lipids. Because of the mounting evidence of the relationship of obesity to health risk, especially risk for heart disease, the American Heart Association classifies obesity as a primary risk factor, along with high blood lipids, high blood pressure, tobacco use, and sedentary living.

Physical fitness provides protection from the health risks of obesity. www.mhhe.com/phys_fit/web15 Click 06. Recent research suggests that people who are above normal standards for BMI are not especially at

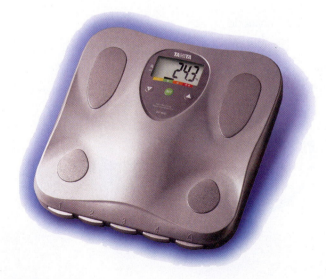

Bioelectric impedance scale.

risk if they participate in regular physical activity and possess relatively high levels of cardiovascular fitness (see Figure 3). In fact, active people who have a high BMI are at less risk than inactive people with normal BMI levels. Even high levels of body fatness may not be especially likely to increase disease risk if a person has good metabolic fitness as indicated by healthy blood fat levels, normal blood pressure, and normal blood sugar levels. It is when several of these factors are present at the same time that risk levels increase dramatically. For this reason, it is important to consider your cardiovascular and metabolic fitness levels before drawing conclusions about the effects of high body weight or high body fat levels on health and wellness. This information also points out the importance of periodically assessing your cardiovascular and metabolic fitness levels.

Overfatness and obesity can contribute to degenerative diseases, health problems, and even shortened life. Some diseases and health problems are associated with overfatness and obesity. In addition to the higher incidence of certain diseases and health problems, evidence shows that people who are moderately overfat have a 40 percent higher than normal risk of shortening their life span. More severe obesity results in a 70 percent higher than normal death rate. This is evidenced by the very high life insurance premiums paid by obese individuals.

Heart disease is not the only disease that is associated with obesity. Diabetes is another leading killer that is associated with all components of metabolic fitness, including obesity. The incidence of diagnosis of this disease has increased sixfold in the past 40 years. Recent studies also indicate a significant increase in risk for breast cancer among the obese. High blood pressure, asthma, and back pain are other conditions associated with obesity.

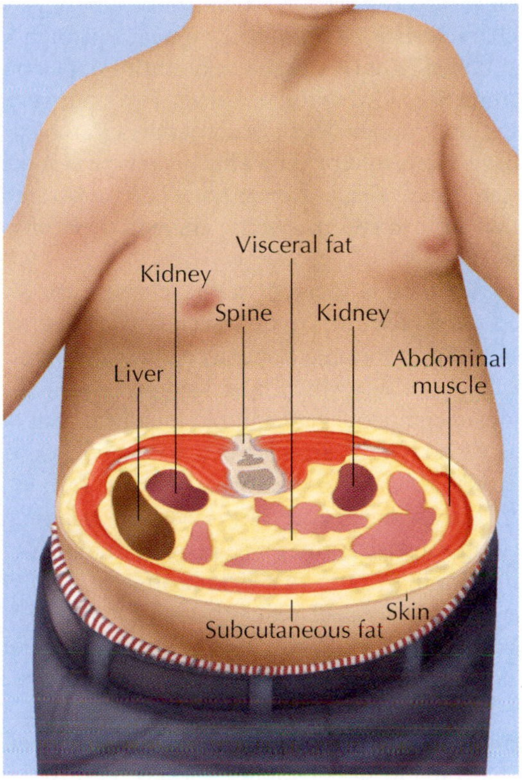

Figure 4 ▶ Visceral, or abdominal, fat is associated with increased disease risk.

Statistics indicate that underweight people also have a higher than normal risk for premature death. Though adequate evidence shows extreme leanness (e.g., anorexia nervosa) can be life threatening, many underweight people included in these studies have lost weight because of a medical condition such as cancer. It appears that the medical problems are often the reason for low body weight rather than low body weight being the source of the medical problem. Most experts agree that people who are free from disease and who have lower than average amounts of body fat have a lower than average risk for premature death.

Excessive abdominal fat and excessive fatness of the upper body can increase the risk of various diseases. The location of body fat can influence the health risks associated with obesity. A variety of terms are associated with the location of body fat. Fat in the upper part of the body is sometimes referred to as "Northern Hemisphere" fat and a body type high in this type of fat is sometimes called the "apple" shape (see Figure 4). Upper

Overweight Weight in excess of normal; not harmful unless it is accompanied by overfatness.

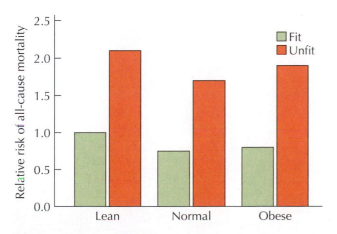

Figure 3 ▶ Risks of fatness vs. fitness.
Source: Lee, C. D., et al.

body fat is also referred to as android fat because is it is more characteristic of men than women. Postmenopausal women typically have a higher amount of upper body fat than premenopausal women. Lower body fat, such as in the hips and upper legs, is sometimes referred to as "Southern Hemisphere" fat. This body type is sometimes called the "pear" shape. Lower body fat is also referred to as gynoid fat because it is more characteristic of women than men.

Body fat that is located in the core of the body is referred to as central fat or visceral fat. Visceral fat is located in the abdominal cavity (see Figure 4), as opposed to subcutaneous fat, which is located just under the skin. Though subcutaneous fat (skinfold measures) can be used to estimate body fatness, it is not a good indicator of central fatness. A useful indicator of fat distribution is the waist-to-hip circumference ratio (see *Lab Resource Materials*). A high waist circumference relative to hip circumference yields a high ratio that is indicative of high visceral fat. Visceral fat is associated with high blood fat levels as well as other metabolic problems. It is also associated with high incidence of heart attack, stroke, chest pain, breast cancer, and early death. The ratio provides an indicator of both upper body fatness and visceral fatness. As you grow older, central and upper body fat levels tend to increase. Recent evidence indicates that people who exercise regularly accumulate less visceral fat and less upper body fat as they grow older. This suggests that regular physical activity throughout life will result in smaller waist-to-hip ratios and reduced risk for various chronic diseases.

Health Risks Associated with Excessively Low Body Fatness

Excessive desire to be thin or low in body weight can result in health problems. www. mhhe.com/phys_fit/web15 Click 07. In Western society, the near obsession with thinness has been, at least in part, responsible for eating disorders. Eating disorders, or altered eating habits, involve extreme restriction of food intake and/or regurgitation of food to avoid digestion. The most common disorders are anorexia nervosa, bulimia, and anorexia athletica. All of these disorders are most common among highly achievement-oriented girls and young women, although they affect virtually all segments of the population.

Anorexia nervosa is the most severe eating disorder. If untreated, it is life-threatening. Anorexics restrict food intake so severely that their bodies become emaciated. Among the many characteristics of anorexia nervosa are fear of maturity and inaccurate body image. The anorexic starves himself or herself and may exercise compulsively or use laxatives to prevent the digestion of food in an attempt to attain excessive leanness. The anorexic's self-image is one of being too fat, even when the person is too lean for good health. Assessing body fatness using procedures such as skinfolds and observation of the eating habits may help identify people with anorexia. Among anorexic girls and women, development of an adult figure is often feared. People with this disorder must obtain medical and psychological help immediately, as the consequences are severe. About 25 percent of those with anorexia do compulsive exercise in an attempt to stay lean.

Bulimia is a common eating disorder characterized by bingeing and purging. Disordered eating patterns become habitual for many people with bulimia. They alternate between bingeing and purging. Bingeing means the periodic eating of large amounts of food at one time. A binge might occur after a relatively long period of dieting and often consists of junk foods containing empty calories. After a binge, the bulimic purges the body of the food by forced regurgitation or the use of laxatives. Another form of bulimia is bingeing on one day and starving on the next. The consequences of bulimia are not as severe as anorexia, but they can result in serious mental, gastrointestinal, and dental problems. Bulimics may or may not be anorexic. It may not be possible to use measures of body fatness to identify bulimia, as the bulimic may be lean, normal, or excessively fat.

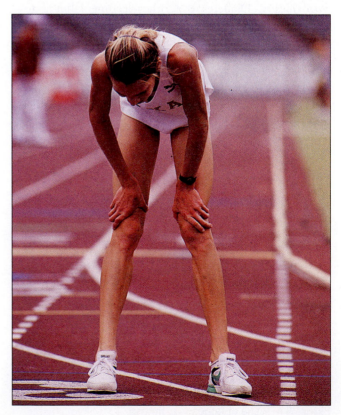

Excessively low levels of body fatness pose health problems.

Anorexia athletica is a recently identified eating disorder that appears to be related to participation in sports and activities that emphasize body leanness. Studies show that participants in sports such as gymnastics, wrestling, and bodybuilding and activities such as ballet and cheerleading are most likely to develop anorexia athletica. This disorder has many of the symptoms of anorexia nervosa, but not of the same severity. In some cases, anorexia athletica leads to anorexia nervosa.

Female athlete triad is an increasingly common condition among female athletes. www.mhhe.com/phys_fit/web15 Click 08. Female athlete triad is an increasingly common condition among female athletes. The three health concerns (the triad) that characterize the condition are eating disorders, amenorrhea, and osteoporosis. The disordered eating patterns may be extreme, as in anorexia or bulimia, or less severe, as evidenced by poor eating habits. Because they are athletes, females with this condition are very active. Together, the poor eating habits and high levels of activity typically result in low body fat levels. The triad of symptoms is often accompanied by considerable pressure to perform well, resulting in high stress levels. In addition to the triad of symptoms, the combination of poor eating, overexercise, and competitive stress can result in other problems, such as depression and anxiety, and even risk of suicide. Many female athletes train extensively and have relatively low body fat levels but experience none of the symptoms of the triad. Eating well, training properly, using stress-management techniques, and monitoring health symptoms are the keys to their success.

Fear of obesity is a less severe condition, but it can still have negative health consequences. *Fear of obesity* is a less severe condition, but it can still have negative health consequences. This condition is most common among achievement-oriented teenagers who impose a self-restriction on caloric intake because they fear obesity. Consequences include stunting of growth, delayed puberty, delayed sexual development, and decreased physical attractiveness. It is important to avoid excessive eating and inactivity to prevent the problems associated with overfatness and obesity; however, an excessive concern for leanness can also result in serious health problems.

Society can help reduce the incidence of the problems associated with disordered eating and desire to be thin by changing its image of attractiveness, especially among young women. Many of the models and movie stars who convey the "ideal" image are anorexic or are exceptionally thin. Teachers and athletic coaches can help by educating people about these disorders, by not placing too much emphasis on leanness, and by screening students for extreme leanness using procedures such as skinfolds and body mass index. Parents and friends can help by

looking for excessive changes in body weight and lack of eating. Once an eating disorder is identified, it is important to help the individual obtain treatment for the problem. Although regular physical activity is good, excessive activity can be harmful. It is important to help athletes learn not to overdo it and to keep competition in perspective, so that it does not become excessively stressful.

Conflicting news reports should not deter efforts to maintain a healthy body fat level. One recent headline said "Excess pounds deadly." One week later, the headline read "It may be better to be a little fat." Adding to the confusion is that BMI standards have been lowered in recent years, so that more people are now classified as overweight using this measurement technique. At the same time, some of the standards for body fatness are now more lenient than they were in the past. In both cases, the changes are made based on new scientific evidence.

Sometimes people read conflicting headlines and adopt a defeatist attitude. Do not let one headline influence your overall plan of fat control. The debate will continue in the years ahead as to just how much you should weigh or how much fat you should have for your good health and wellness. In the meantime, the message is clear. If possible, make several different assessments and consider all of the results before making decisions (see the charts in *Lab Resource Materials*). For some people, meeting the standards described in this book may be difficult. It is far better to be close to the standard than to say, "I can't meet the standard, so I won't even try." Some experts feel that many people are overfat because they have repeatedly failed to meet unrealistic body fatness or weight goals. Adopting a realistic personal standard of fatness is very important. Using many different self-assessments and adopting realistic goals based on personal information rather than comparisons with others can help you make informed decisions about your body composition (see Concept 6).

The Origin of Fatness

Heredity plays a role in fatness. Some people have suggested that every individual is born with a predetermined weight (sometimes called your set-point). This implies that you have little control over your weight or body fat levels. In fact, you do have considerable control over your weight and level of fatness, as evidenced by the fact that **calories** taken in (diet) and calories expended (activity) are the two most important factors

Calories Unit of energy supplied by food; the quantity of heat necessary to raise the temperature of a kilogram of water 1°C (actually, a kilocalorie, but usually called a calorie for weight control purposes).

associated with fat control. Nevertheless, research suggests that people are born with a predisposition toward fatness or leanness. For years, some scholars have suggested that your body type, or **somatotype,** is inherited. Clearly, some people will have more difficulty than others controlling fatness because of their body types and because they come from families with a history of obesity. In fact, recent research by a well-respected team of scholars indicates the body has a "natural" fatness range, which is influenced by heredity. If you deviate more than 10 to 15 percent from this range, your body may actually alter its metabolism in an attempt to maintain your "natural" fatness level. But even these changes are temporary. If you continue the behavior that caused the weight gain (eating more or exercising less), after a period of time your body accepts your new weight as your "natural" level. Scientists caution people not to overgeneralize the importance of heredity to body fatness. Such overgeneralizations could lead to incorrect conclusions about the regulation of body fat levels.

Recently, the "ob-gene" (or gene responsible for obesity) was discovered. It is true that this is an important scientific discovery, but it is unlikely that it will result in a cure for overfatness in the near future. In the meantime, more conventional methods of fat control must be used. Even if you come from a family with a history of obesity, you should not conclude that nothing can be done to prevent obesity. Virtually all people have a natural fatness level below obese levels. Those with a predisposition to high fatness will have a harder time having a low body fat level, but with healthy lifestyles, even these people can maintain body fat levels within normal ranges. Research shows that regular physical activity is especially effective in the control of genetically determined predispositions to fatness.

Glandular disorders are not a cause of overfatness for most people.
Glandular disorders can cause or contribute to overfatness. For example, thyroid problems can cause a low metabolic rate that results in fat gain. However, most experts suggest that only 1 to 2 percent of all overfatness is directly caused by problems of this type. Medical treatment is necessary for people suffering from these problems.

Fatness early in life leads to adult fatness.
Research studies have documented that body composition levels tend to track through the life span. Although there are exceptions, individuals that are overweight or obese as children are more likely to be overweight or obese as adults. One explanation for this is that overfatness in children causes the body to produce more fat cells. Although it was once thought that only children could add fat cells as a result of overfatness, evidence now suggests that obesity can result in new fat cell production, even into adulthood. Still, the increase in the size of existing fat cells is the principal factor influencing body fat levels among adults. Since adults can only increase or decrease the size of existing fat cells, the number of cells becomes an important factor influencing fat levels.

Maintaining healthy levels of body fat is an important objective for children and adults. It was previously thought that only adult obesity was related to health problems, but it is now apparent that teens who are overfat are at a greater risk for heart problems and cancer than leaner peers. Obese children have been found to have symptoms of "adult-onset diabetes," indicating that the effects of obesity can impair health even for young people.

Changes in basal metabolic rate can be the cause of obesity.
The amount of energy you expend each day must be balanced by your energy intake if you are to maintain your body fat and body weight over time (see Figure 5). Your energy intake is determined by the calories you eat. Expenditure is determined by a combination of several factors. You expend calories just to exist, even when you are inactive. Your **basal metabolic rate (BMR)** is the indicator of your energy expenditure when you are totally inactive. You also expend calories digesting food and, of course, in the activities of daily living.

BMR is highest during the growing years. The amount of food eaten increases to support this increased energy expenditure. When growing ceases, if eating does not decrease or activity level increase, fatness can result. Basal metabolism also decreases gradually as you grow older. One major reason for this is the loss of muscle mass associated with inactivity. Regular physical activity throughout life helps keep the muscle mass higher, resulting in a higher BMR. Recent evidence suggests that regular exercise can contribute in other ways to increased BMR. The higher BMR of active people helps them prevent overfatness, particularly in later life.

Excess caloric intake results in an increase in fat cell size.
Overfatness can result in an increase in the number of fat cells among children. For adults, overfatness is a result of the increase in size of fat cells (hypertrophy). When fat cells near the skin become excessively large, they can cause dimples or lumps under the skin. Some people refer to these large fat cells as cellulite. Quacks say that this type of fat is different from other types of fat and is removed from the body in different ways than regular fat. This is not true. All fatness among adults is a result of enlarged fat cells. All fat is lost as a result of reduction in fat cell size.

"Creeping obesity" is a problem as you grow older.
People become less active and their BMR gradually decreases with age. Caloric intake does seem to decrease somewhat with age, but the decrease does not adequately compensate for the decreases in BMR and activity levels. For this reason, body fat increases gradually for the typical person with age (see Figure 6). This increase in fatness

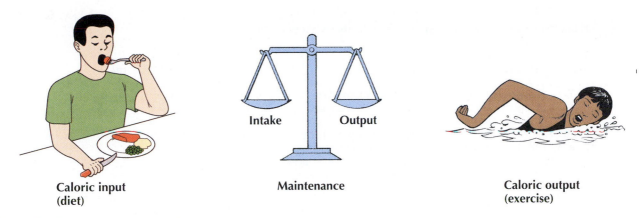

Figure 5 ▶ Balancing caloric input and output.

over time is commonly referred to as "creeping obesity" because the increase in fatness is gradual. For a typical person, creeping obesity can result in a gain of 1/2 to 1 pound per year. People who stay active can keep muscle mass high and delay changes in BMR. For those who are not active, it is suggested that caloric intake decrease by 3 percent each decade after twenty-five, so that, by age sixty-five, caloric intake is at least 10 percent less than it was at age twenty-five. The decrease in caloric intake for active people need not be as great.

The Relationship among Diet, Physical Activity, and Fatness

🌐 **A combination of regular physical activity and dietary restriction is the most effective means of losing body fat.** www.mhhe.com/phys_fit/ web15 Click 09. Studies indicate that regular physical

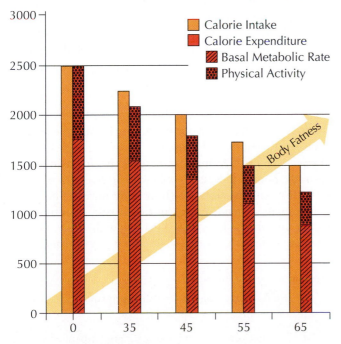

Figure 6 ▶ Creeping obesity.

activity combined with dietary restriction is the most effective method of losing fat. Diet alone can contribute to weight loss, but much of this loss is actually lean tissue. When physical activity and diet are both used in a weight-loss program, the same amount of weight may be lost but more of it is from fat. This is obviously beneficial for appearance and for participation in physical activity, but it can also help to maintain resting metabolic rate at a higher level. This can contribute to further weight loss or facilitate weight maintenance. For optimal results, all weight loss programs should combine a lower caloric intake with a good physical exercise program (see Figure 5). Thresholds of training and target zones for body fat reduction, including information for both physical activity and **diet** are presented in Table 3.

Good physical activity and diet habits can be useful in maintaining desirable body composition. Though physical activity or exercise will not result in immediate and large decreases in body fat levels, there is evidence that fat loss resulting from physical activity may be more lasting than fat loss from dieting. However, not all people want to lose fat. For those who wish to maintain their current body composition, a **caloric balance** between intake and output is essential. For people who want to increase their lean body weight, increased caloric intake with increased exercise can result in the desired changes.

Physical activity that can be sustained for relatively long periods is considered the most effective for losing body fat. Physical activities from virtually any level of the physical activity pyramid can be effective

Somatotype Inherent body build: ectomorph (thin), mesomorph (muscular), and endomorph (fat).

Basal Metabolic Rate (BMR) Your energy expenditure in a basic or rested state.

Diet The usual food and drink for a person or an animal.

Table 3 ▶ Threshold of Training and Target Zones for Body Fat Reduction

| | Threshold of Training* | | Target Zones* | |
	Physical Activity	Diet	Physical Activity	Diet
Frequency	• To be effective, activity must be regular, preferably daily, though fat can be lost over the long term with almost any frequency that results in increased caloric expenditure.	• Reduce caloric intake consistently and daily. To restrict calories only on certain days is not best, though fat can be lost over a period of time by reducing caloric intake at any time.	• Daily moderate activity is recommended. For people who do regular vigorous activity, 3 to 6 days per week may be best.	• It is best to diet consistently and daily.
Intensity	• To lose 1 pound of fat, you must expend 3,500 calories more than you normally expend.	• To lose 1 pound of fat, you must eat 3,500 calories fewer than you normally eat.	• Slow, low-intensity aerobic exercise that results in no more than 1 to 2 pounds of fat loss per week is best.	• Modest caloric restriction resulting in no more than 1 to 2 pounds of fat loss per week is best.
Time	• To be effective, exercise must be sustained long enough to expend a considerable number of calories. At least 15 minutes per exercise bout are necessary to result in consistent fat loss.	• Eating moderate meals is best. Do not skip meals.	• Exercise durations similar to those for achieving aerobic cardiovascular fitness seem best. Exercise of 30 to 60 minutes in duration is recommended.	• Eating moderate meals is best. Skipping meals or fasting is not most effective.

*It is best to combine exercise and diet to achieve the 3,500-calorie imbalance necessary to lose a pound of fat. Using both exercise and diet in the target zone is most effective.

in controlling body fatness because all physical activities expend calories. Among the most effective activities are those in the aerobic activity section of the pyramid because they can be done for relatively long periods of time. Lifestyle activities are also effective, if performed regularly for extended periods of time. Table 4 shows the caloric expenditures for 1 hour of involvement in various physical activities. Heavier people expend more calories than lighter people because more work is required to move larger bodies.

Popular books have claimed that vigorous activities are not effective in helping with body fat loss because they say vigorous activities burn less fat than less intense activities. Although this is true in theory, it has little practical meaning for most people. It is the total calories expended in your activity that counts. If you run for the same period of time that you walk, you will expend more calories in running.

Even though vigorous activity can be effective, it will not work if you do not do it regularly. For this reason, more vigorous activity may not be as effective as some less vigorous activities for certain people. For example, running at 10 miles per hour (a 6-minute mile) will cause a 150-pound person to expend 900 calories in 1 hour. Jogging about half as fast, or at 5 1/2 miles per hour (approximately an 11-minute mile), will result in an expenditure of about 650 calories in the same amount of time. At first glance, the more vigorous exercise seems to be a better choice. But how many people can continue to run at a

10-mile-per-hour pace for a full hour? Each mile run at 10 miles per hour results in an expenditure of 90 calories, whereas each mile run at 5 1/2 miles per hour results in an expenditure of 118 calories. Per mile, you expend more calories in slow running. It takes longer to run a mile, but by the same token, you can also persist longer. The key is to expend as many calories as possible during each regular exercise period. Doing less vigorous activity for longer periods is better for fat control than doing very vigorous activities that can be done only for short periods. Nevertheless, several studies have shown that vigorous activity can be very effective for some people.

Strength training can be effective in maintaining a desirable body composition. Performing exercises from the strength and muscular endurance level of the physical activity pyramid can be effective in maintaining desirable body fat levels. People who do strength training increase their muscle mass (lean body mass). This extra muscle mass expends extra calories at rest, resulting in a higher metabolic rate. Also, people with more muscle mass expend more calories when doing physical activity.

Caloric Balance Consuming calories in amounts equal to the number of calories expended.

METs Multiples of the amount of energy expended at rest.

Table 4 ▶ Calories Expended per Hour in Various Physical Activities (Performed at a Recreational Level)*

Activity	100 lb. (46 kg)	120 lb. (55 kg)	Calories Used per Hour 150 lb. (68 kg)	180 lb. (82 kg)	200 lb. (91 kg)
Archery	180	204	240	276	300
Backpacking (40-lb. pack)	307	348	410	472	513
Badminton	255	289	340	391	425
Baseball	210	238	280	322	350
Basketball (half-court)	225	255	300	345	375
Bicycling (normal speed)	157	178	210	242	263
Bowling	155	176	208	240	261
Canoeing (4 mph)	276	344	414	504	558
Circuit training	247	280	330	380	413
Dance, aerobics	315	357	420	483	525
Dance, ballet (choreographed)	240	300	360	432	480
Dance, modern (choreographed)	240	300	360	432	480
Dance, social	174	222	264	318	348
Fencing	225	255	300	345	375
Fitness calisthenics	232	263	310	357	388
Football	225	255	300	345	375
Golf (walking)	187	212	250	288	313
Gymnastics	232	263	310	357	388
Handball	450	510	600	690	750
Hiking	225	255	300	345	375
Horseback riding	180	204	240	276	300
Interval training	487	552	650	748	833
Jogging (5 1/2 mph)	487	552	650	748	833
Judo/karate	232	263	310	357	388
Mountain climbing	450	510	600	690	750
Pool; billiards	97	110	130	150	163
Racquetball; paddleball	450	510	600	690	750
Rope jumping (continuous)	525	595	700	805	875
Rowing, crew	615	697	820	943	1025
Running (10 mph)	625	765	900	1035	1125
Sailing (pleasure)	135	153	180	207	225
Skating, ice	262	297	350	403	438
Skating, roller/inline	262	297	350	403	438
Skiing, cross-country	525	595	700	805	875
Skiing, downhill	450	510	600	690	750
Soccer	405	459	540	621	775
Softball (fast-pitch)	210	238	280	322	350
Softball (slow-pitch)	217	246	290	334	363
Surfing	416	467	550	633	684
Swimming (fast laps)	420	530	630	768	846
Swimming (slow laps)	240	272	320	368	400
Table tennis	180	204	240	276	300
Tennis	315	357	420	483	525
Volleyball	262	297	350	403	483
Walking	204	258	318	372	426
Waterskiing	306	390	468	564	636
Weight training	352	399	470	541	558

Source: Corbin, C. B., and R. Lindsey.

*Locate your weight to determine the calories expended per hour in each of the activities shown in the table based on recreational involvement. More vigorous activity, as occurs in competitive athletics, may result in greater caloric expenditures.

Appetite is not necessarily increased through exercise. The human animal was intended to be an active animal. For this reason, the human "appetite thermostat" (called the "appestat" by some) is set as if all people were active. Those who are inactive do not have a decreased appetite. Likewise, if a person is sedentary and then begins regular exercise, the appetite does not necessarily increase because this appetite thermostat expects activity. Very vigorous activity does not necessarily cause an appetite increase that is proportional to the calories expended in the vigorous exercise.

Strategies for Action

Making a variety of self-assessments can help you make informed decisions about body composition. www.mhhe.com/phys_fit/web15 Click 10. In Labs 15A and 15B, you will take various body composition self-assessments. It is important that you take all of the measurements and consider all of the information before making final decisions about your body composition. Each of the self-assessment techniques has its strengths and weaknesses, and you should be aware of these when making personal decisions. The importance you place on one particular measure may be different from the importance another person places on that measure because you are a unique individual and should use information that is more relevant for you personally.

Self-assessment information—especially body composition information—is personal and confidential. Body composition self-assessment information is personal and should be confidential. When performing the self-assessments, be aware of the following:

1. If doing a self-assessment around other people makes you self-conscious, do the measurement in private.
2. If the measurement requires the assistance of another person, choose a person you trust and feel comfortable with. If you have someone help you make measurements, identify a person who will be available over time. This will allow the same person to make the measurements each time you make assessments. For Lab 15A, get the assistance of an expert and/or a partner to do skinfold measures. Of course, doing your own measurements when possible is the best way to make sure that the same person does the measures each time you do them. Recent studies show that self-measurements can be relatively accurate if done consistently with the same set of calipers and after practicing to become skilled.
3. The formulas used to determine body fatness from skinfolds and other procedures are based on normal distributions of people. The more a person differs from normal, the less accurate the measurements will be. For this reason, most measurements are less accurate for the very lean and people with higher than normal levels of fat. Special procedures are available for athletes, and techniques such as under-

water weighing, the BodPod, or bioelectrical impedance are best for those with exceptionally high levels of body fatness.

4. Some measurements, such as the thigh skinfold, are hard to make on some people. This is one reason two different skinfold procedures are presented.
5. Self-assessments require skill. With practice, you can become skillful in making measurements. Your first few attempts will, no doubt, lack accuracy.
6. Use the same measuring device each time you measure (scale, calipers, measuring tape, etc.). This will assure that any measurement error is constant and will allow you to track your progress over time. For example, your scale may be off by 2 pounds, but if you use the same scale every time you always know the amount of the error and you can correct for it. If you use a different scale each time you weigh, the error is variable. It is difficult to correct for variable errors.
7. Once you have tried all of the self-assessments in Lab 15A, choose the ones you want to continue to do and use the same measurement techniques each time you do the measurements.

Estimating your BMR can help you determine the number of calories you expend each day. In Lab 15C, you can estimate your BMR. This will give you an idea of how much energy you expend when you are resting. You can use this information together with the information about the energy you expend to help you balance the calories you consume with the calories you expend each day.

Logging your daily activities can help you determine the number of calories you expend each day. In Lab 15C, you will also log the activities you perform in a day. You can then determine your energy expenditure in these activities. You can combine this information with the information about your basal metabolism to determine your total daily energy expenditure.

Counting the calories you consume each day can help you balance the calories you expend with the calories you consume. In the concept on nutrition, you will learn how to count the number of calories you consume each day. You can use this information with the information in Lab 15C to determine if there is a balance in calories consumed and calories expended.

Those interested in weight loss should consider recently approved guidelines. Physical activity is critical in maintaining the weight loss over time. For optimal results, weight loss programs should combine a lower caloric intake with a good physical activity program. The

ACSM has recently released recommendations for weight loss treatment that indicate when weight loss is appropriate and what guidelines should be followed in treatment. The recommendations are intended more for clinical use by physicians, dietitians, and exercise specialists. Guidelines for nonprofessionals based on the ACSM recommendations are outlined in Table 5.

Table 5 ▶ Guidelines for Weight Loss Treatment

Questions about Weight Loss	Recommendations
Who should consider weight loss?	Individuals with a BMI of >25 or in the marginal or overfat zone *should consider* reducing their body weight—especially if it is accompanied by abdominal obesity. Individuals with a BMI of >30 *are encouraged to seek* weight loss treatment.
What types of goals should be established?	Overweight and obese individuals should target reducing their body weight by a minimum of 5–10% and should aim to maintain this long-term weight loss.
What about maintenance?	Individuals should strive for long-term weight maintenance and the prevention of weight regain over the long-term, especially when weight loss is not desired or when attainment of ideal body weight is not achievable.
What should be targeted in a weight loss program?	Weight loss programs should target both eating and exercise behaviors, as sustained changes in both behaviors has been associated with significant long-term weight loss.
How should diet be changed?	Overweight and obese individuals should reduce their current intake by 500–1000 kcal/day to achieve weight loss (<30% of calories from fat). Individualized level of caloric intake should be established to prevent weight regain after initial loss.
How should activity be changed?	Overweight and obese individuals should progressively increase to a minimum of 150 minutes of moderate-intensity physical activity per week for health benefits. However, for long-term weight loss, the program should progress to higher amounts of activity (e.g., 200–300 minutes per week or >2,000 kcal/week).
What about resistance exercise?	Resistance exercise should supplement the endurance exercise program for individuals who are undertaking modest reductions in energy intake to lose weight.
What about using drugs for weight loss?	Pharmocotherapy (medicine/drugs) for weight loss should only be used by individuals with a BMI >30 or those with excessive body fatness. Weight loss medications should only be used in combination with a strong behavioral intervention that focuses on modifying eating and exercise behaviors.

Source: Based on ACSM recommendations; see *Suggested Readings.*

Study Resources

Check out additional online study resources for this concept in the Student Edition of the Online Learning Center at www.mhhe.com/corbin13e.

Web Resources

American Anorexia/Bulimia Association **www.aabainc.org**
FDA Consumer **www.fda.gov/fdac**
National Center for Health Statistics **www.cdc.gov/nchs**
North American Association for the Study of Obesity (NAASO) **www.naaso.org**

Shape Up America **www.shapeup.org**
Fat Control Inc., makers of calipers **wellfarm@nfdc.net**

Suggested Readings

 Additional reference materials for Concept 15 are available at **www.mhhe.com/phys_fit/web15 Click 11.**

American College of Sports Medicine. 2001. Appropriate intervention strategies for weight loss and prevention of weight regain for adults. *Medicine and Science in Sports and Exercise* 33(12):2145–2156.

Bray, G. A. 2004. Obesity and the metabolic syndrome: Implications for dietetics practitioners. *Journal of the American Dietetics Association* 104(1).

Critser, G. 2003. *Fatland: How We Became the Fattest People in the World.* Boston: Houghton Mifflin.

Fairburn, C. G., and K. D. Brownell (eds.). 2002. *Eating Disorders and Obesity: A Comprehensive Handbook.* 2nd ed. New York: Guilford Press.

Finkelstein, E. A., et al. 2003. National medical spending attributable to overweight and obesity: How much and who's paying? *Health Affairs* May 14:1–7, available at www.healthaffairs.org.

Finkelson, E. A., et al. 2004. State-level estimates of annual medical expenditures attributable to obesity. *Obesity Research* 12(1):18–24.

Institute of Medicine. 2004. *Preventing Childhood Obesity: Health in the Balance.* Washington, DC: Institute of Medicine.

Irwin, M. L., et al. 2003. Effect of exercise on total and intra-abdominal body fat in post-menopausal women. *Journal of the American Medical Association* 289(3):323–330.

Janssen, I., et al. 2004. Fitness alters the association of BMI and waist circumference with total and abdominal fat. *Obesity Research* 12(3):525–537.

Lohman, T. G. 2004. Seeing ourselves through the obesity epidemic. *President's Council on Physical Fitness and Sports Research Digest* 5(3):1–8.

Manore, M. M. 2003. Dietary supplements for weight loss: Do they work? Are they safe? *ACSM's Health and Fitness Journal* 7(4):17–21.

Mayo, M. J. 2003. Exercise induced weight loss preferentially reduces abdominal fat. *Medicine and Science in Sports and Exercise* 35(2):207–213.

Mokdad, A. H., et al. 2003. Prevalence of obesity, diabetes, and obesity-related health risk factors. *Journal of the American Medical Association* 289(1):76–79.

Mokdad, A. H., et al. 2004. Actual causes of death in the United States. *Journal of the American Medical Association* 29(10):1238–1246.

Ogden, C. L. et al. 2004. Mean body weight, height, and BMI in the United States—1960–2002. *Advance Data from Vital Health Statistics* 347:1–20. (www.cdc.gov/nchs)

Peeters, A., et al. 2003. Obesity in adulthood and its consequences for life expectancy: A life table analysis. *Annals of Internal Medicine* 138:24–32

Ribisl, P. M. 2004. Toxic "waist" dump: Our abdominal visceral fat. *ACSM's Health and Fitness Journal* 8(4):22–25.

Sacker, I. M., and M. A. Zimmer. 2002. *Dying to Be Thin: Understanding and Defeating Anorexia Nervosa and Bulimia—a Practical, Lifesaving Guide.* New York: Time Warner Bookmark.

Sanborn, C. F., et al. 2000. Disordered eating and the female athlete triad. *Clinics in Sports Medicine* 19(2):199–213.

Thompson, S. R., M. M. Weber, and L. B. Brown. 2001. The relationship between health and fitness magazine readings and eating-disordered weight-loss methods among high school girls. *American Journal of Health Education* 32(3):133–138.

Wong, G., and W. H. Dietz. 2002. Economic burden of obesity in youths aged 6 to 17 years: 1979–1999. *Pediatrics* 109:381.

World Health Organization. 2000. *Obesity: Preventing and Managing the Global Epidemic.* Geneva, Switzerland: WHO.

World Health Organization. 2004. *Global Strategy on Diet, Physical Activity and Health.* Geneva, Switzerland: WHO.

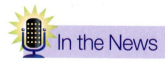 In the News

The Epidemic/Pandemic of Obesity

A highly publicized article in the *Journal of the American Medical Association* reported that it was likely that obesity would overtake tobacco as the leading cause of preventable mortality (see Mokdad et al. 2004). The projection was based on statistics indicating a 33 percent increase in deaths attributable to obesity over the past 10 years. The results of this paper fit with many other published reports, but follow-up analyses revealed that these projections may have been overestimated. The CDC recently released a revised statement suggesting that the actual increases in deaths due to obesity may actually be closer to 10 percent. This change may cause confusion in the public since the findings of the original study were widely circulated. While the actual health implications of obesity are hard to quantify it is clear that obesity has become one of our greatest public health challenges.

Several recent statistics strongly support this contention:

- According to the National Center for Health Statistics, the body weight for the average American has increased by nearly 25 pounds from 1960 to the present.
- The direct economic costs of treating obesity in the United States has been estimated at over $70 billion.
- Recent estimates from the World Health Organization suggest that over 2.6 million deaths worldwide can be attributed to a high BMI.
- Data from the well-known Framingham Heart Study suggest that obese individuals have a reduced life expectancy of between 6 and 7 years.

Lab Resource Materials: Evaluating Body Fat

General Information about Skinfold Measurements

It is important to use a consistent procedure for "drawing up" or "pinching up" a skinfold and making the measurement with the calipers. The following procedures should be used for each skinfold site.

1. Lay the calipers down on a nearby table. Use the thumbs and index fingers of both hands to draw up a skinfold, or layer of skin and fat. The fingers and thumbs of the two hands should be about 1 inch apart, or 1/2 inch on either side of the location where the measurement is to be made.

2. The skinfolds are normally drawn up in a vertical line rather than a horizontal line. However, if the natural tendency of the skin aligns itself less than vertical, the measurement should be done on the natural line of the skinfold, rather than on the vertical.

3. Do not pinch the skinfold too hard. Draw it up so that your thumbs and fingers are not compressing the skinfold.

4. Once the skinfold is drawn up, let go with your right hand and pick up the calipers. Open the jaws of the caliper and place it over the location of the skinfold to be measured and 1/2 inch from your left index finger and thumb. Allow the tips, or jaw faces, of the caliper to close on the skinfold at a level about where the skin would be normally.

5. Let the reading on the calipers settle for 2 or 3 seconds; then note the thickness of the skinfold in millimeters.

6. Three measurements should be taken at each location. Use the middle of the three values to determine your measurement. For example, if you had values of 10, 11, and 9, your measurement for that location would be 10. If the three measures vary by more than 3 millimeters from the lowest to the highest, you may want to take additional measurements.

Skinfold Locations for Women

Triceps skinfold—Make a mark on the back of the right arm, one-half the distance between the tip of the shoulder and the tip of the elbow. Make the measurement at this location.

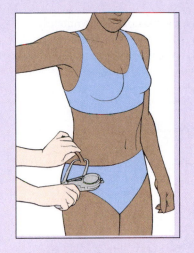

Iliac crest skinfold— Make a mark at the top front of the iliac crest. This skinfold is taken slightly diagonally because of the natural line of the skin.

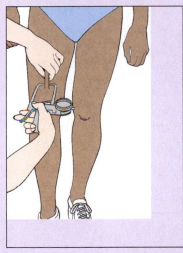

Thigh skinfold— Make a mark on the front of the thigh midway between the hip and the knee. Make the measurement vertically at this location.

Abdominal skinfold—Make a mark on the skin approximately 1 inch to the right of the navel. Make a horizontal measurement at this location for the Fitness-gram Method and a vertical measure for the Jackson-Pollock Method. (See page 291.)

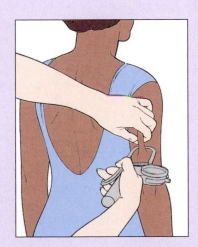

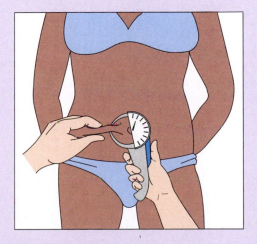

Calf skinfold—Same as for men.

289

Skinfold Locations for Men

Chest skinfold—Make a mark above and to the right of the right nipple (one-half the distance from the midline of the side and the nipple). The measurement at this location is often done on the diagonal because of the natural line of the skin.

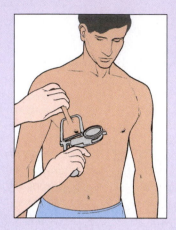

Abdominal skinfold—Make a mark on the skin approximately 1 inch to the right of the navel. Make a vertical measurement at that location for the Jackson-Pollock Method and horizontally for the Fitnessgram Method. (See page 293.)

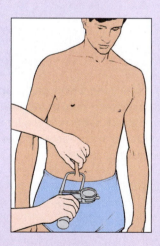

Thigh skinfold—Same as for women (see previous page).

Calf skinfold—Make a mark on the inside of the calf of the right leg at the level of the largest calf size (girth). Place the foot on a chair or other elevation so that the knee is kept at approximately 90 degrees. Make a vertical measurement at the mark.

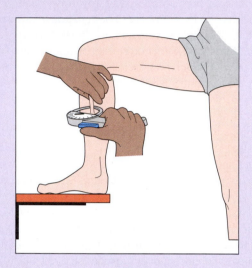

Self-Measured Tricep Skinfold for Both Men and Women

This measurement is made on the left arm so that the caliper can easily be read. Hold the arm straight at shoulder height. Make a fist with the thumb faced upward. Place the fist against a wall. With the right hand, place the caliper over the skinfold as it "hangs freely" on the back of the tricep (halfway from the tip of the shoulder to the elbow).

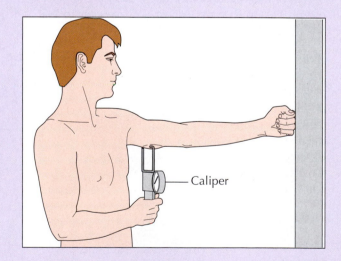

Caliper

Calculating Fatness from Skinfolds (Jackson-Pollock Method)

1. Sum three skinfolds (triceps, iliac crest, and thigh for women; chest, abdominal [vertical], and thigh for men).
2. Use the skinfold sum and your age to determine your percent fat using Chart 1 for men and Chart 2 for women. Locate your sum of skinfold in the left column and your age at the top of the chart. Your estimated body fat percentage is located where the values intersect.
3. Use the Standards for Body Fatness (Chart 4) to determine your fatness rating.

Chart 1 ▶ Percent Fat Estimates for Men (Sum of Thigh, Chest, and Abdominal Skinfolds)

Sum of Skinfolds (mm)	Age to the Last Year								
	22 and Under	23 to 27	28 to 32	33 to 37	38 to 42	43 to 47	48 to 52	53 to 57	Over 57
8–10	1.3	1.8	2.3	2.9	3.4	3.9	4.5	5.0	5.5
11–13	2.2	2.8	3.3	3.9	4.4	4.9	5.5	6.0	6.5
14–16	3.2	3.8	4.3	4.8	5.4	5.9	6.4	7.0	7.5
17–19	4.2	4.7	5.3	5.8	6.3	6.9	7.4	8.0	8.5
20–22	5.1	5.7	6.2	6.8	7.3	7.9	8.4	8.9	9.5
23–25	6.1	6.6	7.2	7.7	8.3	8.8	9.4	9.9	10.5
26–28	7.0	7.6	8.1	8.7	9.2	9.8	10.3	10.9	11.4
29–31	8.0	8.5	9.1	9.6	10.2	10.7	11.3	11.8	12.4
32–34	8.9	9.4	10.0	10.5	11.1	11.6	12.2	12.8	13.3
35–37	9.8	10.4	10.9	11.5	12.0	12.6	13.1	13.7	14.3
38–40	10.7	11.3	11.8	12.4	12.9	13.5	14.1	14.6	15.2
41–43	11.6	12.2	12.7	13.3	13.8	14.4	15.0	15.5	16.1
44–46	12.5	13.1	13.6	14.2	14.7	15.3	15.9	16.4	17.0
47–49	13.4	13.9	14.5	15.1	15.6	16.2	16.8	17.3	17.9
50–52	14.3	14.8	15.4	15.9	16.5	17.1	17.6	18.1	18.8
53–55	15.1	15.7	16.2	16.8	17.4	17.9	18.5	18.2	19.7
56–58	16.0	16.5	17.1	17.7	18.2	18.8	19.4	20.0	20.5
59–61	16.9	17.4	17.9	18.5	19.1	19.7	20.2	20.8	21.4
62–64	17.6	18.2	18.8	19.4	19.9	20.5	21.1	21.7	22.2
65–67	18.5	19.0	19.6	20.2	20.8	21.3	21.9	22.5	23.1
68–70	19.3	19.9	20.4	21.0	21.6	22.2	22.7	23.3	23.9
71–73	20.1	20.7	21.2	21.8	22.4	23.0	23.6	24.1	24.7
74–76	20.9	21.5	22.0	22.6	23.2	23.8	24.4	25.0	25.5
77–79	21.7	22.2	22.8	23.4	24.0	24.6	25.2	25.8	26.3
80–82	22.4	23.0	23.6	24.2	24.8	25.4	25.9	26.5	27.1
83–85	23.2	23.8	24.4	25.0	25.5	26.1	26.7	27.3	27.9
86–88	24.0	24.5	25.1	25.5	26.3	26.9	27.5	28.1	28.7
89–91	24.7	25.3	25.9	25.7	27.1	27.6	28.2	28.8	29.4
92–94	25.4	26.0	26.6	27.2	27.8	28.4	29.0	29.6	30.2
95–97	26.1	26.7	27.3	27.9	28.5	29.1	29.7	30.3	30.9
98–100	26.9	27.4	28.0	28.6	29.2	29.8	30.4	31.0	31.6
101–103	27.5	28.1	28.7	29.3	29.9	30.5	31.1	31.7	32.3
104–106	28.2	28.8	29.4	30.0	30.6	31.2	31.8	32.4	33.0
107–109	28.9	29.5	30.1	30.7	31.3	31.9	32.5	33.1	33.7
110–112	29.6	30.2	30.8	31.4	32.0	32.6	33.2	33.8	34.4
113–115	30.2	30.8	31.4	32.0	32.6	33.2	33.8	34.5	35.1
116–118	30.9	31.5	32.1	32.7	33.3	33.9	34.5	35.1	35.7
119–121	31.5	32.1	32.7	33.3	33.9	34.5	35.1	35.7	36.4
122–124	32.1	32.7	33.3	33.9	34.5	35.1	35.8	36.4	37.0
125–127	32.7	33.3	33.9	34.5	35.1	35.8	36.4	37.0	37.6

Source: Baumgartner, T. A., and Jackson, A. S.

Note: Percent fat calculated by the formula by Siri. Percent fat = $[(4.95/BD) - 4.5] \times 100$, where BD = body density.

Chart 2 ▶ Percent Fat Estimates for Women (Sum of Triceps, Iliac Crest, and Thigh Skinfolds)

Sum of Skinfolds (mm)	Age to the Last Year								
	22 and Under	23 to 27	28 to 32	33 to 37	38 to 42	43 to 47	48 to 52	53 to 57	Over 57
23–25	9.7	9.9	10.2	10.4	10.7	10.9	11.2	11.4	11.7
26–28	11.0	11.2	11.5	11.7	12.0	12.3	12.5	12.7	13.0
29–31	12.3	12.5	12.8	13.0	13.3	13.5	13.8	14.0	14.3
32–34	13.6	13.8	14.0	14.3	14.5	14.8	15.0	15.3	15.5
35–37	14.8	15.0	15.3	15.5	15.8	16.0	16.3	16.5	16.8
38–40	16.0	16.3	16.5	16.7	17.0	17.2	17.5	17.7	18.0
41–43	17.2	17.4	17.7	17.9	18.2	18.4	18.7	18.9	19.2
44–46	18.3	18.6	18.8	19.1	19.3	19.6	19.8	20.1	20.3
47–49	19.5	19.7	20.0	20.2	20.5	20.7	21.0	21.2	21.5
50–52	20.6	20.8	21.1	21.3	21.6	21.8	22.1	22.3	22.6
53–55	21.7	21.9	22.1	22.4	22.6	22.9	23.1	23.4	23.6
56–58	22.7	23.0	23.2	23.4	23.7	23.9	24.2	24.4	24.7
59–61	23.7	24.0	24.2	24.5	24.7	25.0	25.2	25.5	25.7
62–64	24.7	25.0	25.2	25.5	25.7	26.0	26.2	26.4	26.7
65–67	25.7	25.9	26.2	26.4	26.7	26.9	27.2	27.4	27.7
68–70	26.6	26.9	27.1	27.4	27.6	27.9	28.1	28.4	28.6
71–73	27.5	27.8	28.0	28.3	28.5	28.8	28.0	29.3	29.5
74–76	28.4	28.7	28.9	29.2	29.4	29.7	29.9	30.2	30.4
77–79	29.3	29.5	29.8	30.0	30.3	30.5	30.8	31.0	31.3
80–82	30.1	30.4	30.6	30.9	31.1	31.4	31.6	31.9	32.1
83–85	30.9	31.2	31.4	31.7	31.9	32.2	32.4	32.7	32.9
86–88	31.7	32.0	32.2	32.5	32.7	32.9	33.2	33.4	33.7
89–91	32.5	32.7	33.0	33.2	33.5	33.7	33.9	34.2	34.4
92–94	33.2	33.4	33.7	33.9	34.2	34.4	34.7	34.9	35.2
95–97	33.9	34.1	34.4	34.6	34.9	35.1	35.4	35.6	35.9
98–100	34.6	34.8	35.21	35.3	35.5	35.8	36.0	36.3	36.5
101–103	35.3	35.4	35.7	35.9	36.2	36.4	36.7	36.9	37.2
104–106	35.8	36.1	36.3	36.6	36.8	37.1	37.3	37.5	37.8
107–109	36.4	36.7	36.9	37.1	37.4	37.6	37.9	38.1	38.4
110–112	37.0	37.2	37.5	37.7	38.0	38.2	38.5	38.7	38.9
113–115	37.5	37.8	38.0	38.2	38.5	38.7	39.0	39.2	39.5
116–118	38.0	38.3	38.5	38.8	39.0	39.3	39.5	39.7	40.0
119–121	38.5	38.7	39.0	39.2	39.5	39.7	40.0	40.2	40.5
122–124	39.0	39.2	39.4	39.7	39.9	40.2	40.4	40.7	40.9
125–127	39.4	39.6	39.9	40.1	40.4	40.6	40.9	41.1	41.4
128–130	39.8	40.0	40.3	40.5	40.8	41.0	41.3	41.5	41.8

Source: Baumgartner, T. A., and A. S. Jackson.

Note: Percent fat calculated by the formula by Siri. Percent fat = $[(4.95/BD) - 4.5] \times 100$, where BD = body density.

Chart 3 ▶ Percent Fat Estimates for Sum of Triceps, Abdominal, and Calf Skinfolds

Men		Women	
Sum of Skinfolds	Percent Fat	Sum of Skinfolds	Percent Fat
8–10	3.2	23–25	16.8
11–13	4.1	26–28	17.7
14–46	5.0	29–31	18.5
17–19	6.0	32–34	19.4
20–22	6.0	35–37	20.2
23–25	7.8	38–40	21.0
26–28	8.7	41–43	21.9
29–31	9.7	44–46	22.7
32–34	10.6	47–49	23.5
35–37	11.5	50–52	24.4
38–40	12.5	53–55	25.2
41–43	13.4	56–58	26.1
44–46	14.3	59–61	26.9
47–49	15.2	62–64	27.7
50–52	16.2	65–67	28.6
53–55	17.1	68–70	29.4
56–58	18.0	71–73	30.2
59–61	18.9	74–76	31.1
62–64	19.9	77–79	31.9
65–67	20.8	80–82	32.7
68–70	21.7	83–85	33.6
71–73	22.6	86–88	34.4
74–76	23.6	89–91	35.5
77–79	24.5	92–94	36.1
80–82	25.4	95–97	36.9
83–85	26.4	98–100	37.8
86–88	27.3	101–103	38.6
89–91	28.2	104–106	39.4
92–94	29.1	107–109	40.3
95–97	30.1	110–112	41.1
98–100	31.0	113–115	42.0
101–103	31.9	116–118	42.8
104–106	32.8	119–121	43.6
107–109	33.8	122–124	44.5
110–112	34.7	125–127	45.3
113–115	35.6	128–130	46.1
116–118	36.6	131–133	47.0
119–121	37.5	134–136	47.8
122–124	38.4	137–139	48.7
125–127	39.3	140–142	49.5

Calculating Fatness from Skinfolds (Fitnessgram Method)

1. Sum the three skinfolds (triceps, abdominal, and calf) for men and women. Use horizontal abdominal measure. (See page 289.)
2. Use the skinfold sum and your age to determine your percent fat using Chart 3. Locate your sum of skinfold in the left column at the top of the chart. Your estimated body fat percentage is located where the values intersect.
3. Use the Standards for Body Fatness (Chart 4) to determine your fatness rating.

Calculating Fatness from Self-Measured Skinfolds

1. Use either the Jackson-Pollock or Fitnessgram method but make the measures on yourself rather than have a partner do the measures. When doing the tricep measure, use the self-measurement technique for men and women. (See page 290.)
2. Calculate fatness using the methods described previously.
3. Use Chart 4 to determine ratings.

Chart 4 ▶ Standards for Body Fatness (Percent Body Fat)

	Too Low	Borderline	Good Fitness (Healthy)	Marginal	Overfat
	Below Essential Fat Levels	Unhealthy for Many People	Optimal for Good Health	Associated with Some Health Problems	Unhealthy
Males	No less than 5%	6–9%	10–20%	21–25%	>25%
Females	No less than 10%	11–16%	17–28%	29–35%	>35%

Height-Weight Measurements

1. *Height*—Measure your height in inches or centimeters. Take the measurement without shoes, but add 2.5 centimeters or 1 inch to measurements, as the charts include heel height.

2. *Weight*—Measure your weight in pounds or kilograms without clothes. Add 3 pounds or 1.4 kilograms because the charts include weight of clothes. If weight must be taken with clothes on, wear indoor clothing that weighs 3 pounds or 1.4 kilograms.

3. Determine your frame size using the elbow breadth. The measurement is most accurate when done with a broad-based sliding caliper. However, it can be done using a skinfold caliper or can be estimated with a metric ruler. The right arm is measured when it is elevated with the elbow bent at 90 degrees and the upper arm horizontal. The back of the hand should face the person making the measurement. Using the caliper, measure the distance between the epicondyles of the humerus (inside and outside bony points of the elbow). Measure to the nearest millimeter (1/10 of a centimeter). If a caliper is not available, place the thumb and the index finger of the left hand on the epicondyles of the humerus and measure the distance between the fingers with a metric ruler. Use your height and elbow breadth in centimeters to determine your frame size (Chart 5); you need not repeat this procedure each time you use a height and weight chart.

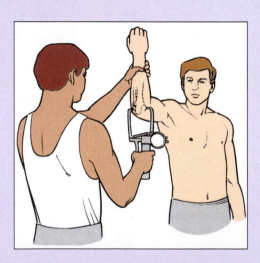

4. Use Chart 6 to determine your healthy weight range. The new healthy weight range charts do not account for frame size. However, you may want to consider frame size when determining a personal weight within the healthy weight range. People with a larger frame size typically can carry more weight within the range than can those with a smaller frame size.

Chart 5 ▶ Frame Size Determined from Elbow Breadth (mm)

	Elbow Breadth (mm)		
Height	Small Frame	Medium Frame	Large Frame
Males			
5′2″ or less	<64	64–72	>72
5′3″–5′6 1/2″	<67	67–74	>74
5′7″–5′10 1/2″	<69	69–76	>76
5′11″–6′2 1/2″	<71	71–78	>78
6′3″ or less	<74	74–81	>81
Females			
4′10 1/2″ or less	<56	56–64	>64
4′11″–5′2 1/2″	<58	58–65	>65
5′3″–5′6 1/2″	<59	59–66	>66
5′7″–5′10 1/2″	<61	61–68	>69
5′11″ or less	<62	62–69	>69

Source: Metropolitan Life Insurance Company.

Height is given including 1-inch heels.

Chart 6 ▶ Healthy Weight Ranges for Adult Women and Men

Women			Men		
Height			Height		
Feet	Inches	Pounds	Feet	Inches	Pounds
4	10	91–119	5	9	129–169
4	11	94–124	5	10	132–174
5	0	97–128	5	11	136–179
5	1	101–132	6	0	140–184
5	2	104–137	6	1	144–189
5	3	107–141	6	2	148–195
5	4	111–146	6	3	152–200
5	5	114–150	6	4	156–205
5	6	118–155	6	5	160–211
5	7	121–160	6	6	164–216
5	8	125–164			

Source: U.S. Department of Agriculture and Department of Health and Human Services.

Chart 7 ▶ Body Mass Index (BMI)

Height	100	105	110	115	120	125	130	135	140	145	150	155	160	165	170	175	180	185	190	195	200	205	210	215	220	225	230	235	240	245	250
5'0"	20	21	21	22	23	24	25	26	27	28	29	30	31	32	33	34	35	36	37	38	39	40	41	42	43	44	45	46	47	48	49
5'1"	19	20	21	22	23	24	25	26	26	27	28	29	30	31	32	33	33	34	35	36	37	38	39	40	41	42	43	43	44	45	46
5'2"	18	19	20	21	22	23	24	25	26	27	27	28	29	30	31	32	33	34	35	36	37	37	38	39	40	41	42	43	44	45	46
5'3"	18	19	19	20	21	22	23	24	25	26	27	27	28	29	30	31	32	33	34	35	35	36	37	38	39	40	41	42	43	43	44
5'4"	17	18	19	20	21	21	22	23	24	25	26	27	27	28	29	30	31	32	33	33	34	35	36	37	38	39	39	40	41	42	43
5'5"	17	17	18	19	20	21	22	22	23	24	25	26	27	27	28	29	30	31	32	32	33	34	35	36	37	37	38	39	40	41	42
5'6"	16	17	18	19	19	20	21	22	23	23	24	25	26	27	27	28	29	30	31	31	32	33	34	35	36	36	37	38	39	40	40
5'7"	16	16	17	18	19	20	20	21	22	23	23	24	25	26	27	27	28	29	30	31	31	32	33	34	34	35	36	37	38	38	39
5'8"	15	16	17	17	18	19	20	21	21	22	23	24	24	25	26	27	27	28	29	30	30	31	32	33	33	34	35	36	36	37	38
5'9"	15	16	16	17	18	18	19	20	21	21	22	23	24	24	25	26	27	27	28	29	30	30	31	32	32	33	34	35	35	36	37
5'10"	14	15	16	17	17	18	19	19	20	21	22	22	23	24	24	25	26	27	27	28	29	29	30	31	32	32	33	34	34	35	36
5'11"	14	15	15	16	17	17	18	19	20	20	21	22	22	23	24	24	25	26	26	27	28	29	29	30	31	31	32	33	33	34	35
6'0"	14	14	15	16	16	17	18	18	19	20	20	21	22	22	23	24	24	25	26	26	27	28	28	29	30	31	31	32	33	33	34
6'1"	13	14	15	15	16	16	17	18	18	19	20	20	21	22	22	23	24	24	25	26	26	27	28	28	29	30	30	31	32	32	33
6'2"	13	13	14	15	15	16	17	17	18	19	19	20	21	21	22	22	23	24	24	25	26	26	27	28	28	29	30	30	31	31	32
6'3"	12	13	14	14	15	16	16	17	17	18	19	19	20	21	21	22	22	23	24	24	25	26	26	27	27	28	29	29	30	31	31
6'4"	12	13	13	14	15	15	16	16	17	18	18	19	20	21	21	22	23	23	24	24	25	26	26	27	27	28	29	29	30	30	30

Weight

■ Low   ■ Good fitness zone   ■ Marginal   ■ Obese

Body Mass Index (BMI)

Use the steps listed below or use Chart 7 to calculate your BMI.

1. Divide your weight in pounds by 2.2 to determine your weight in kilograms.
2. Multiply your height in inches by 0.0254 to determine your height in meters.
3. Square your height in meters (multiply your height in meters by your height in meters).
4. Divide your weight in kilograms from step 1 by your height in meters squared from step 3.
5. If you use these steps to determine your BMI, use the Rating Scale for Body Mass Index (Chart 8) to obtain a rating for your BMI.

Formula

$$BMI = \frac{\text{weight in kilograms}}{(\text{height in meters})^2}$$

Chart 8 ▶ Rating Scale for Body Mass Index (BMI)

Classification	BMI
Obese (high risk)	Over 30
Marginal	25–30
Good fitness zone	17–24.9
Low	Less than 17

Note: An excessively low BMI is not desirable. Low BMI values can be indicative of eating disorders and other health problems. The government rating for marginal is overweight.

Determining the Waist-to-Hip Circumference Ratio

The waist-to-hip circumference ratio is recommended as the best available index for determining risk and disease associated with fat and weight distribution. Disease and death risk are associated with abdominal and upper body fatness. When a person has high fatness and a high waist-to-hip ratio, additional risks exist. The following steps should be taken in making measurements and calculating the waist-to-hip ratio.

1. Both measurements should be done with a nonelastic tape. Make the measurements while standing with the feet together and the arms at the sides, elevated only high enough to allow the measurements. Be sure the tape is horizontal and around the entire circumference. Record scores to the nearest millimeter or 1/16th of an inch. Use the same units of measure for both circumferences (millimeters or 1/16th of an inch). The tape should be pulled snugly but not to the point of causing an indentation in the skin.

2. *Waist measurement*—Measure at the natural waist (smallest waist circumference). If no natural waist exists, the measurement should be made at the level of the umbilicus. Measure at the end of a normal inspiration.

3. *Hip measurement*—Measure at the maximum circumference of the buttocks. It is recommended that you wear thin-layered clothing (such as a swimming suit or underwear) that will not add significantly to the measurement.

4. Divide the hip measurement into the waist measurement or use the waist-to-hip nomogram (Chart 9) to determine your waist-to-hip ratio.

5. Use the Waist-to-Hip Ratio Rating Scale (Chart 10) to determine your rating for the waist-to-hip ratio.

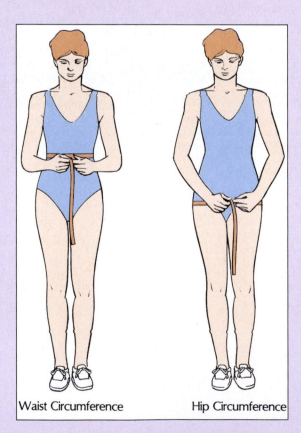

Waist Circumference   Hip Circumference

Note: Using a partner or a mirror will aid you in keeping the tape horizontal.

Chart 9 ▶ Waist-to-Hip Ratio Nomogram

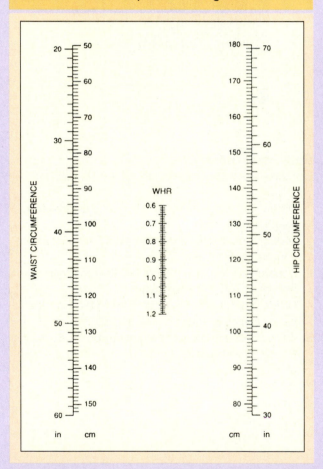

Chart 10 ▶ Waist-to-Hip Ratio Rating Scale

Classification	Men	Women
High risk	>1.0	>0.85
Moderately high risk	0.90–1.0	0.80–0.85
Lower risk	<0.90	<0.80

Lab 15A Evaluating Body Composition: Skinfold Measures

Name	**Section**	**Date**

Purpose: To estimate body fatness using two different skinfold procedures; to compare measures made by an expert, by a partner, and by self-measurements; to learn the strengths and weaknesses of each technique; and to use the results to establish personal standards for evaluating body composition

General Procedures: Follow the specific procedures for the two different self-assessment techniques. If possible, have one set of measurements made by an expert (instructor) for each of the two techniques. Next, work with a partner you trust. Have the partner make measurements at each site for both techniques. Finally, make self-measurements for each of the sites. If you are just learning a measurement technique, it is important to practice the skills of making the measurement. If you do measurements over time, use the same instrument (if possible) each time you measure. If your measurements vary widely, take more than one set until you get more consistent results.

If you have had an underwater weighing, a bioelectric impedance measurement, a near-infrared interactance measure, or some other body fatness measurement done recently, record your results below.

Measurement Technique	**% Body Fat**	**Rating**
1.		
2.		

Skinfold Measurements (Jackson-Pollock Method)

Procedures for Jackson-Pollock Method

1. Read the directions for the Jackson-Pollock Method measurements in *Lab Resource Materials.*
2. If possible, observe a demonstration of the proper procedures for measuring skinfolds at each of the different locations before doing partner or self-measurements.
3. Make expert, partner, and self-measurements (see *Lab Resource Materials*). When doing the self-measure of the triceps, use the self-measurement technique described in *Lab Resource Materials* (women only).
4. Record each of the measurements in the Results section.
5. Calculate your body fatness from skinfolds by summing the appropriate skinfold values (chest, thigh, and abdominal for men; triceps, iliac crest, and thigh for women). Using your age and the sum of the appropriate skinfolds, determine your body fatness using Charts 1 and 2 in *Lab Resource Materials*.
6. Rate your fatness using Chart 4 in *Lab Resource Materials*.

Results for Jackson-Pollock Method

Skinfolds by an Expert (If Possible)	Skinfolds by Partner	Self-Measurements
Male	*Male*	*Male*
Chest ___	Chest ___	Chest ___
Thigh ___	Thigh ___	Thigh ___
Abdominal ___	Abdominal ___	Abdominal ___
Sum ___	Sum ___	Sum ___
% body fat ___	% body fat ___	% body fat ___
Rating ___	Rating ___	Rating ___
Female	*Female*	*Female*
Triceps ___	Triceps ___	Triceps ___
Iliac crest ___	Iliac crest ___	Iliac crest ___
Thigh ___	Thigh ___	Thigh ___
Sum ___	Sum ___	Sum ___
% body fat ___	% body fat ___	% body fat ___
Rating ___	Rating ___	Rating ___

Make a check by the statements that are true about your measurements.

- [ ] The person doing measurements has experience with these three skinfold measurements.
- [ ] Self-measurements were practiced until measurements became consistent.
- [ ] Results of several trials for each measure are consistent (do not vary more than 2–3 mm).
- [ ] You are not exceptionally low or exceptionally high in body fat.

The more checks you have, the more likely your measurements are accurate.

Skinfold Measurements (Fitnessgram Method)

Procedures for Fitnessgram Method

1. Read the directions for the Fitnessgram measurements in *Lab Resource Materials.*
2. Use the procedures as for the Fitnessgram Method using the triceps, abdominal, and calf sites described in *Lab Resource Materials.* When doing the self-measure of the triceps use the self-measurement technique shown earlier.
3. Calculate your body fatness from skinfolds by summing the appropriate skinfold values (same for both men and women). Using the sum of the appropriate skinfolds, determine your body fatness using Chart 3 in *Lab Resource Materials.*
4. Rate your fatness using Chart 4 in *Lab Resource Materials.*

Results for Fitnessgram Method

Skinfolds by an Expert (If Possible)

Triceps ____

Abdominal ____

Calf ____

Sum ____

% body fat ____

Rating ____

Skinfolds by Partner

Triceps ____

Abdominal ____

Calf ____

Sum ____

% body fat ____

Rating ____

Self-Measurements

Triceps ____

Abdominal ____

Calf ____

Sum ____

% body fat ____

Rating ____

Make a check by the statements that are true about your measurements.

☐ The person doing measurements has experience with these three skinfold measurements.

☐ Self-measurements were practiced until measurements became consistent.

☐ Results of several trials for each measure are consistent (do not vary more than 2–3 mm).

☐ You are not exceptionally low or exceptionally high in body fat.

The more checks you have, the more likely your measurements are accurate.

Conclusions and Implications

In the space provided below, discuss your current body composition based on the two different skinfold procedures and any other measures of body fatness you may have done. Note any discrepancies in the measurements and discuss which of the measurements you think provide the most useful information. To what extent do you think you need to alter your level of body fatness?

Lab 15B Evaluating Body Composition: Height, Weight, and Circumference Measures

Name	Section	Date

Purpose: To assess body composition using a variety of procedures, to learn the strengths and weaknesses of each technique, and to use the results to establish personal standards for evaluating body composition

General Procedures: Follow the specific procedures for the three different self-assessment techniques. If possible, work with a partner you trust to help with measurements that you have difficulty making on yourself. If you are just learning a measurement technique, it is important to practice the skills of making the measurement. If you do measurements over time, use the same instrument (if possible) each time you measure. If your measurements vary widely, take more than one set until you get more consistent results. If possible, have an expert make measurements on you using these procedures.

Height and Weight Measurements

Procedures

1. Read the directions for height and weight measurements in *Lab Resource Materials.*
2. Determine your healthy weight range using Chart 6 in *Lab Resource Materials.* You may want to use your elbow breadth (Chart 5). People with a smaller frame size should typically weigh less than those with a larger frame size within the healthy weight range. You may need the assistance of a partner to make the elbow breadth measurement.
3. Record your scores in the Results section.

Results

Weight [ ]   Healthy weight range [ ]

Height [ ]

Make a check by the statements that are true about your measurements.

[ ] You are confident in the accuracy of the scale you used.

[ ] You are confident that the height technique is accurate.

The more checks you have, the more likely your measurements are accurate.
If you are a very active person with a high amount of muscle, use this method with caution.

Body Mass Index

Procedures

1. Use the height and weight measures from Part 1 above.
2. Determine your BMI score by using Chart 7 or the directions in *Lab Resource Materials.* Determine your rating using Chart 8.
3. Record your score and rating in the Results section.

Results

Body mass index [ ]   Rating [ ]

If you are a very active person with a high amount of muscle, use this method with caution.

Waist-to-Hip Ratio

Procedures

1. Measure your waist and hip circumferences using the procedures in *Lab Resource Materials*.
2. Divide your hip circumference into your waist circumference or use Chart 9 in *Lab Resource Materials* to calculate your waist-to-hip ratio.
3. Determine your rating using Chart 10 in *Lab Resource Materials*.
4. Record your scores in the Results section.

Results

Waist circumference [   ]

Hip circumference [   ]

Waist-to-hip ratio [   ]   Rating [   ]

Make a check by the statements that are true about your measurements.

[ ]   You are confident in the accuracy of the waist-to-hip measurement.

Make a check by the statements that are true about you.

[ ]   I am a male 5′9″ or less and have a waist girth of 34 or more.

[ ]   I am a male 5′10″ to 6′4″ and have a waist girth of 36 or more.

[ ]   I am a male 6′5″ or more and have a waist girth of 38 or more.

[ ]   I am a female 5′2″ or less and have a waist girth of 29 or more.

[ ]   I am a female 5′3″ to 5′10″ and have a waist girth of 31 or more.

[ ]   I am a female 5′11″ or more and have a waist girth of 33 or more.

If you checked one of the boxes above, the waist-to-hip ratio is especially relevant for you.

Conclusions and Implications

In the space provided below, discuss your results for the height, weight, and circumference procedures. Note any discrepancies in the measurements. Indicate the strengths and weaknesses of the various methods. Which of the measures do you think provided you with the most useful information? If you also did the skinfold measures (Lab 15A), discuss your body composition based on all of the information you have collected (skinfolds and height, weight, and circumference measures).

Lab 15C Determining Your Daily Energy Expenditure

Name		Section		Date

Purpose: To learn how many calories you expend in a day

Procedures

1. Estimate your basal metabolism using step 1 in the Results section. First determine the number of minutes you sleep.
2. Monitor your activity expenditure for 1 day using Chart 1 (page 305). Record the number of 5-, 15-, and 30-minute blocks of time that you perform each of the different types of physical activities (e.g., if an activity lasted 20 minutes, you would use one 15-minute block and one 5-minute block). Be sure to distinguish between moderate (Mod) and vigorous (Vig) intensity in your logging. If you perform an activity that is not listed, specify the activity on the line labeled "Other" and estimate if it is moderate or vigorous. You may want to keep copies of Chart 1 for future use. One extra copy is provided.
3. Sum the total number of minutes of moderate and vigorous activity. Determine your calories expended during moderate and vigorous activity using steps 2 and 3.
4. Determine your nonactive minutes using step 4. This is all time that is not spent sleeping or being active.
5. Determine your calories expended in nonactive minutes using step 5.
6. Determine your calories expended in a day using step 6.

Results

Daily Caloric Expenditure Estimates

Step 1:

Basal calories = .0076 × [Body wt. (lbs.)] × [Minutes of sleep] = [Basal calories] (A)

Step 2:

Calories (moderate activity) = .036 × [Body wt. (lbs.)] × [Minutes of moderate activity] = [Calories in moderate activity] (B)

Step 3:

Calories (vigorous activity) = .053 × [Body wt. (lbs.)] × [Minutes of vigorous activity] = [Calories in vigorous activity] (C)

Step 4:

Minutes (nonactive) = 1,440 min − [Minutes of sleep] − [Minutes of moderate activity] − [Minutes of vigorous activity] = [Nonactive minutes]

Step 5:

Calories (rest and light activity) = .011 × [Body wt. (lbs.)] × [Nonactive minutes] = [Calories in other activities] (D)

Step 6:

Calories expended (per day) = [ ] (A) + [ ] (B) + [ ] (C) + [ ] (D) = [ ] **Daily calories**

Answer the following questions about your daily calorie expenditure estimate:

Yes	No	
☐	☐	Were the activities you performed similar to what you normally perform each day?
☐	☐	Do you think your daily estimated caloric expenditure is an accurate estimate?
☐	☐	Do you think you expend the correct number of calories in a typical day to maintain the body composition (body fat level) that is desirable for you?

Conclusions and Interpretations: In several paragraphs, discuss your daily caloric expenditure. Comment on your answers to the preceding questions. In addition, comment on whether you think you should modify your daily caloric expenditure for any reason.

Chart 1 ▶ Daily Activity Log

Day of Monitoring:					
Physical Activity Category		**5 Minutes**	**15 Minutes**	**30 Minutes**	**Minutes**
Lifestyle Activity		1 2 3 4 5 6	1 2 3 4 5 6	1 2 3	
Dancing (general)	Mod				
Gardening	Mod				
Home repair/maintenance	Mod				
Occupation	Mod				
Walking/hiking	Mod				
Other:	Mod				
Aerobic Activity		1 2 3 4 5 6	1 2 3 4 5 6	1 2 3	
Aerobic dance (low-impact)	Mod				
	Vig				
Aerobic machines (rowing, stair, ski)	Mod				
	Vig				
Bicycling	Mod				
	Vig				
Running	Mod				
	Vig				
Skating (roller/ice)	Mod				
	Vig				
Swimming (laps)	Mod				
	Vig				
Other:	Mod				
	Vig				
Sport/Recreation Activity		1 2 3 4 5 6	1 2 3 4 5 6	1 2 3	
Basketball	Mod				
	Vig				
Bowling/billiards	Mod				
Golf	Mod				
Martial arts (judo, karate)	Mod				
	Vig				
Racquetball/tennis	Mod				
	Vig				
Soccer/hockey	Mod				
	Vig				
Softball/baseball	Mod				
Volleyball	Mod				
	Vig				
Other:	Mod				
Flexibility Activity		1 2 3 4 5 6	1 2 3 4 5 6	1 2 3	
Stretching	Mod				
Other:	Mod				
Strengthening Activity		1 2 3 4 5 6	1 2 3 4 5 6	1 2 3	
Calisthenics (push-ups/sit-ups)	Mod				
Resistance exercise	Mod				
Other:	Mod				

Minutes of moderate activity	
Minutes of vigorous activity	
Total minutes of activity	

Chart 2 ▶ Daily Activity Log

Day of Monitoring:					
Physical Activity Category		**5 Minutes**	**15 Minutes**	**30 Minutes**	**Minutes**
Lifestyle Activity		1 2 3 4 5 6	1 2 3 4 5 6	1 2 3	
Dancing (general)	Mod				
Gardening	Mod				
Home repair/maintenance	Mod				
Occupation	Mod				
Walking/hiking	Mod				
Other:	Mod				
Aerobic Activity		1 2 3 4 5 6	1 2 3 4 5 6	1 2 3	
Aerobic dance (low-impact)	Mod				
	Vig				
Aerobic machines (rowing, stair, ski)	Mod				
	Vig				
Bicycling	Mod				
	Vig				
Running	Mod				
	Vig				
Skating (roller/ice)	Mod				
	Vig				
Swimming (laps)	Mod				
	Vig				
Other:	Mod				
	Vig				
Sport/Recreation Activity		1 2 3 4 5 6	1 2 3 4 5 6	1 2 3	
Basketball	Mod				
	Vig				
Bowling/billiards	Mod				
Golf	Mod				
Martial arts (judo, karate)	Mod				
	Vig				
Racquetball/tennis	Mod				
	Vig				
Soccer/hockey	Mod				
	Vig				
Softball/baseball	Mod				
Volleyball	Mod				
	Vig				
Other:	Mod				
Flexibility Activity		1 2 3 4 5 6	1 2 3 4 5 6	1 2 3	
Stretching	Mod				
Other:	Mod				
Strengthening Activity		1 2 3 4 5 6	1 2 3 4 5 6	1 2 3	
Calisthenics (push-ups/sit-ups)	Mod				
Resistance exercise	Mod				
Other:	Mod				

Minutes of moderate activity

Minutes of vigorous activity

Total minutes of activity

Nutrition

The amount and kinds of food you eat affect your health and wellness.

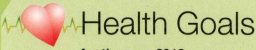

Health Goals

for the year 2010

- Promote health and reduce chronic disease associated with dietary factors and weight.
- Increase proportion of people who eat healthy snacks.
- Increase proportion of people who eat no more than 30 percent of calories as fat.
- Increase proportion of people who eat no more than 10 percent of calories as saturated fat.
- Increase proportion of people who eat at least five servings of vegetables and fruits daily.
- Increase proportion of people who eat at least six servings of grain products daily.
- Increase proportion of people who meet dietary recommendation for calcium.
- Reduce proportion of people who consume excess sodium.
- Reduce incidence of iron deficiency and anemia (especially children and women).
- Increase proportion of worksites that offer nutrition and/or weight-management classes.

The importance of good nutrition for optimal health is well established. Eating patterns have been related to four of the seven leading causes of death, and poor nutrition increases the risks for numerous diseases, including heart disease, obesity, stroke, diabetes, hypertension, osteoporosis, and many cancers (e.g., colon, prostate, mouth, throat, lung, and stomach). The links to cancer are probably not fully appreciated in today's society, but the American Cancer Society estimates that 35 percent of cancer risks are related to nutritional factors. In addition to these health risks, proper nutrition can enhance the quality of life by improving appearance and enhancing the ability to carry out work and leisure-time activity without fatigue.

Most people believe that nutrition is important but still find it difficult to maintain a healthy diet. One reason is that foods are usually developed, marketed, and adver-

tised for convenience and taste rather than for health or nutritional quality. Another reason is that many individuals have misconceptions about what constitutes a healthy diet. Some of these misconceptions are propagated by so-called experts with less than impressive credentials and those with commercial interests. Others are created by the confusing, and often contradictory, news reports about new nutrition research. In spite of the fact that nutrition is an advanced science, many questions remain unanswered.

In this concept, some basic nutrition guidelines are presented to dispel various nutrition myths. A section is presented on nutrition and physical performance to assist those interested in sports and high-level performance. Individuals interested in learning more about nutrition than is covered here are encouraged to seek the advice of a registered dietitian or to study reliable books, journals, and government documents (see *Suggested Readings* and *Web Resources*).

Guidelines for Healthy Eating

National dietary recommendations provide a target zone for healthy eating. www.mhhe.com/phys_fit/web16 Click 01. About forty-five to fifty nutrients in food are believed to be essential for the body's growth, maintenance, and repair. These are classified into six categories: carbohydrates (and fiber), fats, proteins, vitamins, minerals, and water. The first three provide energy, which is measured in calories. Specific dietary recommendations for each of the six nutrients are presented later in this concept.

National guidelines, specifying the nutrient requirements for good health, are developed by the Food and Nutrition Board of the National Academy of Science's Institute of Medicine. **Recommended Dietary Allowance (RDA)** historically were used to set recommendations for nutrients, but the complexity of dietary interactions prompted the board to develop a more comprehensive and functional set of dietary intake recommendations. These broader guidelines, referred to as

Recommended Dietary Allowance (RDA) Dietary guideline that specifies the amount of a nutrient needed for almost all of the healthy individuals in a specific age and gender group.

Table 1 ▶ Dietary Reference Intake (DRI), Recommended Dietary Allowance (RDA), and Tolerable Upper Intake Level (UL) for Major Nutrients

	DRI/RDA Males	DRI/RDA Females	UL	Function
B-Complex Vitamins				
Thiamin (mg/day)	1.2	1.1	ND	Co-enzyme for carbohydrates and amino acid metabolism
Riboflavin (mg/day)	1.3	1.1	ND	Co-enzyme for metabolic reactions
Niacin (mg/day)	16	14	35	Co-enzyme for metabolic reactions
Vitamin B-6 (mg/day)	1.3	1.3	100	Co-enzyme for amino acid and glycogen reactions
Folate (μg/day)	400	400	1,000	Metabolism of amino acids
Vitamin B-12 (μg/day)	2.4	2.4	ND	Co-enzyme for nucleic acid metabolism
Pantothenic acid (mg/day)	5*	5*	ND	Co-enzyme for fat metabolism
Biotin (μg/day)	30*	30*	ND	Synthesis of fat, glycogen, and amino acids
Choline (mg/day)	550*	425*	3,500	Precursor to acetylcholine
Antioxidants and Related Nutrients				
Vitamin C (mg/day)	90	75	2,000	Co-factor for reactions, antioxidant
Vitamin E (mg/day)	15	15	1,000	Undetermined, mainly antioxidant
Selenium (μg/day)	55	55	400	Defense against oxidative stress
Bone-Building Nutrients				
Calcium (mg/day)	1,000*	1,000*	2,500	Muscle contraction, nerve transmission
Phosphorus (mg/day)	700	700	3,000	Maintenance of pH, storage of energy
Magnesium (mg/day)	400–420	310–320	350	Co-factor for enzyme reactions
Vitamin D (μg/day)	5*	5*	50	Maintenance of calcium and phosphorus levels
Flouride (mg/day)	4*	3*	10	Stimulation of new bone formation
Micronutrients and Other Trace Elements				
Vitamin K (μg/day)	120*	90*	ND	Blood clotting and bone metabolism
Vitamin A (μg/day)	900	700	3,000	Vision, immune function
Iron (mg/day)	8	18	45	Component of hemoglobin
Zinc (mg/day)	11	8	40	Component of enzymes and proteins
Energy and Macronutrients				
Carbohydrates (45–65%)	130 g	130 g	ND	Energy (only source of energy for the brain)
Fat (20–35%)	ND	ND	ND	Energy, vitamin carrier
Protein (10–35%)	.8 g/kg	.8 g/kg	ND	Growth and maturation, tissue formation
Fiber (g/day)	38 g/day*	25 g/day*	ND	Digestion, blood profiles

Note: These values reflect the dietary needs generally for adults aged 19–50 years. Specific guidelines for other age groups are available from the Food and Nutrition Board of the National Academy of Sciences (www.iom.edu). Values for fluids and electrolytes have not been released yet. Values labeled with an asterisk (*) are based on Adequate Intake (AI) values rather than the RDA values; ND = not determined.

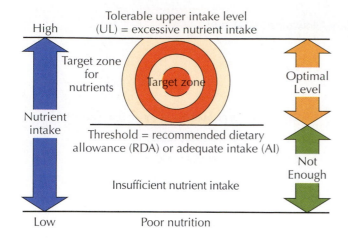

Figure 1 ▶ Dietary Reference Intake: a target zone for healthy eating.

Dietary Reference Intake (DRI), include RDA values when adequate scientific information is available and estimated **Adequate Intake (AI)** values when sufficient data aren't available to establish a firm RDA. The DRI values also include **Tolerable Upper Intake Level (UL),** that reflects the maximum, or highest, level of daily intake a person can consume without adverse effects on health. The guidelines make it clear that, although too little of a nutrient can be harmful to health, so can too much. In many ways, the RDAs can be considered threshold values similar to the threshold of training values for physical activity. The target zone for healthy eating would range from the RDA/AI values to the UL values (see Figure 1).

A unique aspect of the DRI values is that they are categorized by function and classification in order to facilitate awareness of the different roles that nutrients play in the diet. Specific guidelines have been developed for B-complex vitamins, vitamin C and vitamin E, bone-building nutrients such as calcium and vitamin D, micronutrients such as iron and zinc, and the class of macronutrients that includes carbohydrates, fats, proteins, and fiber. Table 1 includes the DRI values (including the UL values) for most of these nutrients, along with examples of food sources of the various nutrients.

The quantity of nutrients recommended varies with age and other considerations; for example, young children need more calcium than adults and pregnant women and postmenopausal women need more calcium than other women. Accordingly, Dietary Reference Intakes, including RDAs, have been established for several age/gender groups. In this book, the values used are appropriate for most adult men and women.

🌐 **National dietary guidelines provide a sound plan for good nutrition.** www.mhhe.com/phys_fit/ web16 Click 03. Federal law requires the publication of national dietary guidelines every 5 years. The most recent

Aim for fitness...

- Aim for a healthy weight.

- Be physically active each day.

Build a healthy base...

- Let the pyramid guide your food choices.

- Choose a variety of grains daily, especially whole grains.

- Choose a variety of fruits and vegetables daily.

- Keep food safe to eat.

Choose sensibly...

- Choose a diet that is low in saturated fat and cholesterol and moderate in total fat.

- Choose beverages and foods to moderate your intake of sugars.

- Choose and prepare foods with less salt.

- If you drink alcoholic beverages, do so in moderation.

Figure 2 ▶ Dietary guidelines for Americans: the ABCs.
Source: U.S. Department of Agriculture.

guidelines were published in 2000 (see Figure 2). These guidelines provide the basis for federal nutrition policy and nutrition education activities. They are also intended to advise Americans on making healthy food choices. The current guidelines include more specific recommendations about maintaining a healthy weight and being physically active every day. The revised guidelines also differ from previous guidelines in making more specific suggestions about food selection. They recommend that consumers use the food pyramid to guide their food choices (as opposed to just eating a variety of foods) and specifically recommend eating a variety of fruits and vegetables *daily*.

The general guidelines from the USDA recommend that the majority of the calories in your diet be comprised of carbohydrates (see Figure 4). Fat and protein provide the other principal sources of energy. The recently

Dietary Reference Intake (DRI) Appropriate amounts of nutrients in the diet (AI, RDA, and UL).

Adequate Intake (AI) Dietary guideline established experimentally to estimate nutrient needs when sufficient data are not available to establish an RDA value.

Tolerable Upper Intake Level (UL) Maximum level of a daily nutrient that will not pose a risk of adverse health effects for most people.

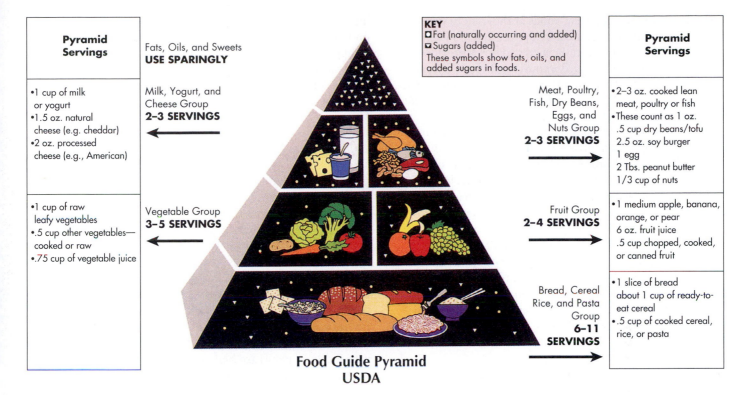

Pyramid Servings			Pyramid Servings

KEY
□ Fat (naturally occurring and added)
▪ Sugars (added)
These symbols show fats, oils, and added sugars in foods.

Pyramid Servings

•1 cup of milk or yogurt
•1.5 oz. natural cheese (e.g. cheddar)
•2 oz. processed cheese (e.g., American)

•1 cup of raw leafy vegetables
•.5 cup other vegetables— cooked or raw
•.75 cup of vegetable juice

Fats, Oils, and Sweets
USE SPARINGLY

Milk, Yogurt, and Cheese Group
2–3 SERVINGS

Vegetable Group
3–5 SERVINGS

Meat, Poultry, Fish, Dry Beans, Eggs, and Nuts Group
2–3 SERVINGS

Fruit Group
2–4 SERVINGS

Bread, Cereal Rice, and Pasta Group
6–11 SERVINGS

Pyramid Servings

•2–3 oz. cooked lean meat, poultry or fish
•These count as 1 oz.
.5 cup dry beans/tofu
2.5 oz. soy burger
1 egg
2 Tbs. peanut butter
1/3 cup of nuts

•1 medium apple, banana, orange, or pear
6 oz. fruit juice
.5 cup chopped, cooked, or canned fruit

•1 slice of bread about 1 cup of ready-to-eat cereal
•.5 cup of cooked cereal, rice, or pasta

**Food Guide Pyramid
USDA**

Figure 3 ► Food guide pyramid and sample serving sizes.

released DRI values of the Food and Nutrition Board of the Institute of Medicine (IOM) for these macronutrients are broader, but like the USDA, the IOM recommends carbohydrates as the principal source of calories followed by fats and proteins (see Figure 4). Both the USDA and IOM guidelines for nutrient intakes are associated with a reduced risk for chronic disease. The reason the IOM provided a slightly broader range of values is to "help people make healthy and more realistic choices based on their own food preferences." An important point in these dietary guidelines is that both the USDA and the IOM now recommend that physical activity be included in balancing energy intake to maintain a healthy body fat level throughout life.

🌐 **The levels of the food guide pyramid provide recommendations for servings of foods.**
www.mhhe.com/phys_fit/web16 Click 02. The food guide pyramid (Figure 3) was designed to guide people in the selection of nutritious food. The typical adult consumes too much fat and too little carbohydrate, especially complex carbohydrate. National health goals suggest that Americans should reduce the amount of dietary fat and increase the amount of complex carbohydrate in the diet. The food guide pyramid provides guidelines for how to fit these foods into an overall diet plan. According to USDA (United States Department of Agriculture) guidelines, carbohydrates should account for 55 to 60 percent of a per-

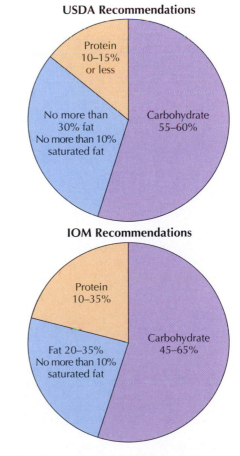

USDA Recommendations

Protein 10–15% or less

No more than 30% fat
No more than 10% saturated fat

Carbohydrate 55–60%

IOM Recommendations

Protein 10–35%

Fat 20–35%
No more than 10% saturated fat

Carbohydrate 45–65%

Figure 4 ► Dietary Reference Intake values.

son's diet, and this represents foods at the bottom two layers of the pyramid. Protein should constitute about 10 to 15 percent of the calories in the diet, and this is provided by meat and dairy products at the third level of the pyramid. Fat should constitute about 30 percent of the calories in the diet and is found mainly in the third and fourth levels of the pyramid.

The U.S. Center for Nutrition Policy and Promotion (CNPP), which promotes the pyramid, has provided clear guidelines on what constitutes a serving. Although the portions of foods that you eat vary, dietary guidelines are based on standard serving sizes (see Figure 2). By following the dietary guidelines and serving recommendations in the pyramid, a person is more likely to obtain the recommended percentages in the diet and to meet the associated nutrient recommendations included in the DRI. Be aware that the guidelines are based on the assumption that a person would be eating a 2,000-calorie diet. Individuals on a low-calorie diet would need to eat nutritionally dense foods to be sure they were getting all of the necessary nutrients needed for good health.

While the food pyramid makes conceptual sense, it has been criticized by some for not clarifying differences in the *quality* of different foods. The U.S. Dietary Guidelines are updated every 5 years but the pyramid is based on Guidelines from 1990. Efforts are currently underway to update the Guidelines for 2005 and it is likely that the pyramid will be revised to better reflect the new recommendations. (See "On the Web" and "In the News" sections for additional information.) The guidelines in the Canadian Food Guide currently recommend consumption of more whole-grain foods and higher-quality fruits and vegetables (see Appendix F).

Food labels provide consumers with detailed information to help them make good food choices. www.mhhe.com/phys_fit/web16 Click 04. Changes in food labeling laws have made it easier for consumers to know what is in the food they are eating (see Figure 5). The labels specify the amount of carbohydrates, fats, and proteins in the food and what percent contribution this food makes to the recommended daily value. The calculations are based on recommendations for people consuming about 2,000 calories per day. The labels also remind individuals that the allotments may vary if caloric needs are higher or lower.

An important aspect of the food labels is that they also provide information about the types of fats (e.g., saturated fat) and carbohydrates (e.g., simple sugars) that should be

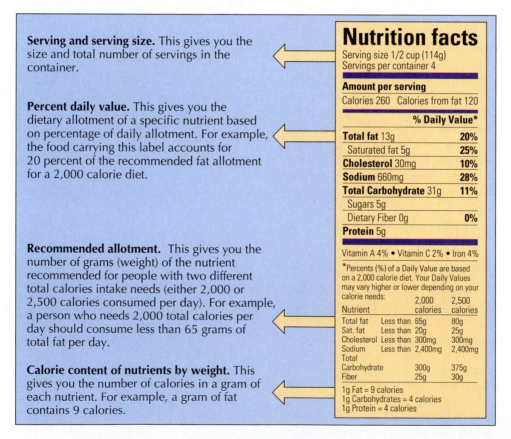

Serving and serving size. This gives you the size and total number of servings in the container.

Percent daily value. This gives you the dietary allotment of a specific nutrient based on percentage of daily allotment. For example, the food carrying this label accounts for 20 percent of the recommended fat allotment for a 2,000 calorie diet.

Recommended allotment. This gives you the number of grams (weight) of the nutrient recommended for people with two different total calories intake needs (either 2,000 or 2,500 calories consumed per day). For example, a person who needs 2,000 total calories per day should consume less than 65 grams of total fat per day.

Calorie content of nutrients by weight. This gives you the number of calories in a gram of each nutrient. For example, a gram of fat contains 9 calories.

Nutrition facts

Serving size 1/2 cup (114g)
Servings per container 4

Amount per serving

Calories 260   Calories from fat 120

	% Daily Value*
Total fat 13g	20%
Saturated fat 5g	25%
Cholesterol 30mg	10%
Sodium 660mg	28%
Total Carbohydrate 31g	11%
Sugars 5g	
Dietary Fiber 0g	0%
Protein 5g	

Vitamin A 4% • Vitamin C 2% • Iron 4%

*Percents (%) of a Daily Value are based on a 2,000 calorie diet. Your Daily Values may vary higher or lower depending on your calorie needs:

Nutrient		2,000 calories	2,500 calories
Total fat	Less than	65g	80g
Sat. fat	Less than	20g	25g
Cholesterol	Less than	300mg	300mg
Sodium	Less than	2,400mg	2,400mg
Total Carbohydrate		300g	375g
Fiber		25g	30g

1g Fat = 9 calories
1g Carbohydrates = 4 calories
1g Protein = 4 calories

Figure 5 ▶ Food label.

Source: U.S. Food and Drug Administration.

minimized in the diet as well as information on cholesterol, sodium, and fiber. Food labeled as "fat-free" on the label must have less than 1/2 a gram of fat per serving (50 grams). Foods labeled as "low-fat" must have less than 3 grams per serving. To be labeled "low in saturated fat," a food must have less than 15 percent of its calories from saturated fat. Additional modifications in the food labels are likely in the future. Over 15 percent of new food products claim to be "low-carb," so guidelines defining requirements for this claim are currently being determined.

Another planned change on food labels is the inclusion of trans fat content. This action is prompted by the evidence that trans fats are more likely to cause atherosclerosis and heart disease than are other types of fat. Companies are actively working to remove excess trans fats from their products and to comply with the labeling law. The FDA estimates that, through greater awareness and changes in food products, the labeling regulations will help to prevent 600 to 1,200 cases of coronary heart disease and 250 to 500 deaths each year.

Reading food labels can help you be more aware of what you are eating and help you make healthier choices in your daily eating.

Dietary Recommendations for Carbohydrates

Complex carbohydrates should be the principal source of calories in the diet. www.mhhe. com/phys_fit/web16 Click 05. Carbohydrates have gotten a bad rap in recent years due to the hype associated with low-carb diet plans. Carbohydrates have been unfairly implicated as a cause of obesity. The suggestion that they cause insulin to be released, and insulin, in turn, causes the body to take up and store excess energy as fat is overly simplistic and doesn't take into account differences in types of carbohydrates. Simple sugars (such as sucrose, glucose, and fructose) found in candy and soda lead to quick increases in blood sugar and tend to promote fat deposition. Complex carbohydrates (e.g., bread, pasta, rice), on the other hand, are broken down more slowly and do not cause the same effect on blood sugar. They contribute valuable nutrients and fiber in the diet and should constitute the bulk of a person's diet. Lumping simple and complex carbohydrates together is not appropriate, since they are processed differently and have different nutrient values.

A number of low-carb diet books have used an index known as the glycemic index (GI) as the basis for determining if foods are appropriate in the diet. Foods with a high GI value produce rapid increases in blood sugar, while foods with a low GI value produce slower increases. While this seems to be a logical way to categorize carbohydrates, it is misleading, since it doesn't take into

account the amount of carbohydrates in different servings of a food. The more appropriate indicator of the effect of foods on blood sugar levels is called the glycemic load. Carrots, for example, are known to have a very high GI value but the overall glycemic load is quite low. The carbohydrates from most fruits and vegetables exhibit similar properties.

While there is merit in trying to reduce excessive consumption of simple sugars, it is important to point out that excess calories are only problematic if caloric intake is larger than caloric expenditure. Carbohydrates are the body's preferred form of energy for physical activity, and the body is well equipped for processing extra carbohydrates. Athletes and active individuals typically have no difficulty burning off extra energy from carbohydrates. Sugar consumption, among people with an adequate diet, is also not associated with major chronic diseases. Increasing carbohydrates in the diet is more desirable than supplementing protein or consuming higher amounts of fat.

Dietary fiber is not considered a separate dietary nutrient, but it is considered to be important for overall good nutrition and health. www.mhhe.com/phys_fit/web16 Click 06. Research studies clearly demonstrate that diets high in complex carbohydrates and **fiber** are associated with a low incidence of coronary heart disease, stroke, and some forms of cancer. Long-term studies indicate that high-fiber diets may also be associated with a lower risk for diabetes mellitus, diverticulosis, hypertension, and gallstone formation. It is not known whether these health benefits are directly attributable to high dietary fiber or other effects associated with the ingestion of vegetables, fruits, and cereals in the diet.

The American Dietetics Association recently released a position statement on dietary fiber that summarizes the health benefits and importance of fiber in a healthy diet. It points out that a fiber-rich diet is lower in energy density, often has a lower fat content, is larger in volume, and is richer in micronutrients, all of which have beneficial health effects. Evidence for health benefits has become strong enough that the FDA has stated that specific beneficial health claims can be made for specific dietary fibers. The National Cholesterol Education Program has also recommended dietary fiber as part of overall strategies for treating high cholesterol in adults.

In the past, clear distinctions were made between soluble fiber and insoluble fiber because they appeared to provide separate effects. Soluble fiber (typically found in

Fiber Indigestible bulk in foods that can be either soluble or insoluble in body fluids.

fruits and oat bran) was more frequently associated with improving blood lipid profiles, whereas insoluble fiber (typically found in grains) was mainly thought to help speed up digestion and reduce risks for colon and rectal cancer. Difficulties in measuring these compounds in typical mixed diets has led a National Academy of Sciences Panel to recommend eliminating distinctions between soluble and insoluble fibers and instead to use a broader definition of fiber.

Currently, few Americans consume the recommended amounts of dietary fiber. The average intake of dietary fiber is about 15 g/day, which is much lower than the recommended 25–35 g/day. Foods in the typical American diet contain little, if any, dietary fiber, and servings of commonly consumed grains, fruits, and vegetables contain only 1–3 g of dietary fiber. Therefore, individuals have to look for specific ways to ensure that they get sufficient fiber in their diet. A number of supplements are available to help consumers increase fiber content in their diet.

🌐 **Fruits and vegetables are increasingly recognized as being essential for good health.** www.mhhe.com/phys_fit/web16 Click 07. Fruits and vegetables are a valuable source of dietary fiber, are packed with vitamins and minerals, and contain many additional "phytochemicals," which may have beneficial effects on health. The International Agency of Research on Cancer (IARC), an affiliate of the World Health Organization, recently completed a comprehensive review on the links between dietary intake of fruits and vegetables and cancer. The group concluded that findings from both human studies and animal experimental studies "indicate that a higher intake of fruits and vegetables is associated with a lower risk of various types of cancer." The clearest evidence of a cancer-protective effect from eating more fruits is for stomach, lung, and oesophageal cancers. A higher intake of vegetables is associated with reduced risks for cancers of the esophagus and colon-rectum. Overall, one in ten cancers are estimated to be due to insufficient intake of fruits and vegetables. This evidence—plus the evidence of the beneficial effects of fruits and vegetables on other major diseases, such as heart disease—indicates that individuals should strive to increase their intake of these foods. The "5 a day" nutrition program sponsored by the National Cancer Institute aims to increase awareness of the importance of eating at least five fruits and vegetables a day. The guidelines in the food guide pyramid recommend up to nine servings for optimal health.

Some recommendations can be followed to assure healthy amounts of carbohydrates in the diet. The following list includes basic recommendations for carbohydrate content in the diet:

- Total carbohydrates in the diet should account for the majority of total calories consumed (see Figure 4).

- Simple carbohydrates should be limited to 15 percent or less of total calories consumed, except for very active people.
- High-fiber foods should be included in the daily diet.

The following guidelines will help you implement these recommendations:

- Consume at least five servings of vegetables and/or fruits each day. Servings of green and yellow vegetables as well as citrus fruits are recommended. A serving of vegetables equals approximately 1/2 cup. A serving of fruit equals one medium-size piece.
- Consume at least six servings a day of complex carbohydrates, such as breads, cereals, and/or legumes. A serving of legumes or cereal equals approximately 1/2 cup. A serving of bread is one slice, one roll, or one muffin.
- Limit intake of desserts, baked goods, and other foods high in simple sugars or empty calories.
- Dietary fiber supplements other than in the form of food (such as oat bran) are not recommended unless prescribed for medical reasons.

Dietary Recommendations for Fat

🌐 **Fat is an essential nutrient and is an important energy source.** www.mhhe.com/phys_fit/web16 Click 08. Humans need some fat in their diet because fats are carriers of vitamins A, D, E, and K. They are a source of essential linoleic acid, make food taste better, and provide a concentrated form of calories, which serve as an important source of energy during moderate to vigorous exercise. Fats have more than twice the calories per gram as carbohydrates.

There are several types of dietary fat. **Saturated fats** come primarily from animal sources, such as red meat, dairy products, and eggs, but they are also found in some vegetable sources, such as coconut and palm oils. **Unsaturated fats** are of two basic types: polyunsaturated and monounsaturated. Polyunsaturated fats are derived principally from vegetable sources, such as safflower, cottonseed, soybean, sunflower, and corn oils (omega-6 fats), and cold-water fish sources, such as salmon and mackerel (omega-3 fats). Monounsaturated fats are derived primarily from vegetable sources, including olive, peanut, and canola oil.

Saturated fat is associated with an increased risk for disease. Excessive total fat in the diet (particularly saturated fat) is associated with atherosclerotic cardiovascular diseases and breast, prostate, and colon cancer, as well as obesity. Excess saturated fat in the diet contributes to increased cholesterol and increased LDL (low-density lipoprotein) cholesterol in the blood. For this reason, no more than 10 percent of your total calories should come from saturated fats.

Unsaturated fats are generally considered to be less likely to contribute to cardiovascular disease, cancer, and obesity than saturated fats. Polyunsaturated fats can reduce total cholesterol and LDL cholesterol, but they also decrease levels of HDL (high-density lipoprotein) cholesterol as well. Monounsaturated fats, on the other hand, have been shown to decrease total cholesterol and LDL cholesterol without an accompanying decrease in the desirable HDL. Omega-3 fatty acids found in cold-water fish have been shown to reduce triglycerides, but it isn't clear if this alters cholesterol levels.

Humans produce their own cholesterol, even when dietary cholesterol is limited. Still, high dietary cholesterol can increase the risk for atherosclerosis and coronary heart disease. Principal sources of dietary cholesterol are organ meats, some shellfish, and egg yolks.

The current Dietary Guidelines recommend a diet low in saturated fat and cholesterol but moderate in total fat. This distinction makes it clear that excess saturated fat is the main concern and acknowledges that some fat is necessary in the diet. Although exceptionally low-fat diets (15 percent or lower) may be appropriate for those individuals at risk for heart disease or other health problems, such diets have been found to be harmful for the majority of the population, especially when used without supervision. For example, the evidence suggests that very low-fat diets may not provide adequate nutrients, may reduce HDL (the good cholesterol), and may increase some of the less desirable blood fats. A recent randomized clinical trial reported better long-term weight maintenance among dieters consuming moderate amounts of fat rather than low amounts. Exceptionally low-fat diets are also considered particularly unhealthy for pregnant women and young children.

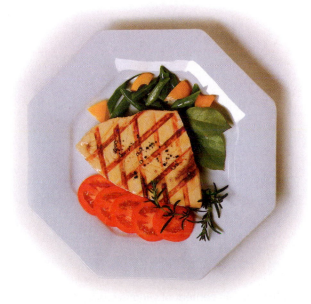

Broiled foods have less fat than fried foods.

 Trans fats and hydrogenated vegetable oils should be minimized in the diet. www.mhhe.com/phys_fit/web16 Click 09. For decades, the public has been cautioned to avoid saturated fats and foods with excessive cholesterol. Many people switched from using butter to margarine because it is made from vegetable oils that are unsaturated and contain no cholesterol. The hydrogenation process used to convert oils into solids, however, is known to produce trans fat, which is just as harmful as saturated fats, if not more so. Trans fats are known to cause increases in LDL cholesterol and have been shown to contribute to the buildup of atherosclerotic plaque. Because of these effects, it is important to try to minimize consumption of trans fats in your diet.

A number of margarines have been developed that have little or no **trans fatty acids** (e.g., Smart Balance). Because food labels will soon include trans fat content, manufacturers are experimenting with ways of cutting the amount of trans fats in other food products that include hydrogenated vegetable oil. New types of soy oils are showing promise because they require little or no hydrogenation.

Fat substitutes and neutraceuticals in food products may reduce fat consumption and lower cholesterol. www.mhhe.com/phys_fit/web16 Click 10. Olestra, approved several years ago by the FDA, is a synthetic fat substitute in foods that passes through the gastrointestinal system without being digested. Thus, foods cooked with Olestra have fewer calories. For example, a chocolate chip cookie cooked in a normal way would have 138 calories, but an Olestra cookie would have 63. To date, studies examining the effects of Olestra use have not noted any harmful effects. Still, some consumer groups warn that promotion of Olestra-containing products may make individuals more likely to snack on less energy-dense snack foods. They also express concern that Olestra inhibits absorption of many naturally occurring antioxidants that have been shown to have many beneficial effects on health.

Several other new products offer potential to modify the amount and effect of dietary fat in our diets. The first

Saturated Fats Dietary fats that are usually solid at room temperature and come primarily from animal sources.

Unsaturated Fats Monounsaturated or polyunsaturated fats that are usually liquid at room temperature and come primarily from vegetable sources.

Trans Fatty Acids Fats that result when liquid oil has hydrogen added to it to make it more solid. Hydrogenation transforms unsaturated fats so that they take on the characteristics of saturated fats, as is the case for margarine and shortening.

is a naturally occurring compound included in several margarines (Benecol and Take Control). The active ingredient in this compound (sitostanol ester) comes from pine trees and has been shown to reduce total and LDL cholesterol in the blood. Several clinical trials have confirmed that these margarines are both safe and effective in lowering cholesterol levels. The products must be used regularly to be effective and may be useful only in individuals with high levels of cholesterol. Food products that contain these medically beneficial compounds are often referred to as neutraceuticals or functional foods because they are a combination of pharmaceuticals and food. Debate continues as to whether this type of product will be regulated by the FDA as a drug or will be classified as a food supplement and not be regulated by FDA. Decisions on these products will, no doubt, influence the way similar neutraceuticals will be regulated in the future.

Some recommendations can be followed to assure healthy amounts of fat in the diet. The following list includes basic recommendations for fat content in the diet:

- Total fat in the diet should consist of no more than one third of total calories consumed (see Figure 4).
- Saturated fat in the diet should be no more than 10 percent of total calories consumed.
- Polyunsaturated and monounsaturated fats should be substituted for saturated fat in the diet.
- Dietary cholesterol should be limited to 300 milligrams per day.

The following guidelines will help you implement these recommendations:

- Substitute lean meat, fish, poultry, nonfat milk, and other low-fat dairy products for high-fat foods.
- Reduce intake of fried foods, especially those cooked in saturated fats (often true of fast-food restaurants), desserts with high levels of fat (many cookies and cakes), and dressings with high-fat ingredients.
- Limit dietary intake of foods high in cholesterol, such as egg yolks, organ meats, and shellfish.
- Use monounsaturated or polyunsaturated fats for cooking.
- Limit the amount of trans fatty acids in the diet and in cooking.
- Though two or three servings of fish per week may be prudent because of its content of omega-3 polyunsaturated oils, there is not sufficient evidence to endorse a fish oil dietary supplement.
- Be careful of the total elimination of a single food source from the diet. For example, the elimination of meat and dairy products could result in iron or calcium deficiency, especially among women and children.

Dietary Recommendations for Proteins

🌐 **Protein is the basic building block for the body, but dietary protein constitutes a relatively small amount of daily caloric intake.** www.mhhe.com/phys_fit/web16 Click 11. Proteins are often referred to as the building blocks of the body because all body cells are made of protein. Proteins are formed from 20 different **amino acids.** More than 100 proteins are made of amino acids. Eleven of these amino acids can be synthesized from other nutrients, but 9 **essential amino acids** must be obtained directly from the diet. Certain foods, called complete proteins, contain all of the essential amino acids, along with most of the others. Examples of complete proteins are meat, dairy products, and fish. Incomplete proteins contain some, but not all, of the essential amino acids. Examples of incomplete proteins are beans, nuts, and rice.

One way to identify amino acids is the *-ine* at the end of their name. For example, arginine and lysine are two of the amino acids that have received recent attention in the press. Only three of the twenty amino acids do not have the *-ine* suffix. They are aspartic acid, glutamic acid, and tryptophan.

All of the amino acids can be obtained from food, and recommended amounts are essential to good health (see Figure 6). Though the IOM recently expanded its recommendation for allowable protein in the diet, most experts agree that there are no known benefits and some possible risks to consuming diets exceptionally high in animal protein. Certain cancers and coronary heart disease risk have been associated with high dietary intake of animal protein. Researchers are not certain whether the increased risk of contracting these diseases is because of the protein itself or because diets high in animal protein are also high in fat.

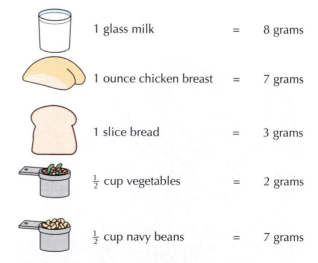

1 glass milk	=	8 grams
1 ounce chicken breast	=	7 grams
1 slice bread	=	3 grams
½ cup vegetables	=	2 grams
½ cup navy beans	=	7 grams

Figure 6 ▶ Protein content of various foods.
Source: Williams, M.

High-protein diets are also damaging on the kidneys, as the body must process a lot of extra nitrogen. Excessive protein intake can lead to urinary calcium loss, which can weaken bones and lead to osteoporosis.

Because of problems associated with excessive protein intake and health problems encountered by people who have used protein supplements, the latter are not recommended. In fact, many of the more serious health problems resulting from the consumption of dietary supplements are associated with excessive protein intake. More information concerning high-protein diets and protein supplements is included later in this concept and in the concept on managing diet and activity.

Vegetarian diets may provide sufficient protein but care must be used. www.mhhe.com/phys_fit/web16 Click 12. Vegetarian diets provide ample sources of protein as long as a variety of protein-rich food sources are included in the diet. The American Dietetics Association recently published a position stand that documents that well-planned vegetarian diets "are appropriate for all stages of the life cycle, including during pregnancy, and lactation," and can "satisfy the nutrient needs of infants, children, and adolescents." You can get enough protein as long as the variety and amounts of foods consumed are adequate. It is noted that **vegans** must supplement the diet with vitamin B-12 because this vitamin's only source is animal foods. **Lacto-ovo vegetarians** do not have the same concerns. The guidelines also emphasize the need for vegans to take care that, especially for children, adequate vitamin D and calcium are contained in the diet because most people get these nutrients from milk products.

People who eat a variety of foods, including meat, dairy products, eggs, and plants rich in protein, virtually always eat more protein than the body needs. Eating various foods assures that all essential amino acids are consumed.

Some recommendations can be followed to assure healthy amounts of protein in the diet. The following list includes basic recommendations for protein content:

- Of the three major nutrients that provide energy, protein should account for the smallest percentage of total calories consumed (see Figure 4).
- Protein in the diet should meet the RDA of 0.8 grams per kilogram (2.2 pounds) of a person's desirable weight. This is about 36 grams for a 100-pound person.
- Generally, protein in the diet should not exceed twice the RDA (1.6 grams per kilogram of a person's desirable weight).
- Vegetarians (people who severely limit the intake of animal products) must be especially careful to eat combinations of foods that assure adequate intake of essential amino acids, and vegans should supplement their diets with vitamin B-12.

The following guidelines will help you implement these recommendations:

- Consume at least two servings a day of lean meat, fish, poultry, and dairy products (especially those low in fat content) or adequate combinations of foods, such as beans, nuts, grains, and rice, in the diet.
- Dietary supplements of protein, such as tablets and powders, are not recommended.

Dietary Recommendations for Vitamins

Adequate vitamin intake is necessary to good health and wellness, but excessive vitamin intake is not necessary and can be harmful. Consuming foods containing the minimum RDA of each of the vitamins is essential to the prevention of disease and maintenance of good health (see Table 1). Consuming foods high in carotinoid and retinoid is recommended because these foods are associated with the reduced risk for some forms of cancer. Carotinoid- and retinoid-rich foods, such as green and yellow vegetables (e.g., carrots and sweet potatoes), contain high amounts of vitamin A. Diets high in vitamin C (e.g., citrus fruits and vegetables) and vitamin E (e.g., green leafy vegetables) are also associated with reduced risk for cancer, and one recent study indicated that diets high in vitamin E are associated with reduced risk for heart disease. It has been hypothesized that vitamins C and E and carotinoid-rich foods act as **antioxidants,** which help prevent cancer and other forms of disease. Most experts point out that selecting more servings from the second level of the food pyramid is

Amino Acids The twenty basic building blocks of the body that make up proteins.

Essential Amino Acids The nine basic amino acids that the human body cannot produce and that must be obtained from food sources.

Vegan Strict vegetarian, who not only excludes all forms of meat from the diet but also excludes dairy products and eggs.

Lacto-Ovo Vegetarian Vegetarian who includes dairy and eggs in the diet.

Antioxidants Vitamins that are thought to inactivate "activated oxygen molecules," sometimes called free radicals. Free radicals are naturally created by human cells but are also caused by environmental factors, such as smoke and radiation. Free radicals may cause cell damage that leads to diseases of various kinds. Antioxidants may inactivate the free radicals before they do their damage.

wise, but they express caution concerning the use of vitamin supplements.

Nevertheless, a number of respected health and wellness publications and popular books have advocated antioxidant supplements, including beta-carotene (a plant product that is converted to vitamin A in the body) and vitamins C and E, to protect the body from cell-damaging free radicals resulting from environmental pollution. These publications also have assumed that supplements of these vitamins have the same health effect as consuming food high in vitamin content. Several very recent large-scale studies have shown either no benefit from beta-carotene supplements or possible negative effects. Another recent study of over 20,000 people failed to find health benefits associated with taking a daily mixture of antioxidants, including vitamin E (600 IU), vitamin C (250 mg), and beta-carotene (20 mg). Individuals in the study had no lower risk for heart disease than participants taking the placebo. Additional studies are needed to confirm these findings in other populations, so some experts still recommend vitamin E supplements.

Although supplements have not proven to be highly effective, the benefits of antioxidants for good health are clear. It is now accepted that there may be other beneficial substances in foods that have not been isolated or that must be consumed naturally. The initial studies suggesting possible benefits of antioxidants were based on studies that compared the amounts of fruits and vegetables consumed, so the best bet is to include more fruits and vegetables in your diet. This is the recommendation in the Dietary Guidelines for Americans, which emphasize "good food" rather than food supplements. Some foods that are especially rich in vitamins and minerals are considered nutritional "all-stars" and make good dietary choices (see Table 2).

Fortification of foods has been used to ensure adequate vitamin intake in the population. National policy requires many foods to be fortified. National policy dictates that milk be fortified with vitamin D, low-fat milk with vitamins A and D, and margarine with vitamin A. These foods were selected because they are common food sources for growing children. Many common grain products are now fortified with folic acid because low folic acid levels increase the risk for birth defects in babies. Fortification is considered essential, since more than half of all women do not consume adequate amounts of folic acid in the diet during the first months of gestation (before most women even realize they are pregnant). Research has clearly demonstrated the value of fortification. One study showed that neural tube defects are 19% less likely today than in 1996 (prior to fortification). Though factors other than fortification may have contributed to this decline, the study supports the benefits of fortification for improving nutritional intakes.

Taking a daily multiple vitamin supplement may be a good idea. www.mhhe.com/phys_fit/ web16 Click 13. Sometimes supplements are needed to meet specific nutrient requirements for specific groups. For example, older people may need a vitamin D supplement if they get little exposure to sunlight, and iron supplements are often recommended for pregnant women. Vitamin

Table 2 ▶ Top Ten Antioxidant All-Stars

	C (mg)	Beta-Carotine (mg)	E (mg)	Folacin (mg)
Broccoli (1/2 cup cooked)	49	0.7	0.9	53
Cantaloupe (1 cup cubed)	68	3.1	0.3	17
Carrot (1 medium)	7	12.2	0.3	10
Kale (1/2 cup cooked)	27	2.9	3.7	9
Mango (1 medium)	57	4.8	2.3	31
Pumpkin (1/2 cup canned)	5	10.5	1.1	15
Red bell pepper (1/2 cup raw)	95	1.7	0.3	8
Spinach (1/2 cup cooked)	9	4.4	2.0	131
Strawberries (1 cup)	86	—	0.3	26
Sweet potato (1 medium, cooked)	28	14.9	5.5	26
Adult RDA or suggested intake	60	5–6	8–10	180–200

Runners-up: Brussels sprouts, all citrus fruits, tomatoes, potatoes, other berries, other leafy greens (dandelion, turnip, and mustard greens; swiss chard; arugula), cauliflower, green pepper, asparagus, peas, beets, and winter squash

Source: *University of California at Berkeley Wellness Letter*

Table 3 ▶ Issues to Consider Regarding the Use of Vitamin and Mineral Supplements

- Limit the use of supplements unless warranted because of a health problem or a specific lack of nutrients in the diet.

- If you decide that supplementation is necessary, select a multivitamin/mineral supplement that contains micronutrients in amounts close to the recommended levels (e.g., "one-a-day"-type supplements).

- If your diet is deficient in a particular mineral (e.g., calcium or iron), it may be necessary to also incorporate dietary sources or an additional mineral supplement since most multivitamins do not contain the recommended daily amount of minerals.

- Choose supplements that provide between 50 and 100 percent of the AI or RDA and avoid those that provide many times the recommended amount. The use of supplements that hype "megadoses" or vitamins and minerals can increase the risk for some unwanted nutrient interactions and possible toxic effects.

- Buy supplements from a reputable company and look for supplements that carry the U.S. Pharmocopoeia (USP) notation (www.usp.org).

Source: Based on recommendations by Manore.

supplements at or below the RDA are considered safe; however, excess doses of vitamins can cause health problems. For example, excessively high amounts of vitamin C are dangerous for the 10 percent of the population who inherit a gene related to health problems. Excessively high amounts of vitamin D are toxic, and mothers who take too much vitamin A risk birth defects in unborn children.

Eating a variety of foods (as recommended in the food guide pyramid) should ensure an adequate amount of vitamins in the diet, but the majority of the population has an inadequate diet. Vitamin intake is especially poor in individuals who avoid certain foods (e.g., limit fats or carbohydrates) or who make poor food choices (e.g., eating a lot of processed foods or few fruits and vegetables). Therefore, a daily multivitamin may be a good way to ensure adequate vitamin intake. A highly publicized article in *JAMA* recently encouraged

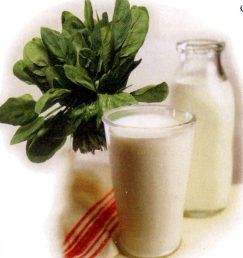

Green leafy vegetables and low-fat milk are good sources of calcium.

physicians to recommend daily multivitamin supplements as a normal part of their counseling. Some guidelines for selecting supplements are presented in Table 3.

Some recommendations can be followed to assure healthy amounts of vitamins in the diet. Vitamins in the amounts equal to the RDAs should be included in the diet each day. The following guidelines will help you implement this recommendation:

- A diet containing the food servings recommended for carbohydrates, proteins, and fats will more than meet the RDA standards.
- Extra servings of green and yellow vegetables, citrus and other fruits, and other nonanimal food sources high in fiber, vitamins, and minerals are wise (especially foods from the nutrition all-stars).
- People who eat a sound diet as described in this concept do not need a vitamin supplement, but taking a daily multivitamin is a sound dietary practice. The guidelines suggested in Table 3 should be considered before taking any supplement.
- People with special needs should seek medical advice before selecting supplements and should inform medical personnel as to the amounts and content of all supplements (vitamin and other).

Dietary Recommendations for Minerals

Adequate mineral intake is necessary for good health and wellness, but excessive mineral intake is not necessary and can be harmful. Like vitamins, minerals have no calories and provide no energy for the body. They are important in regulating various bodily functions. Two particularly important minerals are calcium and iron. Calcium is important to bone, muscle, nerve, blood development, and function and has been associated with reduced risk for heart disease. Iron is necessary for the blood to carry adequate oxygen. Other important minerals are phosphorus, which builds teeth and bones; sodium, which regulates water in the body; zinc, which aids in the healing process; and potassium, which is necessary for proper muscle function.

RDAs for minerals are established to determine the amounts of each necessary for healthy daily functioning. A sound diet provides all of the RDA for minerals. Evidence indicating that some segments of the population may be mineral-deficient have led to the establishment of health goals identifying a need to increase mineral intake for some segments of the population.

A recent National Institutes of Health (NIH) consensus statement indicates that a large percentage of Americans fail to get enough calcium in their diet and emphasizes the need for increased calcium—particularly for pregnant women, postmenopausal women, and people over sixty-five, who need 1,500 mg/day, which is higher than previous RDA amounts. The NIH has indicated that a total intake of 2,000 mg/day of calcium is safe and that adequate vitamin D in the diet is necessary for optimal calcium absorption to take place. Though getting these amounts in a calcium-rich diet is best, calcium supplementation for those not eating properly seems wise. Many multivitamins do not contain enough calcium for some classes of people, so some may want to consider additional calcium. Check with your physician or a dietitian before you consider a supplement because individual needs vary.

One national health goal is to reduce the proportion of people who consume more than recommended amounts of sodium (2,400 mg per day) and sodium chloride or table salt (6 grams a day). Some researchers have questioned the relationship between sodium intake and health, especially among apparently healthy adults. The conventional wisdom is that excessive sodium intake is especially problematic among people with high blood pressure. Salt intake up to recommended amounts is necessary for good health. Beyond those amounts, no apparent benefit exists, so restriction of salt consistent with national goals seems wise. Because many fast foods are high-salt, many people in our culture consume amounts well above the recommended levels. Currently, 79 percent of the population exceeds these amounts.

Another concern is iron deficiency among very young children and women of childbearing age. Low iron levels may be a special problem for women taking birth control pills because the combination of low iron levels and birth control pills has been associated with depression and generalized fatigue. Eating the appropriate number of servings from the food guide pyramid provides all the minerals necessary for meeting the RDA for minerals. Nutrition goals for the nation emphasize the importance of adequate servings of foods rich in calcium, such as green leafy vegetables and milk products; adequate servings of foods rich in iron, such as beans, peas, spinach, and meat; and reduced salt in the diet.

Some recommendations can be followed to assure healthy amounts of minerals in the diet. The following list includes basic recommendations for mineral content in the diet:

- Minerals in amounts equal to the RDAs should be consumed in the diet each day.
- In general, a calcium dietary supplement is not recommended for the general population; however, supplements (up to 1,000 mg/day) may be appropriate for adults who do not eat well. For postmenopausal women, a calcium supplement is recommended (up to

1,500 mg/day for those who do not eat well). A supplement may also be appropriate for people who restrict calories, but RDA values should not be exceeded unless the person consults with a registered dietitian or a physician.

- Salt should be limited in the diet to no more than 4 to 6 grams per day, and even less is desirable (3 grams). Three grams equals 1 teaspoon of table salt.

The following guidelines will help you implement these recommendations:

- A diet containing the food servings recommended for carbohydrates, proteins, and fats will more than meet the RDA standards.
- Extra servings of green and yellow vegetables, citrus and other fruits, and other nonanimal sources of foods high in fiber, vitamins, and minerals are recommended as a substitute for high-fat foods.

Dietary Recommendations for Water and Other Fluids

Water is a critical component of a healthy diet. Though water is not in the food guide pyramid because it contains no calories, provides no energy, and provides no key nutrients, it is crucial to health and survival. Water is a major component of most of the foods you eat, and more than half of all body tissues are composed of it. Regular water intake maintains water balance and is critical to many important bodily functions. Though a variety of fluid-replacement beverages are available for use during and following exercise, replacing water is the primary need.

Beverages other than water are a part of many diets. Some beverages can have an adverse effect on good health. Coffee, tea, soft drinks, and alcoholic beverages are often substituted for water in the diet. Too much caffeine consumption has been shown to cause symptoms such as irregular heartbeat in some people. Tea has not been shown to have similar effects, though this may be because tea drinkers typically consume less volume than coffee drinkers, and tea has less caffeine per cup than coffee. Both beverages contain caffeine, as do many soft drinks, though drip coffee typically contains two to three times the caffeine of a typical cola drink.

Excessive consumption of alcoholic beverages can have negative health implications because the alcohol often replaces nutrients. Excessive alcohol consumption is associated with increased risk for heart disease, high blood pressure, stroke, and osteoporosis. Long-term excessive alcoholic beverage consumption leads to cirrhosis of the liver and to increased risk for hepatitis and cancer. Alcohol consumption during pregnancy can result in low birth weight, fetal alcoholism, and other damage to the fetus. The National Dietary Guidelines indicate that alcohol used in moderation can "enhance the enjoyment of meals" and is associated with a lower risk for coronary heart disease for some individuals.

Some recommendations can be followed to assure healthy amounts of water and other fluids in the diet. The following list includes basic recommendations for water and other fluids in the diet:

- In addition to foods containing water, the average adult needs about eight glasses (8 ounces each) of water every day. Active people and those who exercise in hot environments require additional water.
- Coffee, tea, and soft drinks should not be substituted for sources of key nutrients such as low-fat milk, fruit juices, or foods rich in calcium.
- Limit daily servings of beverages containing caffeine to no more than three.
- Limit sugared soft drinks, they contain empty calories.

Technology Update

Healthy Eating Index

The general public interest in nutrition and advances in computer technology have led to a number of computerized nutrition analysis programs. Unfortunately, most programs have been either too expensive or not comprehensive enough to be of use. The U.S. Department of Agriculture's (USDA) Center for Nutrition Policy and Promotion (CNPP) has recently made its healthy eating index (HEI) available online for free use by consumers. This online dietary assessment uses the most comprehensive database of foods available and features an easy-to-use interface to analyze your foods. After providing a day's worth of dietary information, you will receive a "score" on the overall quality of your diet for that day. This "score" looks at the types and amounts of food you ate, compared with those recommended by the food guide pyramid. It also tells you how much total fat, saturated fat, cholesterol, and sodium you have in your diet. Each HEI score gives you an idea of the quality of your diet from what you ate: for one day or for up to 20 days. The HEI program is based on the healthy eating index developed by the USDA to study how well the American diet complies with the recommendations of the national guidelines and the food guide pyramid. To access this resource, go to the CNPP web page and click on Interactive Eating Index (**www.usda.gov/cnpp**).

- If you are an adult and you choose to drink alcohol, do so in moderation. The latest Dietary Guidelines for Americans indicate that moderation includes no more than one drink per day for women and no more than two drinks per day for men (one drink equals 12 ounces of regular beer, 5 ounces of wine [small glass], or one average-size cocktail [1.5 ounces of 80-proof alcohol]).

Sound Eating Practices

Consistency (with variety) is a good general rule of nutrition. Eating regular meals every day, including a good breakfast, is wise. Many studies have shown breakfast to be an important meal. One-fourth of the day's calories should be consumed at breakfast. Skipping breakfast impairs performance because blood sugar levels drop in the long period between dinner the night before and lunch the following day. Eating every 4 to 6 hours is wise.

Moderation is a good general rule of nutrition. Just as too little food can cause problems, excessive intake of various nutrients can cause problems. More is not always better. Moderation (neither too much nor too little) in choices of foods is advised.

You do not have to permanently eliminate foods that you really enjoy, but some of your favorite foods may not be among the best of choices. Enjoying special foods on occasion is part of moderation. The key is to limit choices of foods high in empty calories.

Considerable evidence has accumulated to indicate that the size of portions has increased in recent years. Large portions are featured in advertising campaigns to lure customers. Cafeteria-style restaurants (and others) sometimes offer all you can eat for a specific price, encouraging large portions. Reducing the size of portions is very important when eating out and at home (see Concept 17 for more information).

Minimizing your reliance on fast foods is a sound eating practice. Many Americans rely on fast foods as part of their normal diet. Unfortunately, many fast foods are poor nutritional choices. Many hamburgers are high in fat. French fries are high in fat because they are usually cooked in saturated fat. Even choices deemed to be more nutritious, such as chicken or fish sandwiches, are often high in fat and calories because they are cooked in fat and covered with high-fat/high-calorie sauces. Become informed about the content of fast foods before you make your selection. Some guidelines for selection of foods are provided in the concept on managing diet. Nutritional analyses for various fast foods are presented in Appendix E. Also fast foods are discussed in more detail in Concept 17.

Table 4 ▶ Fat and Cholesterol Content of Some Typical Restaurant Meals

Food Option	Calories	Total Fat (g)	Saturated Fat (g)
Prime rib, caesar salad, loaded baked potato	2,210	151	78
Fettuccini alfredo, salad with dressing and garlic bread	2,210	146	57
Burger King Double Whopper with cheese, king fries, king soft drink	2,050	95	43
Fried seafood combo with fries, coleslaw, two bisquits	2,170	130	39
BBQ baby back ribs, French fries, coleslaw	1,530	99	36
Starbucks white chocolate mocha (20 oz.), cinnamon scone	1,130	51	31
Lasagna, salad with dressing, garlic bread	1,670	102	30
Denny's meat lovers skillet, two slices of toast with margarine	1,420	105	28
KFC Extra Crisp Chicken, potato wedges, bisquit	1,420	89	28
Beef burrito, refried beans, rice, sour cream, guacamole	1,640	79	28

Source: Adapted from Jacobson and Hurley.

See Table 4 for a list of fat content in restaurant meals. Each of the meals in the table contains over 1,000 calories (about 50% of a daily needs) and more than 1.5 days' worth of saturated fat intake. Minimizing consumption of fast foods can greatly improve overall nutrition patterns.

Minimize your consumption of overly processed foods and foods high in saturated fat or hydrogenated fats. Many foods available in our grocery stores have been highly processed to enhance shelf life and convenience. In many cases, the processing of foods removes valuable food nutrients and includes other additives that may compromise overall nutrition. Processing of grains, for example, typically removes the bran and germ layers, which contain fiber and valuable minerals. In regard to additives, there has been considerable attention on the possible negative effects of high fructose corn syrup, as well as the pervasive use of hydrogenated vegetable oils containing trans fatty acids. One way to enhance overall nutrition is to minimize your reliance on processed foods. Table 5 provides comparisons of less desirable and more desirable options for each of the main food categories. To the extent possible, you should aim to choose foods in the "more desirable" category instead of those in the "less desirable" category.

Healthy snacks can be an important part of good nutrition. Snacking is not necessarily bad. For people interested in losing weight or maintaining their current weight, small snacks of appropriate foods can help fool the appetite. For people interested in gaining weight, snacks can provide additional calories. For people trying to maintain or lose weight, the calories consumed in snacks will probably necessitate limiting the calories consumed at meals. The key is proper selection of the foods for snacking.

Table 5 ▶ Comparing the Quality of Similar Food Products

Food Product	Less Desirable Option	More Desirable Option	Benefit of More Desirable Option in Nutrition Quality
Bread	White bread	Wheat bread	More fiber
Rice	White rice	Brown rice	More fiber
Juice	Sweetened juice	100% juice	More fiber and less fructose corn syrup
Fruit	Canned	Fresh	More vitamins, more fiber, less sugar
Vegetables	Canned	Fresh	More vitamins, less salt
Potatoes	French fries	Baked potato	Less saturated fat
Milk	2% milk	Skim milk	Less saturated fat
Meat	Hamburger	Lean beef	Less saturated fat
Oils	Vegetable oil	Canola oil	More monounsaturated fat
Snack food	Fried chips Crackers	Baked chips Peanuts	Less fat/calorie content, less trans fat Less trans fat

As with your total diet, the best snacks are nutritionally dense. Too many snacks are high in calories, fats, simple sugar, and salt. Check the content of snacks. Even foods sold as "healthy snacks," such as granola bars, are often high in fat and simple sugar. Some common snacks, such as chips, pretzels, and even popcorn, may be high in salt and may be cooked in fat.

Some suggestions for healthy snacks include ice milk (instead of ice cream), fresh fruits, vegetable sticks, popcorn not cooked in fat and with little or no salt, crackers, and nuts with little or no salt.

Nutrition and Physical Performance

Some basic dietary guidelines exist for active people. In general, the nutrition rules described in this concept apply to all people, whether active or sedentary, but some additional nutrition facts are important for exercisers and athletes. Because active people often expend calories in amounts considerably above normal, extra calories are needed in the diet. To avoid excess fat and protein, complex carbohydrates should constitute as much as 70 percent of total caloric intake. A higher amount of protein is generally recommended for active individuals (1.2 grams per kg of body weight) because some protein is used as an energy source during exercise. This extra amount is easily obtained through the additional calories that are consumed. Protein levels above 15 percent of the diet are typically not necessary.

Carbohydrate loading and carbohydrate replacement during exercise can enhance sustained aerobic performances. www.mhhe.com/ phys_fit/web16 Click 14. Athletes and vigorously active people must maintain a high level of readily available fuel, especially in the muscles. Adequate complex carbohydrate consumption is the best way to assure this.

Prior to an activity that will require extended duration of physical performance (more than 1 hour in length, such as a marathon), **carbohydrate loading** can be useful. Carbohydrate loading is accomplished by resting 1 or 2 days before the event and eating a higher than normal amount of complex carbohydrates. This helps to build up maximum levels of stored carbohydrate (**glycogen**) in the muscles and liver so it can be used during exercise. The key in carbohydrate loading is not necessarily to overeat but, rather, to eat a higher percentage of carbohydrates than normal.

Ingesting carbohydrate solutions during sustained exercise can also aid performance by preventing or forestalling muscle glycogen depletion. Drinking fluids that have no more than 6 to 8 percent sugar helps prevent dehydration and replenishes energy stores. Fluid-replacement drinks containing 6 to 8 percent carbohydrates are very helpful in

preventing dehydration and replacing energy stores. A number of companies also make concentrated carbohydrate gels that deliver carbohydrates (generally 80 percent complex, 20 percent simple) in a format that your body can absorb quickly for energy. Examples are PowerGel and Gu. Energy bars, such as Powerbars and Clif bars, are also commonly used during or after exercise to enhance energy stores. The Powerbar version provides about 100 calories of carbohydrates derived from maltodextrin,

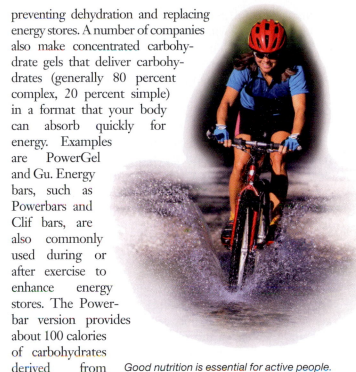
Good nutrition is essential for active people.

brown rice, and oat bran to provide a slow release of energy during exercise. The various carbohydrate supplements have been shown to be effective for exercise sessions lasting over an hour and are good for replacing glycogen stores after exercise. Studies show that consuming carbohydrates 15 to 30 minutes following exercise can aid in rapid replenishment of muscle glycogen, which may enhance future performance or training sessions.

These supplements have little benefit for shorter bouts of exercise. Because they contain considerable calories, they are not recommended for individuals primarily interested in weight control.

The timing may be more important than the makeup of a pre-event meal. If you are racing or doing high-level exercise early in the morning, eat a small meal prior to starting. Eat about 3 hours before competition or heavy exercise to allow time for digestion. Generally, athletes can make their food selections on the basis of past experience, but easily digested carbohydrates are best. Generally, fat intake should be minimal because it digests more slowly; proteins and high-cellulose foods should be kept to a moderate amount prior to prolonged

---

Carbohydrate Loading Extra consumption of complex carbohydrates in the days prior to a long, sustained performance.

Glycogen A source of energy stored in the muscles and liver that is necessary for sustained physical activity.

events to avoid urinary and bowel excretion. Drinking 2 or 3 cups of liquid will ensure adequate hydration.

Consuming simple carbohydrates (sugar, candy) within an hour or two of an event is not recommended because it may cause an insulin response that results in weakness and fatigue, or it may cause stomach distress, cramps, or nausea.

High protein diets for active people and athletes have been questioned by leading health, sports, and nutrition organizations. The American College of Sports Medicine (ACSM), the American Dietetics Association (ADA), and several other groups have challenged the soundness of exceptionally high protein diets for athletes. Most athletes need more carbohydrates in their diet, not fewer. Experts from more than a few organizations suggest that protein amounts equal to 10 to 15 percent of the total calories (as recommended by the USDA) are adequate for active people. Because athletes and active people consume more calories than the typical person, they also get extra protein (more total calories of protein) than the typical person. Contrary to popular opinion, extra protein in the diet (more than 15 percent) does not result in extra muscle development.

Some experts suggest that consuming more than 15 percent of total calories from protein (consistent with IOM recommendations) can be safe when diet is well managed to insure a proper balance of nutrients. Still most experts recommend consuming protein in amounts consistent with USDA recommendations.

People who are interested in enhancing physical performance are especially subject to nutrition quackery. A food or nutrition product thought to enhance performance is considered to be an **ergogenic aid.** Many so-called ergogenic aids can be classified as quack products because they do not enhance performance as promised and are exceptionally expensive. In some cases, so-called performance-enhancing supplements are dangerous to health and wellness (see Concept 7 for more information on ergogenic aids).

Recent legislation designed to regulate food supplements has not been effective in protecting the consumer. The Dietary Supplements Health and Education Act was passed in 1994. It was considered by many experts to be a compromise between health food manufacturers who wanted no regulation of dietary supplements (such as vitamins, minerals, proteins, and herbs) and those who wanted strict control of these substances. Many nutrition experts now feel that the act is responsible for an explosion in sales of products that have not been proven to be effective.

> **Ergogenic Aid** In this concept, a nutritional supplement claimed by its promoters to improve performance.

Strategies for Action

An analysis of your current diet is a good first step in making future decisions about what you eat. Many experts recommend keeping a log of what you eat over an extended period of time, so you can determine the overall quality of your diet. In Lab 16A, you will have an opportunity to analyze your diet over several days. In addition to computing the amount of carbohydrates, fats, and proteins, you will also be able to monitor your consumption of fruits and vegetables. A number of online tools and personal software programs can make dietary calculations for you and provide a more comprehensive report of nutrient intake. It is important to know how to monitor your own diet, but these programs are encouraged for additional information.

Making small changes in diet patterns can have a big impact. Experts in nutrition emphasize the importance of making small changes in your diet over time rather than trying to make comprehensive changes at one time. Try cutting back on sweets or soda. Simply adding a bit more fruit and vegetables to your diet can lead to major changes in overall diet quality. In Lab 16B, you will be given the opportunity to compare a "nutritious diet" to a "favorite diet." Doing the analyses of two different daily meal plans will help you get a more accurate picture as to whether foods you think are nutritious actually meet current healthy lifestyle goals.

Study Resources

Check out additional online study resources for this concept in the Student Edition of the Online Learning Center at www.mhhe.com/corbin13e.

Web Resources

American Dietetic Association **www.eatright.org**
Berkeley Nutrition Services **www.nutritionquest.com**
Center for Nutrition Policy and Promotion
 www.usda.gov/cnpp
Center for Science in the Public Interest **www.cspinet.org**
Food and Drug Administration (FDA) **www.fda.gov**
Food Safety Database **www.foodsafety.gov**
International Food Information Council **www.ific.org**
National Academy of Sciences **www.nas.edu**
National Nutrition Summit Database
 www.nlm.nih.gov/pubs/cbm/nutritionsummit.html
Nutrition.gov **www.nutrition.gov**
Office of Dietary Supplements **http://ods.od.nih.gov**
U.S. Department of Agriculture (USDA) **www.usda.gov**
USDA Food and Nutrition Information Center
 www.nal.usda.gov/fnic

 ## Suggested Readings

Additional reference materials for Concept 16 are available at **www.mhhe.com/phys_fit/web16 Click 15.**

American Dietetic Association 1997. Vegetarian diets: Position of the American Dietetic Association. *Journal of the American Dietetic Association* 97:1317–1321.

American Dietetic Association. 1998. Fat replacers: Position of the American Dietetic Association. *Journal of the American Dietetic Association* 98:463–468.

American Dietetic Association. 2000. *The Health Professional's Guide to Popular Dietary Supplements.* Chicago, IL: ADA.

Fletcher, R. H., and K. M. Fairfield. 2002. Vitamins for chronic disease prevention in adults: Clinical applications. *Journal of the American Medical Association* 287(23):3127–3130.

Food and Nutrition Board, Institute of Medicine. 2002. *Dietary Reference Intakes for Energy, Carbohydrates, Fiber, Fat, Protein, and Amino Acids (Macronutrients).* Washington, DC: National Academy Press.

Gaesser, G. A. (2002). *Big Fat Lies: The Truth about Your Weight and Your Health.* Carlsbad, CA: Gurze Books.

Goldberg, J. P., et al. 2004. The obesity crisis: Don't blame it on the pyramid. *Journal of the American Dietetic Association* 104(7):1141–1147.

Jacobson, M. F., and J. Hurley. 2002. *Restaurant Confidential.* New York: Workman.

Krauss R. M., et al. 2000. AHA dietary guidelines revision 2000: A statement for health-care professionals from the Nutrition Committee of the American Heart Association. *Circulation* 102:2284–2299.

Manore, M. M. 2001. Vitamins and minerals. Part I: How much do you need? *ACSM's Health and Fitness Journal* 5(1):33–36.

Manore, M. M. 2001. Vitamins and minerals. Part II: Who needs supplements? *ACSM's Health and Fitness Journal* 5(3):33–36.

Manore, M. M. 2001. Vitamins and minerals. Part III: Can you get too much? *ACSM's Health and Fitness Journal* 5(5):26–28.

Manore, M. M. 2003. Cultivating good nutrition habits: How can we maintain a healthy body weight throughout life? *ACSM's Health and Fitness Journal* 7(3):24–25.

Manore, M. M. 2003. New Dietary Reference Intakes set for energy, carbohydrates, fiber, fat, fatty acids, cholesterol, proteins, and amino acids. *ACSM's Health and Fitness Journal* 7(1):25–27.

Manore, M. M. 2004. Nutrition and physical activity: Fueling the active individual. *President's Council on Physical Fitness and Sports Research Digest* 5(1):1–8.

Manore, M. M., S. I. Barr, and G. E. Butterfield. 2001. Position of the American Dietetic Association: Nutrition and athletic performance. *Journal of the American Dietetic Association* 5(1):1543–1556.

Millen, A. E., et al. 2004. Use of vitamin, mineral, nonvitamin, and nonmineral supplements in the United States: The 1987, 1992, and 2000 National Health Interview Survey results. *Journal of the American Dietetic Association* 104(8):942–950.

Schlosser, E. 2001. *Fast Food Nation: The Dark Side of the All-American Meal.* New York: Houghton Mifflin.

U.S. Department of Agriculture and U.S. Department of Health and Human Services. 2000. *Report of the Dietary Guidelines Advisory Committee.* Washington, DC: USDA and USDHHS.

U.S. Department of Health and Human Services. 2000. *Healthy People 2010.* 2nd ed. With Understanding and Improving Health and Objectives for Improving Health, 2 vols. Washington, DC: U.S. Government Printing Office.

Vivekananthan, D. P. 2003. Megadoses of E do not work and betacarotine can be dangerous: Use of antioxidant vitamins for the prevention of cardiovascular disease: Meta-analysis of randomised trials. *Lancet* 361(9374):2017–2023.

Weinstein, S. J., et al. 2004. Healthy eating index scores are associated with blood nutrient concentrations in the third national health and nutrition examination survey. *Journal of the American Dietetic Association* 104(4):576–584.

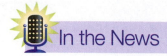

In the News

The Healthy Eating Pyramid

The food guide pyramid has been highly publicized and promoted as a guide to healthy eating. It was intended to serve as a tool to help consumers implement the Dietary Guidelines for Americans, published jointly by the USDA and the U.S. Department of Health and Human Services. As noted earlier, some health experts have questioned some of the underlying premises of the pyramid and it will likely be updated in 2005 as part of the normal 5 year revision process (monitor **www.usda.gov/cnpp/pyramid.html** for details and developments).

The most notable limitation is the lack of attention to the quality of food items at each level of the pyramid. Carbohydrates are considered to be the base of the food pyramid, but emphasis should be placed on high-quality complex carbohydrates rather than simple carbohydrates. Not all fats are equal, either. Many monounsaturated fats are beneficial to your health (by improving blood lipid profiles), while saturated fats are known to increase cholesterol levels (particularly LDL cholesterol).

The Nutrition Source team from the Department of Nutrition at the Harvard School of Public Health has proposed an alternative food guide pyramid that provides a more appropriate, research-based model of healthy eating. The model distinguishes among types of carbohydrates, fats, and proteins and advocates strongly for increased consumption of fruits and vegetables by the American public. A major distinction in the Healthy Eating Pyramid is that it sits atop a foundation of daily physical activity and weight control. This is considered fundamental to diet because they strongly influence your chances of staying healthy and they directly affect what and how you eat and how your food affects you. Other specific "bricks" in the pyramid are

- Whole-grain foods (at most meals)
- Plant oils
- Vegetables (in abundance) and fruits (two to three times per day)
- Fish, poultry, and eggs (zero to two times per day)
- Nuts and legumes (one to three times per day)
- Dairy or calcium supplement (one to two times per day)
- Red meat and butter (use sparingly)
- White rice, white bread, potatoes, pasta, and sweets (use sparingly)
- Multiple vitamin (daily)
- Alcohol (in moderation)

For additional information, visit the Nutrition Source website at **http://www.hsph.harvard.edu/nutritionsource/.**

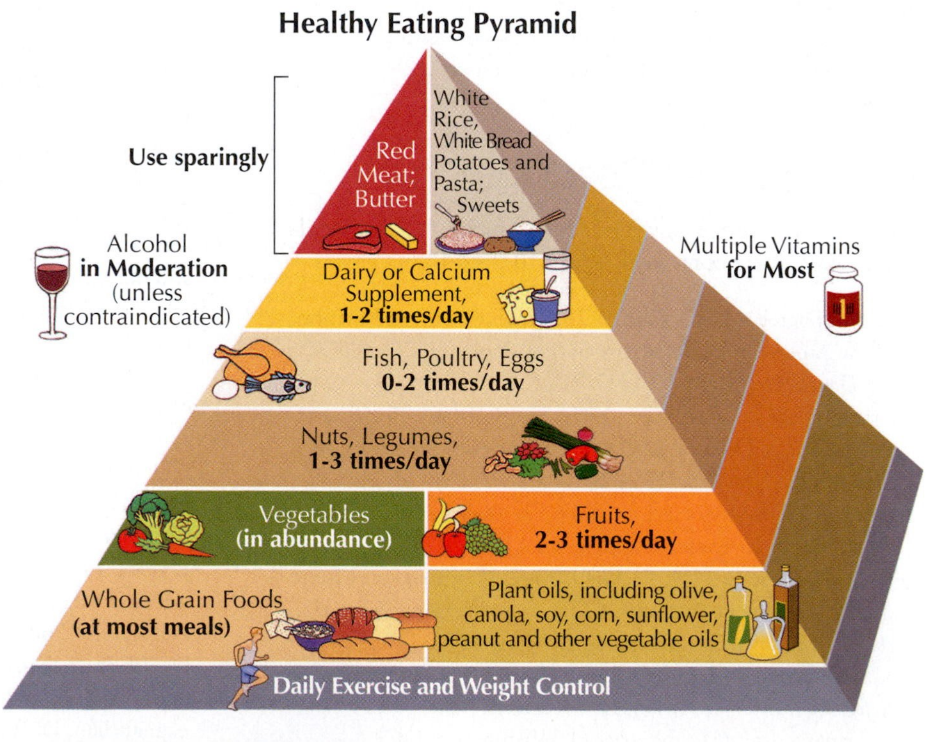

Healthy Eating Pyramid

Figure 7 ▶ Healthy Eating Pyramid
Source: Nutrition Source Harvard School of Public Health.

Late Breaking News: Dietary Guidelines for Americans 2005

On January 12, 2005 the Department of Agriculture (USDA) and the Department of Health and Human Services jointly published new Dietary Guidelines. Like the content of this concept, the new guidelines focus on making smart choices from all food groups, finding a balance between food and physical activity, and getting the most nutrition out of your calories. For more information visit the following website: **www.healthierus.gov/dietaryguidelines**. Additional detail can also be found at the 'On the Web' feature for this concept (**www.mhhe.com/phys_fit/web16, click 01**).

It is expected that the new guidelines will result in changes in the current food guide pyramid since the 2005 guidelines focus on the need for more whole grains, more consumption of fruit, less saturated fat and salt, and increased daily physical activity. All of these are reflected in the Healthy Eating Pyramid above.

Lab 16A Nutrition Analysis

Name	Section	Date

Purpose: To learn to keep a dietary log, to determine the nutritional quality of your diet, to determine your average daily caloric intake, and to determine necessary changes in eating habits

Procedures

1. Record your dietary intake for 2 days using the Daily Diet Record sheets (see page 329). Record intake for one weekday and one weekend day. You may wish to make copies of the Record sheet for future use.
2. Include the actual foods eaten, the amount (size of portion in teaspoons, tablespoons, cups, ounces, or other standard units of measurement). Be sure to include all drinks (coffee, tea, soft drinks, etc.). Include *all* foods eaten, including sauces, gravies, dressings, toppings, spreads, and so on. Determine your calorie consumption for each of the 2 days. Use the Calorie Guide to Common Foods in Appendix C or visit the Healthy Eating Index at **www.usda.gov/CNPP.**
3. List the number of servings from each food group by each food choice.
4. Estimate the proportion of complex carbohydrate, simple carbohydrate, protein, and fat in each meal and in snacks, as well as for the total day.
5. Answer the questions in Chart 1 (page 328), using information for a typical day based on the Daily Diet Record sheets. Score 1 point for each yes answer on Chart 1 (page 328). Use Chart 2 to rate your dietary habits. Circle the appropriate rating.

Results

Record the number of calories consumed for each of the 2 days.

Weekday [   ] calories   Weekend [   ] calories

Conclusions and Implications: In several sentences, discuss your diet as recorded in this lab. Explain any changes in your eating habits that may be necessary. Comment on whether the days you surveyed are typical of your normal diet.

Chart 1 ▶ Dietary Habits Questionnaire

Yes	No	Answer questions based on a typical day (use your Daily Diet Records to help).
◯	◯	1. Do you eat three normal-sized meals?
◯	◯	2. Do you eat a healthy breakfast?
◯	◯	3. Do you eat lunch regularly?
◯	◯	4. Does your diet contain about 55–60 percent carbohydrates with a high concentration of fiber?*
◯	◯	5. Are less than one-fourth of the carbohydrates you eat simple carbohydrates?
◯	◯	6. Does your diet contain 10–15 percent protein?*
◯	◯	7. Does your diet contain no more than 30 percent fat?*
◯	◯	8. Do you limit the amount of saturated fat in your diet (no more than 10 percent)?
◯	◯	9. Do you limit salt intake to acceptable amounts?
◯	◯	10. Do you get adequate amounts of vitamins in your diet without a supplement?
◯	◯	11. Do you typically eat 6 to 11 servings from the bread, cereal, rice, and pasta group of foods?
◯	◯	12. Do you typically eat 3 to 5 servings of vegetables?
◯	◯	13. Do you typically eat 2 to 4 servings of fruits?
◯	◯	14. Do you typically eat 2 to 3 servings from the milk, yogurt, and cheese group of foods?
◯	◯	15. Do you typically eat 2 to 3 servings from the meat, poultry, fish, beans, eggs, and nuts group of foods?
◯	◯	16. Do you drink adequate amounts of water?
◯	◯	17. Do you get adequate minerals in your diet without a supplement?
◯	◯	18. Do you limit your caffeine and alcohol consumption to acceptable levels?
◯	◯	19. Is your average calorie consumption reasonable for your body size and for the amount of calories you normally expend?
		Total number of Yes answers

*Based on USDA standards.

Chart 2 ▶ Dietary Habits Rating Scale

Score	Rating
18–19	Very good
15–17	Good
13–14	Marginal
12 or less	Poor

Daily Diet Record

Day 1

Breakfast Food	Amount (cups, tsp., etc.)	Calories	Food Servings Bread/Cereal	Fruit/Veg.	Milk/Meat	Fat/Sweet	Estimated Meal Calorie %
							☐ % Protein
							☐ % Fat
							☐ % Complex carbohydrate
							☐ % Simple carbohydrate
							100% Total
Meal Total							

Lunch Food	Amount (cups, tsp., etc.)	Calories	Bread/Cereal	Fruit/Veg.	Milk/Meat	Fat/Sweet	Estimated Meal Calorie %
							☐ % Protein
							☐ % Fat
							☐ % Complex carbohydrate
							☐ % Simple carbohydrate
							100% Total
Meal Total							

Dinner Food	Amount (cups, tsp., etc.)	Calories	Bread/Cereal	Fruit/Veg.	Milk/Meat	Fat/Sweet	Estimated Meal Calorie %
							☐ % Protein
							☐ % Fat
							☐ % Complex carbohydrate
							☐ % Simple carbohydrate
							100% Total
Meal Total							

Snack Food	Amount (cups, tsp., etc.)	Calories	Bread/Cereal	Fruit/Veg.	Milk/Meat	Fat/Sweet	Estimated Snack Calorie %
							☐ % Protein
							☐ % Fat
							☐ % Complex carbohydrate
							☐ % Simple carbohydrate
							100% Total
Meal Total							
Daily Totals							
		Calories	Servings	Servings	Servings	Servings	

Estimated Daily Total Calorie %

☐ % Protein
☐ % Fat
☐ % Complex carbohydrate
☐ % Simple carbohydrate
100% Total

Daily Diet Record

Day 2

Breakfast Food	Amount (cups, tsp., etc.)	Calories	Food Servings				Estimated Meal Calorie %
			Bread/Cereal	Fruit/Veg.	Milk/Meat	Fat/Sweet	
							☐ % Protein
							☐ % Fat
							☐ % Complex carbohydrate
							☐ % Simple carbohydrate
							100% Total
Meal Total	✕						

Lunch Food	Amount (cups, tsp., etc.)	Calories	Food Servings				Estimated Meal Calorie %
			Bread/Cereal	Fruit/Veg.	Milk/Meat	Fat/Sweet	
							☐ % Protein
							☐ % Fat
							☐ % Complex carbohydrate
							☐ % Simple carbohydrate
							100% Total
Meal Total	✕						

Dinner Food	Amount (cups, tsp., etc.)	Calories	Food Servings				Estimated Meal Calorie %
			Bread/Cereal	Fruit/Veg.	Milk/Meat	Fat/Sweet	
							☐ % Protein
							☐ % Fat
							☐ % Complex carbohydrate
							☐ % Simple carbohydrate
							100% Total
Meal Total	✕						

Snack Food	Amount (cups, tsp., etc.)	Calories	Food Servings				Estimated Snack Calorie %
			Bread/Cereal	Fruit/Veg.	Milk/Meat	Fat/Sweet	
							☐ % Protein
							☐ % Fat
							☐ % Complex carbohydrate
							☐ % Simple carbohydrate
							100% Total
Meal Total							**Estimated Daily Total Calorie %**
Daily Totals	✕						☐ % Protein
		Calories	Servings	Servings	Servings	Servings	☐ % Fat
							☐ % Complex carbohydrate
							☐ % Simple carbohydrate
							100% Total

Lab 16B Selecting Nutritious Foods

Name	**Section**	**Date**

Purpose: To learn to select a nutritious diet, to determine the nutritive value of favorite foods, and to compare nutritious and favorite foods in terms of nutrient content

Procedures

1. Select a favorite breakfast, lunch, and dinner from the foods list in Appendix D. Include between-meal snacks with the nearest meal. If you cannot find foods you would normally choose, select those most similar to choices you might make.
2. Select a breakfast, lunch, and dinner from foods you feel would make the most nutritious meals. Include between-meal snacks with the nearest meal.
3. Record your "favorite foods" and "nutritious foods" on page 332. Record the calories for proteins, carbohydrates, and fats for each of the foods you choose.
4. Total each column for the "favorite" and the "nutritious" meals.
5. Determine the percentages of your total calories that are protein, carbohydrate, and fat by dividing each column total by the total number of calories consumed.
6. Comment on what you learned in the Conclusions and Implications section.

Results: Record your results below. Calculate percent of calories from each source by dividing total calories into calories from each food source (protein, carbohydrates, or fat).

Food Selection Results

Source	Favorite Foods Calories	Favorite Foods % of Total Calories	Nutritious Foods Calories	Nutritious Foods % of Total Calories
Protein				
Carbohydrates				
Fat				
Total 100%		100%		100%

Conclusions and Implications: In several sentences, discuss differences you found between your nutritious diet and your favorite diet. Discuss the quality of your nutritious diet as well as other things you learned from doing this lab.

"Favorite" versus "Nutritious" Food Choices for Three Daily Meals

Breakfast Favorite					Breakfast Nutritious				
Food No.	Cal.	Pro. Cal.	Car. Cal.	Fat Cal.	**Food No.**	Cal.	Pro. Cal.	Car. Cal.	Fat Cal.
Totals					Totals				

Lunch Favorite					Lunch Nutritious				
Food No.	Cal.	Pro. Cal.	Car. Cal.	Fat Cal.	**Food No.**	Cal.	Pro. Cal.	Car. Cal.	Fat Cal.
Totals					Totals				

Dinner Favorite					Dinner Nutritious				
Food No.	Cal.	Pro. Cal.	Car. Cal.	Fat Cal.	**Food No.**	Cal.	Pro. Cal.	Car. Cal.	Fat Cal.
Totals					Totals				
Daily Totals (Calories)					Daily Totals (Calories)				
Daily % of Total Calories					Daily % of Total Calories				

Managing Diet and Activity for Healthy Body Fatness

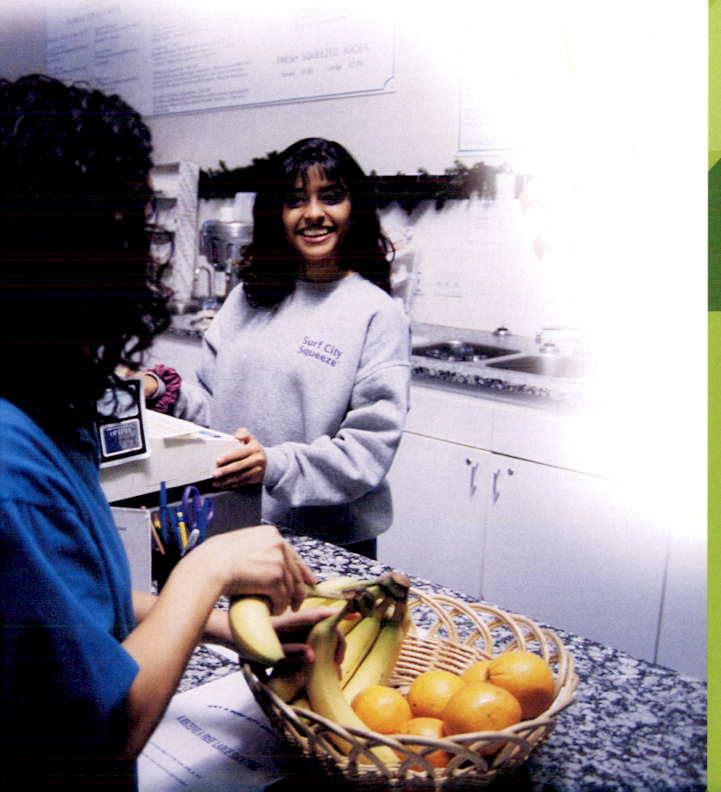

There are various management strategies for eating and performing physical activity that are useful in achieving and maintaining optimal body composition.

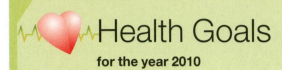

Health Goals

for the year 2010

- Increase prevalence of a healthy weight.

- Reduce prevalence of overweight.

- Increase proportion of people who meet national dietary guidelines.

- Increase adoption and maintenance of daily physical activity.

- Increase teaching about nutrition and physical activity.

With over 60 percent of the population classified as overweight, it is pretty clear that weight control is a vexing problem for most Americans. Experts have concluded that the recent trends in obesity are due in large part to environmental influences that make it difficult to manage body fat levels. The term *obesigenic* has been used to describe the elements of our environment that collectively promote eating and inactivity. The model in Figure 1 shows the various aspects of the obesigenic environment and how they influence the energy balance equation.

The essence of the model is that we are continually confronted with environments that make it easy to consume large quantities of energy-dense food. We also live in an environment in which most physical tasks are no longer necessary and people have less apparent time available for active recreation. Small increases in energy intake combined with decreases in energy expenditure lead to the storage of fat. Awareness of these environmental influences is important if we desire to maintain a healthy body fat level and weight.

It is well documented that many Americans are unhappy with their weight and are on a diet. Too often the focus is on appearance rather than health and on weight loss rather than fat loss. In attempts to lose weight, the dietary (energy intake) side of the energy balance equation is typically emphasized. The best scientific evidence suggests that the energy expenditure side of the equation is equally important. Physical activity results in

true fat loss rather than loss in weight accompanied by loss in muscle mass. In addition physical activity promotes fitness and it has been well established that fitness is more important than being thin if lower risk of chronic disease is the goal. The focus in this concept is on lifestyle patterns that will assist with losing body fat rather than weight. Guidelines for maintaining healthy body fat levels over time are also presented.

Factors Influencing Weight and Fat Control

The first step in fat control is establishing realistic goals. Too many teens and adults, both men and women, establish unrealistic goals for their physical

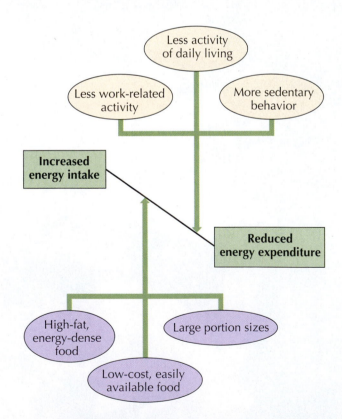

Figure 1 ▶ Factors contributing to increased energy intake and reduced energy expenditure.

Source: Model adapted from Hill et al.

appearance. Fat, weight, and body proportions are all factors that can be changed, but people often set standards for themselves that are difficult, if not impossible, to achieve. Starting with small goals is preferable to establishing goals that seem impossible to accomplish. This necessitates developing an understanding of your own body proportions as well as your body fatness. Unrealistic goals may result in eating disorders, failure to meet goals, or failure to maintain fat loss over time.

Regular physical activity is essential for long-term weight control. One cause of creeping obesity is a reduction in physical activity. By maintaining an active lifestyle, you can burn off extra calories, keep your body's metabolism high, and prevent the decline in basal metabolic rate that typically occurs with aging (due to reduced muscle mass). All types of physical activity can be beneficial for weight control. Since aerobic exercise can be maintained for a long period, it allows you to expend large numbers of calories and therefore is the best type of physical activity for fat loss and maintenance. Strength training can contribute to weight control by increasing muscle mass and helping to increase metabolic rate.

Despite the documented benefits, few people trying to lose weight report being physically active. A recent state-based survey determined that approximately one-half of individuals trying to lose weight do not engage in any physical activity and only 15 percent report exercising regularly. The challenges many people experience with weight control may be an indirect reflection of the challenges people face in trying to be more active. Although being physically active cannot ensure that you will become as thin as you desire, it may allow you to attain a body size that is appropriate for your genetics and body type.

Getting regular activity in our society is sometimes more difficult than it would seem. Numerous labor-saving devices, including garage openers, escalators, moving sidewalks, motorized lawn mowers, and golf carts, have made life, work, and play easier with little or no activity. Even the increase in e-mail in offices has limited the amount of activity that office workers obtain. For effective weight management, you must find ways to keep activity as a regular part of your lifestyle.

Awareness and dietary restraint are needed to avoid excess caloric intake. www.mhhe.com/phys_fit/web17 Click 01. Consumers are able to buy food almost anywhere. For example, convenience stores and food courts in malls allow people to snack more readily during the day. To provide more apparent value to consumers, restaurants and convenience stores have continued to provide larger portion sizes. *Super sizing* and *Value Meals* are commonly used terms "for getting more food for your money." In the 1960s, the average serving of

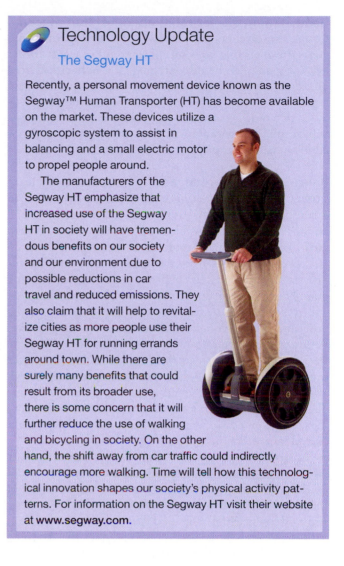

Technology Update

The Segway HT

Recently, a personal movement device known as the Segway™ Human Transporter (HT) has become available on the market. These devices utilize a gyroscopic system to assist in balancing and a small electric motor to propel people around.

The manufacturers of the Segway HT emphasize that increased use of the Segway HT in society will have tremendous benefits on our society and our environment due to possible reductions in car travel and reduced emissions. They also claim that it will help to revitalize cities as more people use their Segway HT for running errands around town. While there are surely many benefits that could result from its broader use, there is some concern that it will further reduce the use of walking and bicycling in society. On the other hand, the shift away from car traffic could indirectly encourage more walking. Time will tell how this technological innovation shapes our society's physical activity patterns. For information on the Segway HT visit their website at **www.segway.com.**

McDonald's French fries was about 200 calories. Today, a large serving provides 540 calories and the "super size" approximately 610 calories. Similarly, consumers can now purchase soft drinks in volumes up to 64 ounces rather than a standard 12- to 16-ounce drink. Choosing normal-sized meals and drinks is one way to avoid excess calories in your diet (see Figure 2).

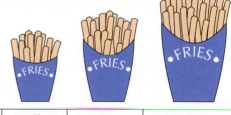

Size	Small	Large	Super Size
Calories (kcal)	450	540	610

Figure 2 ▶ Comparison of added calories in different sizes of French fries.

Behavioral goals are more effective than outcome goals. Researchers have shown that setting **outcome goals,** or goals that set a specific amount of weight or fat loss (or gain), can be discouraging. If a **behavioral goal** of eating a reasonable number of calories per day and expending a reasonable number of calories in exercise is met, outcome goals will be achieved. Most experts believe that behavioral goals work better than weight or fat loss goals, especially in the short term.

Short-term goals can help you reach long-term goals. Individuals wanting to lose weight often want to accomplish their goals too quickly. Losing 20 or 30 pounds can seem impossible, but breaking this long-term goal down into manageable short-term goals is more effective. Guidelines from the ACSM and other organizations recommend maximum weight loss goals of 1 to 2 pounds per week. Efforts to lose weight faster than that will typically lead to frustration or the cessation of the program. The best way to determine if your goals are reasonable is if they can be maintained for a lifetime. Because your weight can fluctuate with the amount of water lost or retained, daily monitoring of weight can also be discouraging. Weight may drop dramatically one day because of water loss and increase the next. Care must be taken not to worry too much about daily weight or fat losses or gains.

To get accurate assessments of true changes in body fatness, weight and body fatness assessments should not be done too frequently. Drinking adequate amounts of water is important to people who are restricting calories and will reduce the risk for false changes in body fat. Measuring weight is best done early in the morning before you have eaten breakfast.

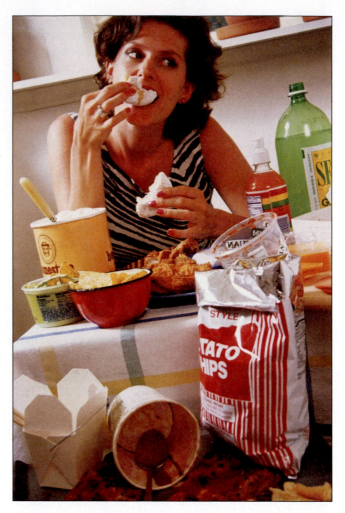

Foods with empty calories have few nutrients and often are relatively high in calorie content.

Guidelines for Losing Body Fat

Changes in eating patterns can be effective in fat loss. www.mhhe.com/phys_fit/web17 Click 02. For successful weight loss or maintenance of healthy weight, it is important to adopt healthy behaviors that can be maintained over time. The following list highlights a few suggested dietary habits that may be helpful.

- Restrict calories in moderate amounts per day rather than make large reductions in daily caloric intake.
- Eat less fat. Research shows that reduction of the fat in the diet not only results in fewer calories consumed (fats have more than twice the calories per gram as carbohydrates or proteins) but in greater body fat loss as well.
- Severely restrict **empty calories,** which provide little nutrition and can account for an excessive amount of your daily caloric intake. Examples of these foods are candy (often high in simple sugar) and potato chips (often fried in saturated fat).

- Increase complex carbohydrates. Foods high in fiber, such as fresh fruits and vegetables, contain few calories for their volume. They are nutritious and filling, and they are especially good foods for a fat loss program.
- Learn the difference between craving and hunger. Hunger is a physiological phenomenon that is a result of the body's need to supply energy to sustain life. A craving is simply a desire to eat something, sometimes a food you do not particularly like. When you feel the urge to eat, you may want to ask yourself, Is this real hunger or a craving? Hunger is accompanied by growling of the stomach and is most likely to occur after long periods without food. If you have the urge to eat soon after a meal, it is probably from craving, not hunger.
- Develop personal habits that can help you make better dietary choices when eating at restaurants, work, and special occasions. Making good selections when purchasing and preparing food are also important. See Table 1 for suggestions.

Table 1 ▶ Guidelines for Healthy Shopping and Eating in a Variety of Settings	
Guidelines for Shopping	• Shop from a list to avoid the purchase of foods that contain empty calories and other foods that will tempt you to overeat. • Shop with a friend to avoid buying unneeded foods. For this technique to work, the other person must be sensitive to your goals. In some cases, a friend can have a bad, rather than a good, influence. • Shop on a full stomach to avoid the temptations of snacking on and buying junk food. • Check the labels for contents of foods to avoid foods that are excessively high in fat or saturated fat.
Guidelines for How You Eat	• When you eat, do nothing else but eat. If you watch television, read, or do some other activity while you eat, you may be unaware of what you have eaten. • Eat slowly. Taste your food. Pause between bites. Chew slowly. Do not take the next bite until you have swallowed what you have in your mouth. Periodically take a longer pause. Be the last one finished eating. • Do not eat food you do not want. Some people do not want to waste food, so they clean their plate even when they feel full. • Follow an eating schedule. Eating at regular meal times can help you avoid snacking. If meals are spaced equally throughout the day, it can help reduce appetite. • Leave the table after eating to avoid taking extra unwanted bites and servings. • Eat meals of equal size. Some people try to restrict calories at one or two meals to save up for a big meal. • Eating several *small* meals helps avoid hunger (fools the appetite) and helps from losing control at one meal. • Avoid second servings. Limit your intake to one moderate serving. If second servings are taken, make them one-half the size of first servings. • Limit servings of salad dressings and condiments (e.g., catsup). These are often high in fat and calories and can amount to greater calorie consumption than is expected.
Guidelines for Controlling the Home Environment	• Store food out of sight. Avoid containers that allow you to see food. It is especially important to limit the accessibility of foods that tempt you and foods with empty calories. Foods that are out of sight are out of mouth. • Do your eating in designated areas only. Designate areas such as the kitchen and dining room as eating areas, so you do not snack elsewhere. It is especially easy to eat too much while watching television. • If you snack, eat foods high in complex carbohydrates and low in fats, such as fresh fruits and carrot sticks. • Freeze leftovers. Leftover foods are often tempting to eat. Freezing them so that it takes preparation to eat them will help you avoid temptation.
Guidelines for Controlling the Work Environment	• Take food from home rather than eating from vending machines or catering trucks. • Do not eat while working but take your lunch as a break. Do something active during other breaks. For example, take a walk. • Avoid sources of food provided by co-workers—for example, food in work rooms, such as birthday cakes, or candy in jars. • Have drinking water or low-calorie drinks available to substitute for snacks.
Guidelines for Eating on Special Occasions	• Practice ways to refuse food. Knowing exactly what to say will help you not get talked into eating something you do not want. • Eat before you go out so you are not as hungry at parties and events. • Do not stand near food sources and distract yourself if tempted to eat when you are not really hungry. • Limit servings of nonbasic parts of the meal. It is easy to consume large numbers of calories on alcohol, soft drinks, appetizers, and desserts. Limit these items.
Guidelines for Eating Out at Restaurants	• Try to make healthy selections from the menu. Choose chicken without skin, fish, or lean cuts of meat. Grilled or broiled options are better than fried. Choose healthier options for dessert, as many decadent desserts can have more calories than the whole dinner. • Limit the use of sauces and condiments, such as butter, margarine, catsup, mayonnaise, and salad dressings. Asking for the condiments on the side allows you to determine how much to put on. • Do not feel compelled to eat everything on your plate. Many restaurants serve exceptionally large portions to try to please the customers. • Order à la carte rather than full meals to avoid multiple courses and servings. • Avoid super sizing your meals if eating at fast-food restaurants, as this can add unwanted calories.

Extreme diets are not likely to be effective. Diets that require severe caloric restriction or exercise programs that require exceptionally large caloric expenditure can be effective in fat loss over a short period but are seldom maintained for a lifetime. Studies show that extreme programs for weight control, designed to "take it off fast," result in long-term success rates of less than 5 percent. Research shows one reason extremely low-calorie diets are ineffective is that they may promote "calorie sparing." When caloric intake is 800 to 1,000 or less, the body protects itself by reducing basal and resting metabolism levels (sparing calories). This results in less fat loss, even though the caloric intake is very low.

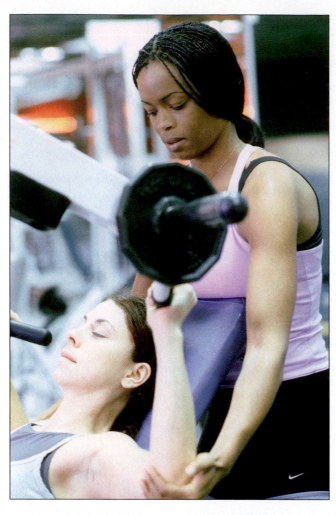

Resistance training helps you gain lean body mass (muscle).

A combination of physical activity and a healthy diet is the best approach for long-term weight control. One major advantage of emphasizing both physical activity and dietary changes is that physical activity can help to maintain the metabolic rate and prevent the decline that occurs with calorie sparing. Studies have shown that programs that include both diet and physical activity promote greater loss of body fat than programs based solely on dietary changes. The total weight loss from the programs may be about the same, but a larger fraction of the weight comes from fat when physical activity is included. In contrast, programs based solely on diet result in greater loss of lean muscle tissue.

A healthy diet and regular physical activity are the keys for long-term weight control. Small changes, such as eating a few hundred calories less per day or walking for 30 minutes every day, can make a big difference over time. The important point is to strive for permanent changes that can be maintained in a normal daily lifestyle. Fad diets cannot be maintained for long periods; therefore, the individual usually regains any weight lost. Constant losing and gaining, known as "yo-yo" dieting, is counterproductive and may lead to negative changes in the person's metabolism and unwanted shifts in sites of fat deposition. When in doubt, avoid programs that promise fast and easy solutions, extreme diets that favor specific foods or eating patterns, and any product that makes unreasonable claims about easy ways to stimulate your metabolism or "melt away fat."

Low-carbohydrate diets are not a good choice for long-term weight control. www.mhhe.com/phys_fit/web17 Click 03. The popularity of high-protein diets is troubling to physicians and public health officials, as most feel that the diet is inconsistent with basic guidelines for good nutrition. Excess protein in the diet can be harmful to the kidneys and liver, since the body must work extra hard to process and remove the unused nitrogen and other metabolites. High-protein diets with an emphasis on animal protein (such as the Atkins diet) may also add excess saturated fat and cholesterol, which can increase risks for coronary heart disease. Last, with low levels of carbohydrate intake, the body enters a state of metabolic ketosis, in which the body starts to break down other substrates for energy. This state has been shown to lead to a loss of appetite, but the long-term effects have not been determined.

Several recent studies of low-carbohydrate (high-protein) diets have shown that they can be effective in reducing weight and blood lipid profiles of extremely obese people. The media have cited these studies widely and, in some cases, have suggested that this is proof that diets work. Experts have been surprised by the findings but still have not supported or endorsed the use of low-carb diets for weight loss by the general population.

There are several factors to consider when interpreting the results of these studies. First, the populations tested in these studies were extremely obese. Results may not generalize to the slightly overweight person

Outcome Goals Statements of intent to achieve a specific test score or a specific standard associated with good health or wellness—for example, "I will lower my body fat level by 3 percent."

Behavioral Goal A statement of intent to perform a specific behavior (changing a lifestyle) for a specific period of time—for example, "I will reduce the calories in my diet by 200 a day for the next four weeks."

Empty Calories Calories in foods considered to have little or no nutritional value.

hoping to lose a few pounds. Second, the actual differences in weight loss between low-carb diets and normal low-fat diets were small and these differences tended to disappear when studies were conducted over longer periods of time. The difficulty in sticking with restrictive low-carb diet plans is a major limitation. Third, effects on cholesterol were often not well described in these studies. Over 30 percent of the low-carb (high-protein) group in one study had significant increases in blood lipids. Last, the weight-loss studies typically included exercise programs to aid in weight-loss efforts. Cutting carbohydrates without incorporating physical activity may yield different results. Without the beneficial effects of physical activity on metabolic fitness, it is likely that the Atkins diet would have much worse effects on blood lipid profiles than reported. The media coverage of these studies tended to portray the results from the low-carb diets in a very positive light, but a more critical analysis shows little advantage over more balanced plans of eating that emphasize healthy food choices and moderation.

Low "glycemic load" diets may be a more sensible alternative to low-carbohydrate diets. Low-carb diets are not the solution to the obesity epidemic but they have sensitized Americans to the problems of consuming too much excess sugar. During the low-fat craze of the early 1990s, people assumed that they could eat anything they wanted as long as it didn't have fat in it. The popularity of "fat-free" cookies and desserts skyrocketed as consumers sought ways to consume snack foods without feeling guilty. Now, the tide has swung the other way and consumers appear to be avoiding carbohydrates with the same vigor. People assume that anything that is "low-carb" is okay to eat, but this is overly simplistic and not the sound basis for a healthy diet. Both low-fat and low-carb diets are probably too restrictive when followed to extremes.

Many experts have begun to recommend less restrictive diets that manage excessive carbohydrate intake without compromising important benefits from other foods. For example, there is overwhelming research documenting important health benefits associated with consuming fruits, vegetables, legumes, and sufficient amounts of fiber. Because these foods have a low glycemic load, they are not prone to the same problems as simple carbohydrates. There is also clear evidence of harm associated with the excessive consumption of saturated fat advocated by some diet plans and potential benefits associated with the consumption of monounsaturated fats. A more sensible diet plan minimizes saturated fats while including heart healthy oils. This type of diet provides the vitamins, minerals, and fiber that are typically lacking in most low-carb diets. The emphasis on healthy forms of polyunsaturated and monounsaturated fats also makes this type of diet easier to adhere to than traditional low-fat diet plans. By emphasizing quality of carbohydrates, fats, and proteins, consumers should be able to make dietary choices that contribute to weight control and good health. See the "On the Web" feature for additional information.

Developing a regular eating plan is important for weight maintenance. A number of recent studies have suggested that individual eating patterns may be associated with obesity. A recent study found that breakfast skipping, meals eaten away from home, and frequent episodes of eating during the day were associated with obesity—even after controlling for total caloric intake. These results highlight the importance of establishing regular patterns of eating.

Some prescription medicines may help some obese individuals curb their appetite. Currently, there are only two prescription drugs that are approved by the Food and Drug Administration for long-term use in the United States. These "pharmacotherapies" are considered to be adjuncts to lifestyle modification and are used only with obese patients (BMI > 30) or overweight individuals with other "comorbidities" (e.g., diabetes, or hypertension). The two medications that are currently being prescribed are sibutramine and orlistat.

Sibutramine is a chemical that acts by inhibiting the reuptake of serotonin and noradrenaline. In research studies, weight loss has been found to be greater among sibutramine-treated participants, compared with those receiving a placebo. Maintenance of weight loss has also been enhanced for 6 to 18 months following initial weight loss if the person continues with the medication. Sibutramine is currently found in the weight loss product Meridia. Studies haven't documented all of the harmful effects to this point, but reports indicate that use can raise blood pressure and lead some people to have irregular heartbeats. The AHA currently cautions consumers to consult their physicians, and consider the relative benefits and risks before using it.

Orlistat (used in Xenical) enhances weight loss by inhibiting the body's absorption of fat. Results from well-controlled studies have shown that patients taking orlistat lose significantly more weight than patients taking a placebo medication. The weight loss is typically accompanied by reductions in total and LDL cholesterol, blood pressure, and glucose/insulin levels, indicating that the changes are related to improvements in metabolic function. A major limitation of the drug is that it also blocks the absorption of fat-soluble vitamins (A, D, E, and K, as well as beta-carotene). Therefore, prolonged use can lead to vitamin deficiencies unless supplementation is included in the diet.

🌐 **Artificial sweeteners and fat substitutes may help but cannot be considered a "sure cure" for body fat problems.** www.mhhe.com/phys_fit/web17 Click 04. Artificial sweeteners are frequently used in soft drinks and food to reduce the calorie content. Because they have few or no calories, these supplements were originally expected to help people with weight control. However, since they were introduced, the general public has not eaten fewer calories and more people are now overweight than before they were introduced. Studies suggest that people consuming these products end up consuming just as many calories per day as people consuming products with real sugar or sweeteners.

New products often referred to as "fake fat" are used as a fat substitute in baking and cooking. Potato chips and other fried foods cooked in these products as well as baked goods using these products have less fat and fewer calories. If you eat no more food than usual and substitute foods made with these products, you will consume fewer calories and less fat. Experts worry that consumers will not eat the same amount of foods with these fake fats but will feel they can eat more because the fake fats contain fewer calories and less fat.

🌐 **Dietary supplements or products containing ephedra should be avoided.** www.mhhe.com/phys_fit/web17 Click 05. Because long-term weight control is difficult, many individuals seek simple solutions from various nonprescription weight loss products. The most common additive in dietary supplements has been the stimulant ephedra (or the herbal equivalent, Ma Huang). Many negative reactions and multiple deaths have been attributed to the use of ephedra, and this led the FDA recently to ban the sale and use of any products containing this compound. This includes the synthetic versions of ephedrine found in commercially available supplements such as Dexatrim and Acutrim. A concern among public health officials is that many products do not accurately label the contents of their supplements. A report in the *Journal of the American Medical Association* indicated that over 50 percent of the ephedra supplements tested by the FDA failed to list the ephedra content or had amounts 20 percent or higher than listed on the label. Manufacturers of supplements have recently started selling "ephedra-free" supplements that use other stimulants. A commonly used alternative compound is known as "bitter orange," and this supplement has also been shown to present similar health risks. Consumers should be wary of dietary supplements, due to the unregulated nature of the industry.

Guidelines for Gaining Muscle Mass

Young people often have difficulty in gaining weight or muscle mass. Typically, those most likely to have difficulty in gaining weight are age ten to twenty. The reason for this is that more calories are required to maintain weight during the growing years than in adulthood. They have probably been told more than once that they will not have trouble gaining weight when they grow older. This is true for most people, but it is of little consolation to those who want to gain weight now. During adolescence, most people begin to gain weight, including muscle mass that can be enhanced with regular exercise. Excessive eating to gain weight (especially during adolescence) is not without its problems. The body requires more caloric intake during the teen years because the body is growing. A person who develops a habit of high caloric intake during this time may have a difficult time controlling fatness when the demands on the body are less. Most people who want to gain weight want to gain lean body tissue. Only those who have body fat percentages less than what is considered to be essential for good health need to gain body fat.

Changes in the frequency and composition of meals are important to gain muscle mass. To increase muscle mass, the body requires a greater caloric intake. The challenge is to provide enough extra calories for the muscle without excess amounts going to fat. An increase of 500 to 1,000 calories a day will help most people gain muscle mass over time. Smaller, more frequent meals are best for weight gain, since they tend to keep the metabolic rate high. The majority of extra calories should come from complex carbohydrates. Breads, pasta, rice, and fruits such as bananas are good sources. Granola, nuts, juices (grape and cranberry), and milk also make good high-calorie, healthy snacks. High-protein diets or diet supplements are not particularly effective if you maintain a normal diet. High-fat diets can result in weight gain but may not be best for good health, especially if they are high in saturated fat. If weight gain does not occur over a period of weeks and months with extra calorie consumption, medical assistance may be necessary.

Physical activity is important in gaining muscle mass. Regular strength training can aid in weight gain. The stimulus from this form of exercise causes the body to increase protein synthesis, which allows the body to gain muscle mass. Of course, the body requires higher caloric intake to form this new muscle tissue.

Excessive aerobic exercise may actually make it difficult to gain weight. Although some regular aerobic exercise is necessary for health and cardiovascular fitness, it may be necessary to limit aerobic exercise if weight gain is the goal. Studies have shown that extensive aerobic training can even cause a reduction in muscle mass. When one is training to gain weight, aerobic exercise expending no more than 3,500 calories per week is probably best.

Strategies for Action

Knowing about guidelines for controlling body fat is not as important as following them. The guidelines presented in this concept are only of value if you use them. In Lab 17A, you will have the opportunity to identify some of the guidelines that you feel will help you the most in the future.

Recordkeeping is important in meeting fat control goals and making moderation a part of your normal lifestyle. Studies have shown that it is easy to fool yourself when determining the amount of food you have eaten or the amount of exercise you have done. Once fat control goals have been set, whether for weight loss, maintenance, or gain, it is important to keep records of your behavior. People often underestimate the amount of food they have eaten, particularly the number of calories consumed. They also tend to overestimate the amount of exercise they do. Keeping a diet log and an exercise log can help you monitor your behavior and maintain the lifestyle necessary to meet your goals. A log can also help you monitor changes in weight and body fat levels. But remember, care should be taken to avoid too much emphasis on short-term weight changes. Lab 17B will help you learn about the actual content of fast foods, so you can learn to make better choices when eating out.

The support of family and friends can be of great importance in balancing caloric intake and caloric expenditure. The importance of family and friends for successful adherence to a regular physical activity program can't be overemphasized. Family and friends can also help you in changing and adhering to healthy eating practices. Parents who overeat often have children who eat more than normal. In these cases, the entire family must participate in a program to control fatness. Family and friends should provide support for the person wanting to gain or lose fat by helping him or her follow the guidelines presented in this concept, rather than tempting the person to eat improperly. Unfortunately, sometimes friends and family members can put too much emphasis on the person's fat loss. This can have the opposite effect of that intended if it is perceived as an attempt to control the person's behavior. The use of extrinsic rewards, such as money or gifts for achieving goals, may be effective in the short term, but it may result in resentment rather than adherence over the long term. Encouragement and support rather than control of behavior is the key.

Group support can be one of the best reinforcers of proper eating and exercise behavior. Group support has been found to be beneficial to many individuals who are attempting to change their behavior. Alcoholics have found that the support of others is critical to their rehabilitation. (Alcoholics Anonymous grew as a result of this need.) If you want to alter your body composition, especially to lose body fat, group support is important if you are to make permanent lifestyle changes in diet and exercise. Groups such as Overeaters Anonymous and Weight Watchers have been organized to help those who need the support of peers in attaining and maintaining desirable fat levels for a lifetime.

Psychological strategies can be of assistance in eating and exercising to attain and maintain a desirable level of body fat. Adopting healthy lifestyle habits often requires use of behavioral skills and some degree of discipline. The following list provides tips on maintaining weight control efforts.

- Avoid food fantasies. Sometimes the thought of food is what causes overeating. Practice restructuring your thought process to something other than food fantasies. Use mental imagery to create a mind's-eye view of something you enjoy other than food. When food fantasies occur, you may want to exercise or engage in some activity that refocuses your attention.

- Avoid weight fantasies. Sometimes the thought of being excessively thin or muscular occurs. By itself, this may not be bad. If, however, it causes you to become discouraged and makes your goals seem unattainable, it is bad. When weight fantasies occur, do some other activity to redirect your focus of attention or imagine something other than the weight fantasy. Altering mental fantasies takes practice.

- Avoid **negative self-talk.** One type of negative self-talk occurs when a person starts self-criticism for not meeting a goal. For example, if a person is determined not to eat more than one serving of food at a party but fails to meet this goal, he or she might say, "It's no use stopping now; I've already blown it." It is not too late. Anyone can fail to meet goals. Negative self-talk makes it easy to fail in the future. A more appropriate response is **positive self-talk,** such as "I'm not going to eat anything else tonight; I can do it."

Negative Self-Talk Self-defeating discussions with yourself focusing on your failures rather than your successes.

Positive Self-Talk Telling yourself positive, encouraging things that help you succeed in accomplishing your goals.

Study Resources

Check out additional online study resources for this concept in the Student Edition of the Online Learning Center at www.mhhe.com/corbin13e.

Web Resources

American Dietetic Association **www.eatright.org**
Berkeley Nutrition Sciences **www.nutritionquest.com**
Center for Science in the Public Interest **www.cspinet.org**
Fast Food Facts: Interactive Food Finder **www.olen.com/food**
Meals Online **www.my-meals.com**
Office of Dietary Supplements **http://ods.od.nih.gov**
USDA Food and Nutrition Information Center
   www.nal.usda.gov/fnic

Suggested Readings

Additional reference materials for Concept 17 are available at **www.mhhe.com/phys_fit/web17 Click 06.**

American College of Sports Medicine. 2001. Appropriate intervention strategies for weight loss and prevention of weight regain for adults. *Medicine and Science in Sports and Exercise* 33(12):2145–2156.

Black, A. K. 2003. The dietary guidelines for Americans 2000: A web based learner application. *American Journal of Health Education* 34(2):105–108.

Blanck, H. M., L. K. Khan, and M. Serdula. 2001. The use of nonprescription weight loss products: Results from a multistate survey. *Journal of the American Medical Association* 286:930–935.

Food and Nutrition Board, Institute of Medicine. 2002. *Dietary Reference Intakes for Energy, Carbohydrates,* *Fiber, Fat, Protein and Amino Acids (Macronutrients).* Washington, DC: National Academy Press.

Foster, G. D., et al. 2003. A randomized trial of a low-carbohydrate diet for obesity. *New England Journal of Medicine* 348(21):2082–2090.

Frank, L. D. 2004. Obesity relationships with community design, physical activity, and time spent in cars. *American Journal of Preventive Medicine* 27(2):87–96.

Goodman, W. C. 2002. *The Invisible Woman: Confronting Weight Prejudice in America.* Carlsbad, CA: Gurze Books.

Jacobson, M. F., and J. Hurley. 2002. *Restaurant Confidential.* New York: Workman.

Lowe, M. R. 2003. Self-regulation of energy intake in the prevention and treatment of obesity: Is it feasible? *Obesity Research* 11 Suppl: 44S–59S.

Ma, Y. 2003. Association between eating patterns and obesity in a free-living US adult population. *American Journal of Epidemiology* 158:85–92.

Manore, M. M., S. I. Barr, and G. E. Butterfield. 2001. Position of the American Dietetic Association: Nutrition and athletic performance. *Journal of the American Dietetic Association* 5(1):1543–1556.

Sacker, I. M., and M. A. Zimmer. 2002. *Dying to Be Thin: Understanding and Defeating Anorexia Nervosa and Bulimia—a Practical, Lifesaving Guide.* New York: Time Warner Bookmark.

Samaha, F. F., et al. 2003. A low-carbohydrate as compared with a low-fat diet in severe obesity. *New England Journal of Medicine* 348(21):2074–2081.

Schlosser, E. 2001. *Fast Food Nation: The Dark Side of the All-American Meal.* New York: Houghton Mifflin.

Shuldiner. A. R. 2003. Genetics of obesity: More complicated than initially thought. *Lipids* 38(2):97–101.

In the News

The Obesity Epidemic

The obesity epidemic has generated considerable media interest in recent years. While the problem has been recognized by health officials for the past 10–15 years, awareness of the issue has reach almost all segments of society. The recent documentary movie *SuperSize Me* brought clear attention to the problem by demonstrating effects of daily consumption of fast food.

The movie clearly exaggerated the problems associated with fast food; however, there have been a number lawsuits made against fast-food companies by individuals, charging that the food at these restaurants has caused them to be overweight or obese. To date, these lawsuits have been thrown out of court—establishing the precedent that individuals are still personally responsible for their food choices. Still, many food companies have taken notice of the allegations and have started to position their products as *part of the solution* rather than *part of the problem.* Kraft Foods, one of the largest food manufacturers, initiated changes in serving sizes and labeling on its products to encourage more sensible eating. McDonald's has also taken major strides to help address the obesity problem. It has water available with some meals and has included pedometers in adult "happy meals" to encourage physical activity.

Lab 17A Selecting Strategies for Managing Eating

Name	**Section**　　**Date**

Purpose: To help you select strategies for managing eating to control body fatness

Procedures

1. Read the strategies listed in Chart 1 below.
2. Make a check in the box beside five to ten of the strategies that you think will be most useful to you.
3. Answer the questions in the Conclusions and Implications section.

Chart 1 ▶ Strategies for Managing Eating to Control Body Fatness

✔	**Check 5 to 10 strategies that you might use in the future.**
	Shopping Strategies
	Shop from a list.
	Shop with a friend.
	Shop on a full stomach.
	Check food labels.
	Consider foods that take some time to prepare.
	Methods of Eating
	When you eat, do nothing but eat. Don't watch television or read.
	Eat slowly.
	Do not eat food you do not want.
	Follow an eating schedule.
	Do your eating in designated areas, such as kitchen or dining room only.
	Leave the table after eating.
	Avoid second servings.
	Limit servings of condiments.
	Limit servings of nonbasics, such as dessert, breads, and soft drinks.
	Eat several meals of equal size rather than one big meal and two small ones.
	Eating in the Work Environment
	Take your own food to work.
	Avoid snack machines.
	If you eat out, plan your meal ahead of time.
	Do not eat while working.
	Avoid sharing foods from co-workers such as birthday cakes.
	Have activity breaks during the day.
	Have water available to substitute for soft drinks.
	Have low-calorie snacks to substitute for office snacks.

✔	**Check 5 to 10 strategies that you might use in the future.**
	Eating on Special Occasions
	Practice ways to refuse food.
	Avoid tempting situations.
	Eat before you go out.
	Don't stand near food sources.
	If you feel the urge to eat, find someone to talk to.
	Strategies for Eating Out
	Limit deep-fat fried foods.
	Ask for information about food content.
	Limit use of condiments.
	Choose low-fat foods (e.g., skim milk, low-fat yogurt).
	Choose chicken, fish, or lean meat.
	Order á la carte.
	If you eat desserts, avoid those with sauces or toppings.
	Eating at Home
	Keep busy at times when you are at risk of overeating.
	Store food out of sight.
	Avoid serving food to others between meals.
	If you snack, choose snacks with complex carbohydrates, such as carrot sticks or apple slices.
	Freeze leftovers to avoid the temptation of eating them between meals.

Conclusions and Implications

1. In several sentences, discuss your need to use strategies for effective eating. Do you need to use them? Why or why not?

2. In several sentences, discuss the effectiveness of the strategies contained in Chart 1. Do you think they can be effective for people who have a problem controlling their body fatness?

3. In several sentences, discuss the value of using behavioral goals versus outcome goals when planning for fat loss.

Lab 17B Evaluating Fast-Food Options

Name	Section	Date

Purpose: To teach you about the energy and fat content of fast food and how to make better choices when eating at fast-food restaurants

Procedures

1. Using Appendix E, select a fast-food restaurant and a typical meal you might order there.
2. Record the total calories, fat calories, saturated fat intake, and cholesterol for each food item.
3. Sum up the totals for the meal in Chart 2 below.
4. Record recommended daily values by selecting an amount from Chart 1. Estimate should be based on your estimated needs for the day.
5. Compute the percentage of the daily recommended amounts that you consume in the meal by dividing recommended amounts (step 4) into meal totals (step 3). Record percent of recommended daily amounts in Chart 2.
6. Answer the questions in the Conclusions and Implications section.

Chart 1 ▶ Recommended Daily Amounts of Fat, Saturated Fat, Cholesterol, and Sodium

	2,000 kcal	3,000 kcal
Total fat	65 g	97.5 g
Saturated fat	20 g	30 g
Cholesterol	300 mg	450 mg
Sodium	2,400 mg	3,600 g

Results

Chart 2 ▶ Listing of Foods Selected for the Meal

Food Item	Total Calories	Total Fat (g)	Saturated Fat (g)	Cholesterol (mg)
1.				
2.				
3.				
4.				
5.				
6.				
Total for meal (sum up each column)				
Recommended daily amount (record your values from Chart 1)				
% of recommended daily amount (record your % of recommended)				

Conclusions and Implications: In several sentences, answer the following questions.

1. Describe how often you eat at fast-food restaurants and indicate whether you would like to reduce how much fast food you consume.

2. Were you surprised at the amount of fat, saturated fat, and cholesterol in the meal you selected?

3. What could you do differently at fast-food restaurants to reduce your intake of fat, saturated fat, and cholesterol?

Stress and Health

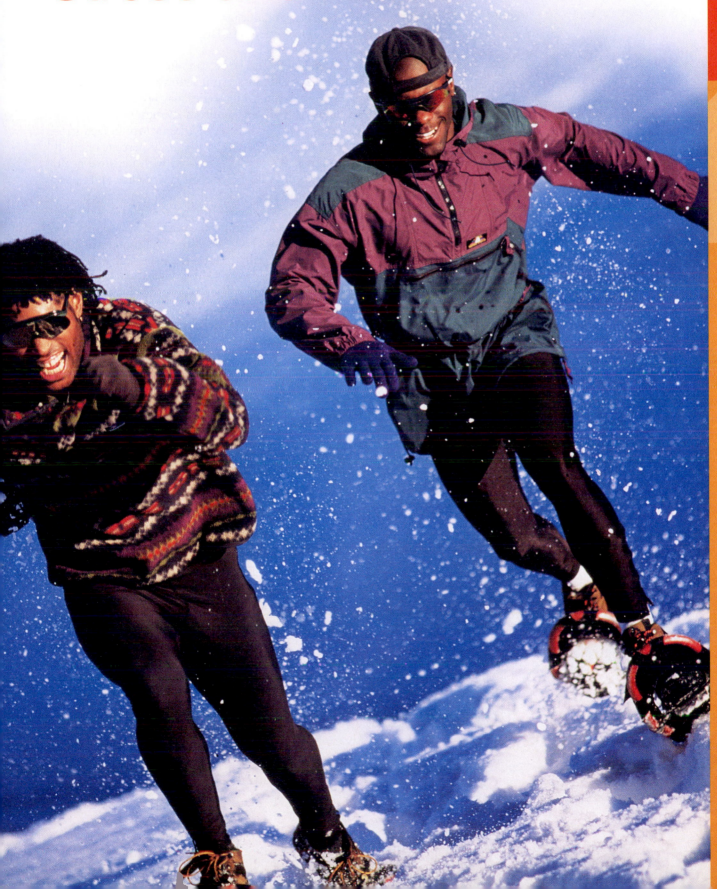

Mental and physical health are affected by an individual's ability to avoid or adapt to stress.

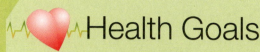

Health Goals

for the year 2010

- Improve mental health and ensure access to appropriate, quality mental health services.

- Increase mental health treatment, including treatment for depression and anxiety disorders.

- Increase mental health screening and assessment.

- Reduce suicide and suicide attempts, especially among young people.

- Increase availability of worksite stress-reduction programs.

Stress affects nearly everyone to some degree. In fact, approximately 67 percent of adults indicate that they experience "great stress" at least 1 day a week. **Stressors** come in many forms, and even positive life events can increase our stress levels. Although all humans have the same physiological system for responding to stress, stress reactivity varies across individuals. In addition, the way we think about or perceive stressful sit-

uations has a significant impact on how our bodies respond. Thus, there are large individual differences in responses to stress.

At moderate levels, stress can motivate us to reach our goals and keep life interesting. However, when stressors are severe or chronic, our bodies may not be able to adapt successfully. Stress can compromise immune functioning, leading to a host of diseases of **adaptation.** In fact, stress has been linked to between 50 and 70 percent of all illnesses. Further, stress is associated with negative health behaviors, such as alcohol and other drug use, and to psychological problems, such as depression and anxiety.

This concept will review the causes and consequences of stress. Figure 1 illustrates the many factors involved in individual reactions to stress. First, the sources of stress (stressors) such as daily hassles and major life events will be described. Then, the physiological and cognitive responses to stressors will be reviewed. Finally, some of the consequences of physiological and cognitive responses, including emotional, physical, and behavioral outcomes will be discussed.

Sources of Stress

The first step in managing stress is to recognize the causes and to be aware of the symptoms. You need to recognize the situations in your life that are the stressors. Identify the things that make you feel "stressed-out."

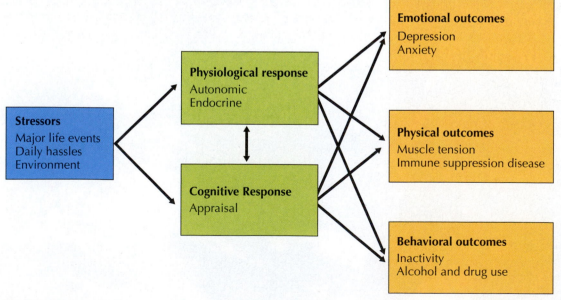

Figure 1 ▶ Reactions to stress.

Everything from minor irritations, such as traffic jams, to major life changes, such as births, deaths, or job loss, can be stressors. A stress overload of too many demands on your time can make you feel that you are no longer in control. You may feel so overwhelmed that you become depressed. The labs at the end of this concept can help you evaluate your current levels of stress and muscle tension and provide a first step in managing stress in your life.

Stress can come from a variety of sources. There are many kinds of stressors. Environmental stressors include heat, noise, overcrowding, climate, and terrain. Physiological stressors are such things as drugs, caffeine, tobacco, injury, infection or disease, and physical effort.

Emotional stressors are the most frequent and important stressors affecting humans. Some people refer to these as psychosocial stressors. These include life-changing events, such as a change in work hours or line of work, family illnesses, problems with superiors, deaths of relatives or friends, and increased responsibilities. In school, pressures such as grades, term papers, and oral presentations may induce stress. A recent national study of daily experiences indicated that more than 60 percent of all stressful experiences fall in a few areas (see Table 1).

Stressors vary in severity. Because stressors vary in magnitude and duration, many experts categorize them by severity. Major stressors create major emotional turmoil or require tremendous amounts of adjustment. This category includes personal crises (e.g., major health problems or death in the family, divorce/separation, financial problems, legal problems) and job/school-related pressures or major age-related transitions (e.g., college, marriage, career, retirement). Minor stressors are generally viewed as shorter-term or less severe. This category includes events or problems such as traffic hassles, peer/work relations, time pressures, and family squabbles, just to name a few. Major stressors can alter our daily patterns of stress and impair our ability to handle the minor stressors or hassles of life. Minor stressors can accumulate and create more significant problems. It is important to be aware of both types of stressors.

Negative, ambiguous, and uncontrollable events are usually the most stressful. Although stress can come from both positive and negative events, negative ones generally cause more distress because negative stressors usually have harsher consequences and little benefit. Positive stressors, on the other hand, usually have enough benefit to make them worthwhile. For example, although the stress of getting ready for a wedding may be tremendous, it is not as bad as the negative stress associated with losing a job.

Ambiguous stressors are harder to accept than more clearly defined problems. In most cases, if the cause of a stressor or problem can be identified, then active measures

Table 1 ▶ Ten Common Stressors in the Lives of College Students and Middle-Aged Adults

College Students	Middle-Aged Adults
1. Troubling thoughts about the future	1. Concerns about weight
2. Not getting enough sleep	2. Health of a family member
3. Wasting time	3. Rising prices of common goods
4. Inconsiderate smokers	4. Home maintenance (interior)
5. Physical appearance	5. Too many things to do
6. Too many things to do	6. Misplacing or losing things
7. Misplacing or losing things	7. Yard work or outside home maintenance
8. Not enough time to do the things you need to do	8. Property, investments, or taxes
9. Concerns about meeting high standards	9. Crime
10. Being lonely	10. Physical appearance

Source: Kanner, A. D. et al.

can be taken to improve the situation. For example, if you are stressed about a project at work or school, you can use specific strategies to help you complete the task on time. Stress brought on by a relationship with friends or co-workers, on the other hand, may be harder to understand. In some cases, it is not possible to determine the primary source or cause of the problem. These situations are more problematic because fewer clear-cut solutions exist.

Another factor that makes events stressful is a lack of control. Stress brought on by illness, accidents, or natural disasters fit into this category. Because little can be done to change the situation, these events leave us feeling powerless. If the stressor is something that can be dealt with more directly, then efforts at minimizing the stress are likely to be effective. This helps us to feel more in control.

🌐 **The nature and magnitude of stressors change during the life span.** www.mhhe.com/phys_fit/web18 Click 01. Depending on your perspective, some periods in life may be more stressful than others, but

Stress The nonspecific response (generalized adaptation) of the body to any demand made upon it in order to maintain physiological equilibrium. This positive or negative response results from emotions that are accompanied by biochemical and physiological changes directed at adaptation.

Stressors Things that place a greater than routine demand on the body or evoke a stress reaction.

Adaptation The body's efforts to restore normalcy.

each phase provides its own challenges and experiences. Some argue that adolescence represents the most stressful time of life. Drastic changes in a person's body and numerous psychosocial challenges must be overcome. College provides additional mental challenges as well as financial pressures and the pressures of living independently. During the early adult years, tremendous pressures and responsibilities force you to juggle career and family obligations. Late adulthood presents still other new challenges, such as coping with declining functioning or illness. Although the nature of the stressor changes, the presence of stress remains consistent. Learning to manage stress can make it easier to handle the changing stresses in life.

College presents unique challenges and stressors.

For college students, schoolwork can be a full-time job, and those who have to work outside of school must handle the stresses of both jobs. Although the college years are often thought of as a break from the stresses of the real world, college life has its own unique stressors. Obvious sources of stress include taking exams, speaking in public, and becoming comfortable with talking to professors. Students are often living independent of family for the first time and at the same time negotiating new relationships—with roommates, dating partners, and so on. Young people entering college are also faced with a less structured environment and simultaneously with the need to control their own schedules. Though this environment has a number of advantages, students are faced with a greater need to manage their stress effectively.

In addition to the traditional challenges of college, the new generation of students faces stressors that were not typical for college students in the past. According to the American Council on Education, only 40 percent of today's college students enroll full-time immediately after high school. Once in college, more students now work to support their studies, and many go back to school after spending time in the working world. These students are likely to have additional pressures not characteristic of the typical college student. Further, more of today's students are the first in their families to go to college. This may place additional pressure on these students to succeed. Perhaps as a result of some of these factors, rates of mental health problems among college students have increased dramatically (see Figure 2). A study from the American College Health Association indicated that 10 percent of college students are diagnosed with depression. In another study, 53 percent of students reported feeling depressed at some point during their college careers and 9 percent reported considering suicide. Although more people are receiving care for mental health problems than have in the past, the vast majority are still not receiving adequate care. University counseling centers are typically understaffed and unable to handle the increasing number of college students seeking mental health services.

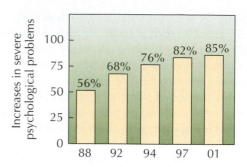

Figure 2 ▶ Colleges reporting increased psychological problems.
Source: R. Gallagher.

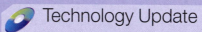

Technology Update

National Mental Health Information Center

The National Institute for Mental Health has an information website that includes a mental health service locator, mental health hot line numbers, a call center that provides answers to mental health questions, and a wide variety of links that provide information about depression, anxiety, and other stress-related disorders. The information center can be accessed at http://www.mentalhealth.samhsa.gov/.

Reactions to Stress

All people have a "general" reaction to stress. As mentioned earlier, all humans have the same type physiological system for responding to stress, leading to certain commonalities in experience. The sympathetic response of the autonomic nervous system (ANS) is associated with a fight-or-flight response, which mobilizes bodily resources when a stressor is identified. Sometimes this alarm reaction of the body is essential to survival, but, when evoked inappropriately or excessively, it may be more harmful than the effects of the original stressor. After the initial sympathetic response, the parasympathetic response takes over in an attempt to restore homeostasis and conserve resources. Hans Selye described the general adaptation syndrome demonstrating how the autonomic system reacts to stressful situations and the conditions under which the system may break down (see Table 2). The term *general* highlights the similarities in responses to stressful situations across individuals.

In addition to the ANS response, several hormones are secreted by the endocrine system. Specifically, the hypothalamus, pituitary, and adrenal glands (HPA) are activated by stress. This endocrine, or HPA, system is slower to respond than the ANS, but takes longer to return to baseline functioning after a stressful event. When presented with a stressor, the hypothalamus produces corticotrophin

Table 2 ▶ The Three Stages in Hans Selye's General Adaptation Syndrome

Stage 1: Alarm Reaction

Any physical or mental trauma will trigger an immediate set of reactions that combat the stress. Because the immune system is initially depressed, normal levels of resistance are lowered, making us more susceptible to infection and disease. If the stress is not severe or long-lasting, we bounce back and recover rapidly.

Stage 2: Resistance

Eventually, sometimes rather quickly, we adapt to stress, and we actually have a tendency to become more resistant to illness and disease. Our immune system works overtime for us during this period, keeping up with the demands placed upon it.

Stage 3: Exhaustion

Because the body is not able to maintain homeostasis and the long-term resistance needed to combat stress, we invariably experience a drop in our resistance level. No one experiences the same resistance and tolerance to stress, but everyone's immunity at some point collapses following prolonged stress reactions. Stress-fighting reserves finally succumb to what Selye called "diseases of adaptation."

Source: Health News Network.

releasing hormone (CRH), and the pituitary gland secretes Adrenocorticotropic Hormone (ACTH). The introduction of ACTH leads to the release of cortisol by the adrenal cortex. Cortisol is often referred to as the "stress hormone." After exposure to chronic stress, the HPA system can become disregulated.

Individuals respond differently to stress. Individuals exposed to high levels of stress are most at risk for negative health consequences. At the same time, not everyone exposed to severe or chronic stress will evidence negative outcomes. Those with positive health outcomes despite high levels of stress are said to be "resilient" and have been the subject of increased attention. There is obviously more to the stress-illness relationship than the total number or severity of stressors. What makes an individual more or less susceptible to negative stress-related outcomes?

Two important areas in which individuals differ are stress reactivity and stress appraisals. Stress reactivity refers to the extent to which the sympathetic nervous system or "fight or flight" system is activated by a stressor, whereas stress appraisals refer to an individual's perception of a stressor and the person's resources for managing a stressful situation. These individual differences are partly due to inherited predispositions and partly due to our unique histories of experiencing and attempting to cope with stress. Recognizing these individual differences has important implications for our well-being because knowledge of our own unique response to stressful situations can increase our awareness of the impact of stress and provide information that may lead to more effective stress management.

Everyone has an optimal level of arousal. We all need sufficient stress to motivate us to engage in activities that make our lives meaningful. Otherwise, we would become apathetic and bored, leading to less than optimal health and wellness. In fact, a certain level of stress, called **eustress,** is experienced positively. In contrast, **distress** is a level of stress that compromises performance and well-being. Each of us possesses a system that allows us to mobilize resources when necessary and that seeks to find a homeostatic level of arousal (see Figure 3). Although we all have an optimal level of arousal, the optimal level varies considerably. What one person finds stressful another may find exhilarating. Stress mobilizes some to greater efficiency, whereas it confuses others. For example, riding a roller coaster is thrilling for some people, but for others it is a stressful and unpleasant experience.

Level of arousal exists on a continuum with all possible gradations, but the extreme ends of the spectrum are illustrative of the marked differences across individuals. At one end of the continuum are those that find even moderate levels of arousal stressful or anxiety-provoking. Behaviorally, these individuals can be identified as early as the first year of life and are generally referred to as temperamentally "inhibited" or "withdrawn." Although an inhibited individual may function quite well in the right environment, such a person is susceptible to a number of emotional disorders, including anxiety and depression. In addition, individuals with a stronger sympathetic response to an acute stressor show a stress-induced increase in cortisol. This is an important finding, given the known relation between cortisol level and immune functioning. Thus, these individuals may be at increased risk for negative physical health consequences by virtue of their stronger sympathetic and cortisol response to stress.

At the other end of the continuum are those who prefer a very high level of arousal. For example, people who

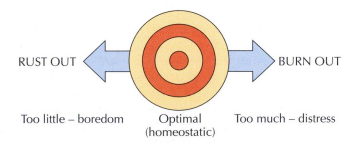

RUST OUT ◀   ▶ BURN OUT

Too little – boredom   Optimal   Too much – distress
                          (homeostatic)

Figure 3 ▶ Stress target zone.

Eustress Positive stress, or stress that is mentally or physically stimulating.

Distress Negative stress, or stress that contributes to health problems.

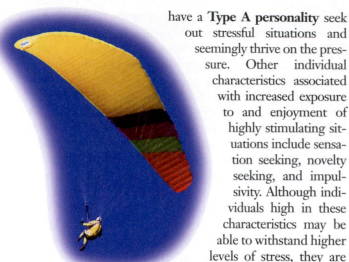

One person's stress is another's pleasure.

have a **Type A personality** seek out stressful situations and seemingly thrive on the pressure. Other individual characteristics associated with increased exposure to and enjoyment of highly stimulating situations include sensation seeking, novelty seeking, and impulsivity. Although individuals high in these characteristics may be able to withstand higher levels of stress, they are also at increased risk for unhealthy lifestyles (e.g., alcohol, nicotine, and other drug use; unprotected sexual behavior; aggressiveness) and the associated health consequences.

Type A personality has been associated with increased risk for heart disease. Although this appears to be the case for some Type A personalities, it is not true for all. Type A individuals who do not express their anger and have hostility associated with stressful situations are more likely to be at risk. A recent study found that these emotions may increase risk for heart disease by increasing cholesterol levels and risk for obesity. In addition to the physical health risks, recent research suggests that individuals who are high in hostility are likely to have poor social support and greater susceptibility to chronic depression.

Reactions to stress depend on one's appraisal of both the event and the subsequent physiological response.
Stressors by themselves generally do not cause problems unless they are perceived as stressful. Appraisal usually involves consideration of the consequences of the situation (primary appraisal), and an evaluation of the resources available to cope with the situation (secondary appraisal). If one sees a stressor as a challenge that can be tackled, one is likely to respond in a more positive manner than if the stressor is viewed as an obstacle that cannot be overcome.

The events that occurred on September 11, 2001, provide a vivid example of the very different reactions that people have to the same or similar stressors. Everyone who witnessed these events, in person or on television, was profoundly impacted. At the same time, individual reactions varied dramatically. Most felt overwhelming sadness, many felt extreme anger, others felt hopeless or desperate, and yet others felt lost or confused. Undoubtedly, there were some that were simply too shocked to process their emotional experience at all. With time, most Americans began to experience a wave of additional emotions, such as

hope, patriotism, community, courage, and determination. Others were less quick to experience these positive emotions and many developed anxiety, depression, or posttraumatic stress disorder. All of these emotions were reactions to the same stressful events. Although a number of factors contributed to these individual differences (e.g., proximity to New York City or personal relationship with someone who lost their life), differences in appraisals of the events were probably responsible for much of the variability.

In addition to the appraisal of the event, one's appraisal of the body's response to an event is important. The way in which bodily sensations are interpreted has a significant impact on how one will react emotionally and behaviorally. For example, public speaking is a situation that leads to significant autonomic arousal for most people. Those who handle these situations well probably recognize that these sensations are normal and may even interpret them as excitement about their upcoming speech. In contrast, those who experience severe and sometimes debilitating anxiety are probably interpreting the same sensations as indicators of fear, panic, and loss of control.

🌐 Hardy individuals appraise stress in an adaptive manner. www.mhhe.com/phys_fit/web18
Click 02. Certain characteristics (collectively referred to as **hardiness**) have been found to influence a person's reaction to stressful situations. Individuals possessing hardiness have been found to appraise and respond to stress in more favorable ways than people without it. Research in a college population indicates that individuals who are high in hardiness are at reduced risk for illness, due to the way they perceive stress and the coping mechanisms they use in response to stressful situations. The dimensions of hardiness are

Commitment: The stressors of everyday life can be overwhelming to many people. Although stress cannot be avoided, a sense of commitment to your life and your aspirations can make stress more tolerable. Hardy individuals possess a strong sense of commitment and are willing to put up with adversity to keep pushing toward their desired goals.

Challenge: Many people experience considerable stress from the high-pressure demands of school and work. Much of the stress is caused by concern about being able to meet these new demands and the fear associated with failure. Hardy individuals see new responsibilities and situations as challenges rather than stressors. With this perspective, new situations become opportunities for growth rather than chances for failure.

Control: As previously mentioned, situations tend to be more stressful when they are out of our control. Rather than easily giving up when situations seem out of control, hardy individuals find ways to assume control over their problems. Being proactive rather than reactive is an effective strategy for combating stress. It is important to acknowledge that many stressors may be out of your control. In these situations, it is important to "go with the flow." Depending on the degree of control that is available, some coping strategies may be more effective than others. Specific recommendations are provided in the next concept.

Stress can have physical effects on the body. Many of the commonly observed symptoms of stress are physical. Increases in heart rate and blood pressure and sweaty palms are some of the many physical changes that are commonly observed following acute stress (see Figure 4).

Chronic exposure to stress can lead to other physical symptoms, such as headaches, indigestion, and stomach cramps. Muscle tension is another common result of stress. One form of this tension is seen in the unnecessary "bracing" or "splinting" action of muscles—for example, the clinched jaw, hunched shoulders, white knuckles, or muscles contracting when not needed. They may stay contracted for long periods without your being aware of it. This tension can cause muscle spasms and pain, which, in turn, becomes an additional stressor.

Fatigue is often a symptom of chronic stress. It can result from lack of sleep, emotional strain, pain, disease, or a combination of these factors. Fatigue can be classified as either **physiological fatigue** or **psychological fatigue,** but both can result in a state of exhaustion.

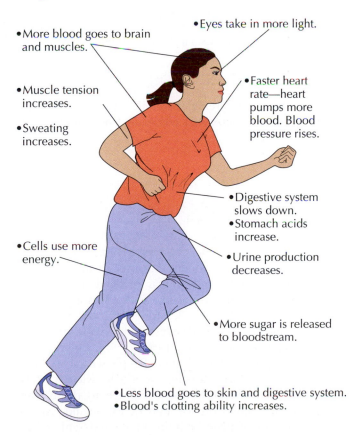

- More blood goes to brain and muscles.
- Eyes take in more light.
- Muscle tension increases.
- Sweating increases.
- Faster heart rate—heart pumps more blood. Blood pressure rises.
- Cells use more energy.
- Digestive system slows down.
- Stomach acids increase.
- Urine production decreases.
- More sugar is released to bloodstream.
- Less blood goes to skin and digestive system.
- Blood's clotting ability increases.

Figure 4 ▶ Physical symptoms of stress.

Stress Responses and Health

Chronic or repetitive acute stress can cause or exacerbate a variety of health problems. Some stress persists only as long as the stressor is present. For example, job-related stress caused by a challenging project generally subsides once that project is complete. In contrast, exposure to chronic stress or repeated exposure to acute stress may lead to a host of long-term negative physical and mental health consequences. Stress has been linked to chronic health maladies that plague individuals on a daily basis, such as headaches, indigestion, insomnia, and the common cold. In fact, a recent study concluded that "out-of-control" stress is the leading preventable source of increased health-care cost in the workforce, roughly equivalent to the costs of the health problems related to smoking.

Even illnesses with a substantial genetic component, such as cardiovascular disease and depression, have been linked to stress. One model (diathesis-stress model) suggests that individuals with a genetic or biological predisposition for a particular illness will express that illness only when environmental stresses are sufficient. Schizophrenia provides a good example. Although there is a strong genetic component to schizophrenia, not all individuals with a genetic risk will experience the disorder. Further, stressful situations typically precede the onset of symptoms.

Excessive stress reduces the effectiveness of the immune system. Research on the immune system indicates that stress compromises the function of the body's immune system. With an inefficient immune system, it is more difficult to fight off bacterial infections and to recover from medical treatments. An altered immune function also increases a person's susceptibility to allergies. Therefore, allergies and asthma attacks may be more severe under periods of high stress. Other autoimmune disorders, such as rheumatoid arthritis, are also worsened by stress.

Type A Personality The personality type characterized by impatience, ambition, and aggression; Type A personalities may be more susceptible to the effects of stress but may also be more able to cope with stress.

Hardiness A collection of personality traits thought to make a person more resistant to stress.

Physiological Fatigue A deterioration in the capacity of the neuromuscular system as a result of physical overwork and strain; also referred to as true fatigue.

Psychological Fatigue A feeling of fatigue, usually caused by such things as lack of exercise, boredom, or mental stress, that results in a lack of energy and depression; also referred to as subjective or false fatigue.

Stress can have mental and emotional effects. The challenges caused by psychosocial stress may lead to a variety of mental and emotional effects. In the short term, stress can impair concentration and attention span. Anxiety is an emotional response to stress that is characterized by apprehension. Because the response usually involves expending a lot of nervous energy, anxiety can lead to fatigue and muscular tension.

Anxiety may persist long after a stressful experience. For example, getting physically or sexually assaulted is an incredibly stressful experience and one that tends to stay with a person long after the crime. In some cases, traumatic experiences may lead to posttraumatic stress disorder (PTSD). Symptoms of PTSD include "flashbacks" of the traumatic event; avoidance of situations that remind the person of the event, emotional numbing, and increased level of arousal.

People who are excessively stressed are also more likely to be depressed than people who have optimal amounts of stress in their lives. Health-care costs for depressed people are 70 percent higher than for those who are not, and costs for people reporting high levels of stress are 50 percent higher than those for their less-stressed counterparts. Recent research has shown that drugs commonly prescribed to reduce depression can be effective in many cases. However, drugs do not get to the source of the life stressors that cause depression and often have negative side effects.

Stress can lead to changes in behavior. Stress can cause people to adopt nervous habits, such as biting their nails. It can also cause normally calm people to become irritable and short-tempered. Other behavioral responses to stress include altered eating and sleeping patterns, smoking, and the use of alcohol and other drugs. In addition to increased tendencies for negative behavior, stress can result in engaging in fewer positive behaviors such as regular physical activity and sufficient sleep.

Strategies for Action

Self-assessments of stressors in your life can be useful in managing stress. You will have the opportunity to evaluate your stress levels using the Life Experience Survey; assess your hardiness, a characteristic associated with effectively coping with stress; and evaluate your neuromuscular tension in the labs that follow.

Study Resources

Check out additional online study resources for this concept in the Student Edition of the Online Learning Center at www.mhhe.com/corbin13e.

Web Resources

Ulifeline: The online behavioral support system for young
    adults **www.ulifeline.org**
American Institute of Stress **www.stress.org**
American Psychological Association **www.apa.org**
International Stress Management Association **www.isma.org**
National Center for Post Traumatic Stress Disorder
    www.ncptsd.org
National Institute of Mental Health **www.nimh.nih.gov**

Suggested Readings

 Additional reference materials for Concept 18 are available at **www.mhhe.com/phys_fit/web18 Click 03.**

 ## In the News

Research Updates

Virtually every day new information is discovered that helps us to better understand the role of stress in our daily lives. Following are some new findings:

- *Genetic predisposition.* Recently, researchers have found evidence that some people have a genetic vulnerability to stress-related disorders such as depression. The researchers note that genetic factors do not soley determine if an individual will develop depression, but genetic variations do make some people more vulnerable and others more resilient.

- *"Tend or befriend" model.* A new paradigm called the "tend or befriend" model suggests a unique stress response for women. Women respond to stress by tending to others (nuturing) and affiliating with a social group (befriending). This response is helpful in protecting offspring and reducing the risk for the negative health consequences of stress.

- *Impatience as a health risk factor.* People who score high on a measure of impatience are nearly twice as likely to have high blood pressure relative to those who score low. Indicators of impatience include stress when caught in a checkout line or at a red light and an exaggerated sense of time urgency.

Lab 18A Evaluating Your Stress Level

Name		Section	Date

Purpose: To evaluate your stress during the past year and determine its implications

Procedures

1. Complete the Life Experience Survey based on your experiences during the past year. This survey lists a number of life events that may be distressful or eustressful. Read all of the items. If you did not experience an event, leave the box blank. In the box after each event that you did experience, write a number ranging from –3 to +3 using the scale described in the directions. Extra blanks are provided to write in positive or negative events not listed. Some items apply only to males or females. Items 48 to 56 are only for current college students.
2. Add all of the negative numbers and record your score (distress) in the Results section. Add the positive numbers and record your score (eustress) in the Results section. Use all of the events in the past year.
3. Find your scores on Chart 1 and record your ratings in the Results section.
4. Interpret the results by discussing the conclusions and implications in the space provided.

Results

Sum of negative scores [____] (distress)   Rating on negative scores [____]

Sum of positive scores [____] (eustress)   Rating on positive scores [____]

Chart 1 ▶ Scale for Life Experiences and Stress

	Sum of Negative Scores (Distress)	Sum of Positive Scores (Eustress)
May need counseling	14+	
Above average	9–13	11+
Average	6–9	9–10
Below average	<6	<9

Scoring the Life Experience Survey

1. Add all of the negative scores to arrive at your own distress score (negative stress).
2. Add all of the positive scores to arrive at a eustress score (positive stress).

Conclusions and Implications: In several sentences, discuss your current stress rating and its implications.

Life Experience Survey

Directions: If you did not experience an event, leave the box next to the event empty. If you experienced an event, enter a number in the box based on how the event impacted your life. Use the scale below:

Extremely negative impact	= −3
Moderately negative impact	= −2
Somewhat negative impact	= −1
Neither positive nor negative impact	= 0
Somewhat positive impact	= +1
Moderately positive impact	= +2
Extremely positive impact	= +3

1. Marriage
2. Detention in jail or comparable institution
3. Death of spouse
4. Major change in sleeping habits (much more or less sleep)
5. Death of close family member:
   a. Mother
   b. Father
   c. Brother
   d. Sister
   e. Child
   f. Grandmother
   g. Grandfather
   h. Other (specify) _____
6. Major change in eating habits (much more or much less food intake)
7. Foreclosure on mortgage or loan
8. Death of a close friend
9. Outstanding personal achievement
10. Minor law violation (traffic ticket, disturbing the peace, etc.)
11. *Male:* Wife's/girlfriend's pregnancy

    Female: Pregnancy
12. Changed work situation (different working conditions, working hours, etc.)
13. New job
14. Serious illness or injury of close family member:
   a. Father
   b. Mother
   c. Sister
   d. Brother
   e. Grandfather
   f. Grandmother
   g. Spouse
   h. Child
   i. Other (specify) _____
15. Sexual difficulties
16. Trouble with employer (in danger of losing job, being suspended, demoted, etc.)
17. Trouble with in-laws
18. Major change in financial status (a lot better off or a lot worse off)
19. Major change in closeness of family members (decreased or increased closeness)

20. Gaining a new family member (through birth, adoption, family member moving in, etc.)
21. Change of residence
22. Marital separation from mate (due to conflict)
23. Major change in church activities (increased or decreased attendance)
24. Marital reconciliation with mate
25. Major change in number of arguments with spouse (a lot more or a lot fewer arguments)
26. *Married male:* Change in wife's work outside the home (beginning work, ceasing work, changing to a new job)

    Married female: Change in husband's work (loss of job, beginning new job, retirement, etc.)
27. Major change in usual type and/or amount of recreation
28. Borrowing more than $10,000 (buying a home, business, etc.)
29. Borrowing less than $10,000 (buying car or TV, getting school loan, etc.)
30. Being fired from job
31. *Male:* Wife/girlfriend having abortion

    Female: Having abortion
32. Major personal illness or injury
33. Major change in social activities, such as parties, movies, visiting (increased or decreased participation)
34. Major change in living conditions of family (building new home, remodeling, deterioration of home or neighborhood, etc.)
35. Divorce
36. Serious injury or illness of close friend
37. Retirement from work
38. Son or daughter leaving home (due to marriage, college, etc.)
39. Ending of formal schooling
40. Separation from spouse (due to work, travel, etc.)
41. Engagement
42. Breaking up with boyfriend/girlfriend
43. Leaving home for the first time
44. Reconciliation with boyfriend/girlfriend

Other recent experiences that have had an impact on your life: list and rate.

45. _____
46. _____
47. _____

For Students Only

48. Beginning new school experience at a higher academic level (college, graduate school, professional school, etc.)
49. Changing to a new school at same academic level (undergraduate, graduate, etc.)
50. Academic probation
51. Being dismissed from dormitory or other residence
52. Failing an important exam
53. Changing a major
54. Failing a course
55. Dropping a course
56. Joining a fraternity/sorority

Source: Sarason, G., Johnson, J. H., and Siegel, J. M.

Lab 18B Evaluating Your Hardiness

Name	**Section**	**Date**

Purpose: To evaluate your level of hardiness and to help you identify the ways in which you appraise and respond to stressful situations

Procedures

1. Complete the Hardiness Questionnaire. Make an X over the circle that best describes what is true for you personally.
2. Summarize your score using the scoring chart.
3. Evaluate your score using the hardiness rating chart (Chart 1) and record your ratings in the Results section.
4. Interpret the results by answering the questions in the Conclusions and Implications section.

Hardiness Questionnaire

	Not True	Rarely True	Sometimes True	Often True	Score
1. I look forward to school and work on most days.	①	②	③	④	
2. Having too many choices in life makes me nervous.	④	③	②	①	
3. I know where my life is going and look forward to the future.	①	②	③	④	
4. I prefer to not get too involved in relationships.	④	③	②	①	
			Commitment Score, Sum 1–4		
5. My efforts at school and work will pay off in the long run.	①	②	③	④	
6. I just have to trust my life to fate to be successful.	④	③	②	①	
7. I believe that I can make a difference in the world.	①	②	③	④	
8. Being successful in life takes more luck and good breaks than effort.	④	③	②	①	
			Control Score, Sum 5–8		
9. I would be willing to work for less money if I could do something really challenging and interesting.	①	②	③	④	
10. I often get frustrated when my daily plans and schedule get altered.	④	③	②	①	
11. Experiencing new situations in life is important to me.	①	②	③	④	
12. I don't mind being bored.	④	③	②	①	
			Challenge Score, Sum 9–12		

357

Results

Commitment score [　　　　]   Commitment rating [　　　　]

Control score [　　　　]   Control rating [　　　　]

Challenge score [　　　　]   Challenge rating [　　　　]

Sum the three scores:

Hardiness score [　　　　]   Hardiness rating [　　　　]

Chart 1 ▶ Hardiness Rating

Rating	Individual Hardiness Scale Scores	Total Hardiness Scores
High hardiness	14–16	40–48
Moderate hardiness	10–13	30–39
Low hardiness	<10	< 30

Conclusions and Implications

1. In several sentences, discuss your three hardiness scores. Commitment scores reflect a dedication to personal goals and life in general. Control scores reflect a belief that events in your life are within your control. Challenge scores reflect an ability to see stressful situations as opportunities for growth. Do you think these scores have implications for you? Are there changes you can make?

2. In several sentences, discuss your total hardiness score. This collection of traits has been referred to as the "stress-resistant personality," since hardy individuals have been found to respond better to stressful situations. Do you think your score is accurate for you? Do you think the score has implications for you?

Lab 18C Evaluating Neuromuscular Tension

Name	Section	Date

Purpose: To learn to recognize the signs of excess muscle tension

Procedures

1. Choose a partner. Designate one partner as the subject and the other as the tester.
2. The subject should lie supine on the floor in a comfortable position and consciously try to relax.
3. The tester should kneel beside the subject's right hand and remain very still and quiet while the subject is concentrating.
4. After 5 minutes have elapsed, the tester should observe the subject for the visual signs of tension listed in Chart 1 (page 360). Check "yes" or "no" for visual symptoms of tension.
5. Quietly and gently, the tester should grasp the subject's right wrist with his or her fingers and slowly raise it about 3 inches from the floor, letting it hinge at the elbow, then let the hand drop, observing for the manual symptoms in Chart 1 (page 360). *Caution:* Make no movement or sound to disturb your partner's concentration and relaxation. Check "yes" or "no" for manual symptoms of tension.
6. You may wish to repeat this after another minute or two.
7. Arouse the subject at the end of the testing and total the number of "yes" checks.
8. Find the rating in Chart 2 (page 360) and record your score and rating.
9. Change roles and repeat the evaluation with a new subject and tester.
10. Answer the questions in the Results and Conclusions and Implications sections.
11. If time permits, perform the exercises from Table 4 in Concept 19.

Results

Check one circle for each of the following questions.

Yes	No	
○	○	Were you aware of your own tension?
○	○	Was it more difficult to relax than you expected?
○	○	Did your awareness of your partner make it more difficult to concentrate?
○	○	Could you concentrate on your breathing without altering its rhythm?
○	○	Could you learn to release muscle tension and help manage your stress with additional practice?
○	○	Could you learn to release tension while sitting or standing with your eyes open?
○	○	Do you think your score today is typical of your normal tension level?

Chart 1 ▶ Signs of Tension Observed by Tester

Visual Symptoms	No	Yes
Frowning	○	○
Twitching	○	○
Eyelids fluttering	○	○
Breathing	○	○
Shallow	○	○
Rapid	○	○
Irregular	○	○
Tight mouth	○	○
Swallowing	○	○

Manual Symptoms	No	Yes
Assistance (subject helps lift arm)	○	○
Resistance (subject resists movement)	○	○
Posturing (subject holds arm in raised position)	○	○
Perseveration (subject continues upward movement)	○	○

Total score equals sum of "yes" checks ☐

Chart 2 ▶ Tension-Relaxation Rating Scale

Classification	Total Score
Excellent (relaxed)	0
Very good (mild tension)	1–3
Good (moderate tension)	4–6
Fair (tense)	7–9
Poor (marked tension)	10–12

Record your tension-relaxation rating: ☐

Conclusions and Implications

In several sentences, describe the implications this lab has for you in terms of your daily life (e.g., sleeping, studying, taking exams, performing on stage).

Stress Management, Relaxation, and Time Management

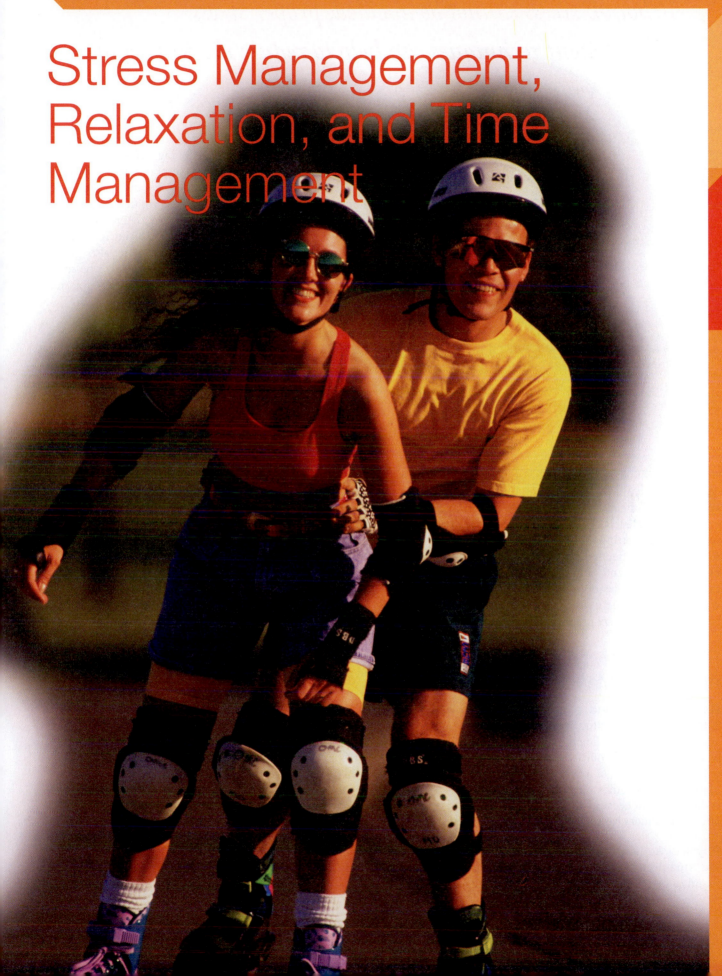

Although stress cannot be avoided, proper stress management techniques can help to reduce the impact of stress in your life.

Health Goals

for the year 2010

- Improve mental health and ensure access to appropriate, quality mental health services.

- Increase mental health treatment, including treatment for depression and anxiety disorders.

- Increase mental health screening and assessment.

- Reduce suicide and suicide attempts, especially among young people.

- Increase availability of worksite stress-reduction programs.

As outlined in Concept 18, we all experience stress on a daily basis and must find ways to manage stress effectively. We can do many things to prevent excessive levels of stress. Examples include exercising regularly, getting sufficient sleep, and allowing time for recreation. Effective time management is essential for balancing work and other activities. Despite our best efforts, stressful situations will occur and we must find a way to deal with them. Later in this concept, three effective methods for managing stress will be described.

Physical Activity and Stress Management

Regular activity and a healthy diet can help you adapt to stressful situations. An individual's capacity to adapt is not a static function but fluctuates as situations change. The better your overall health, the better you can withstand the rigors of tension without becoming susceptible to illness or other disorders. Physical activity is especially important because it conditions your body to function effectively under challenging physiological conditions.

Physical activity can provide relief from stress and aid muscle tension release. Physical activity has been found to be effective at relieving stress, particularly white-collar job stress. Studies show that regular exercise decreases the likelihood of developing stress disorders and reduces the intensity of the stress response. It also shortens the time of recovery from an emotional trauma. Its effect tends to be short-term, so one must continue to exercise regularly for it to have a continuing effect. Aerobic exercise is believed to be especially effective in reducing anxiety and relieving stress (though other activities are also good). Whatever your choice of exercise, it is likely to be more effective as an antidote to stress if it is something you find enjoyable.

The relation between physical activity and the stress response remains unclear. Physical activity is associated with a physiological response that is similar, in many ways, to the body's response to psychosocial stressors. Further, individuals who are physically fit have a reduced physiological response to exercise. Presumably, someone who is physically fit would also have a reduced response to psychosocial stressors. Research supports this hypothesis indicating that chronic exercise reduces physiological reactivity to nonexercise stressors. However, more research is necessary.

Recent studies have attempted to clarify the role of exercise in stress reactivity by more clearly specifying the physiological systems activated by exercise-related stress and nonexercise-related stress. The body's physiological response consists of both a sympathetic nervous system response and an endocrine response. Results of a recent study showed that the sympathetic nervous system response to exercise is immediate, whereas the endocrine response to exercise is delayed. In contrast, the endocrine response to psychosocial stressors is usually immediate. Such differences in responses suggest that more complex models may be necessary to understand the role of exercise in protecting against psychosocial stress.

Physical activity can improve mental health. www.mhhe.com/phys_fit/web19 Click 01. The physical health benefits of exercise have been well established for some time. Recent research suggests that the benefits of exercise extend beyond the physical and into the realm of mental health. Studies have demonstrated that exercise can reduce anxiety, aid in recovery from depression, and assist in efforts to eliminate negative health behaviors such as smoking. More information concerning exercise and stress follows.

- **Physical activity can reduce anxiety.** Evidence shows that physical activity leads to reductions in anxiety in nonclinical samples. One recent study found that exercise may also be effective in reducing anxiety among individuals with panic disorder. An aerobic exercise program led to reductions in panic symptoms relative to a control group. Although exercise was not as effective as medication, it may be a useful addition to other treatment methods for anxiety disorders.
- **Physical activity can reduce depression.** A randomized clinical trial compared antidepressant medication and aerobic exercise with a combined antidepressant and exercise condition in the treatment of major depressive disorder. Results indicated that the aerobic exercise group fared as well as the other two at the end of treatment. In addition, patients who only exercised were less likely to have a remission to depression at a 6-month follow-up. Individuals in the exercise condition possibly felt more responsible for the improvements in their condition and this increase in self-efficacy led to better long-term outcomes. The results of this clinical trial are consistent with evidence reported in a review of thirty studies on exercise and depression. This review found that those who exercise are less depressed than those who do not exercise.
- **Physical activity can aid in changing behaviors related to health.** A recent study tested vigorous physical activity as an adjunct to a cognitive-behavioral smoking cessation program for women. The results indicated that women who received the exercise intervention were able to sustain continuous abstinence from smoking for a longer period of time relative to those who did not receive the exercise intervention. Women in the exercise condition also gained less weight during smoking cessation.

Stress, Sleep, and Recreation

Stress can be both a cause and a consequence of impaired sleep. In order to function effectively and adapt effectively to stressful situations, one must get adequate sleep. In addition to helping you function more effectively in your everyday life, a good night's sleep may increase your life span. In a series of studies among seniors, researchers found that study participants who reported sleep difficulties had higher morbidity at the follow-up data collection. Thus, sleep may improve both the quality and quantity of your life.

Although the number of hours needed varies from person to person, the average adult needs between 7 and 8 hours of sleep per night. Getting enough sleep can be quite difficult, given the hectic schedules that many individuals keep. Furthermore, the effects of stress can impair one's ability to get to sleep or stay asleep. Thus, a

Table 1 ▶ Guidelines for Good Sleep

- Be aware of the effects of your medications. Some medicines, such as weight loss pills and decongestants, contain caffeine, ephedrine, or other ingredients that interfere with sleep.
- Avoid tobacco use. Nicotine is a stimulant and can interfere with sleep.
- Avoid excess alcohol use. Alcohol may make it easier to get to sleep but may be a reason you wake up at night and are unable to get back to sleep.
- You may exercise late in the day, but do not do vigorous activity right before bedtime.
- Sleep in a room that is cooler than normal.
- Avoid hard-to-digest foods late in the day. Fatty and spicy foods should be avoided.
- Avoid large meals late in the day or right before bedtime. A light snack before bedtime should not be a problem for most people.
- Avoid too much liquid before bedtime.
- Avoid naps during the day.
- Go to bed and get up at the same time each day.
- Do not study, read, or engage in other activities in your bed. You want your brain to associate your bed with sleep, not with activity.
- If you are having difficulty falling asleep, do not stay in bed. Get up and find something to do until you begin to feel tired and then go back to bed.

cycle of stress and impaired sleep ensues. Some guidelines for good sleep are presented in Table 1.

All work and no play can lead to poor mental and physical health. The amount of time the average person spends at work has increased rather than decreased in the past two decades. Since 1860, the amount of hours typically spent in work decreased dramatically. The most recent statistics (see Figure 1), however, indicate a trend toward increased work time. A major reason for this increase is that more people now hold second jobs than in the past. Also, some jobs of modern society have increasing rather than decreasing time demands. For example, medical doctors and other professionals often work more

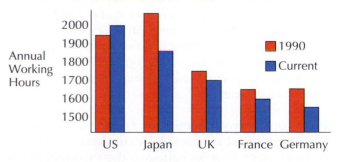

Figure 1 ▶ Average annual working hours of five nations.

Source: Organization for Economic Cooperation and Development.

hours than the 35 to 44 hours that the majority of people work. Nearly three times as many married women with children work full-time now, as compared with 1960.

Experts have referred to young adults as the "over-worked Americans" because they work several jobs and maintain dual roles (full-time employment coupled with normal family chores), or they work extended hours in demanding professional jobs. A recent Gallup poll shows that the great majority of adults have "enough time" for work, chores, and sleep but not enough time for friends, self, spouse, and children. When time is at a premium, the factors most likely to be negatively affected are personal health, relationships with children, and marriage or romantic relationships.

Work pressures can be stressful. This suggests a need to manage time effectively and to find activities that are enjoyable during free time.

Free time is important to the average person. Most people say that **free time** is important, but surveys indicate that more than half of all adults feel that they get too little of it. Many adults report that they get too little time for **recreation** or to simply relax and "do nothing."

 Recreation and leisure are important contributors to wellness (quality of life). www.mhhe.com/phys_fit/web19 Click 02. **Leisure** is time spent "doing things I just want to do" or "doing nothing." Recreation, on the other hand, is often purposeful. Leisure and recreation can contribute to stress reduction and wellness, though leisure activities are not done specifically to achieve these benefits.

The value of recreation and leisure in the busy lives of people in Western culture is evidenced by the emphasis public health officials place on the availability and accessibility of recreational facilities in the future.

To achieve wellness and stress-reduction benefits, recreation should provide a sense of play. **Play** is done of one's own free will and most often done for fun or intrinsic rather than extrinsic reasons. Activities performed for material things, such as trophies and medals, can be considered recreational as long as the principal reason for doing the activity is a sense of fun and playfulness. If the activity is done primarily for extrinsic reasons, it may not provide wellness benefits and is probably not true recreation. For example, playing golf to impress the boss is an extrinsic reason that may increase life stress rather than decrease it.

There are many meaningful types of recreation. Many recreational activities involve moderate to vigorous physical activity. If fitness is the goal, these activities should be chosen. Involvement in nonphysical activities also constitutes recreation. For example, reading is a participation

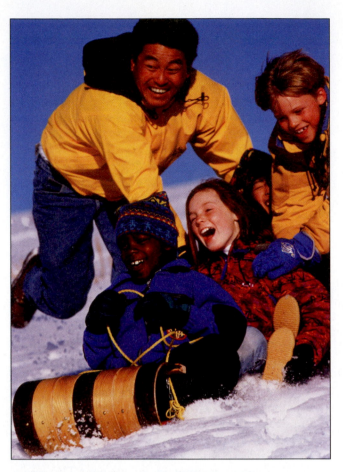

It is important to take time for recreation.

activity that can contribute significantly to other wellness dimensions, such as emotional/mental and spiritual. Passive involvement (spectating) is a third type of participation.

Passive participation has been criticized by some people who feel that active participation is an important ingredient of meaningful recreation. Experts point out that spectating can be refreshing and meaningful. For example, watching a good play at the theater qualifies as meaningful recreation and can be true leisure. Likewise, active participation in community theater can be meaningful recreation. To achieve the wellness benefits of recreation, liberal participation and meaningful passive involvement (spectating) are encouraged.

Time Management

Effective time management aids in adapting to the stresses of modern living. Many people in our culture lead stress-filled lives and see the need for lifestyle changes but fail to carry out their plans for various reasons. Most often mentioned is the lack of time: "I would like to exercise, but I don't have the time." "My two jobs don't allow me as much time as I would like to spend with my family." "I know I need to relax and enjoy myself, but I just can't

Table 2 ▶ Steps for Effective Time Management

Step	Strategies	Example
• Establish priorities.	Analyze what you value in life. Make a list of your priorities to see if you are meeting them.	Would you like to have more time for recreation or to spend with family or friends?
• Monitor your current time use.	Keep a pad and pencil with you so you can record your activities as you do them.	You may find that you are wasting time on unimportant activities, such as surfing the Net.
• Analyze your current time use.	Determine which activities you could spend less time doing. Figure out how to reduce time spent on these activities.	You might like to study less, but is this realistic? You may have to give up other committed time. You might be able to combine recreation with exercise and socializing by exercising with friends.
• Make a schedule.	Make a commitment to reserving time for important recreational activities as well as daily responsibilities. Be structured but flexible enough to allow for spontaneity.	If you have study time scheduled and a friend invites you to a movie, you can replace other recreational time with studying so you don't miss out.
• Evaluate progress.	Continue to monitor your time use to see if you are keeping to your schedule.	If you struggle to keep your schedule, it may require modification so it does not become a new source of stress.

find the time." You may never find time to do all of the things you want to do, but you can learn to manage time more effectively to help you cope with the stresses of daily living. In Lab 19C, you will get the opportunity to practice the time-management skills outlined in Table 2.

Coping with Stress

Unresolved stress poses the greatest physical and emotional danger. Although some stressors are short-lived, many stressors persist over a long period of time. The ability to adapt, or cope with these stressors, largely determines their ultimate effect. If effective **coping** strategies are used, the effects of a stressful situation can be more tolerable. In many cases, reasonable solutions or compromises can be found. On the other hand, if ineffective coping strategies are used, problems may become even worse. This can lead to more stress and more severe outcomes. Although stress cannot be avoided, it can be managed. Effective stress management is a skill that contributes to both health and quality of life.

Coping strategies can be classified into three basic categories. Individuals deal with stress in a variety of ways; however, the methods of coping can generally be classified as **emotion-focused coping, problem-focused coping,** or **appraisal-focused coping** (see Table 3). Emotion-focused coping strategies attempt to regulate the emotions resulting from stressful events. In contrast, problem-focused strategies are aimed at changing the source of the stress. Appraisal-focused coping strategies are based on changing the way one perceives the stressor or changing one's perceptions of resources for effectively managing stress. Whereas each of these strategies is effective in various circumstances, **avoidant coping** strategies, such as ignoring or escaping the problem, are likely to be ineffective for almost everyone.

Free Time Time not committed to work or other duties.

Recreation *Recreation* means creating something anew. In this book, it refers to something that you do for your amusement or for fun to help you divert your attention and to refresh yourself (re-create yourself).

Leisure Time that is free from the demands of work. Leisure is more than free time; it is also an attitude. Leisure activities need not be means to ends (purposeful) but are ends in themselves.

Play Activity done of one's own free will. The play experience is fun, intrinsically rewarding, and a self-absorbing means of self-expression. It is characterized by a sense of freedom or escape from life's normal rules.

Coping A person's constantly changing cognitive and psychological efforts to manage stressful situations.

Emotion-Focused Coping The method of adapting to stress that is based on regulating the emotions that cause or result from stress.

Problem-Focused Coping The method of adapting to stress that is based on changing the source or cause of stress.

Appraisal-Focused Coping The method of adapting to stress that is based on changing your perceptions of stress and your resources for coping.

Avoidant Coping Seeking immediate, temporary relief from stress through distraction or self-indulgence (i.e., drugs, alcohol, tobacco use).

Table 3 ▶ Strategies for Stress Management

Category	Description
Emotion-Focused Strategies	**Strategies That Minimize the Emotional and Physical Effects of the Situation**
• Relaxing	• Using relaxation techniques to reduce the symptoms of stress
• Exercising	• Using physical activity to reduce the symptoms of stress
• Seeking passive social support	• Talking with someone about what you are experiencing or accepting sympathy and understanding
• Praying	• Looking for spiritual guidance to provide comfort
Appraisal-Focused Strategies	**Strategies That Alter Perceptions of the Problem or Your Ability to Cope Effectively with the Problem**
• Cognitive restructuring	• Changing negative or automatic thoughts leading to unnecessary distress
• Seeking knowledge or practicing skills	• Finding ways to increase your confidence in your ability to cope
Problem-Focused Strategies	**Strategies That Directly Seek to Solve or Minimize the Stressful Situation**
• Systematic problem solving	• Making a plan of action to solve the problem and following through to make the situation better
• Being assertive	• Standing up for your own rights and values while respecting the opinions of others
• Seeking active social support	• Getting help or advice from others who can provide specific assistance for your situation
Avoidant Coping Strategies	**Strategies That Attempt to Distract the Individual from the Problem**
• Ignoring	• Refusing to think about the situation or pretending no problem exists
• Escaping	• Looking for ways to feel better or to stop thinking about the problem, including eating or using nicotine, alcohol, or other drugs

Coping with most stress requires a variety of thoughts and actions. Stress forces our bodies to work under less than optimal conditions, yet this is the time when we need to function at our best. Effective coping may require some efforts to regulate the emotional aspects of the stress and other efforts directed toward solving the problem. For example, if you are experiencing stress over grades in school, you have to accept your current grades and take active steps to improve them. Your appraisal of your past performance and the likelihood of improving your performance in the future will significantly impact how you respond to the situation. It does no good to worry about past events. Instead, it is important to look ahead for ways to solve the problems at hand. Coping with this situation may, therefore, require the use of all three effective coping strategies.

Emotion-Focused Coping Strategies

Relaxation technique and/or coping strategies can help in relieving stress. When you are aware of what stress does to your body, you can do something to relieve those symptoms immediately as well as on a regular and more long-term basis. Although there is no magical cure for stress or tension, various therapeutic approaches may be effective in helping you handle stress. These approaches can slow your heart and respiration, relax tense muscles, clear your mind, and help you relax mentally and emotionally. Perhaps most important, these techniques can improve your outlook and help you cope better with the stressful situation. In Lab 19A, you will perform a progressive relaxation program. Performing Lab 19A only once will not prepare you to use relaxation techniques effectively. Remember, you must practice learning to relax.

Some treatments are less desirable than others because they act only as "crutches" or "fire extinguishers" and do not get at the root of the problem. Hypnosis may lead to fantasy and dependency. Alcoholic beverages, tranquilizers, and painkillers may give temporary relief and may be prescribed by a physician as part of the treatment, but they do not resolve the problem and may even mask symptoms or cause further problems, such as addiction. Drugs do not provide a long-term solution to chronic stress or tension, and, contrary to vitamin and mineral advertisements, supplementing the diet with vitamin C or so-called stress vitamin formulations has no proven benefits.

Various conscious relaxation techniques exist. Conscious relaxation techniques reduce stress and tension by directly altering the symptoms. When you are stressed, heart rate, blood pressure, and muscle tension all increase to help your body deal with the challenge. Conscious relaxation techniques reduce these normal effects and bring the body back to a more relaxed state. Most techniques use the "three *R*s" of relaxation to help the body relax: (1) reduce mental activity, (2) recognize tension, and (3) reduce respiration. Because these techniques do not change the nature or impact of a stressor, they are considered to be a passive, or emotion-focused, coping strategy. The following are several examples of these techniques:

- *The Quick Fix.* To get relief from a stressful situation during the day, take a timeout for 5 to 10 minutes by finding a quiet place away from the situation with as few distractions as possible. Sit, loosen your clothes, take off your shoes, and close your eyes. Then follow these steps:

(1) Inhale deeply for about 4 seconds and exhale, letting the air out slowly for about 8 seconds (twice as long as the inhalation). Do this several times. (2) Mentally visualize a pleasant image, such as a peaceful lake or stream. Continue to relax and breathe deeply. (3) When your time is up, breathe deeply and stretch luxuriously. Go back to your work, refreshed and with a changed attitude. You may need to do this several times a day.

- *Jacobson's progressive relaxation method.* You must be able to recognize how a tense muscle feels before you can voluntarily release the tension. In this technique, contract the muscles strongly and then relax. Each of the large muscles is relaxed first and later the small ones. The contractions are gradually reduced in intensity until no movement is visible. Always, the emphasis is placed on detecting the feeling of tension as the first step in "letting go," or "going negative." Jacobson, a pioneer in muscle relaxation research, emphasized the importance of relaxing eye and speech muscles, because he believed these muscles trigger reactions of the total organism more than other muscles. A sample contract-relax exercise routine for relaxation is presented in Lab 19A.

- *Autogenic (self-generated) relaxation training.* Several times daily, sit or lie in a quiet room with eyes closed. Block out distracting thoughts by passively concentrating on preselected words or phrases. This technique has been used to focus on heaviness of limbs, warmth of limbs, heart rate regulation, respiratory rate and depth regulation, and coolness in the forehead. It evokes changes opposite to those produced by stress. Research has shown that people who are skilled in this technique can decrease oxygen consumption, change the electrical activity of the brain, slow the metabolism, decrease blood lactate, lower body temperature, and slow the heart rate.

- *Biofeedback/autogenic relaxation training.* Biofeedback training uses machines that monitor certain physiological processes of the body and that provide visual or auditory evidence of what is happening to normally unconscious bodily functions. The evidence, or feedback, is then used to help you decrease these functions. When combined with autogenic training, subjects have learned to relax and reduce the electrical activity in their muscles, lower blood pressure, decrease heart rate, change their brainwaves, and decrease headaches, asthma attacks, and stomach acid secretion.

- *Stretching and rhythmical exercises.* People who work long hours at a desk can release tension by getting up frequently and stretching, by taking a brisk walk down the hall, or by performing "office exercises." Exercising to music or to a rhythmic beat has been found to be relaxing and even hypnotic. Some exercises designed specifically for relaxation are illustrated in Table 4.

Technology Update

Video Games

Can video games actually be good for your health? The answer is yes, according to NASA. A new system combines biofeedback technology with the fun of video games by having the game respond to the player's body and brain. As the player's brainwaves become closer to optimal functioning, the joystick becomes easier to control. Thus, the player is motivated to optimize his or her brainwaves in order to perform well. In turn, the optimized brainwaves may contribute to improved physical and mental health.

Prayer and positive thinking can help you cope with stress and daily problems. In addition to managing the body's physical response to stress, one must deal with the impact of stress on thoughts and emotions. Although relaxation strategies may also impact these dimensions, additional approaches may be necessary to adequately manage these aspects of the stress response. Examples include prayer, positive thinking, and mindful meditation.

- *Prayer.* Recent studies have shown that prayer can decrease blood pressure for many people and can be a source of internal comfort. It can have other calming effects that are associated with reduced distress. It can also provide confidence to function more effectively, thereby reducing the stresses associated with ineffectiveness at work or in other situations.

- *Positive thinking.* Research supports the idea that optimism relates to psychological well-being. Recent research suggests that positive emotion may also be an effective coping mechanism for managing acute stress. Positive moods seem to help undo the effects of negative emotions. For example, positive moods have been shown to undo some of the cardiovascular effects associated with negative emotions. Positive moods may also help individuals effectively use additional coping strategies to manage stress. The practical

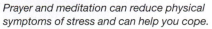

Prayer and meditation can reduce physical symptoms of stress and can help you cope.

Table 4

Table 4 Relaxation Exercises

1. Neck Stretch

Roll the head slowly in a half-circle from 9:00 to 8:00 to 7, 6, 5, 4, 3, and then reverse from 3 to 9. Close your eyes and feel the stretch. Do *not* make a full circle by tipping the head back. Repeat several times.

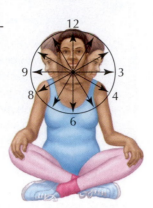

2. Shoulder Lift

Hunch the shoulders as high as possible (contract) and then let them drop (relax). Repeat several times. Inhale on the lift; exhale on the drop.

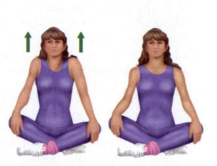

3. Trunk Stretch and Drop

Stand and reach as high as possible; tiptoe and stretch every muscle; then collapse completely, letting knees flex and trunk, head, and arms dangle. Repeat two or three times. Inhale on the stretch and exhale on the collapse.

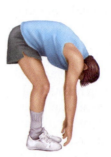

4. Trunk Swings

Following the trunk stretch and drop (see illustration 3), remain in the "drop" position and, with a minimum of muscular effort, set the trunk swinging from side to side by shifting the weight from one foot to the other, letting the heels come off the floor alternately. Keep the entire body (especially the neck) limp.

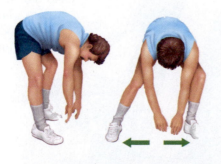

5. Tension Contrast

With arms extended overhead, lie on your side. Tense the body as stiff as a board; then let go and relax, letting the body fall either forward or backward in whatever direction it loses balance. Continue letting go for a few seconds after falling and allow yourself to feel as if you are still sinking. Repeat on the other side.

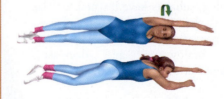

implications are relatively simple. Do whatever you need to do to create a positive mood when you are stressed or upset. The one thing you do not want to do is dwell on your negative mood. This is likely to prolong the negative mood state and the negative physical, cognitive, and behavioral consequences.

- *Mindfulness meditation.* Whereas most relaxation techniques seek to distract attention away from distressing emotions, mindfulness meditation encourages the individual to experience fully his or her emotions in a nonjudgmental way. The individual is encouraged to bring full attention to the internal and external experiences that are occurring "in the moment." John Kabat-Zinn, founder of the Stress Reduction Clinic at the University of Massachusetts, has generated considerable enthusiasm for this technique, which is based on ancient Buddhist philosophy. Mindfulness training has now been incorporated into empirically validated psychotherapies, and a number of self-help books provide additional information about the technique (see *Suggested Readings*).

recognize some of the common types of distorted thinking. If you can learn to recognize distorted thinking, you can change the way you think and often reduce your stress levels. Some common types of distorted thinking are listed in Table 5.

If you have ever used any of the ten types of distorted thinking described in Table 5, you may find it useful to consider different methods of "untwisting" your thinking. Using the strategies for untwisting your thinking can be useful in changing negative thinking to positive thinking (see Table 6).

If you really want to change your way of thinking to avoid stress, you may have to practice the guidelines outlined in Table 6. To do this, you can think of a recent situation that caused stress. Describe the situation on paper, and see if you used distorted thinking in the situation (see Table 5). If so, write down which types of distorted thinking you used. Finally, determine if any of the guidelines in Table 6 would have been useful. If so, write down the strategy you could have used. When a similar situation arises, you will be prepared to deal with the stressful situation. Repeat this technique, using several situations that have recently caused stress.

Appraisal-Focused Coping Strategies (Cognitive Restructuring)

Changing your way of thinking can help you cope. Research suggests you can reduce stress by changing the way you think. At one time or another, virtually all people have distorted thinking, which can create unnecessary stress. Distorted thinking is also referred to as negative or automatic thinking. To alleviate stress, it can be useful to

Problem-Focused Coping Strategies

Problem-focused coping is most effective in dealing with controllable stressors. Whereas emotion- and appraisal-focused coping may be the most effective means for coping with situations beyond one's control, a problem under personal control may be best addressed by taking action to solve the problem. Effective

Table 5 ▶ Types of Distorted Thinking

Type	Description
1. All-or-none thinking	You look at things in absolute, black-and-white categories.
2. Overgeneralization	You view a negative event as a never-ending pattern of defeat.
3. Mental filter	You dwell on the negatives and ignore the positives.
4. Discounting the positives	You insist that your accomplishments and positive qualities don't count.
5. Jumping to conclusions	(A) Mind reading—you assume that others are reacting negatively to you when there is no definite evidence of this. (B) Fortune telling—you arbitrarily predict that things will turn out badly.
6. Magnification or minimization	You blow things out of proportion or shrink their importance inappropriately.
7. Emotional reasoning	You reason from how you feel: "I feel like an idiot, so I must be one." "I don't feel like doing this, so I'll put it off."
8. Should statements	You criticize yourself or other people with "shoulds" or "shouldn'ts." "Musts," "oughts," and "have tos" are similar offenders.
9. Labeling	You identify with your shortcomings. Instead of saying, "I made a mistake," you tell yourself, "I am a jerk," "a fool," or "a loser."
10. Personalization and blame	You blame yourself for something that you weren't entirely responsible for, or you blame other people and overlook ways that your own attitudes and behaviors might have contributed to the problem.

Source: Burns, D. D.

Table 6 ▶ Ten Ways to Untwist Your Thinking	
The Ten Ways	**Description**
1. Identify the distortion.	Write down your negative thoughts, so you can see which of the ten types of distorted thinking you are involved in. This will make it easier to think about the problem in a more positive and realistic way.
2. Examine the evidence.	Instead of assuming that your negative thought is true, if you feel you never do anything right, you can list several things that you have done successfully.
3. Use the double standard method.	Instead of putting yourself down in a harsh, condemning way, talk to yourself in the same compassionate way you would talk to a friend with a similar problem.
4. Use the experimental technique	Do an experiment to test the validity of your negative thought. For example, if during an episode of panic you become terrified that you are about to die of a heart attack, you can jog or run up and down several flights of stairs. This will prove that your heart is healthy and strong.
5. Think in shades of gray.	Although this method might sound drab, the defects can be illuminating. Instead of thinking about your problems in all-or-none extremes, evaluate things on a range from 0 to 100. When things do not work out as well as you had hoped, think about the experience as a partial success, rather than a complete failure. See what you can learn from the situation.
6. Use the survey method.	Ask people questions to find out if your thoughts and attitudes are realistic. For example, if you believe that public speaking anxiety is abnormal and shameful, ask several friends if they ever felt nervous before they gave a talk.
7. Define terms.	When you label yourself "inferior," "a fool," or "a loser," ask, "What is the definition of 'a fool'?" You will feel better when you see that there is no such thing as a fool or a loser.
8. Use the semantic method.	Simply substitute language that is less colorful or emotionally loaded. This method is helpful for "should" statements. Instead of telling yourself "I *shouldn't* have made that mistake," you can say, "It would be better if I hadn't made that mistake."
9. Use re-attribution.	Instead of automatically assuming you are "bad" and blaming yourself entirely for a problem, think about the many factors that may have contributed to it. Focus on solving the problem instead of using up all your energy blaming yourself and feeling guilty.
10. Do a cost-benefit analysis.	List the advantages and disadvantages of a feeling (such as getting angry when your plane is late), a negative thought (such as "No matter how hard I try, I always screw up"), or a behavior pattern (such as overeating and lying around in bed when you are depressed). You can also use the cost-benefit analysis to modify a self-defeating belief, such as "I must always be perfect."

Source: Burns, D. D.

problem-focused coping requires individual beliefs that support action and the skills with which to carry out the desired behavior. Each of these factors is outlined in the following section.

Your locus of control influences your coping responses. In order to engage in problem-focused coping, people must believe that they have some degree of control over the stressor. People with an "internal" locus of control generally believe that they have the capacity to impact the outcomes of stressful events. In contrast, individuals with an external locus of control generally believe that outcomes are determined by factors other than personal control (e.g., luck, fate, powerful others). You can evaluate your own locus of control in Lab 19B.

An individual's locus of control can have a significant impact on how he or she responds to a stressful situation. Research has consistently found that having an internal locus of control is associated with better health outcomes. People with an internal locus of control are more likely to take active steps to address the problems that created the stress, rather than avoiding the problem.

Those with an external locus of control are more likely to use passive methods for managing stress.

Although an internal locus of control generally promotes health, this is not always the case. This truth is apparent in depressed individuals with a pessimistic explanatory style. They believe that their failures are due to internal factors, squarely placing control of these events within themselves. Even though they believe stressors are under their control, they don't believe in their ability to initiate change. Thus, for an internal locus of control to be beneficial to your well-being, it must be combined with the belief that you are capable of making changes to prevent future problems.

Your self-efficacy influences your stress management strategy. Self-efficacy is the belief that one is capable of performing a particular task. For example, a professional golfer would generally have high self-efficacy for making a 5-foot putt. The rest of us would probably have considerably lower self-efficacy for performance on the same task. People's beliefs about their ability to engage in effective coping strategies, or make changes in their lifestyles that will prevent future risk are relevant to health and wellness. They must believe that they can engage successfully in problem solving or stick with an exercise program in order to succeed. One way to increase self-efficacy is to increase your knowledge of the options available for managing stress.

Your outcome expectancies influence your stress-management strategy. In addition to believing in your own ability to manage stress, you must believe that the response will lead to the desired outcome—in this case, stress reduction. These beliefs are called "outcome expectancies," because they represent what you expect to happen as a result of your response.

Problem solving and assertiveness can help you cope. Each stressful situation has its own unique circumstances and meaning to the individual. Thus, providing specific information on how to actively cope with each stressor you may face becomes impossible. However, you can develop a consistent way of responding to difficult situations. A technique called systematic problem solving provides an excellent framework. This approach has been shown to improve the likelihood of problem resolution.

The first step is called brainstorming. This is when you generate every possible solution to the problem. During this stage, you should not limit the solutions you generate in any way. Even silly and impractical solutions should be included. After you have generated a comprehensive list, you can narrow your focus by eliminating any solutions that do not seem reasonable. When you have reduced the number of solutions to a reasonable number (four or five), carefully evaluate each option. You should consider the potential costs and benefits of each approach to aid in making a decision. Once you decide on an approach, it is time to carefully plan the implementation of the strategy. This includes anticipating anything that might go wrong and being prepared to alter your plan as necessary.

In some cases, directly addressing the source of stress involves responding assertively. For example, if the source of stress is an employer placing unreasonable demands on your time, the best solution to the problem may involve talking to your boss about the situation. This type of confrontation is difficult for many people concerned about being overly aggressive. However, you can stand up for yourself without infringing on the rights of others.

Many people confuse assertiveness with aggression, leading to passive responses in difficult situations. An aggressive response intimidates others and fulfills one's own needs at the expense of others. In contrast, an assertive response protects your own rights and values while still respecting the opinions of others.

Once you are comfortable with the idea of responding assertively, you may want to practice or role-play assertive responses before trying them in the real world. Find a friend you trust and practice responding assertively. Your friend may provide valuable feedback about your approach, and the practice may increase your self-efficacy for responding and your expectancies for a positive outcome.

Social Support and Stress Management

Social support is important for effective stress management. **Social support** has been found to play an important role in coping with stress. Social support has been linked to faster recovery from various medical procedures. One study of athletic injuries has shown that people who were the most stressed were injured more often, and those who had the poorest support system were the most likely to be injured. Although the mechanism for these effect is not understood, it is clear that social support plays a major role in stress management. Social support can assist in emotion-focused and problem-focused forms of coping. Friends and family can provide concrete advice that can help solve a problem, and they can provide moral support and encouragement.

Social support can come from various sources. Everyone needs someone to turn to for support when feeling overwhelmed. Support can come from friends, family members, clergy, a teacher, a coach, or a professional counselor. Different sources may provide different forms of support. Even pets have been shown to be a good source of social support, with consequent health and quality of life benefits. The goal is to identify and nurture relationships that can provide this type of support. In turn, it is important to look for ways to support and assist others.

There are many types of social support. Social support can generally be divided into three main components: informational, material, and emotional. Informational (technical) support includes tips, strategies, and advice that can help a person get through a specific stressful situation. For example, a parent, friend, or co-worker may offer insight into how he or she once resolved similar problems. Material support is direct assistance to get a person through a stressful situation—for example, providing a

Social Support The behavior of others that assists a person in addressing a specific need.

loan to help pay off a short-term debt. Emotional support is encouragement or sympathy that a person provides to help another cope with a particular challenge.

Regardless of the type of support you receive, it is important for social support to foster autonomy. Social support that helps you to become more self-reliant because of increased feelings of competence is best for developing autonomy. Social support that is controlling or leads to dependence on another person does not lead to autonomy and may increase rather than decrease stress over time.

Obtaining good social support requires close relationships. Although we live in a social environment, it is often difficult to ask people for help. Sometimes the nature and severity of our problems may not be apparent to others. Other times, friends may not want to offer suggestions or insight because they do not want to appear too pushy. To obtain good support, it is important to develop quality personal relationships with several individuals. Research on the effects of social support indicates that the quality, not the quantity, of social support leads to better health outcomes. A high-quality social support system is particularly important during times of high stress.

Upper respiratory infections are related to stress levels and social interaction. While social support is a protective factor that can reduce the impact of stress on health and wellness, research shows that having a diverse social network and high stress levels may be related to incidence of upper respiratory infections (URI). For people with low levels of stress, having a diverse social network (many friends) is associated with lower URI rates such as colds. On the other hand, high social network diversity was associated with increased incidence of colds for those experiencing a high level of stress. Self-reported cold symptoms were verfied by a physician who performed a thorough examination. So, you may want to focus on the quality social support and limit the quantity of social support when you are feeling stressed.

Strategies for Action

There are several practical steps that can help you to identify and manage your stress. This concept is dedicated to strategies and skills for preventing, managing, and coping with stress. It is important to understand that for strategies to be effective they must be used regularly. Several practical steps that you can take are described in the following list.

- *Self-assess your stress levels.* Making self-assessments such as those in Labs 18A, 18B, and 18C can help you identify the sources and the magnitude of stress in your life.
- *Adopt coping strategies.* Consistent with the information presented in this concept, learning about and using a variety of emotion-focused, appraisal-focused, and problem-focused strategies will help you manage stress in your daily life. Lab 19A will help you to relax tense muscles, an emotion-focused coping strategy.
- *Manage time effectively.* Lab 19C can help you understand your current time use patterns and help you develop a schedule that will allow you to focus on your priorities.
- *Evaluate strategy effectiveness.* Lab 19B will help you evaluate your current social support system and determine the extent to which you feel you have control over factors in your life that cause stress. Lab 19D is designed to help you assess the effectiveness of the various coping strategies you adopt. It will also provide a basis for altering strategies to manage your stress levels more effectively.

Study Resources

Check out additional online study resources for this concept in the Student Edition of the Online Learning Center at www.mhhe.com/corbin13e.

Web Resources

American Institute of Stress **www.stress.org**
American Psychological Association **www.apa.org**
International Stress Management Association
   www.stress-management-isma.org
National Institute of Mental Health **www.nimh.nih.gov**

Suggested Readings

Additional reference materials for Concept 19 are available at **www.mhhe.com/phys_fit/web19 Click 03.**

Bernardi, L., et al. 2001. Effect of rosary prayer and yoga mantras on autonomic cardiovascular rhythms: Comparative study. *British Medical Journal* 323:1446–1449.

Caspi, A., et al. 2003. Influence of life stress on depression. *Science* 301(5631):386–389.

Craft, L. L. 2003. Potential mechanisms for the antidepressant effects of exercise. *Medicine and Science in Sports and Exercise* 35(5):S216.

Diener, E., et al. 2002. Subjective well-being: The science of happiness and life satisfaction. In C. R. Snyder and S. J. Lopez (eds.). *Handbook of Positive Psychology.* New York: Oxford University Press.

Edwards, K. J. 2001. Stress, negative social exchange, and health symptoms in university students. *Journal of American College Health* 50(2):57–80.

Girdano, D., Dosek, D., and G. Everly. 2005. *Controlling Stress and Tension.* 7th ed. Needham Heights, MA: Benjamin Cummings.

Greenberg, J. S. 2004. *Comprehensive Stress Management.* 8th ed. St. Louis: McGraw-Hill.

Hudd, S., et al. 2000. Stress at college: Effects on health habits, health status, and self-esteem. *College Student Journal* 34(2):217–227.

Jacobson, E. 1978. *You Must Relax.* New York: McGraw-Hill.

Jason, L. A., and G. S. Glenwick. 2002. *Innovative Strategies for Promoting Health and Mental Health Across the Life Span.* New York: Springer.

Kubzansky, L. D., et al. 2001. Is the glass half empty or half full? A prospective study of optimism and coronary heart disease in the normative aging study. *Psychosomatic Medicine* 63:910–916.

Maddux, J. E. 2002. Self-efficacy: The power of believing you can. In C. R. Snyder and S. J. Lopez (eds.). *Handbook of Positive Psychology.* New York: Oxford University Press.

Nolen-Hoeksema, S. 2003. *Women Who Think Too Much.* New York: Henry Holt.

Paterson, R. J. 2000. *The Assertiveness Workbook: How to Express Your Ideas and Stand Up for Yourself at Work.* Oakland, CA: New Harbinger.

Romas, J. A., and M. Sharma. 2004. *Practical Stress Management.* 3rd ed. Needham Heights, MA: Benjamin Cummings.

Santrock, J. W. 2005. *Psychology Updated.* 7th ed. St. Louis: McGraw-Hill.

Seligman, M. E. 1998. *Learned Optimism: How to Change Your Mind and Your Life.* New York: Pocket Books.

Selye, H. 1978. *The Stress of Life.* 2nd ed. New York: McGraw-Hill.

Shapiro, S. L., et al. 2002. Meditation and positive psychology. In C. R. Snyder and S. J. Lopez (eds.). *Handbook of Positive Psychology.* New York: Oxford University Press.

Smith, J. C. 2002. *Stress Management: A Comprehensive Handbook of Techniques and Strategies.* New York: Springer.

Snyder, C. R. (ed.). 2001. *Coping with Stress: Effective People and Processes.* New York: Oxford University Press.

Snyder, C. R., and S. J. Lopez (eds.). 2002. *Handbook of Positive Psychology.* New York: Oxford University Press.

Taylor, S. E. 2002. *The Tending Instinct: How Nurturing Is Essential for Who We Are and How We Live.* New York: Times Books.

Tsigos, C., and G. P. Chrousos. 2002. Hypothalamic-pituitary-adrenal axis, neuroendocrine factors and stress. *Journal of Psychosomatic Research* 53(4):865–871.

U.S. Department of Health and Human Services. November 2000. *Healthy People 2010.* 2nd ed. With *Understanding and Improving Health and Objectives for Improving Health.* 2 vols. Washington, DC: U.S. Government Printing Office.

U.S. Food and Drug Administration. 2004. Worsening depression and suicidality in patients being treated with antidepressant medications. *FDA Public Health Advisory* March 22.

Williams, R., and V. Williams. 1999. *Anger Kills: 17 Strategies for Controlling Hostility That Can Harm You.* New York: Harper Collins Publishers, Inc.

Yan, L. L., et al. 2003. Psychosocial factors and risk of hypertension. *Journal of the American Medical Association* 290(16):2138–2148.

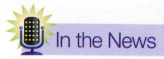

In the News

Research on Depression and Sleep

In attempt to help people manage and cope with stress health professionals use a variety of techniques. In some cases medicine is prescribed. New evidence suggests that some of these medicines can have dangerous side effects. New information about these drugs is presented below. In addition, we are aware that the amount of sleep you get is related to stress levels. Facts about side some dangerous side effects of depressions drugs and the relationship of sleep to stress levels are presented below.

- *FDA recommends warning labels for antidepressants.* The United States Food and Drug Administration (FDA) has asked drug companies to add strong warnings to ten of the most widely used antidepressant drugs. Millions of people take these drugs (e.g., Prozac/fluoxetine, Zoloft/sertraline, Paxil/paroxetine). In issuing the statement, the FDA noted that patients on these drugs should be watched for suicidal behavior and anxiety. The warning applies to people of all ages, but there is special concern that the drugs may increase suicide risk among children using the drugs.

- *The need for sleep.* A recent study found that the groups needing the most sleep are teenagers and those in their early twenties. The researchers who conducted the study found that these age groups need over 9 hours of sleep, as compared with the 7 or 8 that most adults need. Unfortunately, these age groups are unlikely to get anywhere close to this ideal amount of sleep and are likely to use caffeine to stay awake. This, in turn, may lead to disturbed sleep. Thus, an endless cycle of deficient sleep and caffeine use may develop. College students often stay up late at night, sometimes "pulling an all-nighter" to prepare for exams. The result may be impaired scholastic performance and compromised health.

- *Sleep and Obesity.* New evidence suggests that people who do not get enough sleep are at risk for obesity. Those who get 7–9 hours of sleep are at no extra risk for obesity. Those who get 6 hours of sleep increase obesity risk by 50% and those who sleep for 4 hours of less increase risk of obesity by 73%. College students who do not get enough sleep increase their odds of gaining weight. This in turn can lead to higher stress evels associated with concerns for increasing body weight. Getting enough sleep can help keep weight under control, help reduce stress levels, and lead to increased productivity.

- *More on sleep.* Not getting enough sleep can be harmful to health but the same may be true of getting too much sleep. Several studies have shown that adults who sleep an average of 10 hours or more and night have a higher overall death rate than those who sleep fewer hours.

Lab 19A Relaxing Tense Muscles

Name	Section	Date

Purpose: To learn how to relax tense muscles

Procedures

Part I

1. Lie on your back in a quiet, nondistracting atmosphere while you are learning this relaxation technique. (Later, you will want to be able to use the technique in public, in everyday situations, at work, or at any time you are under stress.) Get as comfortable as possible. Close your eyes.
2. Do the Contract-Relax Exercise Routine for Relaxation. Contract the muscles to a moderate level of tension (do not use maximum contractions) as you inhale for 5 to 7 seconds. Study where you are feeling the tension. Try to keep the tension isolated to the designated muscle group without allowing it to spill over to other muscles. Use the dominant side of the body first (right or left); repeat on the nondominant side (other side).
3. Next, release the tension completely, instantly relaxing the muscles, and exhale. Extend the feeling of relaxation throughout your muscles for 20 to 30 seconds before contracting again. Think of relaxation words such as *warm, calm, peaceful,* and *serene.*
4. If time permits, practice each muscle group two to five times (until tension is gone) before proceeding to the next group. In a class, you may have time for only one trial. For home practice, do the routine twice a day for 15 minutes.

Contract-Relax Exercise Routine for Relaxation

1. Hand and forearm—Contract your right hand, making a fist; hold 3 counts. Relax and keep letting go 6–10 counts. Repeat; then do left fist, then both fists.
2. Biceps—Flex elbows and contract your biceps; hold 3 counts. Relax and continue relaxing 6–10 counts. Repeat.
3. Triceps—Straighten the arm, contract the triceps on the back of the arms. Hold 3 counts. Relax 6–10 counts. Repeat.
4. Relax hands, forearms, and upper arms.
5. Forehead—Raise your eyebrows and wrinkle your forehead; hold 3 counts. Relax and continue relaxing 6–10 counts.
6. Cheeks and nose—Make a face. Wrinkle your nose and squint. Hold 3 counts. Relax and continue relaxing 6–10 counts.
7. Jaws—Clench your teeth 3 counts. Relax 6–10 counts.
8. Lips and tongue—With teeth apart, press lips together and press tongue to roof of mouth. Hold 3 counts. Relax 6–10 counts.
9. Neck and throat—Push head backward while tucking chin, pushing against floor or pillow if lying down. If sitting, push against high chairback. Hold 3 counts. Relax for 6–10 counts.
10. Relax forehead, cheeks, nose, jaws, lips, tongue, neck, and throat. Relax hands, forearms, and upper arms.
11. Shoulder and upper back—Hunch shoulders to ears. Hold 3 counts. Relax 6–10 counts.
12. Relax lips, tongue, neck, throat, shoulders, and upper back.
13. Abdomen—Suck in abdomen. Hold 3 counts. Relax 6–10 counts.
14. Lower back—Contract and arch the back. Hold 3 counts. Relax 6–10 counts.
15. Thighs and buttocks—Squeeze your buttocks together and push your heels into the floor (if lying down) or against a chair rung (if sitting). Hold 3 counts. Relax 6–10 counts.
16. Relax shoulders and upper back, abdomen, lower back, thighs, and buttocks.
17. Calves—Pull instep and toes toward shins. Hold 3 counts. Relax 6–10 counts.
18. Toes—Curl toes; hold 3 counts. Relax 6–10 counts.
19. Relax every muscle in your body.

Note: Eventually, you should progress to a combination of muscle groups and gradually eliminate the "contract" phase of the program.

Part II Perform each of the relaxation exercises that follow (see page 368 for pictures).

1. **Neck stretch**—Roll the head slowly in a half-circle from 9:00 to 8:00 to 7, 6, 5, 4, and 3. Then reverse from 3 to 9. Close your eyes and feel the stretch. Do *not* make a full circle by tipping the head back. Repeat several times.

2. **Shoulder lift**—Hunch the shoulders as high as possible (contract) and then let them drop (relax). Repeat several times. Inhale on the lift; exhale on the drop.

3. **Trunk stretch and drop**—Stand and reach as high as possible; tiptoe and stretch every muscle; then collapse completely, letting knees flex and trunk, head, and arms dangle. Repeat two or three times. Inhale on the stretch and exhale on the collapse.

4. **Trunk swings**—Following the trunk stretch and drop, remain in the "drop" position and, with a minimum of muscular effort, set the trunk swinging from side to side by shifting the weight from one foot to the other, letting the heels come off the floor alternately. Keep the entire body (especially the neck) limp.

5. **Tension contrast**—With arms extended overhead, lie on your side. Tense the body as stiff as a board; then let go and relax, letting the body fall either forward or backward in whatever direction it loses balance. Continue letting go for a few seconds after falling and allow yourself to feel as if you were still sinking. Repeat on the other side.

Results

 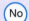 Did you find the relaxation exercises effective?

 No Do you think you would find them useful as part of your normal daily routine or as a quick fix for stress?

  Did you find the contract-relax exercise routine relaxing?

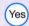 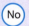 Do you think you would find it useful as part of your normal daily routine or as a quick fix for stress?

Conclusions and Implications

In several sentences, discuss whether or not you feel that relaxation exercises will be a part of your wellness program.

Lab 19B Evaluating Levels of Social Support and Locus of Control

Name	**Section**	**Date**

Purpose: To evaluate your level of social support and to identify ways that you can find additional support, as well as to assess your perceptions of locus of control (perception that you control your own life)

Procedures

1. Use Chart 1 to get personal social support and locus of control scores. Answer each question by placing a check below Not True, Somewhat True, or Very True. Place the number value for each answer in the score box to the right. Sum scores in smaller boxes to get subscale scores for the three bands of social support and for locus of control.
2. In the Results section, record your scores and determine your ratings (use Charts 2 and 3 for ratings).
3. Answer the questions in the Conclusions and Implications section.

Chart 1 ▶ Social Support and Locus of Control Questionnaire

The first nine questions assess various aspects of social support. Base your answer on your actual degree of support, not on the type of support that you would like to have. Answer questions 10–16 to determine your locus of control. Place a check in the space that best represents what is true for you.

Social Support Questions	Not True 1	Somewhat True 2	Very True 3	Score
1. I have close personal ties with my relatives.				
2. I have close relationships with a number of friends.				
3. I have a deep and meaningful relationship with a spouse or close friend.				
Access to social support score:				
4. I have parents and relatives who take the time to listen and understand me.				
5. I have friends or co-workers whom I can confide in and trust when problems come up.				
6. I have a nonjudgmental spouse or close friend who supports me when I need help.				
Degree of social support score:				
7. I feel comfortable asking others for advice or assistance.				
8. I have confidence in my social skills and enjoy opportunities for new social contacts.				
9. I am willing to open up and discuss my personal life with others.				
Getting social support score:				
Locus of Control Questions				
10. Hard work usually pays off.				
11. Buying a lottery ticket is not worth the money.				
12. Even when I fail I keep trying.				
13. I am usually successful in what I do.				
14. I am in control of my own life.				
15. I make plans to be sure that I am successful.				
16. I know where I stand with my friends.				
Locus of control score:				

Results

Scores and Ratings

(Use Chart 2 to obtain ratings)

Access to social support score [ ]   Rating [ ]

Degree of social support score [ ]   Rating [ ]

Getting social support score [ ]   Rating [ ]

Total social support score [ ]   Rating [ ]
(sum of three scores)

Locus of control score [ ]   Rating [ ]

Chart 2 ▶ Rating Scale for Social Support

Rating	Item Scores	Total Score
High	8–9	24–27
Moderate	6–7	18–23
Low	Below 6	Below 18

Chart 3 ▶ Rating Scale for Locus of Control

Rating	Score
High	19–21
Moderate	12–19
Low	Below 12

Conclusions and Implications

1. In several sentences, discuss your overall social support and locus of control. Do you think your scores and ratings are a true representation of your social support? Do you think you are in control of your own life? Does your locus of control score seem accurate?

2. In several sentences, describe any changes you think you should make to improve your social support system or your own perceptions of the control you have over your life. If you do not think change is necessary, explain why.

Lab 19C Time Management

Name	**Section**	**Date**

Purpose: To help you learn to manage time to meet personal priorities

Procedures

1. Follow the four steps outlined below.
2. Complete the Conclusions and Implications section.

Results

Step 1: Establishing Priorities

1. Check the circles that reflect your priorities in the list below. Add priorities as necessary.

2. Rate each of the priorities you checked. Use a 1 for highest priority, 2 for moderate priority, and 3 for low priority.

Check Priorities	Rating	Check Priorities	Rating	Check Priorities	Rating
◯ More time with family	☐	◯ More time with boy/girlfriend	☐	◯ More time with spouse	
◯ More time for leisure	☐	◯ More time to relax	☐	◯ More time to study	
◯ More time for work success	☐	◯ More time for physical activity	☐	◯ More time to improve myself	☐
◯ More time for other recreation	☐	◯ Other _____	☐	◯ Other _____	☐
					☐
					☐

Step 2: Monitor Current Time Use

1. On the following daily calendar, keep track of daily time expenditure.

2. Write in exactly what you did for each time block.

7–9 A.M.	9–11 A.M.	11 A.M.–1 P.M.	1–3 P.M.
3–5 P.M.	**5–7 P.M.**	**7–9 P.M.**	**9–11 P.M.**

Step 3: Analyze Your Current Time Use

Where can I spend less time? (write below)

Where do I need to spend more time? (write below)

Step 4: Make a Schedule: Write in Your Planned Activities for the Day

7–9 A.M.	9–11 A.M.	11 A.M.–1 P.M.	1–3 P.M.
3–5 P.M.	5–7 P.M.	7–9 P.M.	9–11 P.M.

Conclusions and Implications

In several sentences, discuss how you might modify your schedule to find more time for important priorities.

Lab 19D Evaluating Coping Strategies

Name	**Section**	**Date**

Purpose: To learn how to use appropriate coping strategies that work best for you

Procedures

1. Think of five recent stressful experiences that caused you some concern, anxiety, or distress. Describe these situations in Chart 1. Then use Chart 2 to make a rating for changeability, severity, and duration. Assign one number for each category for each situation.
2. In Chart 3, place a check for each coping strategy that you used in coping with each of the five situations you described.
3. Answer the questions in the Conclusions and Implications section.

Results

Chart 1 ▶ Stressful Situations

Think of five different stressful situations. Appraise each situation and assign a score (changeability, severity, duration) using the scale in Chart 2.

Briefly describe the situation.	Changeability	Severity	Duration
1.			
2.			
3.			
4.			
5.			

Chart 2 ▶ Appraisal of the Stressful Situations

Use this chart to rate the five situations you described in Chart 1. Assign a number for changeability, severity, and duration for each situation in Chart 1.

	1	2	3	4	5
Was the situation changeable?	Completely within my control	Mostly within my control	Both in and out of my control	Mostly out of my control	Completely outside of my control
What was the severity of the stress?	Very minor	Fairly minor	Moderate	Fairly major	Very major
What was the duration of the stress?	Short-term (weeks)	Moderately short	Moderate (months)	Moderately long	Long (months to year)

Chart 3 ▶ Coping Strategies

Directions: Think about your response to the five stressful situations you recently experienced and check the strategies that you used in each situation.

Coping Strategy	Situation 1	Situation 2	Situation 3	Situation 4	Situation 5
1. I apologized or corrected the problem as best I could.					
2. I ignored the problem and hoped that it would go away.					
3. I told myself to forget about it and grew as a person from the experience.					
4. I tried to make myself feel better by eating, drinking, or smoking.					
5. I prayed or sought spiritual meaning from the situation.					
6. I expressed anger to try to change the situation.					
7. I took active steps to make things work out better.					
8. I used music, images, or deep breathing to help me relax.					
9. I tried to keep my feelings to myself and kept moving forward.					
10. I pursued leisure or recreational activity to help me feel better.					
11. I talked to someone who could provide advice or help me with the problem.					
12. I talked to someone about what I was feeling or experiencing.					

Conclusions and Implications

In several sentences, discuss the coping strategies you used. Were they the ones you used the most? The ones you typically use? Were they effective? Would you consider other strategies in the future?

Recognizing Quackery: Becoming an Informed Consumer

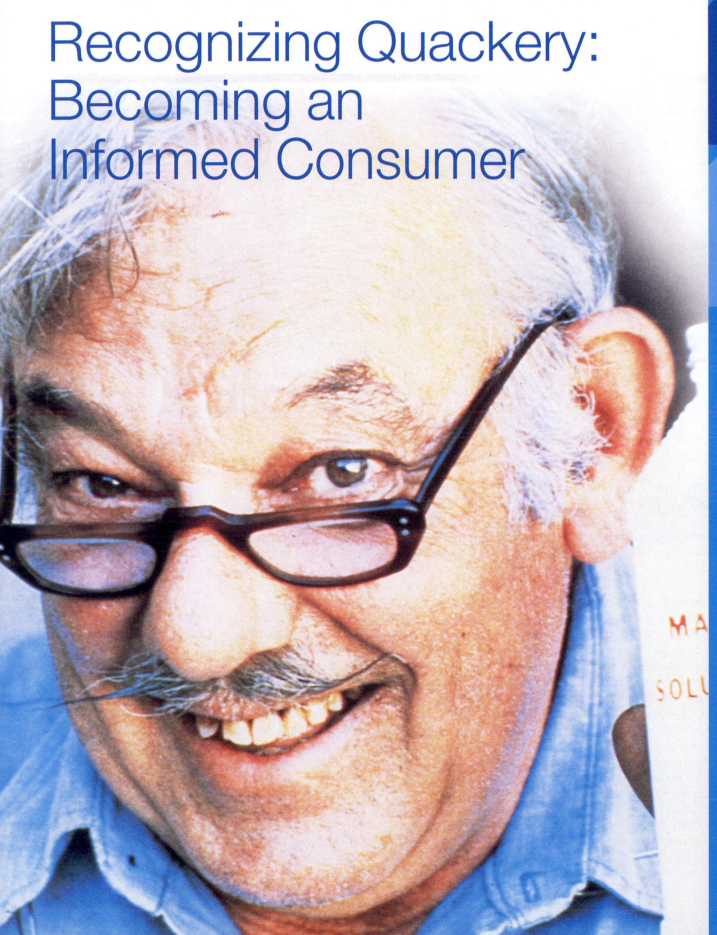

"Let the buyer beware" is a good motto for the consumer seeking advice or planning a program for developing or maintaining fitness, health, or wellness.

Health Goals

for the year 2010

- Increase number of college and university students who receive information on priority health-risk behaviors.

- Improve health literacy and increase access to public health information.

- Increase health communication activities that include research and evaluation.

- Increase adoption and maintenance of appropriate daily physical activity.

- Increase proportion of people who meet national dietary guidelines.

- Promote healthy and safe communities.

People have always searched for the fountain of youth and the easy, quick, and miraculous route to health and happiness. In current society, this search often focuses on fitness, nutrition, weight loss, or appearance. A variety of products are available that promise weight loss, improved health, or improved fitness with little or no effort. Sale of these products can typically be classified as either quackery or fraud, since in nearly all cases they do not work.

The dictionary definition of *quack* is "a pretender of medical skill" or "one who talks pretentiously without sound knowledge of the subject discussed." These definitions imply that the promotion of quackery involves deliberate deception, but quacks often believe in what they are doing. A consumer watchdog group called Quackwatch defines quackery more broadly as "anything involving overpromotion in the field of health." This definition encompasses questionable ideas as well as questionable products and services. The word *fraud* is reserved for situations in which deliberate deception is involved. This concept discusses common myths and provides important guidelines to help you be a more informed consumer of health, fitness, and nutrition products.

Common Myths about Exercise, Nutrition, and Health

There is no easy way to get the benefits from physical activity. Contrary to the hype from some fitness commercials and products, the benefits associated with regular activity require real effort maintained over time. Advertisements for some fitness devices claim that 10 minutes on their product is as good as 30 minutes on another product—this is simply not true. The benefits of any activity depend on the relative intensity and duration, not on the equipment. Some products promise to enhance the metabolism in the same way as exercise and these are just stimulants that have little or no effect on energy expenditure and certainly no effect on fitness.

It is NOT true that if a little of something is "good" more is "better." Marketing of nutrition products often relies on convincing people that additional vitamins, minerals, or enzymes are beneficial. It is true that deficiency of certain compounds may be harmful but extra amounts don't always provide added protection or improved health. The myth that vitamin C can cure the common cold is based on the fact that deficiencies of vitamin C can lead to scurvy. The same hype is used to sell consumers many unnecessary exercise, diet, and nutrition supplements. For example, protein supplements are marketed with convincing (and honest) claims that the body needs amino acids to form muscle. The hidden truth is that the body cannot store or use more than it needs.

Getting rid of cellulite does not require a special exercise, diet, cream, or device, as some books and advertisements insist. Cellulite is ordinary fat with a fancy name. You do not need a special treatment or device to get rid of it. In fact, it has no special remedy. Fat is fat. To decrease fat, reduce calories and do more physical activity.

Spot-reducing, or losing fat from a specific location on the body, is not possible. It is a fallacy. When you do physical activity, calories are burned and fat is recruited from all over the body in a genetically determined pattern. You cannot selectively exercise, bump, vibrate, or squeeze the fat from a particular spot. If you were flabby to begin with, local exercise could strengthen the local muscles, causing a change in the contour and the girth of that body part. But exercise affects the muscles, not the fat on that body part. General aerobic exercises are the most effective for burning fat, but you cannot control where the fat comes off.

Surgically sculpting the body with implants and liposuction to acquire physical beauty will not give you physical fitness and may be harmful. Rather than doing it the hard way, an increasing number of people are having their love handles removed surgically and fake calf and pectoral muscles implanted to improve their physique. Liposuction is not a weight loss technique but, rather, a contouring procedure. Like any surgery, it is not without risks. There have been fatalities and there is a risk for infection, hematoma, skin slough, and other conditions.

Muscle implants give a muscular appearance, but they do not make you stronger or more fit. The implants are not really muscle tissue but, rather, silicon gel or saline such as that used in breast implants or a hard substitute. Some complications can occur, such as infection and bleeding, and some physicians believe that calf implants may put pressure on the calf muscles and cause them to atrophy. A better way to improve physique and fitness is proper exercise.

The use of hand weights and wrist weights while walking, running, dancing, or bench-stepping can increase the energy expended but requires caution. Various devices have been marketed for increasing the energy expenditure in activities such as walking, running, and other forms of aerobic exercise. Examples include wrist, arm, or ankle weights and small hand-held weights. Step benches are another device that can be used to increase energy expenditure for aerobic exercise.

The practice of carrying weights is controversial. Carrying weights (not more than 1 to 3 pounds) while doing aerobic dance, walking, and other aerobic activities has been shown to increase energy expenditure, but the effect is negligible unless the arms are pumped (bending the elbow and raising the weight to shoulder height and then extending the elbow as the arm swings down). When the arms are pumped, the energy output is comparable to a slow jog. Some experts caution that pumping the arms using weight can increase the risk for injury and suggest that the benefit of added energy expenditure is not worth the added risk for injury. Also, gripping weights while exercising can cause an increase in blood pressure.

Those who choose to use weights while doing aerobic activity are at less risk for injury if they use wrist weights rather than hand-held weights. Arm movements should be limited to a range of motion below the shoulder level. Coronary patients and people with shoulder or elbow joint problems, such as arthritis, are advised not to use hand or wrist weights. Ankle weights are not recommended because they may alter your gait pattern in a way that is stressful to the knees.

Herbal products are often assumed to be safer or better than other products and this isn't true. A number of herbal products contain no useful ingredients, and some even lack the principal ingredient for which people buy them. Herbs may seem safe because they are purported to be "natural." However, it is important to recognize that a large percentage of medicines are extracted from plants. The fact that it comes from nature does not imply that it is safe. Improper use of herbs may lead to a number of harmful side effects and even death.

Claims for many forms of exercise are overstated or unsubstantiated. New exercise programs or routines are often promoted as the complete answer for total fitness or a **panacea** for health. Claims for Hatha Yoga suggest it will help you lose weight, trim inches, strengthen glands and organs, or cure health problems, such as the common cold or arthritis. Hatha Yoga can be useful in reducing stress, promoting relaxation, and improving flexibility but the other claims are overstated.

Similar hype may be used for promoting new pieces of exercise equipment. Each piece of equipment claims to be fun, easy to use, and more effective than other forms of exercise. The benefits from exercise are dependent on the relative intensity and duration of the activity—and whether it is done regularly over time. The best form of exercise is clearly the one that you are willing and able to do!

Contrary to claims, passive exercises do not provide any benefits for fitness or weight loss. For exercise to be beneficial the actual work must be done by contracting skeletal muscles. A variety of **passive exercise** forms have been promoted to try to reduce the effort required to perform regular exercise. These devices employ a variety of approaches to convince people of possible benefits, but without active involvement of muscles in the movement they cannot be of any real value. The fallacies associated with many past forms of passive exercise such as fat rolling machines (purported to break up and redistribute fat) would seem obvious today but new approaches come out all the time with different marketing and promotions. The list that follows highlights some of the common forms of passive exercise.

Panacea A cure-all; a remedy for all ills.

Passive Exercise Exercise in which no voluntary muscle contraction occurs; an outside force moves the body part with no effort by the person.

- *Vibrating belts.* These wide canvas or leather belts may be designed for the chin, hips, thighs, or abdomen. Driven by an electric motor, they jerk back and forth, causing loose tissue of the body part to shake. They have no beneficial effect on fitness, fat, or figure, and they are potentially harmful if used on the abdomen (especially if used by women during pregnancy, during menstruation, or while an IUD is in place). They might also aggravate a back problem.

- *Vibrating tables and pillows.* Some of these quack devices are actually called toning tables. Contrary to advertisements, these passive devices will not improve posture, trim the body, reduce weight, or develop muscle **tonus.**

- *Continuous passive motion (CPM) tables.* The motor-driven CPM table, unlike the vibrating table, moves body parts repeatedly through a range of motion. Tables are designed to do such things as passively extend the leg at the hip joint or raise the upper trunk in a sit-up-like motion. Many of the same false claims are made for it as for the vibrating table. It also claims to remove cellulite, increase circulation and oxygen flow, and eliminate excess water retention. All of these claims are false, but the table might be justified in claiming to maintain the range of motion in certain body parts for people who cannot move themselves. Hospitals and rehabilitation centers use a similar machine to maintain range of motion in the legs of knee surgery patients, maintain integrity of the cartilage, and decrease the incidence of blood clots. Certainly, the normal, healthy person has nothing to gain from using such a device.

- *Motor-driven cycles and rowing machines.* Like all mechanical devices that do the work for the individual, these motor-driven machines are not effective in a fitness program. They may help increase circulation, and some may even help maintain flexibility, but they are not as effective as active exercise. *Nonmotorized cycles and rowing machines* are good equipment for use in a fitness program.

- *Massage.* Whether done by a masseur/masseuse or by a mechanical device, massage is passive, requiring no effort on the part of the individual. It can help increase circulation, induce relaxation, prevent or loosen adhesions, retard muscle atrophy, and serve other therapeutic uses when administered in the clinical setting for medical reasons. However, massage has no useful role in a physical fitness program and will not alter your shape. There is no scientific evidence that it can hasten nerve growth, remove subcutaneous fat, or increase athletic performance. Some athletes (e.g., cyclists) find that it aids in recovery from exercise.

- *Magnets.* The law requires magnets marketed with medical claims to obtain clearance from the **Food and Drug Administration (FDA).** To date, the FDA has not approved the marketing of any magnets for med-

ical use, and sellers making medical claims for magnets are in violation of the law.

- *Electrical muscle stimulators.* Neuromuscular electrical stimulators cause the muscle to contract involuntarily. In the hands of qualified medical personnel, muscle stimulators are valuable therapeutic devices. They can increase muscle strength and endurance selectively and aid in the treatment of edema. They can also help prevent atrophy in a patient who is unable to move, and they may decrease muscle spasms, but in a healthy person they do not have the same value as exercise. The Federal Trade Commission (FTC) recently filed a false advertising complaint against three firms that market exercise stimulators that promise to build six-pack abs and tone muscles without exercise. These devices, worn over the abdomen, are heavily advertised in infomercials and have been shown to be ineffective and potentially hazardous to health. Electrical stimulators placed on the chest, back, or abdomen can interfere with the normal rhythm of the heart, even for normally healthy people. For those with heart, gastrointestinal, orthopedic, kidney, and other health problems, such as epilepsy, hernia, and varicose veins, they can be especially dangerous. These devices are ineffective and potentially harmful for personal use. Also beware of spas and clinics that use these devices and make claims of fitness enhancement for normally healthy people.

- *Weighted belts.* Claims have been made that these belts reduce waists, thighs, and hips when worn for several hours under the clothing. In reality, they do none of these things and have been reported to cause physical harm. However, when used in a progressive resistance program, wristlet, anklet, or laced-on weights can help produce an overload and, therefore, develop strength or endurance.

- *Inflated, constricting, or nonporous garments.* These garments include rubberized inflated devices (sauna belts and sauna shorts) and paraphernalia that are airtight plastic or rubberized. Evidence indicates that their girth-reducing claims are *unwarranted.* If exercise is performed while wearing such garments, the exercise, not the garment, may be beneficial. You cannot squeeze fat out of the pores, nor can you melt it.

- *Body wrapping.* Some reducing salons, gyms, or clubs advertise that wrapping the body in bandages soaked in a magic solution will cause a permanent reduction in body girth. This so-called treatment is pure quackery. Tight, constricting bands can temporarily indent the skin and squeeze body fluids into other parts of the body, but the skin or body will regain its original size within minutes or hours. The solution is usually similar to epsom salts, which can cause fluid to be drawn from tissue. The fluid is water, not fat, and is quickly replaced. Body wrapping may be dangerous to your health; at least one fatality has been documented.

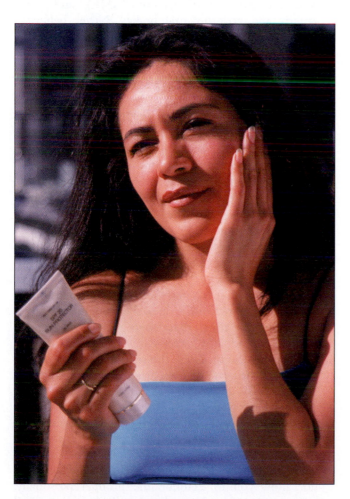

Having a good tan is often associated with being fit and looking good, but getting tanned can be risky business. www.mhhe.com/phys_fit/web20 Click 01. Tanning salons may claim their lamps are safe because they emit only UV-A rays, but these rays can age the skin prematurely and make it look wrinkled and leathery. They may also increase the cancer-producing potential of UV-B rays and cause eye damage. Since there is no warning sign of redness, overdosing can occur. Thirty minutes of exposure to UV-A can suppress the immune system. Tanning devices can also aggravate certain skin diseases. The Food and Drug Administration (FDA) advises against the use of any suntan lamp. It is dangerous to use tanning accelerator lotions with the lamps because they can promote burning of the skin. Tanning pills are an even worse choice. They can cause itching, welts, hives, stomach cramps, and diarrhea and can decrease night vision. Tanning in the sun is also hazardous because it damages the skin, making it age prematurely. It may cause skin cancer. It is best to use products with sun blockers if you must spend long periods in the sun (SPF 15 or higher).

Wearing sunscreen (SPF 15 or higher) is recommended by the American Cancer Society.

Saunas, steam baths, whirlpools, and hot tubs provide no significant health benefits, and guidelines must be followed to ensure safety. Baths do not melt off fat; fat must be metabolized. The heat and humidity from baths may make you perspire, but it is water, not fat, oozing from the pores.

The effect of such baths is largely psychological, although some temporary relief from aches and pains may result from the heat. The same relief can be had by sitting in a tub of hot water in your bathroom. The following guidelines/precautions should be considered when using a sauna, steam bath, whirlpool, or hot tub:

- Take a soap shower before and after entering the bath.
- Do not wear makeup or skin lotion/oil.
- Wait at least an hour after eating before bathing.
- Cool down after exercise before entering the bath to avoid overheating.
- Drink plenty of water before or during the bath to avoid dehydration.
- Do not wear jewelry.
- Do not sit on a metal stool; do sit on a towel in the steam or sauna bath.
- Do not bathe alone.
- Do not drink alcohol before bathing.
- Get out immediately if you become dizzy; feel hot, chilled, or nauseous; or get a headache.
- Get approval from your physician if you have heart disease, low or high blood pressure, a fever, kidney disease, or diabetes; are obese; are pregnant or think you might be pregnant; or are on medications (especially anticoagulants, stimulants, or tranquilizers).
- Limit use for the elderly and for children.
- Do not exercise in a sauna or steam bath.
- Skin infections can be spread in a bath; make certain it is cleaned regularly and that the hot tub or whirlpool has proper pH and chlorination.
- Follow appropriate guidelines:

  Sauna: should not exceed 190°F (88°C) and duration should not exceed 10 to 15 minutes

  Steam bath: should not exceed 120°F (49°C) and duration should not exceed 6 to 12 minutes

  Whirlpool/hot tub: should not exceed 100°F (37°C) and duration should not exceed 5 to 10 minutes

Tonus Tonus (or tone) is the most frequently misused and abused term in fitness vocabularies. Tonus is the tension developed in a muscle as a result of passive muscle stretch. Tonus cannot be determined by feeling or inspecting a muscle. It has little or nothing to do with the strength of a muscle.

Food and Drug Administration (FDA) The federal agency that recommends and enforces government regulations regarding certain foods and drugs.

Beware of energy drinks with "boosts" sold at health bars in fitness clubs. Many health bars that sell food and drinks of various types. Some drinks contain "boosts" consisting of a tablespoon or two of a food supplement. Pharmacies were developed to prevent medical practioners from selling their own medicines rather than the best available medicine. Health clubs that sell drinks with supplements are susceptible to the claim that they are selling products for financial gain rather than the best interest of clients. Even if supplements are effecitve, which most are not, taking one dose in a drink would be ineffective and a waste of money.

Quacks

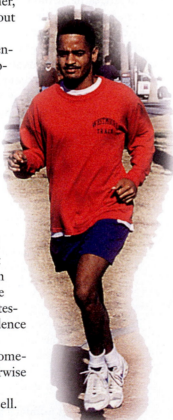 **You can usually tell the difference between an expert and a quack because a quack does not use scientific methods.** www.mhhe.com/ phys_fit/web20 Click 02. A good example of this fact is seen in a study that attempted to obtain documentation for products claiming to enhance athletic performance. The study found that no published scientific evidence existed to support the promotional claims of 42 percent of the products. Thirty-two percent had some scientific documentation but were marketed in a misleading manner, and 21 percent were without any human clinical trials.

Some of the ways to identify quacks, frauds, and rip-offs are to look for these clues:

- They do not use the scientific method of controlled experimentation that can be verified by other scientists.
- To a large extent, they use testimonials and anecdotes to support their claims rather than scientific methods. There is no such thing as a valid testimonial. Anecdotal evidence is no evidence at all.
- They advise you to buy something you would not otherwise have bought.
- They have something to sell.

Changing your lifestyle, rather than quick solutions, is the key to health, fitness, and wellness.

- They claim everyone can benefit from the product or service they are selling. There is no such thing as a simple, quick, easy, painless remedy/tonic or other concoction that is effective for ailments or conditions for which medical science has not yet found a remedy.
- They promise quick, miraculous results. A perfect, no-risk treatment does not exist.
- The claims for benefits are broad, covering a wide variety of conditions.
- They may offer a money-back guarantee. A guarantee is only as good as the company.
- They may claim the treatment or product is approved by the FDA. Note: Federal law does not permit the mention of the FDA in any way that suggests marketing approval.
- They may claim the support of experts, but the experts are not identified.
- The ingredients or materials in the product may not be identified.
- They may claim there is a conspiracy against them by "bureaucrats," "organized medicine," the FDA, the American Medical Association (AMA), and other experts and governmental bodies. Never believe a doctor who claims the medical community is persecuting him or her or that the government is suppressing a wonderful discovery.
- Their credentials may be irrelevant to the area in which they claim expertise.
- They use scare tactics, such as "If you don't do this, you will die of a heart attack."
- They may appear to be a sympathetic friend who wants to share a new discovery with you.
- They may quote from a scientific journal or another legitimate source, but they misquote or quote out of context to mislead you; they may also mix a little bit of truth with a lot of fiction.
- They may cite research or quote from individuals or institutions that have questionable reputations for scientific truth.
- They may claim it is a new discovery (usually it is said to have originated in Europe). There is never a great medical breakthrough that debuts in an obscure magazine or tabloid. No secret cures or magic formulas have been recognized by the scientific community, a picture on the cover of *Time* magazine, nomination for a Nobel Prize, and so on.
- The product or organization named is often similar to that of a famous person or creditable institution (e.g., the Mayo diet had no connection with the Mayo Clinic).
- They often sell products through the mail, which does not allow you to examine the product personally. There are no miracle products available only by mail order or from a single source.

You can reduce your susceptibility to quackery by being an informed consumer. The three key characteristics that predispose people to health-related quackery are a concern about appearance, health, or performance; a lack of knowledge; and a desire for immediate results. Understanding the principles of exercise and nutrition presented in this book will help you know when something sounds "too good to be true."

When evaluating health-related products or information, carefully consider the quality of your source. Common sources of misinformation are magazines, health food stores, and TV infomercials. These entities all have an economic incentive in promoting the purchase and use of exercise, diet, and weight loss products. Because of freedom of speech laws, it is legal to state opinion through these media. Note, however, that few companies make claims on product labels, since this is false advertising. Follow these additional guidelines to avoid being a victim of quackery:

- Read the ad carefully, especially the small print.
- Do not send cash; use a check, money order, or credit card so you will have a receipt.
- Do not order from a company with only a post office box, unless you know the company.
- Do not let high-pressure sales tactics make you rush into a decision.
- When in doubt, check out the company through your Better Business Bureau (BBB).

Equipment

Home exercise equipment can be helpful, but care should be used when selecting and purchasing equipment. There are many types of home exercise equipment available on the market. Because they are often expensive, care should be used when making a decision. To determine if a piece of equipment is worthwhile, ask yourself the following four questions. *Do you need it? Will you use it? Does it work? Does it work for you?* For it to be a worthwhile purchase, the answer to all four questions should be yes. Many people wonder about the relative advantages and disadvantages of different pieces of equipment. The answer to the question "What is the best piece of exercise equipment?" is the one that you will use.

It is best to buy your equipment from reputable dealers or companies. When considering several models of the same type of device, remember that you get what you pay for. Higher-end models may last longer and may promote more use, since they may be quieter or feel better to use than lower-priced models. Consult an expert if you want to know more about the quality and effectiveness of different products. Individuals with a college degree in physical education, physical therapy, or kinesiology should be able to give you good advice.

Health Clubs

Health and fitness clubs provide access to equipment and support but it is important to consider a number of factors before deciding to join. The first question to ask yourself is whether access to the facility is essential for you to begin or maintain your exercise program. The second question is whether the facility is convenient enough for you to access regularly. The distance of the gym from home or work will greatly influence your potential use of the facility. If you are serious about joining a club, consider the following points:

- Determine the qualifications of the personnel, especially of the individual responsible for your program. Is he or she an expert, as defined previously?
- Check to see if your membership can be sold or transferred to another person if you move. Check to see if you can cancel the contract if you prove you are moving outside the community.
- Choose a no-contract or monthly payment option if it is available so you can change your mind. Be prepared to resist options for long-term contracts.
- Check for hidden costs associated with membership (e.g., costs for testing, use of personal training).
- Do not be swayed by promises of quick results.
- Check the equipment to be sure that it is up to date and well maintained.
- Check to see that towels are provided to wipe machines after use and that weights are replaced after use. If not, it is good indication that supervision is not adequate.
- Check to see if rules are posted. For example, is there a time limit for using machines and is there a dress code?
- Speak with other members to get an insider's perspective regarding how they have been treated.
- Make a trial visit to the establishment during the hours when you would normally expect to use the facility to determine if it is open, if it is overcrowded, and if you would enjoy the company of the other patrons.

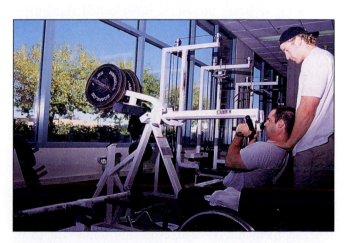

Visit a health club before you join.

- Make certain the club is a well-established facility that will not disappear overnight.
- Check its reputation with the Better Business Bureau. Be aware, however, that the BBB can only tell you if complaints have been made against a company. It does not endorse companies and may lack information on new companies.
- Investigate programs offered by the YMCA/YWCA, local colleges and universities, and municipal park and recreation departments. These agencies often have excellent fitness classes at lower prices than commercial establishments and usually employ qualified personnel.

Dietary Supplements

The burden of proof about the effectiveness of food supplements rests with the consumer. www.mhhe.com/phys_fit/web20 Click 03. The passage of the Dietary Supplements Health and Education Act in 1994 shifted the burden of providing assurances of product effectiveness from the FDA to the food supplement industry, which really means it shifted to you—the consumer. Food supplements are typically not considered to be drugs, so they are not regulated. Unlike drugs and medicines, food supplements need not be proven effective or even safe to be sold in stores. To be removed from stores, they must be proven ineffective or unsafe. This leaves consumers vulnerable to false claims. Many experts suggest that quackery has increased significantly since 1994, when the act was passed.

The act had at least one positive effect. Food supplement labeling must now be truthful and not misleading. Claims concerning disease prevention, treatment, or diagnosis must be substantiated in order to appear on the product. Unfortunately, the act did not limit false claims if they are not on the product label. The result has been the removal of claims from labels in favor of claims on separate literature, often called third-party literature, because the label makes no claims, and the seller makes no written claims (second party). Rather, the seller provides claims in literature by other people (third party). The literature is distributed separately from the product, thus allowing sellers to make unsubstantiated claims for products. Also, the law does not prohibit unproven verbal claims by salespeople. A highly respected medical journal indicates that "alternative treatments should be subjected to scientific testing no less rigorous than that required for advocating unproven and potentially harmful treatments." However, as things currently stand, it is up to the consumer to make decisions about the safety and effectiveness of food supplements, so it is especially important to be well informed.

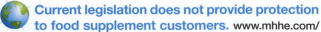 **Current legislation does not provide protection to food supplement customers.** www.mhhe.com/phys_fit/web20 Click 04. Since the Dietary Supplements Health and Education Act was passed in 1994, food supplement sales have doubled (from $8 billion to more than $16 billion a year). A wide variety of supplements include ergogenic aids, vitamins and minerals, and herbals and botanicals. Ergogenic aids associated with muscle fitness are discussed in other concepts. Vitamin and mineral supplements are discussed in the nutrition concept, and herbals and botanicals are discussed here.

Recently, the sales of supplements has leveled off, primarily because of the increasing evidence of the danger of some supplements and the evidence showing the ineffectiveness of others. Evidence supports the value of some supplements. As noted earlier in this book, folic acid, calcium, vitamin E, and a daily multiple vitamin supplement can be beneficial for many people. Also, aspirin can be important for the prevention of heart disease and some forms of cancer, and evidence shows that glucosomine supplements can relieve joint pain for some people. On the other hand, over the past few years, the FDA has received thousands of complaints of adverse events (resulting in approximately 200 deaths). An editorial in a leading national newspaper suggests that "troubling side effects mount" and that "putting customers' health at risk is a high price to pay for a free market in diet supplements." Some of the problems associated with supplements are described in Table 1. Among the adverse effects reported are lead poisoning, nausea, vomiting, diarrhea, abnormal heart rhythm, fainting, impotence, and lethargy. Over a 6-year period, 2,621 adverse events were reported to the FDA and 184 resulted in death. Also, one study showed that 15 to 20 percent of over 1,600 supplements tested included substances that would cause a positive test for drugs banned by sports organizations.

More than one-half of American adults are unaware that food supplements are unregulated by the FDA or any governmental agency. Because they are unregulated, there is no guarantee that a supplement contains the ingredients it claims to contain. Further, many have been shown to contain contaminants. Even when a supplement is what it claims to be, the effects can vary widely from one person to another. Many supplements have dangerous interactions with prescribed and over-the-counter medicines and can be very dangerous.

In spite of the problems associated with lack of supplement regulations, a recent study indicates that nearly half of Americans routinely take supplements and slightly more than half believe in the value of the supplements. Interestingly, 44 percent believe that physicians know little or nothing about supplements.

Most adults (80 percent) believe that the FDA should review supplements before they are offered for sale. More than 60 percent believe that there are not enough

Table 1 ▶ Problems Associated with Supplements
Postsurgical problems, including bleeding, irregular heartbeat, and stroke. Examples: echinacea, ephedra, ginkgo, kava, St. John's wort, ginseng.
Dangerous interactions with medicines. Examples: ephedra, St. John's wort (interact with birth control pills and HIV pills).
FDA warnings concerning unsubstantiated claims about herbs added to foods, such as energy bars and water. Examples: ginkgo, ginseng, echinacea.
Allergic and other physiological reactions; negative effect on decision making. Example: GHB.
Known ill effects to health. Examples: comfrey (kidneys), kava (liver), ephedra (54 deaths associated with use).
Possible slow bone mending. Example: Vioxx.
Recall because of dangerous effects associated with contamination. Examples: PC SPES, Lipokinetix.
Action by the FTC because of deceptive advertisements. Examples: Exercise in a Bottle, Fat Trapper.
Banned by several sporting groups, including the International Olympic Committee, NCAA, and NFL. Examples: steroids, androstendione, ephedra, THC.
Contents may not be what they appear to be and dosage information is unknown. Example: The government does not guarantee contents of supplements and there is little evidence concerning dosage for most supplements.

rules to ensure purity and accurate dosage. A similar number of adults want more regulation on advertising claims. More than a few critics point out that self-regulation within the industry has not worked well. They suggest that the public will have more confidence in supplements if the FDA was watching out for their best interest. Table 2 presents some questions that should be asked about food supplements.

Fitness Books, Magazines, and Articles

Not all fitness books provide scientifically sound, accurate, and reliable information. Because publishers are motivated by profit and publishing is a highly competitive field, the choice of material to be printed is often selected on the basis of how popular, famous, or attractive the author is or how sensational or unusual his or her ideas are. Movie stars, models, TV personalities, and even Olympic athletes are rarely experts in biomechanics, anatomy and physiology, exercise, and other foundations of physical fitness. Having a good figure/physique, being fit, or having gone through a training program does not, in itself, qualify a person to advise others.

After reading the facts presented in this book you should be able to evaluate whether or not a book, a magazine, or an article on exercise and fitness is valid, reliable, and scientifically sound. To assist you further, however, ten guidelines are listed in Lab 20A.

Health Information on the Internet

 Not all Internet websites provide scientifically sound, accurate, and reliable information. www. mhhe.com/phys_fit/web20 Click 05. The development of the Internet (World Wide Web) has made information more and more accessible to the masses. Since 1995, Internet saturation has increased from 9 percent to 66 percent. Nearly three-fourths of teens and young adult computer users seek health information on the Web. Leading topics of information are cancer, diabetes, sexually transmitted diseases, and weight control. A health goal for the nation—as outlined in *Healthy People 2010*—is to increase the proportion of households with access to the Internet with the intent of making reliable health information available to as many people as possible. The Internet has made an almost unlimited amount of health information accessible, it has also been the source of much misinformation and even fraud.

The FTC is a federal government agency charged with making sure that advertising claims for products are not false or misleading. In an effort to clean up websites, the FTC initiated "Operation Cure-All." As part of this operation, the FTC conducted two "Health Claim Surf Days," during which they identified 800 websites and usenet newsgroups with questionable content. The FTC sent mailers to these sites, and 28 percent either removed the claims or the website completely. In spite of the FTC efforts, there is still much health misinformation on the Web, leading one FTC official to suggest that "miracle cures, once thought to have been laughed out of existence, have now found a new medium . . . on the Internet" (see *Web Resources*).

Another research study randomly selected 400 websites from 27,000 available on four different well-known search engines for a study of cancer. Nearly half had unverified information and 6 percent had major inaccuracies. Clearly, Internet users must be careful in selecting websites for obtaining fitness, health, and wellness information. One of the most useful rules is always get a second opinion. Consult at least two or more sources to confirm information. Getting confirmation of information from non-Web sources is also a good idea.

You can follow some general rules to help when you use the Web to obtain fitness, health, and wellness information. In general, government websites are good sources that contain sound information prepared by experts and based on scientific research. Government sites typically include

Table 2 ► Questions and Comments about Food Supplements

Questions	Comments
Does the government regulate this product to be sure that it is safe and effective?	Since 1994, food supplements can be sold without proof that they are effective. The government does not test food supplements to ensure effectiveness or safety. The FDA must prove the product to be harmful or ineffective to remove it from the market. It is much harder to prove a product ineffective than to provide evidence that it is effective.
Do claims for the supplement have supporting evidence?	The evidence should be based on research with normal people, not evidence based on a population of subjects who have medical problems or nutritional deficiencies. Third-party information often cites research out-of-context or refers to weak studies that use inappropriate research techniques.
What are the active ingredients?	If the active ingredient really works, research will show its effectiveness. Of course, if it works, then it is much like a medicine and has similar side effects. Sellers of supplements often suggest the product works but that it has no side effects that are associated with medicines. Both cannot be true. For example, Cholestin is a variety of red yeast—a natural product. It contains lovastatin, the same active ingredients in medicines for lowering cholesterol. Though the product works, it has now been banned by the FDA as an over-the-counter supplement because it has the same active ingredient as medicine and has the same side effects. The regulation of this product by the FDA has been challenged in the courts by the supplement industry. The decision of the courts will have consequences for future regulation of supplements.
What are the possible side effects and risks of taking the supplement?	As noted above, if a product works as well as a medicine, it probably has the same side effects. If you know the active ingredient, you will know more about the side effects.
Are there possible interactions associated with taking the supplement?	When you take a medicine, you consult a physician or pharmacist about drug interactions. Supplements may interact with other supplements or medicines.
What are the long-term effects of taking the supplement?	Because supplements are not regulated, there has been little research about long-term effects of products. For example, melatonin is a hormone that is used for insomnia. Hormones have strong effects on the body and little is known about melatonin's long-term effects. Consider alternative solutions to long-term use of an unstudied supplement.
Are you sure the product is what it claims to be and that the size of the dose is appropriate?	U.S. Pharmacopeia (USP) is a private nonprofit organization that tests vitamins, minerals, and other supplements, to assure quality and purity as well as appropriate size and strength of a standard unit of the product (dose size and strength). The USP label ensures that the product is what it says it is. As many as two or three dozen herbal products are currently being evaluated to determine appropriate dose size. Products with the USP label that fail to meet standards will be removed from stores. Without the USP label, you are at the mercy of the company that produces the product. The deaths associated with L-tryptophan, an amino acid supplement, occurred because of contaminants (Peak-X) in the unregulated product.
Who makes the product?	In the absence of regulations, the reputation of the company that makes the product is crucial. Have complaints been made against the company? Have there been health problems with their products? How long has the company been in business? Large pharmaceutical companies are now beginning to sell supplements because of the high profit margin. Using a product from a large drug company is more likely to ensure that a product is what it is supposed to be, but it does not ensure that the product is effective.
Is the cost worth the potential benefits?	The costs of dietary supplements are typically quite high. For example, protein supplements may cost as much as $1.00 a gram. The cost per gram in good food, such as protein in a chicken breast, is typically a few cents per gram. Most experts suggest that even the most effective supplements have relatively small effects at a high cost.
Is the source of your information about the supplement reliable and accurate?	Avoid verbal information about products, especially information from the seller. Be wary of third-party literature or research in obscure journals. Be wary of those who discredit sound medical advice or information from regulatory agencies, such as the FDA.

"gov" as part of the address. Professional organizations and universities can also be good sources of information. Organizations typically have "org" and universities typically have "edu" as part of the address. However, caution should still be used with organizations because it is easy to start an organization and obtain an "org" Web address. Your greatest trust can be placed in the sites of stable organizations of long standing, such as the AMA, the American Cancer Society, the American Heart Association, the American College of Sports Medicine, the National Council against Health Fraud, and the American Alliance for Health, Physical Education, Recreation and Dance, among others listed in this text. The AMA has recently developed extensive guidelines for health information on the Web (see *Suggested Readings*). The great majority of websites promoting health products have "com" in the title because these are commercial sites that are in business to make a profit. Because they are in business to make a profit, they are more inclined to contain information that is suspect or totally incorrect. Some "com" sites contain good information—for example, those listed at the end of each concept of this book. Nevertheless, it is important to evaluate, with special care, information found at "com" sites. The Tufts University School of Nutrition Science and Policy has developed a website that rates diet and health sites on the Internet. You may want to consult this website (http://navigator.tufts.edu). In Lab 20A, you can rate a website, using a checklist.

When selecting websites for inclusion at the end of each concept of the book, we used the same checklist as in Lab 20A. You will see that a majority of the sites listed are governmental and organizational sites. We do include some commercial sites but with some reservation. What we see when we evaluate a site may not be what you see when you use the site at a later date. It is important that you evaluate all websites, using the criteria suggested here.

Study Resources

Check out additional online study resources for this concept in the Student Edition of the Online Learning Center at www.mhhe.com/corbin13e.

Web Resources

Agency for Health Care Policy and Research **www.ahcpr.gov**
American Dietetics Association **www.eatright.org**
AMA Health Insight **www.ama-assn.org**
Center for Science in the Public Interest **www.cspinet.org**
Federal Trade Commission **www.ftc.gov**
Food and Drug Administration **www.fda.gov**
Healthfinder **www.healthfinder.gov**
Medwatch **www.fda.gov/medwatch/**
National Council against Health Fraud **www.ncahf.org**

Technology Update

Medwatch

Medwatch is a website of the FDA. This website provides a variety of consumer information, including safety alerts for drugs, product recall advisories, changes in drug safety labeling, warnings and safety information concerning dietary supplements, and health advisories concerning medical devices. This is an excellent source relating to quackery (**www.fda.gov/medwatch**).

Strategies for Action

Being a good consumer requires time, information, and effort. www.mhhe.com/phys_fit/web20 Click 06. With time and effort, you can gain the information you need to make good decisions about products and services that you purchase. In Lab 20A, you will evaluate an exercise device, a food supplement, a magazine article, or a website. In Lab 20B, you will evaluate a health/wellness or fitness club. Taking the time to investigate a product will help you save money and help you avoid making poor decisions that affect your health, fitness, and wellness. When you are making decisions about products or services, it is a good idea to begin your investigation well in advance of the day when a decision is to be made. Salespeople often suggest that "this offer is only good today." They know that people often make poor decisions when under time pressure, and they want you to make a decision today so that they will not lose a sale.

Office of Dietary Supplements **http://ods.od.nih.gov**
Quackwatch **www.familyinternet.com/quackwatch/**
Tufts University Nutrition Navigator
   http://navigator.tufts.edu
U.S. Consumer Information Center **www.pueblo.gsa.gov**

Suggested Readings

Additional reference materials for Concept 20 are available at **www.mhhe.com/phys_fit/web20 Click 07**.

Blendon, R. J., et al. 2001. Americans' views on the use and regulation of dietary supplements. *Archives of Internal Medicine* 161(6):805–810.

Catlin, D. H., et al. 2000. Trace contamination of over-the-counter androstenedione and positive urine test results for a nandrolone metabolite. *Journal of the American Medical Association* 284(20):2618–2621.

Consumer Reports. June 2003. Regular reports on exercise machines. For example treadmills and heart rate monitors.

Drazen, J. M. 2003. Inappropriate advertising of dietary supplements. *New England Journal of Medicine* 348(9):777–778.

Ernst, E., and K. Schmidt. 2002. Alternative cancer cures via the Internet. *British Journal of Cancer* 87(5):479–480.

Fairfield, K. M., and R. H. Fletcher. 2002. Vitamins for chronic disease prevention in adults: Scientific review. *Journal of the American Medical Association* 287(23): 3116–3126.

Fletcher, R. H., and K. M. Fairfield. 2002. Vitamins for chronic disease prevention in adults: Clinical applications. *Journal of the American Medical Association* 287(23):3127–3129.

Fontanarosa, P. B., et al. 2003. The need for regulation of dietary supplements—lessons from ephedra. *Journal of the American Medical Association* 289(12):1568–1570.

Krone, C. 2004. Nutritional supplements: Friend or foe? *New Zealand Medical Journal* 117(1196):U937–U945.

National Council against Health Fraud Newsletter. Published every other month, it contains articles about health products and food supplements. NCAHF, P.O. Box 1276, Loma Linda, CA 92354.

Park, R. L. 2000. *Voodoo Science: The Road from Foolishness to Fraud.* New York: Oxford University Press.

Soloman, P. R., et al. 2002. Ginkgo for memory enhancement: A randomized controlled trial. *Journal of the American Medical Association* 288(7):835–840.

Tekin, K. A., and L. Kravitz. 2004. The growing trend of ergogenic aids and supplements. *ACSM's Health and Fitness Journal* 8(2):15–18.

USA Today. April 15, 2002. Dietary supplement use: Troubling side effects. *USA Today* 11A.

USA Today. May 10, 2001. Herbal drug bust. *USA Today* A14.

Winker, M. A., et al. 2000. Guidelines for medical and health information sites on the Internet: Principles governing AMA web sites. *Journal of the American Medical Association* 283(12):1600–1606.

 In the News

Increased Regulation of Dietary Supplements

There are over 29,000 dietary supplements available to consumers and sales have topped $16 billion. Because the Dietary Supplement Health and Education Act (DSHEA) shifted the burden of proof to the FDA, there has been rampant quackery and fraud in this industry. Recent efforts by a number of organizations are aiming to address the problem. The following list summarizes some of the recent initiatives.

• The FDA recently published regulations that would strengthen the manufacturing requirements of dietary supplements. If finalized, this rule would give consumers greater confidence that the dietary supplements they choose to use will have the purity, strength, quality, and potency claimed on the label. This will help to reduce problems such as superpotency, subpotency, contamination, and improper packaging that have been reported in recent years.

• The Federal Trade Commission (FTC) and the FDA have tightened links that will help to detect and deter health fraud. The FDA is responsible for the safety, manufacturing, and labeling of supplements. The FTC is responsible for regulating the advertising of the products. The revised arrangements will improve communication and provide a clearer jurisdiction of authority between the two organizations.

• The Institute of Medicine released a recent report (*Dietary Supplements: A Framework for Evaluating Safety*), which proposes solutions to the loopholes that were created after the release of the 1994 Dietary Supplement Health and Education Act (DSHEA). The document highlights ways in which the FDA can set priorities for evaluating potentially harmful products. For additional information, visit **http://nap.edu.**

• The *Consumer Health Information for Better Nutrition Initiative* of the FDA is designed to provide more science-based, FDA-regulated information on food labels. The idea is to provide information on the product that will allow the consumer to know the level of agreement of scientists concerning various claims. The following are the new informational labels:

  • A, significant scientific agreement for the claim
  • B, good scientific evidence but not entirely conclusive
  • C, evidence is limited and inconclusive
  • D, there is little scientific evidence support the claim

By providing clearer information about the health consequences of foods and dietary supplements the FDA hopes that consumers can make better nutritional choices. The initiative ultimately hopes that consumer demand for healthier products will stimulate changes in the food service industry. A system in which companies have to compete to provide healthier products to Americans would greatly improve the quality of products available to consumers. For additional information, visit the website at **www.fda.gov/oc/mcclellan/chbn.html.**

Lab 20A Practicing Consumer Skills: Evaluating Products

Name	Section	Date

Purpose: To evaluate an exercise device, a book, a magazine article, a food supplement, or an Internet site

Procedures

1. Evaluate an exercise device, book or article, food supplement or Internet site. Place an X in the circle by the item you choose to evaluate.
2. Read each of the 10 evaluation factors for the item you selected. Place an X in the circle by the factors that describe the item you are evaluating.
3. Total number of X marks to determine a score for the item being evaluated. The higher the score the more likely it is to be safe and/or effective.
4. Answer the questions in the Conclusions and Implications section.

Results

Directions: Place an X by the product you evaluated. Place an X over each true statement. Provide information about the product in the space provided.

Exercise Device

1. The exercise device requires effort consistent with the FIT formula.

2. The exercise device is safe and the exercise done using the device is safe.

3. There are no claims that the device uses exercise that is effortless.

4. Exercise using the device is fun or is a type that you might do regularly.

5. There are no claims using gimmick words such as *tone, cellulite, quick,* or *spot fat reduction.*

6. The seller's credentials are sound.

7. The product does something for you that cannot be done without it.

8. You can return the device if you do not like it (the seller has been in business for a long time).

9. The cost of the product is justified by the potential benefits.

10. The device is easy to store or you have a place to permanently use the equipment without storing it.

Exercise Device

Name of device: _____
_____
_____

Description and manufacturer:
_____
_____
_____
_____
_____
_____
_____

Book or Article

Author(s): _____
_____
_____

Journal article or book title: _____
_____
_____

Journal name or name of publisher:
_____
_____

Date of publication: _____
_____
_____

Book/Article

1. The credentials of the author are sound. He or she has a degree in an area related to the content of the book or magazine.

2. The facts in the article are consistent with the facts described in this book.

3. The authors do not claim "quick" or "miraculous" results.

4. There are no claims about the spot reduction of fat.

5. The author is not selling a product described in the article.

6. Reputable experts are cited.

7. The article does not promote unsafe exercises or products.

8. New discoveries from exotic places are not cited.

9. The article does not rely on testimonials by nonexpert, famous people.

10. The author does not make claims that the AMA, the FDA, or another legitimate organization is trying to suppress information.

Food Supplement

1. The seller is not the prime source of product information.

2. The seller has been in business for a long time and has a good reputation.

3. There is scientific evidence of product effectiveness.

4. There is clear evidence about the side effects of the active ingredients.

5. The long-term effectiveness and safety of the product are cited.

6. You are sure of the content of the product.

7. You have information that the manufacturer is reputable.

8. The known benefits are worth the cost.

9. There is evidence that you can get benefits from this product that cannot be obtained from good food.

10. There are no claims that use quack words or claims about conspiracies against the product by reputable organizations.

Food Supplement

Name: _____

_____

_____

Purported benefit: _____

_____

_____

Manufacturer/seller: _____

_____

_____

Dose and active ingredient: _____

_____

_____

Internet Site

Web address: _____

_____

_____

Type of information provided: ____

_____

_____

Organization or person responsible for information: _____

_____

_____

Internet Site

1. The site does not sell products associated with information provided.

2. The provider is a person, an organization (org), or a governmental agency (gov) with a sound reputation.

3. The site does not use quack words.

4. The site does not try to discredit well-established organizations or government agencies.

5. The site does not rely on testimonials, celebrities, or people with unknown credentials.

6. The site is well regarded by experts, and has a high rating at http://navigator.tufts.edu.

7. The site has a history of providing good information.

8. The site provides complete information that is documented by research.

9. No claims of quick cures or miracle results are made.

10. The site provides information consistent with information provided in this text.

Conclusions and Implications

Total number of Xs for device, book/magazine, food supplement, or website: [   ]

In several sentences, give your assessment of the product. Did it score well? Would you use/buy the product? Explain.

Lab 20B Evaluating a Health/Wellness or Fitness Club

Name	Section	Date

Purpose: To practice evaluating a health club (various combinations of the words *health, wellness,* and *fitness* are often used for these clubs)

Procedures

1. Choose a club and make a visit.
2. Listen carefully to all that is said and ask lots of questions.
3. Look carefully all around you as you are given the tour of the facilities; ask what the exercises or the equipment does for you or ask leading questions, such as "Will this take inches off my hips?"
4. As soon as you leave the club, rate it, using Chart 1. Space is provided for notes in Chart 1.

Chart 1 ▶ Health Club Evaluation Questionnaire

Directions: Place an X over a yes or no answer. Make notes as necessary.	Yes	No	Notes
1. Were claims for improvement in weight, figure/physique, or fitness realistic?	◯	◯	
2. Was a long-term contract (1 to 3 years) encouraged?	◯	◯	
3. Was the sales pitch high-pressure to make an immediate decision?	◯	◯	
4. Were you given a copy of the contract to read at home?	◯	◯	
5. Did the fine print include objectionable clauses?	◯	◯	
6. Did they ask you about medical readiness?	◯	◯	
7. Did they sell diet supplements as a sideline?	◯	◯	
8. Did they have passive equipment?	◯	◯	
9. Did they have cardiovascular training equipment or facilities (cycles, track, pool, aerobic dance)?	◯	◯	
10. Did they make unscientific claims for the equipment, exercise, baths, or diet supplements?	◯	◯	
11. Were the facilities clean?	◯	◯	
12. Were the facilities crowded?	◯	◯	
13. Were there days and hours when the facilities were open but would not be available to you?	◯	◯	
14. Were there limits on the number of minutes you could use a piece of equipment?	◯	◯	
15. Did the floor personnel closely supervise and assist clients?	◯	◯	
16. Were the floor personnel qualified experts?	◯	◯	
17. Were the managers/owners qualified experts?	◯	◯	
18. Has the club been in business at this location for a year or more?	◯	◯	

Results

1. Score the chart as follows:

   A. Give 1 point for each no answer for items 2, 3, 5, 7, 8, 10, 12, 13, and 14 and place the score in the box.   Total A   [ ]

   B. Give 1 point for each yes answer for items 1, 4, 6, 9, 11, and 18 and place the score in the box.   Total B   [ ]

   Total A and B above and place the score in the box.   Total A and B   [ ]

   C. Give 1 point for each yes answer for items 15, 16, and 17 and place the score in the box.   Total C   [ ]

2. A total score of 12–15 points on items A and B suggests the club rates at least fair, compared with other clubs.

3. A score of 3 on item C indicates that the personnel are qualified and suggests that you could expect to get accurate technical advice from the staff.

4. Regardless of the total scores, you would have to decide the importance of each item to you personally, as well as evaluate other considerations, such as cost, location, personalities of the clients and the personnel, and so on, to decide if this would be a good place for you or your friends to join.

Conclusions and Implications: In the space below, use several sentences to discuss your conclusion about the quality of this club and whether you think it would fit your needs if you wanted to belong.

Toward Optimal Health and Wellness: Planning for Healthy Lifestyle Change

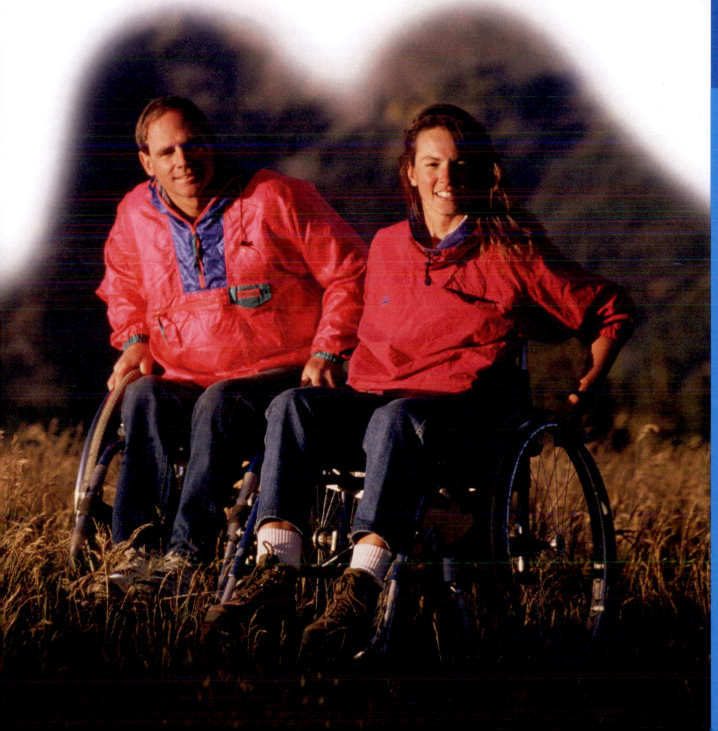

In addition to healthy lifestyles, other factors such as heredity, health care, the environment, and personal actions and interactions contribute to good health, wellness, and fitness.

Health Goals

for the year 2010

- Increase quality and years of healthy life.

- Increase healthy days.

- Eliminate health disparities.

- Increase adoption and maintenance of appropriate daily physical activity.

- Promote health by improving dietary factors and nutritional status.

- Promote healthy and safe communities.

- Promote availability of high-quality health information.

- Increase availability of health care and counseling for mental health problems.

- Avoid destructive behaviors.

The two primary health goals for the nation for the year 2010 are increasing the quality and years of life and eliminating health disparities so that all people can attain and maintain lifelong health, wellness, and fitness. The focus of this book is making a healthy lifestyle change, such as performing adequate physical activity, eating well, managing stress, and avoiding destructive behaviors. This concept provides information about other factors that can increase quality and years of life, including other lifestyle factors, the environment, the health-care system, and hereditary factors. The *Strategies for Action* at the end of this concept will help you use the self-management skills you learned in Concept 2 and the self-planning skills you learned in Concept 6. You will have the opportunity to tie together all of the information in this book, so that you can plan for a lifetime of healthy, active living.

A Model for Achieving and Maintaining Lifelong Health, Wellness, and Fitness

Many factors are important in developing lifetime health, wellness, and fitness, and some are more in your control than others. In Concept 1, you were exposed to a simplified model describing the factors important in achieving lifetime health, wellness and fitness. In this concept, that model (see Figure 1) will be developed in more detail to help you in lifetime planning.

Central to the model are health, wellness and fitness because these are the states of being (shaded in green and yellow) that each of us wants to achieve. Around the periphery (see Figure 1) are the factors that influence these states of being. Those shaded in blue are the factors over which you have less control (heredity, health-care systems, and environment). Those shaded in red are the factors over which you have greater control (healthy lifestyles and personal actions/interactions).

Factors Influencing Health, Wellness, and Fitness

Heredity (human biology) is a factor over which you have little control. Experts estimate that human biology or heredity accounts for 16 percent of all health problems, including early death. You have already learned that heredity influences each of the parts of health-related physical fitness, including your tendencies to build muscle and to deposit body fat. You also know that each of us reaps different benefits from the same healthy lifestyles, based on our hereditary tendencies. Even more important is that predispositions to disease are inherited. For example, some early deaths are a result of hereditary conditions (e.g., congenital heart defects) that are untreatable. Obviously, some inherited conditions are manageable (e.g., diabetes) with proper medical supervision and appropriate lifestyles. Heredity is a factor over which we have little control and is, therefore, illustrated in dark blue in Figure 1. Each of us can limit the effects of heredity by being aware of personal family history and making efforts to best manage those factors over which we do have control.

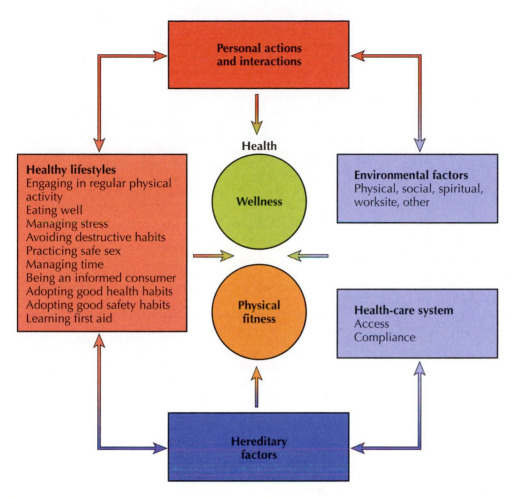

Figure 1 ▶ Factors influencing physical fitness, health, and wellness.

🌐 **The health-care system affects our ability to overcome illness and improve our quality of life.** www.mhhe.com/phys_fit/web21 Click 01. Approximately 10 percent of unnecessary deaths occur as a result of disparities in the health-care system. The quality of life for those who are sick and those who tend to be sick is influenced greatly by the type of medical care received. Access to health care is not equally available to all. A recent study by the Institute of Medicine, entitled "Care without Coverage: Too Little, Too Late," indicates that 18,000 people die unnecessarily in the United States each year because they lack health insurance. Those without health insurance are more likely to go but less likely to be admitted to emergency rooms, are less likely to get high-quality medical care, and are at greater risk for complications from illness than those with insurance. Those without insurance often have chronic conditions that go undetected and as a result become untreatable. One of the great health inequities is that those with lower income are less likely to be insured.

Many people fail to seek medical help even though care is accessible. Others seek medical help but fail to comply. For example, they do not take prescribed medicine or do not follow up with treatments. As noted earlier in this book, men are less likely to seek medical advice than women. For this reason, treatable conditions sometimes become untreatable. Once men seek medical care, evidence reveals they get better care than women. Also, more of the medical research has been done on men. This is of concern, since treatments for men and women often vary for similar conditions.

Wellness as evidenced by **quality of life** is also influenced by the health-care system. Traditional medicine, sometimes referred to as the **medical model,** has focused primarily on the treatment of illness with medicine rather than illness prevention and wellness promotion. Efforts to educate medical and health-care personnel about techniques for promoting wellness have been initiated in recent years. Still, it is often up to the patient to find information about health promotion. For example, a patient with risk factors for heart disease might be advised to eat better or to exercise more, but little specific information may be offered.

In Figure 1, the health-care system is colored in a light shade of blue to illustrate the fact that it is a factor over which you may have limited control. There are some things that you can do to assume more control, and they will be discussed in *Strategies for Action* at the end of this concept.

Quality of Life Wellness. An individual with quality of life can enjoy the activities of life with little or no limitation and can function independently. Individual quality of life requires a pleasant and supportive community quality of life.

Medical Model The focus of the health-care system on treating illness with medicine, with little emphasis on prevention or wellness promotion.

Table 1 ▶ Environmental Factors Influencing Health, Wellness, and Fitness

Physical environment. Many factors that influence the physical environment interact with each other. Urban sprawl and population growth, for example, are responsible for increased auto travel, and automobiles are the leading source of air pollution. Autos are also a cause of many accidental deaths (safety concern). Air and water pollution results in a variety of health problems and lowered quality of life. Pollution and sanitation problems are associated with population density and are much more likely to cause health problems for low-income people than for those in the middle class. Urban sprawl has also been associated with the heat island effect (the increase in temperature in industrial and inner-city areas) associated with increases in roadways and rooftops, as well as decreased vegetation.

- *Pollution.* Of particular concern is air pollution (increased ozone, hydrocarbons, and particulates). Carbon dioxide is a greenhouse gas that accounts for 80 percent of global warming. Urban sprawl negatively impacts water quantity and quality because water in populated areas is diverted to sewers rather than returning naturally to aquifers. Industrial pollution is another threat to air and water quality. Smoking in public places is a source of pollution.
- *Loss of natural resources.* High gas, oil, and mineral use risks early depletion of resources and can result in disfiguring the landscape and contribute to environmental hazards.
- *Urban sprawl and population growth.* Sprawl reduces opportunities for healthy lifestyles, such as walking and biking, and increases the need for auto travel. Population growth results in greater housing density and can result in less community and home safety.
- *Sanitation.* Urban growth places great demands on sanitation systems and contributes to land pollution.

Social environment. A healthy social environment offers opportunities for friendly interactions in a supportive environment. Not all social environments are healthy, and sometimes you must remove yourself, especially if relationships become abusive. Social environments interact with physical environments. For example, crowded roadways often lead to negative social interactions known as road rage. Drivers with road rage depersonalize other drivers and display behaviors they would never consider under normal circumstances.

- *Sense of community.* Being a part of the greater community is important to social and mental health.
- *Opportunities for personal relationships.* We all need friendly personal interactions. These relationships contribute to all aspects of health and wellness.
- *Family and peer support.* Support by others, especially family members, is important to all of us.
- *Time availability.* We tend to take time for what we think is important. Social interactions require that time be spent with other people.
- *Removal from abusive environments.* If relationships become abusive, you may have to remove yourself and others at risk and to seek help from others.

Spiritual environment. A positive environment provides each person with opportunities to find spiritual fulfillment. Whether interpreted as a belief in a higher power or a personal sense of wholeness associated with something greater than self, spiritual wellness is most likely to occur in a supportive environment (see column 2). Additional information is presented in the *Strategies for Action* section of this concept.

- *Opportunities for spiritual development.* Reading spiritual materials, prayer, meditation, and discussions with others (of similar and dissimilar beliefs) all provide opportunities to clarify and solidify spiritual beliefs.
- *Access to spiritual community.* Finding a community for worship and/or spiritual support has been shown to be comforting and a path to fulfillment for many.
- *Available spiritual leadership.* Like many other life experiences, spiritual fulfillment may benefit from consultation with those with experience and expertise.

Intellectual environment. Environments that foster learning and sound critical thinking are important to intellectual wellness. Evidence shows that people with more education are more likely to practice healthy lifestyles, to seek medical help, and to live in healthy environments than those with less education.

- *Access to accurate information.* Whether the source is formal education or self-learning, access to accurate information is essential. Of course, good information is beneficial only if used.
- *Stimulation for effective thinking.* Sometimes, we can become lazy, failing to evaluate information effectively. Seeking environments that stimulate critical thinking is important.

Work environment. The work environment is a combination of the physical, social, intellectual, and spiritual environments discussed earlier. Work environments are discussed separately because so many people spend so much time at work. Changing the work environment has been shown to be possible with cooperative efforts among workers and management. Many people now consider a healthy work environment to be as important as financial compensation.

- *Healthy physical environment.* A healthy work environment includes an adequate, well-lit, pollution-free workspace and reasonable work hours.
- *Healthy social environment.* Good relationships with bosses and co-workers and adequate work breaks are key elements of a healthy social work environment.
- *Opportunity and support for healthy lifestyles.* Many companies now have worksite wellness programs, which include opportunities for physical activity and other healthy lifestyle change. Programs that have quality professional leadership have been shown to produce reduced absenteeism, reduced health-care costs, and increased job satisfaction.

Environment supporting healthy lifestyles. When we think of a toxic environment, we often think of a toxic physical environment. In recent years, experts have suggested that environments that reduce opportunities for adopting healthy lifestyles are also toxic. For example, the easy availability of fast food and junk food in vending machines creates a toxic environment for unhealthy eating.

- *Toxin-free environments.* If we are to promote healthy lifestyles at home, work, and school, it is important to create environments that encourage active lifestyles. Examples include providing safe, open recreational areas and worksite wellness programs.
- *People working together.* Changes designed to promote healthy lifestyles require the efforts of many people. Cooperative efforts by groups with well-defined goals are most likely to be successful.

The environment is a major factor affecting our health, wellness, and fitness. Environmental factors account for nearly one-fourth of all early deaths and affect quality of life in many ways. We do have more control over environmental factors than heredity, but they are not totally under our control. For this reason, the environment box is depicted in Figure 1 with a lighter shade of blue than the heredity box.

Some of the more important environmental factors are described in Table 1. You can exert personal control by selecting healthy environments rather than by exposing yourself to unhealthy or unsafe environments. This includes your choice of living and work location, as well as the social, spiritual, and intellectual environments. On the other hand, circumstances may make it impossible to make the choices you would prefer. Those who work in cities are typically more exposed to pollution and environmental risks than those who live in rural areas, including the heat island effect described in Table 1. Some suggestions for how you can work to alter the environment in a positive way are discussed later in this concept.

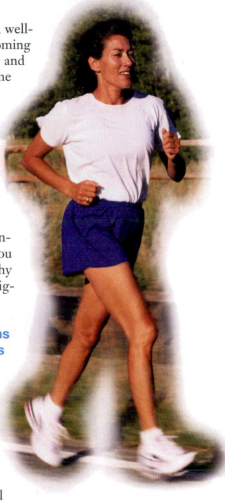

Healthy lifestyles are the greatest contributor to living a long, healthy life. www.mhhe.com/phys_fit/web21 Click 02. Statistics show that more than half of early deaths are caused by unhealthy lifestyles. For this reason, changing lifestyle is the focus of this book. Lifestyles are depicted in red (Figure 1) because they are much more in your control than the factors previously discussed and depicted in blue.

We have focused on adopting priority healthy lifestyles such as being regularly active, eating well, and managing stress because they are all factors over which we have some control and, if adopted, they have considerable impact on health, wellness, and fitness. Becoming an informed consumer and learning to manage time were also discussed in detail in earlier concepts. Other healthy lifestyles not emphasized in this book are described in Table 2. We hope you will adopt a new way of thinking and that you will use the self-management skills to help you adopt the ten healthy lifestyles depicted in Figure 1.

Personal actions and interactions are under your control and greatly influence your lifetime fitness, health, and wellness. www.mhhe.com/phys_fit/web21 Click 03. In the final analysis, you can learn all about heredity, health care, the environment, and healthy lifestyles; if you do not use what you

Making one lifestyle change, such as becoming more physically active, can lead to other healthy lifestyle changes.

Table 2 ▶ Other Healthy Lifestyles	
Lifestyle	**Examples**
Adopting good personal health habits. Many of these habits, important to optimal health, are considered to be elementary because they are often taught in school or in the home at an early age. In spite of their importance, many adults regularly fail to adopt these behaviors.	• Brushing and flossing teeth • Regular bathing and hand washing • Adequate sleep • Care of ears, eyes, and skin
Adopting good safety habits. Unintentional injuries cost Canadians about $8.7 billion per year and, in the United States, the cost of injury and violence is $224 billion a year. Thousands of people die each year and thousands more suffer disabilities or problems that detract from good health and wellness. Not all accidents can be prevented, but we can adopt habits to reduce risk.	• *Automobile accidents.* Wear seat belts, avoid using the phone while driving, and do not drink and drive. • *Water accidents.* Learn to swim, learn CPR, wear life jackets while boating, do not drink while boating. • *Others.* Store guns safely, use smoke alarms, use ladders and electrical equipment safely, and maintain cars, bikes, and motorcycles properly.
Learning first aid. Many deaths could be prevented and the severity of injury could be reduced if those at the sites of emergencies were able to administer first aid.	• Learn cardiopulmonary resuscitation (CPR). • Learn the Heimlich maneuver to assist people who are choking, and learn basic first aid.
Avoid destructive habits. For those who practice these habits, changes in behaviors could reduce disease and early death risk as well improve quality of life.	• Do not abuse drugs including alcohol. • Do not use tobacco. • Practice safe sex.

learn, it will not help you. You are ultimately responsible for your personal actions. For this reason, the box illustrating personal actions and interactions (Figure 1) is depicted in red. You can learn about your family history and use the information to limit the negative influence of heredity. You can do research about the health-care system and the environment to minimize the problems associated with them. Perhaps most important of all, you can learn self-management skills to help you in adopting healthy lifestyles.

Some people think that good health is totally out of personal control. Others think that they are totally in control of personal health. Neither statement is entirely true. It would seem wise to learn as much about what you cannot control and use that information to make wise decisions.

Your interactions also influence your health, wellness, and fitness. You are not in this world alone. To be sure, your various environments influence you greatly. More important, however, is how you interact in these environments (see Table 1). You have a choice about the environments in which you place yourself, the people with whom you interact in these environments, and how you interact with the environments themselves.

None of us makes perfect decisions all of the time. Sometimes, we take actions and make choices with faulty or inadequate information. The more we learn, the less likely we are to repeat mistakes. From a positive point of view, well-informed people are healthier, happier, and more fulfilled than those who are less careful choosing a course of action.

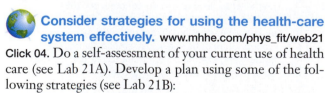

Strategies for Action

Consider strategies for taking advantage of your heredity. You are aware that heredity is a factor that affects all aspects of fitness as well as your health and wellness. You can use several strategies to overcome negative predispositions and to take advantage of positive ones:

- *Learn about your family history.* If members of your family have had specific diseases or health problems, make sure you inform your physician. Investigate to see if the conditions could affect you.
- *Take action to diminish risk factors for which you have a predisposition.* For example, if you have a family history of Type II diabetes, you must do regular activity, eat well, and keep your body fat level in the good fitness zone.
- *Take advantage of your hereditary strengths.* Self-assessments can help you see where you have strength and account for weaknesses. Build on your strengths and find ways to compensate for your weaknesses. For example, people who have fewer fast-twitch muscle fibers will probably not be great sprinters but often have more slow-twitch fibers, which favor endurance performances, such as distance running.

 Consider strategies for using the health-care system effectively. www.mhhe.com/phys_fit/web21 **Click 04.** Do a self-assessment of your current use of health care (see Lab 21A). Develop a plan using some of the following strategies (see Lab 21B):

- *Get periodic medical exams.* Do not wait until something is wrong before you seek medical advice. After 40 years of age, a yearly preventive physical exam is recommended. Younger people should have an exam at least every 2 years. Mammograms for women and prostate

tests (PSA) for men are recommended. Breast and testicular self-exams are also important.
- *Get medical insurance.* Find a way to get health insurance. Young people who save money by avoiding the payment of insurance premiums are placing themselves (and families) at risk.
- *Immunize.* Pneumonia and the flu are the sixth leading cause of death. With immunization, death, hospitalization, and loss of healthy days decrease dramatically. Many children go without immunizations that could prevent illness.
- *Identify a regular doctor and a convenient emergency care center.*
- *Become familiar with the symptoms of common medical problems.*
- *If symptoms persist, seek medical help.* Many deaths can be prevented if early warning signs of medical problems are heeded.
- *If medical advice is given, comply.* People commonly stop taking medicine when symptoms stop rather than taking the full amount of medicine prescribed.
- *If you have doubts about medical advice, get a second opinion.*
- *Be cautious when using the Internet for health information.* If you use the Internet for health information, be sure to use reliable websites (see Concept 20). Seek information from more than one source.
- *Make your wishes for health care known.* Have a medical power of attorney. This document spells out the treatments you desire in the case of severe illness. Without such a document, your loved ones may not be able to make decisions consistent with your wishes. Be sure your loved ones have a similar document so that you can help them carry out their wishes.

Consider strategies for improving your environment.
Do a self-assessment to determine the quality of your environment (see Lab 21A). Develop a plan for improving your environment using the following practical strategies (Lab 21B):

- *Strategies for improving the physical environment.* Recycle; carpool; use public transportation; safely dispose of hazardous waste; conserve water; use fuel-efficient cooling, heating, and appliances; buy environmentally friendly products; do not litter; work with others to seek public policy change; join a zoning board.
- *Strategies for interacting with the physical environment.* Avoid polluted environments, such as smoke-filled establishments; choose a living location low in pollution (see Figure 2); keep your home free of pollutants (regularly check filters, avoid use of toxic products); and stay inside on days with high pollution.
- *Strategies for the social environment.* Find a social community that accommodates your personal and family needs; get involved in community affairs including those that affect the environment; build relationships with family and friends; provide support for others so that the support of others will be there for you when you need it; use time-management strategies to help you allocate time for social interactions.
- *Strategies for the spiritual environment.* Pray, meditate, read spiritual materials, participate in spiritual discussions, find a place to worship, provide spiritual support for others, seek spiritual guidance from those with experience and expertise, keep a journal, experience nature, honor relationships, help others.
- *Strategies for the intellectual environment.* Make decisions based on sound information, question simple solutions to complex problems, seek environments that stimulate critical thinking.

- *Strategies for the work environment.* Choose a job that has a healthy physical environment, including adequate space, lighting, and freedom from pollution (tobacco smoke) as well as a healthy social, spiritual, and intellectual environment and one that has a worksite wellness program led by professionals.
- *Strategies for finding an environment that supports healthy lifestyles.* Choose a place to live that is near parks and playgrounds and has sidewalks, bike paths, jogging trails, and swimming facilities; join a gym or health club; avoid environments that limit choices to fast food and food with empty calories; find a social environment that reinforces healthy lifestyles.

Consider strategies for adopting healthy lifestyles.
As noted earlier in this concept, healthy lifestyles are the greatest contributor to a long and quality life. For this reason, find ways to incorporate each of the health lifestyles (described in Figure 1) into your life plan. The following list includes other strategies you can use to implement healthy lifestyles:

- *Use the six steps to help you plan lifestyle programs.* In Concept 6, you learned about six steps in planning a physical activity program. The same six steps (see Table 3) can be used to plan for each of the many healthy lifestyles. The labs at the end of this concept are designed to help you use the six steps in program planning. Labs 21A and 21B relate to a broad range of lifestyles, whereas Lab 21C helps you use the six steps to plan a lifetime physical activity program.
- *Use self-management skills.* Learning and using self-management skills, discussed in Concept 2 and throughout the book, can help you to adopt and maintain healthy lifestyles.

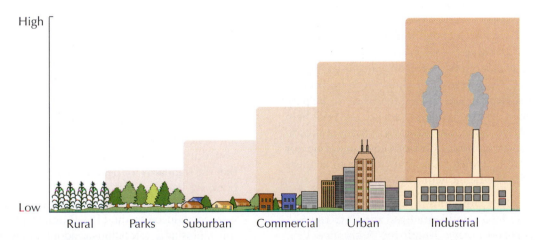

Figure 2 ▶ The effects of urban sprawl and industrial development on the physical environment.

Note: Darker shades reflect greater pollution, greater automobile density, higher temperature (heat effect), and more pavement.

• *Formal steps can become less formal with experience.* Few of us will go through life doing formal fitness assessments every month, writing down goals weekly, or self-monitoring activity daily. However, the more a person does self-assessments, the more he or she is aware of personal fitness status. This awareness reduces the need for frequent testing. For example, a person who does regular heart rate monitoring knows when he or she is in the target zone without counting heart rate every minute. A person who has frequently used skinfold measures to self-assess fatness can develop a good sense of body fatness with less frequent measurements. The same is true of other self-management skills. With experience, you can use the techniques less formally.

Consider strategies for taking action and benefitting from interactions. In the end, it is what you do that counts. You can learn everything there is to know about fitness, health, and wellness, but if you do not take action and take advantage of your interactions with people and your environments, you will not benefit (see Figure 1). The following are some strategies for taking action and interacting effectively:

• *Collect and evaluate information before you act.* Become informed before you make important decisions. Get information from good sources and consult with others you trust.

• *Plan your actions and interactions.* Use the information in this book to plan your actions. Seek environments that produce positive interactions. People who plan are not only more likely to act but also more likely to act effectively.

• *Put your plans into action.* Do not put off until tomorrow what you can do today. For good plans to be effective, they must be implemented. Actions and interactions that influence various dimensions of wellness are described in Table 3.

• *Honor your beliefs and relationships.* Actions and interactions that are inconsistent with basic beliefs and that fail to honor important relationships can result in reduced quality of life.

• *Seek the help of others and provide support for others who need your help.* As already noted, support by friends, family, and significant others can be critical in helping you to achieve health, wellness, and fitness. Seek help for failing and abusive relationships. If your attempts to change meet with failure, do not set yourself up for repeated failure. Get help! Do what you can to be there for others who need your help.

Most colleges have programs through their health centers that provide free, confidential assistance or referral. Many businesses now have Employee Assistance Programs (EAP). The programs have counselors who will help you or your family members find help with a particu-

Table 3 ▶ Factors Influencing Wellness

Dimension of Wellness	Influential Factors
Physical wellness	Pursuing behaviors that are conducive to good physical health (being physically active and maintaining a healthy diet)
Social wellness	Being supportive of family, friends, and co-workers and practicing good communication skills
Emotional wellness	Balancing work and leisure and responding proactively to challenging or stressful situations
Intellectual wellness	Challenging yourself to continually learn and improve in your work and personal life
Spiritual wellness	Praying, meditating, or reflecting on life
Total wellness	Taking responsibility for your own health and happiness

lar problem. The EAP staff are dedicated to help you without revealing personal information to your employer. These programs have a strong record for helping people with problems ranging from small to very serious, such as drug addiction or smoking cessation. Many other programs and support groups are now available to help you change your lifestyle. For example, most hospitals and many health organizations now have hot lines that provide you with referral services for establishing healthy lifestyles.

Consider your personal beliefs and philosophy when making decisions. Though science can help you make good decisions and solve problems, most experts tell you that there is more to it than that. Your personal philosophy and beliefs play a role. The following are factors to consider:

• *Clarify your personal philosophy and consider a new way of thinking.* The determination as to whether a person is healthy, well, or fit is often subjective. Many make comparisons with other people, and such comparisons often result in setting personal standards impossible to achieve. Achieving the body fat of a model seen on television is not realistic or healthy for most people. Expecting to be able to perform as a professional athlete is not something most of us can achieve. It is for this reason that the standards for health, wellness, and fitness in this book are based on health criteria rather than comparative criteria. As you began your study on this book, you were introduced to the HELP philosophy. Adhering to this philosophy can help you adopt a new way of thinking. This philosophy suggests that each person should use health (H) as the basis for making decisions rather than comparisons with others. This is something that everyone (E) can do for a lifetime (L). This allows each of us to set personal (P) goals that are realistic and possible for each person to attain. You may adopt all or parts of this philosophy. Whether you do or do not, you should have a clear idea of your own personal philosophy.

The new way of thinking simply allows each of us to be successful on our own terms rather than comparing ourselves with others in ways that make success impossible. As you set personal health, wellness, and fitness goals, consider using a new way of thinking:

- *Allow for spontaneity.* The reliance on science emphasized in this book can help you make good choices.

But if you are to live life fully you sometimes must allow yourself to be spontaneous. In doing so, the key is to be consistent with your personal philosophy, so that your spontaneous actions will be enriching rather than a source of future regret.

- *Believe that you can make a difference.* As noted previously, you make your own choices. Though heredity and several other factors are out of your control, the choices that you make are yours. Believing that your actions make a difference is critical to taking action and making changes when necessary. We hope the information presented in this book helps you make choices that allow you to be healthy, well, and fit for a lifetime.

Study Resources

Check out additional online study resources for this concept in the Student Edition of the Online Learning Center at www.mhhe.com/corbin13e.

Web Resources

American College Health Association **www.acha.org**
American Dietetics Association **www.eatright.org**
Health Canada Online **www.hc_sc.gc.ca**
Health Canada–Physical Activity Guide
    www.hc_sc.gc.ca/hppb/paguide
Healthfinder **www.healthfinder.gov**
Healthy People 2010 **www.health.gov/healthypeople**
Mayo Clinic **www.mayoclinic.com**
Morbidity and Mortality Weekly Reports **www.cdc.gov/mmwr**
National Institute of Alcohol Abuse and Alcoholism
    www.niaaa.nih.gov
National Institute of Drug Abuse **www.nida.nih.gov**
National Institute of Environmental Health Sciences
    www.niehs.nih.gov
U.S. Consumer Information Center **www.pueblo.gsa.gov**
World Health Organization **www.who.int**

Suggested Readings

Additional reference materials for Concept 21 are available at **www.mhhe.com/phys_fit/web21 Click 05.**

Booth, F. W., and M. W. Chakravarthy. 2002. Cost and consequences of sedentary living: New battleground for an old enemy. *President's Council on Physical Fitness and Sports* 3(16):1–8.

Corbin, C. B., and R. P. Pangrazi. 2001. Toward a uniform definition of wellness: A commentary. *President's Council on Physical Fitness and Sports* 3(15):1–8.

Diener, E., R. E. Lucas, and S. Oishi. 2002. Subjective well-being: The science of happiness and life satisfaction.

Technology Update

Your Fitness Profile

Computer programs provide an effective way to track and monitor your fitness results over time. A customized software program called Interactive Personal Trainer is available to users of the book. Go to the *On the Web* site for Concept 6 (www.mhhe.com/phys_fit/web06) and click on the link labeled Fitness Profile to learn how to download and use the program. Once you install it, you can enter your scores for the various fitness self-assessments in the book. The program will generate a personal Fitness Profile, which rates each component of fitness testing using the criterion referenced standards in this book.

In C. R. Snyder and S. J. Lopez (eds.). *Handbook of Positive Psychology.* New York: Oxford University Press.

Donatelle, R. J., and L. G. Davis. 2005. *Health: The Basics.* 6th ed. Boston: Addison-Wesley.

Ewing, R. 2004. Relationship between urban sprawl and physical activity, obesity, and morbidity. *American Journal of Health Promotion* 18(1):47–57.

Fields, R. 2004. *Drugs in Perspective.* 5th ed. St. Louis: McGraw-Hill.

Frumkin, H. 2002. Urban sprawl and public health. *Public Health Reports* 117(3):201–217.

Glanz, K., et al. (eds.). 2002. *Health Behavior and Health Education: Theory, Research and Practice.* 3rd ed. San Francisco: Jossey-Bass.

Greenberg, J. S. 2004. *Health Education and Health Promotion.* 5th ed. St. Louis: McGraw-Hill.

Hahn, D. B., and W. A. Payne. 2005. *Focus on Health.* 7th ed. St. Louis: McGraw-Hill.

Institute of Medicine. 2002. *Care without Coverage: Too Little, Too Late.* Washington, DC: National Academy Press.

Isaacs, S. L., and J. R. Knickman. 2004. *Generalist Medicine and the U.S. Health Care System*. San Francisco: Jossey-Bass.

Keyes, C. L., and S. J. Lopez. 2002. Toward a science of mental health. In C. R. Snyder and S. J. Lopez (eds.). *Handbook of Positive Psychology*. New York: Oxford University Press.

Pargament, K. I., and A. Manhoney. 2002. Spirituality: Discovering and conserving the sacred. In C. R. Snyder and S. J. Lopez (eds.). *Handbook of Positive Psychology*. New York: Oxford University Press.

Payne, W. A., and D. B. Hahn. 2002. *Understanding Your Health*. 7th ed. St. Louis: McGraw-Hill.

Sallis, J. F., and N. Owen. 2002. Ecological models. In K. Glanz, et al. (eds.). *Health Behavior and Health Education: Theory, Research and Practice*. 3rd ed. San Francisco: Jossey-Bass.

Sanmartin, C., et al. 2004. *Joint Canada/United States Survey of Health, 2002–2003*. Atlanta, GA: CDC.

Snyder, C. R., and S. J. Lopez. 2002. *Handbook of Positive Psychology*. New York: Oxford University Press.

Taylor, S. 2003. *Health Psychology*. 5th ed. St. Louis: McGraw-Hill.

U.S. Department of Health and Human Services. Nov. 2000. *Healthy People 2010*. 2nd ed. With *Understanding and Improving Health and Objectives for Improving Health*. 2 vols. Washington, DC: U.S. Government Printing Office.

Wanda, G. C. 2004. Factors of the physical environment associated with walking and bicycling. *Medicine and Science in Sports and Exercise* 36(4):725–730.

World Health Organization. 2004. *World Health Report 2003: Shaping the Future*. Geneva: WHO. Available at www.who.int/whr/2003/en/.

 In the News

Policies and Environmental Changes for Health

Environmental influences on health have received considerable attention from public health officials and researchers in recent years. Characteristics in the environment that contribute to increases in energy intake and decreases in energy expenditure have been blamed for the increasing prevalence of obesity. While individuals still have to accept personal responsibility, it is difficult for people to act on their good intentions when confronted with an environment that is not conducive to good health. To reverse these trends there have been major efforts to develop environmental interventions that promote changes in economic, social, and physical settings. These interventions have complemented traditional public health efforts to change individual behaviors. Declines in

smoking in the United States have been attributed in large part to successful policy and environmental interventions that have restricted access and changed the social norm. Similar efforts are being planned for lifestyle behaviors such as physical activity and nutrition. The Cardiovascular Health Branch of the Centers for Disease Control and Prevention recently released a tool that will be used by state and local public health agencies to promote environmental and policy changes to decrease cardiovascular diseases. The document, called *Taking Action for Heart-Healthy and Stroke-Free States: A Communication Guide for Policy and Environmental Change*, provides a number of examples of how to link policy and environmental change interventions (see conceptual model). For additional information, visit the CDC website: www.cdc.gov/cvh/library/heart_stroke_guide/index.htm.

Lab 21A Assessing Factors That Influence Health, Wellness, and Fitness

Name	**Section**	**Date**

Purpose: To assess the factors that relate to health, wellness, and fitness

Chart 1 ▶ Assessment Questionnaire: Factors That Influence Health, Wellness, and Fitness

Factor	Very True	Somewhat True	Not True At All	Score
Heredity				
1. I have checked my family history for medical problems.	③	②	①	
2. I have taken steps to overcome hereditary predispositions.	③	②	①	
			Heredity Score =	
Health Care				
3. I have health insurance.	③	②	①	
4. I get regular medical exams and have my own doctor.	③	②	①	
5. I get treatment early, rather than waiting until problems get serious	③	②	①	
6. I carefully investigate my health problems before making decisions.	③	②	①	
			Health-Care Score =	
Environment				
7. My physical environment is healthy.	③	②	①	
8. My social environment is healthy.	③	②	①	
9. My spiritual environment is healthy.	③	②	①	
10. My intellectual environment is healthy.	③	②	①	
11. My work environment is healthy.	③	②	①	
12. My environment fosters healthy lifestyles.	③	②	①	
			Environment Score =	
Lifestyles				
13. I am physically active on a regular basis.	③	②	①	
14. I eat well.	③	②	①	
15. I use effective techniques for managing stress.	③	②	①	
16. I avoid destructive behaviors.	③	②	①	
17. I practice safe sex.	③	②	①	
18. I manage my time effectively.	③	②	①	
19. I evaluate information carefully and am an informed consumer.	③	②	①	
20. My personal health habits are good.	③	②	①	
21. My safety habits are good.	③	②	①	
22. I know first aid and can use it if needed.	③	②	①	
			Lifestyles Score =	
Personal Actions and Interactions				
23. I collect and evaluate information before I act.	③	②	①	
24. I plan before I take action.	③	②	①	
25. I am good about taking action when I know it is good for me.	③	②	①	
26. I honor my beliefs and relationships.	③	②	①	
27. I seek help when I need it.	③	②	①	
			Personal Actions/Interactions Score =	

Procedures

1. Answer each of the questions in Chart 1 on page 409. Consider the information in this concept as you answer each question.
2. Calculate the scores for heredity (sum items 1 and 2), health care (sum items 3–6), environment (sum items 7–12), lifestyles (sum items 13–22), and actions/interactions (sum items 23–27).
3. Determine ratings for each of the scores using the Rating Chart.
4. Record your scores and ratings in the Results chart. Record your comments in the Conclusions and Implications section.

Results

Factor	Score	Rating
Heredity		
Health care		
Environment		
Lifestyles		
Actions/interactions		

Rating Chart

Factor	Healthy	Marginal	Needs Attention
Heredity	6	4–5	Below 4
Health care	11–12	9–10	Below 9
Environment	16–18	13–15	Below 13
Lifestyles	26–30	20–25	Below 20
Actions/interactions	13–15	10–12	Below 10

Conclusions and Implications

1. In the space below, discuss your scores for the five factors (sums of several questions) identified in Chart 1. Use several sentences to identify specific areas that need attention and changes that you could make to improve.

2. For any individual item on Chart 1, a score of 1 is considered low. You might have a high score on a set of questions and still have a low score in one area that indicates a need for attention. In several sentences, discuss actions you could take to make changes related to individual questions.

Lab 21B Planning for Improved Health, Wellness, and Fitness

Name	**Section**	**Date**

Purpose: To make plans to make changes in areas that can most contribute to improved health, wellness, and fitness

Procedures

1. Experts agree that it is best not to make too many changes all at once. Focusing attention on one or two things at a time will produce better results. Based on your assessments made in Lab 21A, select two areas in which you would like to make changes. Choose one from the list related to environments and health care and one related to lifestyle change. Place a check by those areas in Chart 1 in the Results section. Because Lab 21C is devoted to physical activity, it is not included in the list. You may want to make additional copies of this lab for future use in making other changes in the future.
2. Use Chart 2 to determine your Stage of Change for the changes you have identified. Since you have identified these as an area of need, it is unlikely that you would identify the stage of maintenance. If you are at maintenance, you could select a different area of changes that would be more useful.
3. In the appropriate locations, record the change you want to make related to your environment or health care. State your reasons, your specific goal(s), your written statement of the plan for change, and a statement about how you will self-monitor and evaluate the effectiveness of the changes made. In Chart 3, record similar information for the lifestyle change you identified.

Results

Chart 1 ▶

Check one in each column.

Area of Change	✔	Area of Change	✔
Health insurance		Eating well	
Medical checkups		Managing stress	
Selecting a doctor		Avoiding destructive habits	
Physical environment		Practicing safe sex	
Social environment		Managing time	
Spiritual environment		Becoming a better consumer	
Intellectual environment		Improving health habits	
Work environment		Improving safety habits	
Environment for lifestyles		Learning first aid	

Chart 2 ▶

List the two areas of change identified in Chart 1. Make a rating using the diagram at the right.

Identified Area of Change	Stage of Change Rating
1.	
2.	

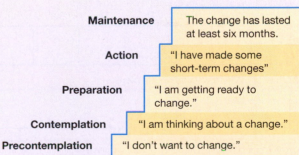

Maintenance — The change has lasted at least six months.

Action — "I have made some short-term changes"

Preparation — "I am getting ready to change."

Contemplation — "I am thinking about a change."

Precontemplation — "I don't want to change."

Note: Some of the areas identified in this assignment relate to personal information. It is appropriate not to divulge personal information to others (including your instructor) if you choose not to. For this reason, you may choose not to address certain problems in this assignment. You are encouraged to take steps to make changes independent of this assignment and to consult privately with your instructor to get assistance.

Chart 3 ▶ Making Changes for Improved Health, Wellness, and Fitness

Describe First Area of Change (from Chart 1)	Describe Second Area of Change (from Chart 1)

Step 1: State Reasons for Making Change

Step 1: State Reasons for Making Change

Step 2: Self-Assessment of Need for Change
List your stage from Chart 2.

Step 2: Self-Assessment of Need for Change
List your stage from Chart 2.

Step 3: State Your Specific Goals for Change
State several specific and realistic goals.

Step 3: State Your Specific Goals for Change
State several specific and realistic goals.

Step 4: Identify Activities or Actions for Change
List specific activities you will do or actions you will take to meet your goals.

Step 4: Identify Activities or Actions for Change
List specific activities you will do or actions you will take to meet your goals.

Step 5: Write a Plan; Include a Timetable
Expected start date:

Expected finish date:

Days of week and times: List times below days.

Mon.	Tue.	Wed.	Th.	Fri.	Sat.	Sun.

Location: Where will you do the plan?

Step 5: Write a Plan; Include a Timetable
Expected start date:

Expected finish date:

Days of week and times: List times below days.

Mon.	Tue.	Wed.	Th.	Fri.	Sat.	Sun.

Location: Where will you do the plan?

Step 6: Evaluate Your Plan
How will you self-monitor and evaluate to determine if the plan is working?

Step 6: Evaluate Your Plan
How will you self-monitor and evaluate to determine if the plan is working?

Lab 21C Planning Your Personal Physical Activity Program

Name	Section	Date

Purpose: To establish a comprehensive plan of lifestyle physical activity and to self-monitor progress in your plan (note: you may want to reread the concept on planning for physical activity before completing this lab)

Procedures

Step 1. Establishing Your Reasons

In the spaces provided below, list several of your principal reasons for doing a comprehensive activity plan.

1.
2.
3.

4.
5.
6.

Step 2. Identify Your Needs Using Fitness Self-Assessments and Ratings of Stage of Change for Various Activities

In Chart 1, rate your fitness by placing an X over the circle by the appropriate rating for each part of fitness. Use your results obtained from previous labs or perform the self-assessments again to determine your ratings. If you took more than one self-assessment for one component of physical fitness, select the rating that you think best describes your true fitness for that fitness component. If you were unable to do a self-assessment for some reason, check the "No Results" circle.

Chart 1 ▶ Rating for Self-Assessments

Health-Related Fitness Tests	High-Performance Zone	Good Fitness Zone	Rating Marginal Zone	Low Zone	No Results
1. Cardiovascular: 12-minute run (Chart 6, page 119)	○	○	○	○	○
2. Cardiovascular: step test (Chart 2, page 117)	○	○	○	○	○
3. Cardiovascular: bicycle test (Chart 5, page 119)	○	○	○	○	○
4. Cardiovascular: walking test (Chart 1, page 117)	○	○	○	○	○
5. Cardiovascular: swim test (Chart 7, page 120)	○	○	○	○	○
6. Flexibility: sit and reach (Chart 1, page 160)	○	○	○	○	○
7. Flexibility: shoulder flexibility (Chart 1, page 160)	○	○	○	○	○
8. Flexibility: hamstring/hip flexibility (Chart 1, page 160)	○	○	○	○	○
9. Flexibility: trunk rotation (Chart 1, page 160)	○	○	○	○	○
10. Strength: isometric grip (Chart 3, page 198)	○	○	○	○	○
11. Strength: 1 RM upper body (Chart 2, page 197)	○	○	○	○	○

Chart 1 ▶ Rating for Self-Assessments, *continued*

Health-Related Fitness Tests	High-Performance Zone	Good Fitness Zone	Rating Marginal Zone	Low Zone	No Results
12. Strength: 1 RM lower body (Chart 2, page 197)	○	○	○	○	○
13. Muscular endurance: curl-up (Chart 4, page 198)	○	○	○	○	○
14. Muscular endurance: 90-degree push-up (Chart 4, page 198)	○	○	○	○	○
15. Muscular endurance: flexed arm support (Chart 5, page 198)	○	○	○	○	○
16. Fitness rating: skinfold (Chart 4, page 293)	○	○	○	○	○
17. Body mass index (Chart 8, page 295)	○	○	○	○	○

Skill-Related Fitness and Other Self-Assessments	High-Performance Zone	Good Fitness Zone	Rating Marginal Zone	Low Zone	No Results
1. Agility (Chart 1, page 265)	○	○	○	○	○
2. Balance (Chart 2, page 266)	○	○	○	○	○
3. Coordination (Chart 3, page 266)	○	○	○	○	○
4. Power (Chart 4, page 267)	○	○	○	○	○
5. Reaction Time (Chart 5, page 267)	○	○	○	○	○
6. Speed (Chart 6, page 268)	○	○	○	○	○
7. Fitness of the back (Chart 2, page 242)	○	○	○	○	○
8. Posture (Chart 2, page 245)	○	○	○	○	○

Summarize Your Fitness Ratings Using the Results Above	High-Performance Zone	Good Fitness Zone	Rating Marginal Zone	Low Zone	No Results
Cardiovascular	○	○	○	○	○
Endurance	○	○	○	○	○
Strength	○	○	○	○	○
Flexibility	○	○	○	○	○
Body fatness	○	○	○	○	○
Skill-related fitness	○	○	○	○	○
Posture and fitness of the back	○	○	○	○	○

Rate your stage of change for each of the different types of activities from the physical activity pyramid. Make an X over the circle beside the stage that best represents your behavior for each of the five types of activity in the lower three levels of the pyramid. A description of the various stages is provided below to help you make your ratings.

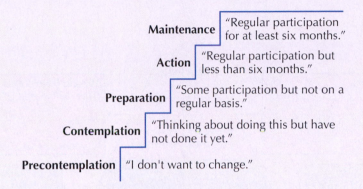

Maintenance — "Regular participation for at least six months."

Action — "Regular participation but less than six months."

Preparation — "Some participation but not on a regular basis."

Contemplation — "Thinking about doing this but have not done it yet."

Precontemplation — "I don't want to change."

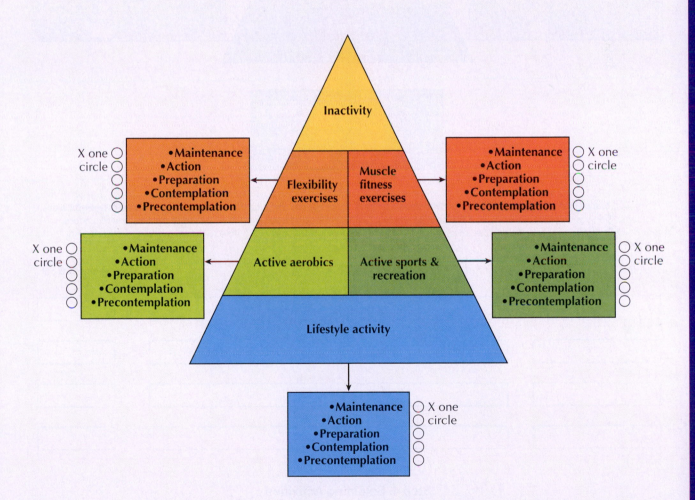

In step 1, you wrote down some general reasons for developing your physical activity plan. Setting goals requires more specific statements of goals that are realistic and achievable. For people who are at the contemplation or preparation stage for a specific type of activity, it is recommended that you write only short-term physical activity goals (no more than 4 weeks). Those at the action or maintenance level may choose short-term goals to start with or, if you have a good history of adherence, choose long-term goals (longer than 4 weeks). Precontemplators are not considered, because they would not be doing this activity.

Step 3. Set Specific Goals

Chart 2 ▶ Setting Goals

Physical Activity Goals. Place an X over the appropriate circle for the number of days of the week and the number of weeks for each type of activity. Write the number of exercises or activities you plan in each of the five areas.

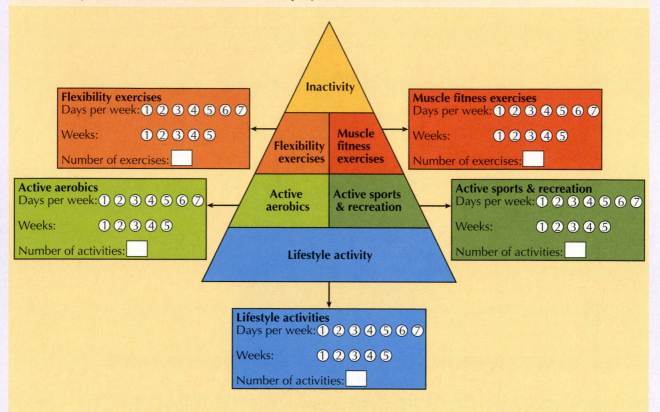

Physical Fitness Goals (for People at Action or Maintenance Only). Write specific physical fitness goals in the spaces provided below. Indicate when you expect to accomplish the goal (in weeks). Examples include improving the 12-minute run to a specific score, being able to perform a specific number of push-ups, attaining a specific BMI, and being able to achieve a specific score on a flexibility test.

Part of Fitness	Description of Specific Performance	Weeks to Goal

Step 4. Selecting Activities

In Chart 3, indicate the specific activities you plan to perform from each area of the physical activity pyramid. If the activity you expect to perform is listed, note the number of minutes or reps/sets you plan to perform. If the activity you want to perform is not listed, write the name of the activity or exercise in the space designated as "Other." For lifestyle activities, active aerobics, and active sports and recreation, indicate the length of time the activity will be performed each day. For flexibility, muscle fitness exercises, and exercises for back and neck, indicate the number of repetitions for each exercise.

Chart 3 ▶ Lifetime Physical Activity Selections

✔	Lifestyle Activities	Min./Day	✔	Active Aerobics	Min./Day	✔	Active Sports and Recreation	Min./Day
	Walking			Aerobic exercise machines			Basketball	
	Yard work			Bicycling			Bowling	
	Active housework			Circuit training or calisthenics			Golf	
	Gardening			Dance or step aerobics			Karate/judo	
	Social dancing			Hiking or backpacking			Mountain climbing	
	Occupational activity			Jogging or running (or walking)			Racquetball	
	Wheeling in wheelchair			Skating/cross-country skiing			Skating	
	Bicycling to work or store			Swimming			Softball	
	Other:			Water activity			Skiing	
	Other:			Other:			Soccer	
	Other:			Other:			Volleyball	
	Other:			Other:			Other:	
	Other:			Other:			Other:	
	Other:			Other:			Other:	
	Other:			Other:			Other:	

✔	Flexibility Exercises	Reps/Sets	✔	Muscle Fitness Exercises	Reps/Sets	✔	Exercises for Back and Neck	Reps/Sets
	Calf stretch			Bench or seated press			Back saver stretch	
	Hip and thigh stretch			Biceps curl			Single knee to chest	
	Sitting stretch			Triceps curl			Low back stretch	
	Hamstring stretch			Lat pull down			Hip/thigh stretch	
	Back stretch (leg hug)			Seated rowing			Pelvic tilt	
	Trunk twist			Wrist curl			Bridging	
	Pectoral stretch			Knee extension			Wall slide	
	Arm stretch			Heel raise			Pelvic stabilizer	
	Other:			Half-squat skiing			Neck rotation	
	Other:			Lunge			Isometric neck exercise	
	Other:			Toe press			Chin tuck	
	Other:			Crunch or reverse curl			Trapezius stretch	
	Other:			Other:			Other:	
	Other:			Other:			Other:	
	Other:			Other:			Other:	

Step 5. Preparing a Written Plan

In Chart 4, place a check in the shaded boxes for each activity you will perform for each day you will do it. Indicate the time of day you expect to perform the activity or exercise (Example: 7:30 to 8 A.M. or 6 to 6:30 P.M.). In the spaces labeled "Warm-Up Exercises" and "Cool-Down Exercises," check the warm-up and cool-down exercises you expect to perform. Indicate the number of reps you will use for each exercise.

Chart 4 ▶ My Physical Activity Plan

✔ Monday	Time	✔ Tuesday	Time	✔ Wednesday	Time
Lifestyle activity		Lifestyle activity		Lifestyle activity	
Active aerobics		Active aerobics		Active aerobics	
Active sports/rec.		Active sports/rec.		Active sports/rec.	
Flexibility exercises*		Flexibility exercises*		Flexibility exercises*	
Muscle fitness exercises*		Muscle fitness exercises*		Muscle fitness exercises*	
Back/neck exercises*		Back/neck exercises*		Back/neck exercises*	
Warm-up exercises		Warm-up exercises		Warm-up exercises	
Other:		Other:		Other:	

✔ Thursday	Time	✔ Friday	Time	✔ Saturday	Time
Lifestyle activity		Lifestyle activity		Lifestyle activity	
Active aerobics		Active aerobics		Active aerobics	
Active sports/rec.		Active sports/rec.		Active sports/rec.	
Flexibility exercises*		Flexibility exercises*		Flexibility exercises*	
Muscle fitness exercises*		Muscle fitness exercises*		Muscle fitness exercises*	
Back/neck exercises*		Back/neck exercises*		Back/neck exercises*	
Warm-up exercises		Warm-up exercises		Warm-up exercises	
Other:		Other:		Other:	

✔ Sunday	Time	✔ Warm-Up Exercises	Reps	✔ Cool-Down Exercises	Reps
Lifestyle activity		Walk or jog 1–2 min.		Walk or jog 1–2 min.	
Active aerobics		Calf stretch		Calf stretch	
Active sports/rec.		Hamstring stretch		Hamstring stretch	
Flexibility exercises*		Leg hug		Leg hug	
Muscle fitness exercises*		Sitting side stretch		Sitting side stretch	
Back/neck exercises*		Zipper		Zipper	
Warm-up exercises		Other:		Other:	
Other:		Other:		Other:	

*Perform the specific exercises you checked in Chart 3.

Step 6. Keeping Records of Progress and Evaluating Your Plan

Make copies of Chart 4 (one for each week that you plan to keep records). Each day, make a check by the activities you actually performed. Include the times when you actually did the activities in your plan. Periodically check your goals to see if they have been accomplished. At some point, it will be necessary to reestablish your goals and create a revised activity plan.

Results

After performing your plan for a specific period of time, answer the question in the space provided.

How long have you been performing the plan?

Conclusions and Implications

1. In several sentences, discuss your adherence to the plan. Have you been able to stick with the plan? If so, do you think it is a plan you can do for a lifetime? If not, why do you think you are unable to do your plan?

2. In several sentences, discuss how you might modify your plan in the future.

3. In several sentences, discuss your goals for your program. Do you think you will meet your goals? Why or why not?

Appendix A
Metric Conversion Chart

Approximate Conversions from Metric to Traditional Measures

Length

centimeters to inches: $cm \times .39 = in.$

meters to feet: $m \times 3.3 = ft.$

meters to yards: $m \times 1.09 = yd.$

kilometers to miles: $km \times 0.6 = mi.$

Mass (Weight)

grams to ounces: $g \times 0.0352 = oz.$

kilograms to pounds: $kg \times 2.2 = lb.$

Area

square centimeters to square inches: $cm^2 \times 0.16 = in.^2$

square meters to square feet: $m^2 \times 11.11 = ft.^2$

square meters to square yards: $m^2 \times 1.02 = yd.^2$

Volume

milliliters to fluid ounces: $ml \times 0.03 = fl.\ oz.$

liters to quarts: $1 \times 1.06 = qt.$

liters to gallons: $1 \times 0.264 = gal.$

Approximate Conversions from Traditional to Metric Measures

Length

inches to centimeters: $in. \times 2.54 = cm$

feet to meters: $ft. \times .3048 = m$

yards to meters: $yd. \times 0.92 = m$

miles to kilometers: $mi. \times 1.6 = km$

Mass (Weight)

ounces to grams: $oz. \times 28.41 = gm$

pounds to kilograms: $lb. \times 0.45 = kg$

Area

square inches to square centimeters: $in.^2 \times 6.5 = cm^2$

square feet to square meters: $ft.^2 \times 0.09 = m^2$

square yards to square meters: $yd.^2 \times 0.76 = m^2$

Volume

fluid ounces to milliliters: $fl.\ oz. \times 29.573 = ml$

quarts to liters: $qt. \times 0.95 = 1$

gallons to liters: $gal. \times 3.8 = 1$

Appendix B
Metric Conversions of Selected Charts and Tables

Chart 1 ▶ 12-Minute Run Test (Scores in Meters)

Classification	Men (Age)			
	17–26	27–39	40–49	50+
High-performance zone	2,880+	2,560+	2,400+	2,240+
Good fitness zone	2,480–2,779	2,320–2,559	2,240–2,399	2,000–2,239
Marginal zone	2,160–2,479	2,080–2,319	2,000–2,239	1,760–1,999
Low zone	<2,160	<2,080	<2,000	<1,760

Classification	Women (Age)			
	17–26	27–39	40–49	50+
High-performance zone	2,320+	2,160+	2,000+	1,840+
Good fitness zone	2,000–2,319	1,920–2,159	1,840–1,999	1,680–1,839
Marginal zone	1,840–1,999	1,680–1,919	1,600–1,839	1,520–1,679
Low zone	<1,840	<1,680	<1,600	<1,520

Chart 2 ▶ 12-Minute Swim Rating Chart (Score in Meters)

Classification	Men (Age)			
	17–26	27–39	40–49	50+
High-performance zone	644+	598+	552+	506+
Good fitness zone	552–643	506–597	460–551	413–505
Marginal zone	460–551	414–505	368–459	322–412
Low zone	<460	<414	<368	<322

Classification	Women (age)			
	17–26	27–39	40–49	50+
High-performance zone	552+	506+	460+	414+
Good fitness zone	460–551	414–505	367–459	321–413
Marginal zone	367–459	321–413	276–366	230–320
Low zone	<367	<321	<276	<230

Chart 3 ▶ Isometric Strength Rating Scale (kg)

Classification Men	Left Grip	Right Grip	Total Score
High-performance zone	57+	61+	118+
Good fitness zone	45–56	50–60	95–117
Marginal zone	41–44	43–49	84–94
Low zone	<41	<43	<84

Women			
High-performance zone	34+	39+	73+
Good fitness zone	27–33	32–38	59–72
Marginal zone	20–26	23–31	43–58
Low zone	<20	<23	<43

Suitable for use by young adults between 18 and 30 years of age. After 30, an adjustment of 0.5 of 1 percent per year is appropriate because some loss of muscle tissue typically occurs as you grow older.

Chart 4 ▶ Power Rating Scale

Classification	Men	Women
Excellent	68 cm+	60 cm+
Very good	53–67 cm	48–59 cm
Good	42–52 cm	37–47 cm
Fair	31–41 cm	27–36 cm
Poor	<32 cm	<27 cm

Chart 5 ▶ Reaction Time Rating Scale

Classification	Score in Inches	Score in Centimeters
Excellent	>21"	>52
Very good	19"–21"	48–52
Good	16"–18 3/4"	41–47
Fair	13"–15 3/4"	33–40
Poor	<13"	<33

Chart 6 ▶ Speed Rating Scale

Classification	Men Yards	Men Meters	Women Yards	Women Meters
Excellent	24+	22+	22+	20+
Very good	22–23	20–21.9	20–21	18–19.9
Good	18–21	16.5–19.9	16–19	14.5–17.9
Fair	16–17	14.5–16.4	14–15	13–14.4
Poor	<16	<14.5	<14	<13

Appendix C
Calorie Guide to Common Foods

Beverages

Coffee (black)	0
Coke (12 oz.)	137
Hot chocolate, milk (1 cup)	247
Lemonade (1 cup)	100
Limeade, diluted to serve (1 cup)	110
Soda, fruit-flavored (12 oz.)	161
Tea (clear)	0

Breads and Cereals

Bagel (1 half)	76
Biscuit (2" × 2")	135
Bread, pita (1 oz.)	80
Bread, raisin (1/2" thick)	65
Bread, rye	55
Bread, white enriched (1/2" thick)	68
Bread, whole-wheat (1/2" thick)	67
Bun (hamburger)	120
Cereals, cooked (1/2 cup)	80
Corn flakes (1 cup)	96
Corn grits (1 cup)	125
Corn muffin (2 1/2" diam.)	103
Crackers, graham (1 med.)	28
Crackers, soda (1 plain)	24
English muffin (1 half)	74
Macaroni, with cheese (1 cup)	464
Muffin, plain	135
Noodles (1 cup)	200
Oatmeal (1 cup)	150
Pancakes (1–4" diam.)	59
Pizza (1 section)	180
Popped corn (1 cup)	54
Potato chips (10 med.)	108
Pretzels (5 small sticks)	18
Rice (1 cup)	225
Roll, plain (1 med.)	118
Roll, sweet (1 med.)	178
Shredded wheat (1 med. biscuit)	79
Spaghetti, plain cooked (1 cup)	218
Tortilla (1 corn)	70
Waffle (4 1/2" × 5")	216

Dairy Products

Butter, 1 pat (1 1/2 tsp.)	50
Cheese, cheddar (1 oz.)	113
Cheese, cottage (1 cup)	270
Cheese, cream (1 oz.)	106
Cheese, Parmesan (1 tbsp.)	29
Cheese, Swiss natural (1 oz.)	105
Cream, sour (1 tbsp.)	31
Frozen custard (1 cup)	375
Frozen yogurt, vanilla (1 cup)	180
Ice cream, plain (prem.) (1 cup)	350
Ice cream soda, choc. (large glass)	455
Ice milk (1 cup)	184
Ices (1 cup)	177
Milk, chocolate (1 cup)	185
Milk, half-and-half (1 tbsp.)	20
Milk, malted (1 cup)	281
Milk, skim (1 cup)	88
Milk, skim dry (1 tbsp.)	28

Milk, whole (1 cup)	166
Sherbet (1 cup)	270
Softserve cone (med.)	335
Whipped topping (1 tbsp.)	14
Yogurt (1 cup)	150

Desserts and Sweets

Cake, angel (2" wedge)	108
Cake, chocolate (2" × 3" × 1")	150
Cake, plain (3" × 2 1/2")	180
Chocolate, bar	200–300
Chocolate, bitter (1 oz.)	142
Chocolate, sweet (1 oz.)	133
Chocolate, syrup (1 tbsp.)	42
Cocoa (1 tbsp.)	21
Cookies, plain (1 med.)	75
Custard, baked (1 cup)	283
Donut (1 large)	250
Gelatin, dessert (1 cup)	155
Gelatin, with fruit (1 cup)	170
Gingerbread (2" × 2" × 2")	180
Jams, jellies (1 tbsp.)	55
Pie, apple (1/7 of 9" pie)	345
Pie, cherry (1/7 of 9" pie)	355
Pie, chocolate (1/7 of 9" pie)	360
Pie, coconut (1/7 of 9" pie)	266
Pie, lemon meringue (1/7 of 9" pie)	302
Sugar, granulated (1 tsp.)	27
Syrup, table (1 tbsp.)	57

Fruit

Apple, fresh (med.)	76
Applesauce, unsweetened (1 cup)	184
Avocado, raw (1/2 peeled)	279
Banana, fresh (med.)	88
Cantaloupe, raw (1/2, 5" diam.)	60
Cherries (10 sweet)	50
Cranberry sauce, unsweetened (1 tbsp.)	25
Fruit cocktail, canned (1 cup)	170
Grapefruit, fresh (1/2)	60
Grapefruit juice, raw (1 cup)	95
Grape juice, bottled (1/2 cup)	80
Grapes (20–25)	75
Nectarine (1 med.)	88
Olives, green	72
Olives, ripe (10)	105
Orange, fresh (med.)	60
Orange juice, frozen diluted (1 cup)	110
Peach, fresh (med.)	46
Peach, canned in syrup (2 halves)	79
Pear, fresh (med.)	95
Pears, canned in syrup (2 halves)	79
Pineapple, crushed in syrup (1 cup)	204
Pineapple (1/2 cup fresh)	50
Prune juice (1 cup)	170
Raisins, dry (1 tbsp.)	26
Strawberries, fresh (1 cup)	54
Strawberries, frozen (3 oz.)	90
Tangerine (2 1/2" diam.)	40
Watermelon, wedge (4" × 8")	120

Meat, Fish, Eggs

Bacon, drained (2 slices)	97
Bacon, Canadian (1 oz.)	62
Beef, hamburger chuck (3 oz.)	316
Beef pot pie	560
Beef steak, sirloin or T-bone (3 oz.)	257
Beef and vegetable stew (1 cup)	185
Chicken, fried breast (8 oz.)	210
Chicken, fried (1 leg and thigh)	305
Chicken, roasted breast (2 slices)	100
Chili, with meat (1 cup)	510
Chili, with beans (1 cup)	335
Egg, boiled	77
Egg, fried	125
Egg, scrambled	100
Fish and chips (2 pcs. fish; 4 oz. chips)	275
Fish, broiled (3" × 3" × 1/2")	112
Fish stick	40
Frankfurter, boiled	124
Ham (4" × 4")	338
Lamb (3 oz. roast, lean)	158
Liver (3" × 3")	150
Luncheon meat (2 oz.)	135
Pork chop, loin (3" × 5")	284
Salmon, canned (1 cup)	145
Sausage, pork (4 oz.)	510
Shrimp, canned (3 oz.)	108
Tuna, canned (1/2 cup)	185
Veal, cutlet (3" × 4")	175

Nuts and Seeds

Cashews (1 cup)	770
Coconut (1 cup)	450
Peanut butter (1 tbsp.)	92
Peanuts, roasted, no skin (1 cup)	805
Pecans (1 cup)	752
Sunflower seeds (1 tbsp.)	50

Sandwiches (2 Slices of White Bread)

Bologna	214
Cheeseburger (small McDonald's)	300
Chicken salad	185
Egg salad	240
Fish fillet (McDonald's)	400
Ham	360
Ham and cheese	360
Hamburger (small McDonald's)	260
Hamburger, Burger King Whopper	600
Hamburger, Big Mac	550
Hamburger (McDonald's Quarter Pounder)	420
Peanut butter	250
Roast beef (Arby's Regular)	425

Sauces, Fats, Oils

Catsup, tomato (1 tbsp.)	17
Chili sauce (1 tbsp.)	17
French dressing (1 tbsp.)	59
Margarine (1 pat)	50
Mayonnaise (1 tbsp.)	92
Mayonnaise-type (1 tbsp.)	65

Vegetable, sunflower, safflower oils (1 tbsp.)	120	Beans, pork and molasses (1 cup)	325	Peas, green (1 cup)	145
		Broccoli, fresh, cooked (1 cup)	60	Pickles, dill (med.)	15
Soup, Ready-to-Serve (1 Cup)		Cabbage, cooked (1 cup)	40	Pickles, sweet (med.)	22
Bean	190	Cauliflower (1 cup)	25	Potato, baked (med.)	97
Beef noodle	100	Carrot, raw (med.)	21	Potato, French fried (8 sticks)	155
Cream	200	Carrots, canned (1 cup)	44	Potato, mashed (1 cup)	185
Tomato	90	Celery, diced raw (1 cup)	20	Radish, raw (small)	1
Vegetable	80	Coleslaw (1 cup)	102	Sauerkraut, drained (1 cup)	32
		Corn, sweet, canned (1 cup)	140	Spinach, fresh, cooked (1 cup)	46
Vegetables		Corn, sweet (med. ear)	84	Squash, summer (1 cup)	30
Alfalfa sprouts ($^1/_2$ cup)	19	Cucumber, raw (6 slices)	6	Sweet pepper (med.)	15
Asparagus (6 spears)	22	Lettuce (2 large leaves)	7	Sweet potato, candied (small)	314
Bean sprouts (1 cup)	37	Mushrooms, canned (1 cup)	28	Tomato, cooked (1 cup)	50
Beans, green (1 cup)	27	Onion, raw (med.)	25	Tomato, raw (med.)	30
Beans, lima (1 cup)	152	Onions, French fried (10 rings)	75		
Beans, navy (1 cup)	642	Peas, field ($^1/_2$ cup)	90		

Due to space limitations, it is not possible to list the nutrient content of all commercially available foods. You can access many valuable Web-based resources to obtain more detailed lists of foods or complete dietary analyses. The Nutrition Department at Tufts University has developed a webpage called Nutrition Navigators (www.navigator.tufts.edu/), which reviews the quality of various nutrition-related websites. The following list highlights a few of the dietary analysis programs that received favorable reviews from the Nutrition Navigator website. These resources are recommended for students interested in learning about the nutrient content of foods not listed in Appendices C and D. Directly consulting the Nutrition Navigator site may bring up additional sites that may be useful as well.

Cyberdiet www.cyberdiet.com/

This website, developed by a team of registered dietitians, offers a variety of information about nutrition. The database of commonly used foods (www.cyberdiet.com/ni/htdocs/index.html) can be quickly searched for dietary information. An advantage of this database is that it allows you to search by various categories of foods and quickly view and compare foods in a similar category.

Diet Analysis website dawp.anet.com/

This diet analysis site lets you enter the foods you've eaten over the course of a day and then, based on the RDA, reports a complete nutritional review of your diet. Tufts' Nutrition Navigator gives this site a rating of "better than most."

Fast Food Finder www.olen.com/food/

This online analysis program, developed with support from the Minnesota Attorney General's Office, allows you to obtain dietary information about nearly all items available from fast-food chains.

Nutrition Analysis Tool www.nat.uiuc.edu

This diet analysis program, developed by the University of Illinois Department of Food Science/Nutrition, provides a nutrient analysis of foods by searching foods within the USDA database.

Sante Food Database www.nightcrew.com/sante7000/sante7000_search.cfm

This website program provides a nutrient analysis of over 7,248 foods that are listed in the USDA database. The report provides a listing of over twenty-nine nutrients for each food.

Appendix D

Calories of Protein, Carbohydrates, and Fats in Foods

Food No./Food Choice	Total Calories	Protein Calories	Carbohydrate Calories	Fat Calories	Food No./Food Choice	Total Calories	Protein Calories	Carbohydrate Calories	Fat Calories
Breakfast					*Lunch*				
1. Scrambled egg (1 lg.)	111	29	7	75	1. Hamburger (reg. FF[1])	255	48	120	89
2. Fried egg (1 lg.)	99	26	1	72	2. Cheeseburger (reg. FF)	307	61	120	126
3. Pancake (1-6)	146	19	67	58	3. Doubleburger (FF)	563	101	163	299
4. Syrup (1 T[4])	60	0	60	0	4. $^1/_4$ lb. burger (FF)	427	73	137	217
5. French toast (1 slice)	180	23	49	108	5. Doublecheese burger (FF)	670	174	134	362
6. Waffle (7-inch)	245	28	100	117	6. Doublecheese baconburger (FF)	724	138	174	340
7. Biscuit (medium)	104	8	52	44	7. Hot dog (FF)	214	36	54	124
8. Bran muffin (medium)	104	11	63	31	8. Chili dog (FF)	320	51	90	179
9. White toast (slice)	68	9	52	7	9. Pizza, cheese (slice FF)	290	116	116	58
10. Wheat toast (slice)	67	14	52	6	10. Pizza, meat (slice FF)	360	126	126	108
11. Peanut butter (1 T)	94	15	11	68	11. Pizza, everything (slice FF)	510	179	173	158
12. Yogurt (8 oz. plain)	227	39	161	27	12. Sandwich, roast beef (FF)	350	88	126	137
13. Orange juice (8 oz.)	114	8	100	6	13. Sandwich, bologna	313	44	106	163
14. Apple juice (8 oz.)	117	1	116	0	14. Sandwich, bologna-cheese	428	69	158	201
15. Soft drink (12 oz.)	144	0	144	0	15. Sandwich, ham-cheese (FF)	380	91	133	156
16. Bacon (2 slices)	86	15	2	70	16. Sandwich, peanut butter	281	39	118	124
17. Sausage (1 link)	141	11	0	130	17. Sandwich, PB and jelly	330	40	168	122
18. Sausage (1 patty)	284	23	0	261	18. Sandwich, egg salad	330	40	109	181
19. Grits (8 oz.)	125	11	110	4	19. Sandwich, tuna salad	390	101	109	180
20. Hash browns (8 oz.)	355	18	178	159	20. Sandwich, fish (FF)	432	56	147	229
21. French fries (reg.)	239	12	115	112	21. French fries (reg. FF)	239	12	115	112
22. Donut, cake	125	4	61	60	22. French fries (lg. FF)	406	20	195	191
23. Donut, glazed	164	8	87	69	23. Onion rings (reg. FF)	274	14	112	148
24. Sweet roll	317	22	136	159	24. Chili (8 oz.)	260	49	62	148
25. Cake (medium slice)	274	14	175	85	25. Bean soup (8 oz.)	355	67	181	107
26. Ice cream (8 oz.)	257	15	108	134	26. Beef noodle soup (8 oz.)	140	32	59	49
27. Cream cheese (T)	52	4	1	47	27. Tomato soup (8 oz.)	180	14	121	45
28. Jelly (T)	49	0	49	0	28. Vegetable soup (8 oz.)	160	21	107	32
29. Jam (T)	54	0	54	0	29. Small salad, plain	37	6	27	4
30. Coffee (cup)	0	0	0	0	30. Small salad, French dressing	152	8	50	94
31. Tea (cup)	0	0	0	0	31. Small salad, Italian dressing	162	8	28	126
32. Cream (T)	32	2	2	28	32. Small salad, bleu cheese	184	13	28	143
33. Sugar (t)	15	0	15	0	33. Potato salad (8 oz.)	248	27	159	62
34. Corn flakes (8 oz.)	97	8	87	2	34. Cole slaw (8 oz.)	180	0	25	155
35. Wheat flakes (8 oz.)	106	12	90	4	35. Macaroni and cheese (8 oz.)	230	37	103	90
36. Oatmeal (8 oz.)	132	19	92	21	36. Taco beef (FF)	186	59	56	71
37. Strawberries (8 oz.)	55	4	46	5	37. Bean burrito (FF)	343	45	192	106
38. Orange (medium)	64	6	57	1	38. Meat burrito (FF)	466	158	196	112
39. Apple (medium)	96	1	86	9	39. Mexican rice (FF)	213	17	160	36
40. Banana (medium)	101	4	95	2	40. Mexican beans (FF)	168	42	82	44
41. Cantaloupe (half)	82	7	73	2	41. Fried chicken breast (FF)	436	262	13	161
42. Grapefruit (half)	40	2	37	1	42. Broiled chicken breast	284	224	0	60
43. Custard pie (slice)	285	20	188	77	43. Broiled fish	228	82	32	114
44. Fruit pie (slice)	350	14	259	77	44. Fish stick (1 stick FF)	50	18	8	24
45. Fritter (medium)	132	11	54	67	45. Fried egg	99	26	1	72
46. Skim milk (8 oz.)	88	36	52	0	46. Donut	125	4	61	60
47. Whole milk (8 oz.)	159	33	48	78	47. Potato chips (small bag)	115	3	39	73
48. Butter (pat)	36	0	0	36	48. Soft drink (12 oz.)	144	0	144	0
49. Margarine (pat)	36	0	0	36					

The principal reference for the calculation of values used in this appendix was the *Nutritive Value of Foods*, published by the United States Department of Agriculture, Washington, DC, Home and Gardens Bulletin, No. 72, although other published sources were consulted, including Jacobson, M., and S. Fritschner. *The Fast-Food Guide* (an excellent source of information about fast foods). New York: Workman.

Notes:
1. FF by a food indicates that it is typical of a food served in a fast food restaurant.
2. Your portions of foods may be larger or smaller than those listed here. For this reason, you may wish to select a food more than once (e.g., two hamburgers) or select only a portion of a serving (i.e., divide the calories in half for a half portion).
3. An oz. equals 28.35 grams.
4. T = tablespoon and t = teaspoon.

Food No./Food Choice	Total Calories	Protein Calories	Carbohydrate Calories	Fat Calories	Food No./Food Choice	Total Calories	Protein Calories	Carbohydrate Calories	Fat Calories
49. Apple juice (8 oz.)	117	1	116	0	45. Broiled chicken breast	284	224	0	60
50. Skim milk (8 oz.)	88	36	52	0	46. Broiled fish	228	82	32	114
51. Whole milk (8 oz.)	159	33	48	78	47. Fish stick (1 stick FF)	50	18	8	24
52. Diet drink (12 oz.)	0	0	0	0	48. Soft drink (12 oz.)	144	0	144	0
53. Mustard (t)	4	0	4	0	49. Apple juice (8 oz.)	117	1	116	0
54. Catsup (t)	6	0	6	0	50. Skim milk (8 oz.)	88	36	52	0
55. Mayonnaise (T)	100	0	0	100	51. Whole milk (8 oz.)	159	33	48	78
56. Fruit pie	350	14	259	77	52. Diet drink (12 oz.)	0	0	0	0
57. Cheesecake (slice)	400	56	132	212	53. Mustard (t)	4	0	4	0
58. Ice cream (8 oz.)	257	15	108	134	54. Catsup (t)	6	0	6	0
59. Coffee (8 oz.)	0	0	0	0	55. Mayonnaise (T)	100	0	0	100
60. Tea (8 oz.)	0	0	0	0	56. Fruit pie (slice)	350	14	259	77
					57. Cheesecake (slice)	400	56	132	212
Dinner					58. Ice cream (8 oz.)	257	15	108	134
1. Hamburger (reg. FF)	255	48	120	89	59. Custard pie (slice)	285	20	188	77
2. Cheeseburger (reg. FF)	307	61	120	126	60. Cake (slice)	274	14	175	85
3. Doubleburger (FF)	563	101	163	299					
4. ¼ lb. burger (FF)	427	73	137	217	*Snacks*				
5. Doublecheese burger (FF)	670	174	134	362	1. Peanut butter (1 T)	94	15	11	68
6. Doublecheese baconburger (FF)	724	138	174	412	2. Yogurt (8 oz. plain)	227	39	161	27
7. Hot dog (FF)	214	36	54	124	3. Orange juice (8 oz.)	114	8	100	6
8. Chili dog (FF)	320	51	90	179	4. Apple juice (8 oz.)	117	1	116	0
9. Pizza, cheese (slice FF)	290	116	116	58	5. Soft drink (12 oz.)	144	0	144	0
10. Pizza, meat (slice FF)	360	126	126	108	6. Donut, cake	125	4	61	60
11. Pizza, everything (slice FF)	510	179	173	158	7. Donut, glazed	164	8	87	69
12. Steak (8 oz.)	880	290	0	590	8. Sweet roll	317	22	136	159
13. French fried shrimp (6 oz.)	360	133	68	158	9. Cake (medium slice)	274	14	175	85
14. Roast beef (8 oz.)	440	268	0	172	10. Ice cream (8 oz.)	257	15	108	134
15. Liver (8 oz.)	520	250	52	218	11. Softserve cone (reg.)	240	10	89	134
16. Corned beef (8 oz.)	493	242	0	251	12. Ice cream sandwich bar	210	40	82	88
17. Meat loaf (8 oz.)	711	228	35	448	13. Strawberries (8 oz.)	55	4	46	5
18. Ham (8 oz.)	540	178	0	362	14. Orange (medium)	64	6	57	1
19. Spaghetti, no meat (13 oz.)	400	56	220	124	15. Apple (medium)	96	1	86	9
20. Spaghetti, meat (13 oz.)	500	115	230	155	16. Banana (medium)	101	4	95	2
21. Baked potato (medium)	90	12	78	0	17. Cantaloupe (half)	82	7	73	2
22. Cooked carrots (8 oz.)	71	12	59	0	18. Grapefruit (half)	40	2	37	1
23. Cooked spinach (8 oz.)	50	18	18	14	19. Celery stick	5	2	3	0
24. Corn (1 ear)	70	10	52	8	20. Carrot (medium)	20	3	17	0
25. Cooked green beans (8 oz.)	54	11	43	0	21. Raisins (4 oz.)	210	6	204	0
26. Cooked broccoli (8 oz.)	60	19	26	15	22. Watermelon (4" × 6" slice)	115	8	99	8
27. Cooked cabbage	47	12	35	0	23. Chocolate chip cookie	60	3	9	48
28. French fries (reg. FF)	239	12	115	112	24. Brownie	145	6	26	113
29. French fries (lg. FF)	406	20	195	191	25. Oatmeal cookie	65	3	13	49
30. Onion rings (reg. FF)	274	14	112	148	26. Sandwich cookie	200	8	112	80
31. Chili (8 oz.)	260	49	62	148	27. Custard pie (slice)	285	20	188	77
32. Small salad, plain	37	6	27	4	28. Fruit pie (slice)	350	14	259	77
33. Small salad, French dressing	152	8	50	94	29. Gelatin (4 oz.)	70	4	32	34
34. Small salad, Italian dressing	162	8	28	126	30. Fritter (medium)	132	11	54	67
35. Small salad, bleu cheese	184	13	28	143	31. Skim milk (8 oz.)	88	36	52	0
36. Potato salad (8 oz.)	248	27	159	62	32. Diet drink	0	0	0	0
37. Cole slaw (8 oz.)	180	0	25	155	33. Potato chips (small bag)	115	3	39	73
38. Macaroni and cheese (8 oz.)	230	37	103	90	34. Roasted peanuts (1.3 oz.)	210	34	25	151
39. Taco beef (FF)	186	59	56	71	35. Chocolate candy bar (1 oz.)	145	7	61	77
40. Bean burrito (FF)	343	45	192	106	36. Choc. almond candy bar (1 oz.)	265	38	74	164
41. Meat burrito (FF)	466	158	196	112	37. Saltine cracker	18	1	1	16
42. Mexican rice (FF)	213	17	160	36	38. Popped corn	40	7	33	0
43. Mexican beans (FF)	168	42	82	44	39. Cheese nachos	471	63	194	214
44. Fried chicken breast (FF)	436	262	13	161					

See Appendix C for additional nutrition information on the Web.

Calorie, Fat, Saturated Fat, Cholesterol, and Sodium Content of Selected Fast-Food Items

Burger King	Calories	Total Fat	Sat. Fat	Chol.	Sodium
Hamburger	320	14	7	45	530
Whopper Jr.	410	23	8	50	520
Whopper	680	39	13	80	940
Chicken sandwich	660	39	11	70	1,330
Double cheeseburger	570	34	19	110	1,020
Bacon double cheeseburger	780	47	19	105	1,390
Double whopper	920	57	22	150	1,020
Double whopper with cheese	1,020	65	27	170	1,460
Fries (small—2.25 oz.)	230	11	60	0	530
Fries (medium—4 oz.)	360	18	10	0	690
Fries (large—5.5 oz.)	500	25	13	0	940
Fries (king—6 oz.)	600	30	16	0	1,140
Onion rings (medium—3.5 oz.)	320	16	8	0	460
Onion rings (king—5.5 oz.)	550	27	13	0	N/A
Coca-Cola classic (small—16 oz.)	160	0	0	0	N/A
Coca-Cola classic (med.—22 oz.)	230	0	0	0	N/A
Coca-Cola classic (large—32 oz.)	330	0	0	0	N/A
Coca-Cola classic (king—42 oz.)	430	0	0	0	N/A
Shake (medium—14 oz.)	460	8	5	30	320
Apple pie	340	14	6	0	470
Sundae pie	310	18	15	10	140

Taco Bell	Calories	Total Fat	Sat. Fat	Chol.	Sodium
Chicken fiesta burrito	370	12	4	35	1,000
Bean burrito	370	12	4	10	1,080
Chili cheese burrito	330	13	5	24	900
Chicken burrito supreme	410	16	6	45	1,120
Steak burrito supreme	420	16	6	35	1,140
7-layer burrito	520	22	7	25	1,270
Grilled stuft chicken burrito	690	29	8	70	1,900
Grilled stuft steak burrito	690	30	8	60	1,970
Chicken chalupa nacho cheese	350	19	5	25	640
Chicken chalupa baja	400	24	5	40	660
Beef chalupa nacho cheese	370	22	6	25	740
Steak chalupa baja	400	24	6	30	680
Chicken gordita supreme	300	13	5	45	530
Steak gordita supreme	300	14	5	35	550
Beef gordita supreme	300	14	5	35	550
Chicken soft taco	190	7	3	35	480
Beef soft taco	210	10	4	30	570
Steak soft taco	280	17	4	35	630
Taco supreme	260	16	6	40	350
Double decker taco supreme	420	21	8	40	760
Pintos and cheese	180	8	4	15	640
Nachos	320	18	4	5	560
Nachos supreme	440	24	7	35	800
Nachos bell grande	760	39	11	35	1,300
Chicken quesadilla	540	30	12	80	1,270
Taco salad with salsa	850	52	14	70	2,250
Shake (large—32 oz.)	1,010	29	19	115	530
Cola (small—16 oz.)	100	0	0	0	10
Cola (medium—20 oz.)	130	0	0	0	10

McDonald's	Calories	Total Fat	Sat. Fat	Chol.	Sodium
Hamburger	280	10	4	30	590
Fillet o-fish	470	26	5	50	890
Crispy chicken	550	27	5	50	1,180
Cheeseburger	330	14	6	50	830
Quarter pounder	430	21	8	70	840
Big Mac	590	34	11	85	1,090
Quarter pounder with cheese	590	30	13	95	1,310
French fries (small—2.5 oz.)	210	10	3	0	140
French fries (medium—5 oz.)	450	22	8	0	290
French fries (large—6 oz.)	540	26	9	0	350
French fries (supersize—7 oz.)	610	29	10	0	390
Grilled chicken caesar salad	100	3	2	40	240
Garden salad	100	6	3	75	120
Chef salad	150	8	4	95	740
Caesar dressing	150	13	3	10	400
Thousand island dressing	130	9	2	15	350
Honey mustard	160	11	2	15	260
Coca-Cola classic (small—16 oz.)	150	0	0	0	N/A
Coca-Cola classic (med.—21 oz.)	210	0	0	0	N/A
Coca-Cola classic (large—32 oz.)	310	0	0	0	N/A
Coca-Cola classic (supersize—42 oz.)	410	0	0	0	N/A
Shake (small—14 oz.)	360	9	6	40	230
Hot fudge sundae	340	12	9	30	170
McFlurry	610	22	14	75	250
Shake (large—32 oz.)	1,010	29	19	115	530

Wendy's	Calories	Total Fat	Sat. Fat	Chol.	Sodium
Grilled chicken sandwich	300	7	2	55	740
Spicy chicken sandwich	410	14	3	65	1,280
Chicken breast fillet sandwich	430	16	3	55	750
Chicken club sandwich	470	20	5	65	940
Jr. cheeseburger	310	12	6	45	800
Jr. cheeseburger deluxe	350	16	6	45	800
Jr. bacon cheeseburger	380	19	7	55	870
Classic single with everything	410	19	7	70	920
Big bacon classic	580	30	12	100	1,460
Classic double with everything	760	45	19	175	1,730
Classic triple with everything	1,030	65	29	245	2,280
Chicken nuggets	230	16	3	30	470
French fries (small—3 oz.)	270	13	4	0	90
French fries (med.—5 oz.)	420	20	6	0	130
French fries (biggie—5.5 oz.)	470	23	7	0	150
French fries (great biggie—6.5 oz.)	570	27	8	0	180
Plain baked potato	310	0	0	0	30
Chili	210	7	3	30	800
Broccoli and cheese potato	470	14	3	5	470
Bacon and cheese potato	530	17	4	25	820
Cola (small—16 oz.)	100	0	0	0	10
Cola (med.—20 oz.)	130	0	0	0	10
Cola (biggie—32 oz.)	210	0	0	0	20
Frosty (small)	170	4	3	20	100
Frosty (large)	330	8	5	35	200

Jacobson, M. F. and Hurley, J.

Canada's Food Guide to Healthy Eating

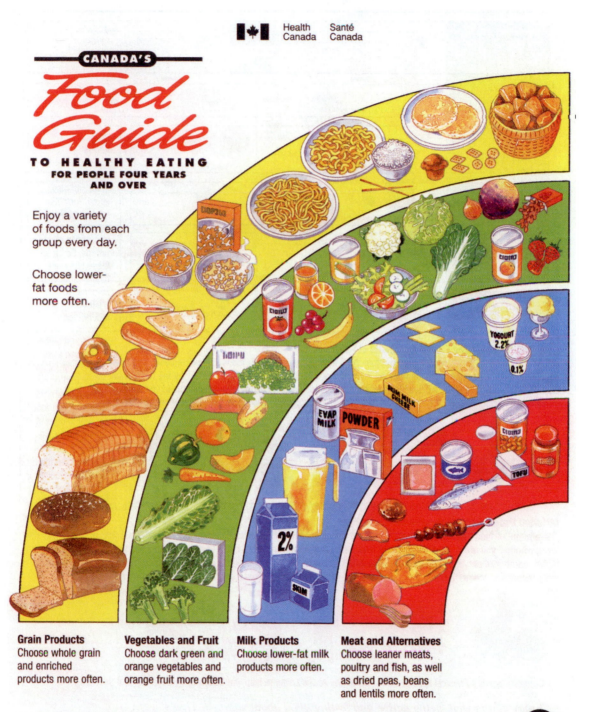

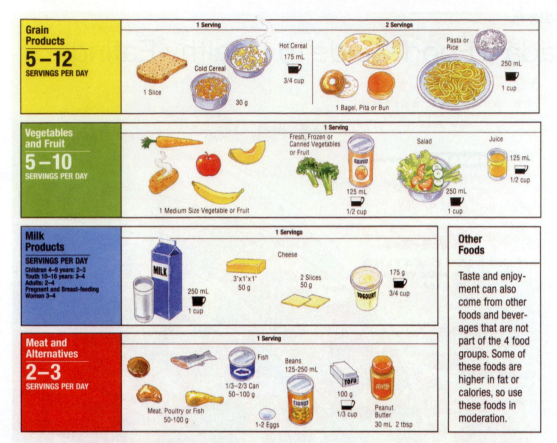

Grain Products
5–12 SERVINGS PER DAY

1 Serving — 1 Slice, Cold Cereal 30 g, Hot Cereal 175 mL 3/4 cup

2 Servings — 1 Bagel, Pita or Bun, Pasta or Rice 250 mL 1 cup

Vegetables and Fruit
5–10 SERVINGS PER DAY

1 Serving — 1 Medium Size Vegetable or Fruit, Fresh, Frozen or Canned Vegetables or Fruit 125 mL 1/2 cup, Salad 250 mL 1 cup, Juice 125 mL 1/2 cup

Milk Products
SERVINGS PER DAY
Children 4–9 years: 2–3
Youth 10–16 years: 3–4
Adults: 2–4
Pregnant and Breast-feeding Women 3–4

1 Servings — MILK 250 mL 1 cup, Cheese 3"x1"x1" 50 g, 2 Slices 50 g, YOGOURT 175 g 3/4 cup

Meat and Alternatives
2–3 SERVINGS PER DAY

1 Serving — Meat, Poultry or Fish 50-100 g, Fish 1/3–2/3 Can 50–100 g, 1-2 Eggs, Beans 125–250 mL, TOFU 100 g 1/3 cup, Peanut Butter 30 mL 2 tbsp

Other Foods

Taste and enjoyment can also come from other foods and beverages that are not part of the 4 food groups. Some of these foods are higher in fat or calories, so use these foods in moderation.

Different People Need Different Amounts of Food

The amount of food you need every day from the 4 food groups and other foods depends on your age, body size, activity level, whether you are male or female and if you are pregnant or breast-feeding. That's why the Food Guide gives a lower and higher number of servings for each food group. For example, young children can choose the lower number of servings, while male teenagers can go to the higher number. Most other people can choose servings somewhere in between.

Consult *Canada's Physical Activity Guide to Healthy Active Living* to help you build physical activity into your daily life.

Enjoy eating well, being active and feeling good about yourself. That's VITALIT*e*

© Minister of Public Works and Government Services Canada, 1997
Cat. No. H39-252/1992E   ISBN 0-662-19648-1
No changes permitted. Reprint permission not required.

Selected References

This list includes references new to the thirteenth edition of Concepts of Physical Fitness. *For a complete listing of all references, please go to the Online Learning Center at* **www.mhhe.com/corbin13e.**

Addy, C. L. et al. Association of perceived social and physical environmental supports with physical activity and walking behavior. *American Journal of Public Health* 94(3): 440–443.

Akalan, C. et al. 2004. VO2 Max: Essentials of the most widely used test in exercise physiology. *ACSM's Health and Fitness Journal* 8(3): 5–9.

Alter, M. J. 2004. *Science of Stretch* (3rd Ed.) Champaign, IL: Human Kinetics.

Alan Guttmacher Institute. 2004. Washington, D.C. *Adding It Up: The Benefits of Investing in Sexual and Reproductive Health Care.* Available on the web at **www.agi-usa.org/pubs/**

American College of Sports Medicine. 2004. *ACSM's Health-Related Physical Fitness Assessment Manual.* Philadelphia, PA: Lippinicott, Williams, & Wilkins.

Barnes, D. E., Yaffe, K., Satariano, W. A., et al. 2003. A longitudinal study of cardiovascular fitness and cognitive function in healthy older adults. *Journal of the American Geriatric Society* 51(4): 459–465.

Barnes, P. M. and C. A. Schoenhorn. 2003. Physical Activity Among Adults. *Advance Data from Vital and Health Statistics* 333(May 14): 1–23.

Bassuk, S. S. and Manson, J. E. Physical activity and cardiovascular disease prevention in women: How much is good enough? *Exercise and Sport Sciences Reviews* 31(4): 176–181.

Blair, S. N. 2004. Modifiable behavioral factors as causes of death. *Journal of the American Medical Association* 291(24)2942.

Bracko, M. R. 2004. Can we prevent back injuries? *ACSM's Health and Fitness Journal* 8(4): 5–11.

Bray, G. A. 2004. Obesity and the metabolic syndrome: Implications for dietetics practitioners. *Journal of the American Dietetics Association* 104(1):

Bray, S. A. and H. A. Born.. 2004. Transition to university and vigorous physical activity: implications for health and psychological well-being. *Journal of American College Health* 52(4): 181–188.

British Department of Health, Physical Activity, Helath Improvement and Prevention. 2004. *At Least Five a Week: Evidence on the Impact of Physical Activity and Its Relationship to Health.* London: British Department of Health.

Brown, D. W. et al. 2004. Associations between physical activity dose and health-related quality of life. *Medicine and Science in Sports and Exercise* 36(5): 890–896.

Brown, S. L. 2004. Reducing subclinical symptoms of anxiety and depression: A comparison of two college courses. *American Journal of Health Education* 35(3): 158–164.

Burke, D. G. et al. 2003. Effects of creatine and weight training on muscle creatine and performance in vegetarians. *Medicine and Science in Sports and Exercise* 35(11): 1946–1955.

California Department of Helath Services. 2004. California's adult smoking declines to historic low. *California Department of Health Services News release* Number 04-30, May 26, **http://www.dhs.ca.gov.**

Cardinal, B. J. and M. Kosma. 2004. Self-efficacy and the stages and processes of change associated with adopting and maintaining muscular fitness-promoting behaviors. *Research Quarterly for Exercise and Sport* 75(2): 186–196.

Carnethon, M. R. et al. 2003. Cardiorespiratory fitness of young adults and the development of cardiovascular disease risk factors. *Journal of the American Medical Association* 290(23): 3092–3100.

Caspi, A. et al. 2003. Influence of life stress on depression. *Science* 301(5631): 386–389.

Chesson, H. W. et al. 2004. The Estimated Direct Medical Cost of Sexually Transmitted Diseases Among American Youth. *PPerspecitves on Sexual and Reproductive Health* 36(1): 11–19.

Chong, C. L. et al. 2003. Predictors of college students' use of complementary and alternative medicine. *American Journal of Health Education* 34(5): 267–271.

Cobb, K. L. 2003. Disordered eating, menstrual irregularity and bone density in female runners. *Medicine and Science in Sports and Exercise* 35(5):711–719.

Corbin, C. B. et al. 2004. Physical activity for children: Current patterns and guidelines. *President's Council on Physical Fitness and Sports Research Digest* 4(6): 1–8.

Craft, L. L. 2003. Potential mechanisms for the antidepressant effects of exercise. *Medicine and Science in Sports and Exercise* 35(5):S216.

Dennis, D. L. and B. G. Dennis. 2003. **Spirituality@work.health**. *American Journal of Health Education* 34(5): 297–301.

Doll, R. et al. 2004. Mortality in relation to smoking. *British Medical Journal* 328(7455): 1519–1528.

Dohle, G. et al. 2003. Androgens and male fertility. *World Journal of Urology* 21: 341–345.

Donatelle, R. J. and L. G. Davis. 2005. *Health: The Basics.* (6th ed.) Boston: Addison-Wesley.

Dutto, D. J. and W. A. Braun. 2004. DOMS-associated changes in ankle and knee joint dynamics during running. *Medicine and Science in Sports and Exercise* 36(4): 560–566.

Dziura, J. et al. 2004. Physical activity reduces Type 2 Diabetes risk in aging independent of body weight change. *Journal of Physical Activity and Helath* 1(1): 19–28.

Earnest, E. P. et al. 2004. Effects of a commercial herbal-based formula on exercise performance in cyclists. *Medicine and Science in Sports and Exercise* 35(11): 504–509.

Ezzati, M. and A. D. Lopez. 2003. Estimates of global mortality attributed to smoking. *Lancet* 362(9387): 847–852.

Farrell S. W., Braun L., Barlow C. E., et al. 2002. The relation of body mass index, cardiorespiratory fitness, and all-cause mortality in women. *Obesity Research* 10: 417–423.

Fawzi, W. W. 2004. A randomized trial of multivitamin supplements and HIV disease progression and mortality. *New England Journal of Medicine* 351(1): 23–32.

FDA. 2004. FDA approves first oral fluid based rapid HIV test kit. *FDA News* March 26.

Fields, R. 2004. *Drugs in Perspective.* (5th ed.) St. Louis: McGraw-Hill Higher Education.

Finkelson, E. A. et al. 2004. State-level estimates of annual medical expenditures attributable to obesity *Obesity Research* 12(1): 18–24.

FitzGerald, S. J. et al. 2004. Muscular fitness and all-cause mortality: Prospective observations. *Journal of Physical Activity and Health* 1(1): 7–18.

Foote, J. et al. 2004. A national survey of alcohol screenings and referrals in college health centers. *Journal of American College Health* 52(4): 149–157.

Frank, L. D. 2004. Obesity relationships with community design, physical activity, and time spent in cars. *American Journal of Preventive Medicine* 27(2): 87–96.

Franks, P. W. et al. 2004. Does the association of habitual physical activity with the metabolic syndrome differ by level of cardiorespiratory fitness *Diabetes Care* 27(5): 1187–1193

Graves, B. S. and Welsh, R. L. 2004. Recognizing the signs of body dysmorphic disorder and muscle dysmorphia. *ACSM's Helath and Fitness Journal* 8(1): 11–13.

Greenberg, J. S. 2004. *Health Education and Helath Promotion.* (5th ed.) St. Louis: McGraw-Hill Higher Education.

Greenland, P. et al. 2003. Major risk factors as antecedents of fatal and nonfatal coronary heart disease events. *Journal of the American Medical Association* 290: 891–897.

Goldberg, J. P. et al. 2004. The obesity crisis: don't blame it on the pyramid. *Journal of the American Dietetic Association* 104(7): 1141–1147.

Hahn, D. B. and W. A. Payne. 2005. *Focus on Health.* (7th ed.) St. Louis: McGraw-Hill Higher Education.

Hamaoui, A. et al. 2004 Postural sway increase in low back pain subjects is not related to reduced spine range of motion. *Neuroscience Letters* 357(2): 135–138.

Heath, G. W. 2003. Increasing physical activity in communities: What really works? *President's Council on Physical Fitness and Sports Research Digest* 4(4): 1–8.

Hingson, R. et al. 2003. Age of first intoxication, heavy drinking, driving after drinking and risk of unintentional injury among U.S. college students. *Journal of Studies on Alcohol* 64(1): 23–31.

Hootman, J. M., Macera, C. A., Ainsorth, B. E. 2001. Association among physical activity level, cardiorespiratory fitness, and risk of musculoskeletal injury. *American Journal of Epidemiology* 154(3): 251–258.

Institute of Medicine. 2004. *Preventing Childhood Obesity: Health in the Balance.* Washington, DC: Institute of Medicine.

Issacs, S. L. and J. R. Knickman. 2004. *Generalist Medicine and the U.S. Health Care System.* San Fransisco, CA: Jossey-Bass.

Janssen, I. et al. 2004. Fitness alters the association of BMI and waist circumference with total and abdominal fat. *Obesity Research* 12(3): 525–537.

Jason, L. A. and G. S. Glenwick. 2002. *Innovative Strategies for Promoting Health and Mental Health Across the Life Span.* New York: Springer Publishing.

Johansson, A. K. et al. 2004. How should parents protect their children from

environmental tobacco smoke exposure in the home? *Pediatrics* 113(4): e291–e295.

Jones, A. M. 2002. Running economy is negatively related to sit and reach test performance in international-standard distance runners. *International Journal of Sports Medicine* 23(1): 40–43.

Journal of the American Dental Association. 2004. Defibrillators. *Journal of the American Dental Association* 135(3): 366–367.

Khot, U. N. et al. 2003. Prevalence of conventional risk factors in patients with coronary artery disease. *Journal of the American Medical Association* 290(7): 898–904.

Kraemer, W. J. and N. A. Ratamess. 2004. Fundamentals of Resistance Training: Progression and Exercise Prescription. *Medicine and Science in Sports and Exercise* 36(4): 674–688.

Kraus, V. 2004. Joint flexibility may lessen wear and tear on joints. *Arthritis & Rheumatism* 50: 2178–2183.

Lakka, T. A. 2003. Sedentary lifestyle, poor cardiorespiratory fitness, and the metabolic syndrome. *Medicine and Science in Sports and Exercise* 35(8): 1279–1286.

Lappe, J. M., Stegman, M. R., Recker, R. R. 2001. The impact of lifestyle factors on stress fractures in female Army recruits. *Osteoporos International* 12(1): 35–42.

Lawrence, J. et al. 2003. Structured treatment interruption in patients with multidrug-resistant human immuno-deficiency virus. *New England Journal of Medicine* 349(9): 837–846.

Lee, C. D., S. N. Blair, and A. S. Jackson. 1999 Cardiorespiratory fitness, body composition, and all-cause and cardiovascular disease mortality in men. *American Journal of Clinical Nutrition* 69: 373–380.

Lee, I-Min 2003. Physical activity and cancer prevention: Data from epidemiological studies. *Medicine and Science in Sports and Exercise* 35(11): 1823–1827.

Le Masurier, G. C. 2004. Walk this way? *ACSM's Health and Fitness Journal* 8(1): 7–10.

Lemmink, K. A. et al. 2003. The validity of the sit-and-reach test and the modified sit-and-reach test in middle-aged to older men and women *Research Quarterly for Exercise and Sport* 74(3): 331–336.

Li, J. X. et al. 2001. Tai chi: Physiological characteristics and beneficial effects on health. *British Journal of Sports Medicine* 35(3): 148–156.

Leimohn, W. et al. 2004. Questionable exercises. In Corbin, C. B. et al. (eds.) 2004 Toward an Understanding of Physical Fitness and Activity, Vol. II Scottsdale, AZ: Holcomb Hathaway Publishers.

Lohman, T. G. 2004. Seeing ourselves through the obesity epidemic. *President's Council on Physical Fitness and Sports Research Digest* 5(3): 1–8.

Lowe, M. R. 2003. Self-regulation of energy intake in the prevention and treatment of obesity: is it feasible? *Obesity Research* 11 Suppl: 44S–59S.

Ma Y. 2003. Association between eating patterns and obesity in a free-living US adult population. *American Journal of Epidemiology* 158: 85–92.

Magill, R. A. 2004. *Motor Learning: Concepts and Applications.* 7th ed. St. Louis. McGraw-Hill.

Manore, M. M. 2004. Nutrition and physical activity: Fueling the active individual. *President's Council on Physical Fitness and Sports Research Digest* 5(1): 1–8.

Manore, M. M. 2004. Keeping the weight off: How can you maintain your weight loss after the diet is over? *ACSM's Health and Fitness Journal* 8(3): 23–24.

Meyer, M. 2004. Wiggle your toes, save your life. *AARP Bulletin* 45(6): 18.

Millen, A. E. et al. 2004. Use of vitamin, mineral, nonvitamin, and nonmineral supplements in the United States: The 1987, 1992, and 2000 National Health Interview Survey results. *Journal of the American Dietetic Association* 104(8): 942–950.

Miller, W. C. et al. 2004. Prevalence of Chlamydial and gonococcal infections among young adults in the United States. *Journal of the American Medical Association* 291(18): 2229–2236.

Milliaropoulos, N. et al. 2004. The role of stretching in rehabilitiation of hamstring injuries: 80 athletes follow-up. *Medicine and Science in Sports and Exercise* 36(5): 756–759.

Mokdad, A. H. et al. 2004. Actual causes of death in the United States. *Journal of the American Medical Association* 291(10): 1238–1246.

Morbidity and Mortality Weekly Report. 2004. Cigarette smoking among adults. *Morbidity and Mortality Weekly Report* 53(29): 427–431.

National Association for Sports and Physical Education. 2004. *Physical Activity for Children: A Statement of Guidelines* Reston, VA: National Association for Sports and Physical Education.

National Center on Addiction and Substance Abuse. 2004. *You've got drugs! Prescription drug pushers on the internet.* New York: National Center on Addiction and Substance Abuse. Available on the internet at **www.casacolumbia.org**.

National Center on Addiction and Substance Abuse. 2003. *CASA National Survey of American Attitudes on Substance Abuse VIII: Teens and Parents.* New York: National Center on Addiction and Substance Abuse. Available on the internet at **www.casacolumbia.org**.

National Center on Addiction and Substance Abuse. 2003. *Depression, Substance Abuse and College Student Engagement: A Review of the Literature.* New York: National Center on Addiction and Substance Abuse. Available on the internet at **www.casacolumbia.org**.

Noonan, P. J. (2004). Do you suffer from Syndrome X? *USA Weekend.* April 23–25.

Office of the Surgeon General. 2004. *The health consequence of smoking: A report of the Surgeon General.* Atlanta, GA: United States Department of Health and Human Services.

Ogden, C. L. et al. 2004. Mean body weight, height, and BMI in the United States—1960–2002. *Advance Data from Vital and Health Statistics* 247: 1–20. (**www.cdc.gov/nchs**)

Rainville, J. et al. 2004 Exercise as treatment for chronic low back pain. *Spine* 4(1): 106–115.

Reifman, A. et al. 2003. Binge drinking during the first semester of college: Continuation and desistance from high school patterns. *Journal of American College Health* 52(2): 173–182.

Reynolds, S. J. et al. 2004. Male circumcision and risk of HIV-1 and other sexually transmitted infections in India. *Lancet* 363(9414):

Rhea, M. R., Ball, S. D., Phillips, W. T. et al. 2002. A comparison of linear and daily undulating periodized programs with equated volume and intensity for strength. *Journal of Strength and Conditioning Research* 16(2): 250–255.

Ries LAG, Eisner MP, Kosary CL, Hankey BF, Miller BA, Clegg L, Mariotto A, Feuer EJ, Edwards BK (eds). 2004. *SEER Cancer Statistics Review, 1975–2001*, National Cancer Institute. Bethesda, MD, **http://seer.cancer.gov/csr/1975_2001/,2004**.

Ribisl, P. M. 2004. Toxic "waist" dump: Our abdominal visceral fat. *ACSM's Health and Fitness Journal* 8(4): 22–25.

Romas, J. A. and M. Sharma. 2004. *Practical Stress Management (3rd ed.)* Needham Heights, MA: Benjamin Cummings.

Sanmartin, C. et al. 2004. *Joint Canada/United States Survey of Health, 2002–2003.* Atlanta, GA: CDC.

Santrock, J. W. 2005. *Psychology Updated* (7th ed.) St. Louis: McGraw-Hill Higher Education.

Sargent, R. P. et al. 2004. Reduced incidence of admissions for myocardial infarction associated with public smoking ban: before and after study. *British Medical Journal* 328(7446): 977–980.

Schneider Institute for Health Policy. 2001. *Substance Abuse: The Nation's Number One Health Problem.* Princeton, N.J.: Robert Wood Johnson Foundation. Available on the web at **www.rwjf.org**.

Schoenborn, C. A. and P. M. Barnes. 2002. Leisure-Time Physical Activity Status Among American Adults. *Advance Data from Vital and Helath Statistics* 325(April 7): 1–24.

Scurr, J. H. et al. 2001. Frequency and prevention of symptomless deep-vein thrombosis in long haul flights. *Lancet* 357(9275): 9–15.

Shuldiner, A. R. 2003. Genetics of obesity: more complicated than initially thought. *Lipids* 38(2) 97–101.

Sidman, C. L. et al. 2004. Promoting physical activity among sedentary women using pedometers. *Research Quarterly for Exercise and Sport* 75(2): 122–129.

Smith, J. C. 2002. *Stress Management: A Comprehensive Handbook of Techniques and Strategies.* New York: Springer Publishing.

Smith, T. W. et al. 2004. Prevention and health promotion: Decades of progress, new challenges, and an emerging agenda. *Health Psychology* 223(2): 126–131.

Stewart, D. E. 2004. What about men's health? A chair of women's health perspective. *Journal of Men's Health and Gender* 1(1): 20–21.

Stone, W. J. and D. A. Klein. 2004. Long-term exercisers: What can we learn from them? *ACSM's Health and Fitness Journal* 8(2): 11–14.

Task Force of the National Advisory Council on Alcohol Abuse and Alcoholism. 2002. *A Call to Action: Changing the Culture of Drinking at U.S. Colleges* Bethesda, MD: National Institutes of Health.

Tekin, K. A. and L. Kravitz. 2004. The growing trend of ergogenic drugs and supplements. *ACSM's Health and Fitness Journal* 8(1): 15–18.

Thacker, S. B. et al. 2004. The impact of stretching on sports injury risk: A systematic review of the literature. *Medicine and Science in Sports and Exercise* 36(3): 371–378.

Thompson IM (2004). Prevalence of prostate cancer among men with a prostate-specific antigen level < or = 4.0 ng per milliliter. *New England Journal of Medicine* 350(22): 2239–46.

USDHHS. 2004. *Guidelines for the Use Antiretroviral Agents in HIV-1 Infected Adults and Adolescents.* Washington, DC: USDHHS. Available on the web at **www.aidsinfo.nih.gov/guidelines**.

USDHHS. 2004. *HIV and Its Treatment: What You Should Know.* Washington, DC: USDHHS. Available on the internet at **www.aidsinfo.nih.gov/other/cbrochure/english/cbrochure_en.html**.

United States Food and Drug Administration. 2004. Worsening depression and suicidality in patients being treated with antidepressant medications. *FDA Public Health Advisory* March 22. Available on the internet at **www.aidsinfo.nih.gov/guidelines**.

Urhausen, A. et al. 2004. Are the cardiac effects of anabolic steroids abuse in strength athletes reversible? *Heart* 90: 496–501.

Uusitalo, A. L., Uusitalo, A. J., Rusko, H. K. 2000. Heart rate and blood pressure variability during heavy training and overtraining in the female athlete. *International Journal of Sports Medicine* 21(1): 45–53.

Volek, J. S. 2004. Influence of nutrition on responses to resistance training. *Medicine and Science in SPorts and Exercise* 36(4): 689–696.

Wechsler, H. et al. 2004. Colleges respond to student binge drinking: Reducing student demand or limiting access. *Journal of American College Health* 52(4): 159–168.

Weinstein, S. J. et al. 2004. Healthy eating index scores are associated with blood nutrient concentrations in the third national health and nutrition examination survey. *Journal of the American Dietetic Association* 104(4) 576–584.

Weinstock, H. et al. 2004. Sexually transmitted diseases among American youth: Incidence and prevalence estimates. *Perspectives on Sexual and Reproductive Health* 36(1): 6–10.

Weitzman, E. R. 2004. Poor mental health, depression and associations with alcohol consumption, harm and abuse in a national sample of young adults in college. *Journal of Nervous and Mental Disease* 192(4): 269–277.

Williams, G. C. 2004. Testing a self-determination theory process model for promoting glycemic control through diabetes self-management. *Health Psychology* 8(1):

Wilson, G. S. et al. 2004. Athletic status and drinking behavior in college students: The influence of gender and coping styles. *Journal of American College Health* 52(6): 269–274.

Winner, P. and D. Rothner. 2001. *Headache in Children and Adolescents* Hamilton, ON (Canada): B C Decker Inc.

Wong, S. H. S. and S. Chung. 2003. Glycemic index: An educational tool for health and fitness professionals. *ACSM's Health and Fitness Journal* 7(6): 13–19.

Wong, S. L. et al. 2004. Cardiorespiratory fitness is associated with lower abdominal fat independent of body mass index. *Medicine and Science in Sports and Exercise* 36(2): 286–291.

World Health Association. 2004. *Global Strategy on Diet, Physical Activity and Health* Geneva, Switzerland: WHO.

World Health Association. 2004. *World Helath Report 2003: Shaping the Future.* Geneva, Switzerland: WHO. (available on the web at **http://www.who.int/whr/2003/en/**)

Yan, L. L. et al. 2003. Psychosocial factors and risk of hypertension. *Journal of the American Medical Association* 290(16): 2138–2148.

Yesalis, C. E. and M. S. Bahrke. 2004. Anabolic and androgenic steroids: Incidence of use and health implicatons. *President's Council on Physical Fitness and Sports Research Digest* 6(1): 10–8.

Credits

Photos, Figures, and Tables

Concept 1

CO1: © Charles B. Corbin; p. 6: © Jim Cummins/Getty Images/Taxi; p. 8 top left: © Charles B. Corbin; p. 8 bottom right: © David Young Wolff/Photo Edit; p. 8 bottom left: © PhotoDisc/Getty Images; p. 8 top right: © Myrleen Cate/Index Stock Imagery; p. 8 middle left: © Bonnie Kamin/Photo Edit; p. 9 top left & right: © PhotoDisc/Getty Images; p. 9 bottom left: Corel; p. 9 middle top: © PhotoDisc/Getty Images; p. 9 middle bottom: Corel; p. 9 bottom right: © David R. Frazier Photolibrary; p. 12: © Michael Brinson/Index Stock Imagery.

Concept 2

CO2: © Brian Bailey/Getty Images/Stone; p. 24: © BSIP Agency/Index Stock Imagery; p. 26: © Courtesy of Vivonics; p. 28: © Jose Luis Pelaez, Inc./Corbis.

Concept 3

CO3: © Charles B. Corbin; p. 36 Table 1: American College of Sports Medicine. *ACSM's Guidelines for Exercise Testing and Prescription* (6th ed.), Philadelphia: Lippencott, Williams, and Wilkins, 2000.

Concept 4

CO4: © John Kelly/Getty Images/The Image Bank; p. 82 Table 2: National Institute for Health. The Sixth Report of the Joint Committee on Detection, Evaluation and Treatment of High Blood Pressure. NIH Publication Number 98-4080, 1997; p. 60: © Charles B. Corbin; p. 61: © Lori Adamski Peek/Getty Images/Stone.

Concept 5

CO5: © Randy M. Ury/Corbis; p. 69: © David Young Wolff/Photo Edit.

Concept 6

CO6: © PhotoDisc/Getty Images; p. 80: © PhotoDisc/Getty Images; p. 81: © Jim McGuire/Index Stock Imagery; p. 86: Bob Winsett/Corbis.

Concept 7

CO7: © Brand X Pictures; p. 94: Cara Sherman.

Concept 8

CO8: © PhotoDisc/Getty Images; p. 107 Table 1 and Figure 6: Blair, S. N. et al. "Influences of Cardiorespiratory Fitness and Other Precursors on Cardiovascular Disease and All-Cause Mortality in Men and Women." *Journal of the American Medical Association.* 276(3)(1996): 205; p. 108: Bouchard, C. "Heredity and Health-Related Physical Fitness." In Corbin, C. B. and Pangrazi, R. P. *Toward a Better Understanding of Physical Fitness and Activity.* Scottsdale, AZ: Holcomb-Hataway, 1999; p. 111 left: © Jeff Greenberg/Index Stock Imagery; p. 111 right: © PhotoDisc/Getty Images; p. 113: Courtesy of Polar®; p. 114 Table 7: Borg, G. "Psychological Bases of Perceived Exertion." *Medicine and Science in Sports and Exercise.* 14(1982):377; p. 117 Chart 1: Adapted from the *One Mile Walk Test* with permission from the author, James M. Rippe, M. D.; p. 117 Chart 2: Data from Kasch, F. W. and Boyer, J. L. *Adult Fitness: Principles and Practices.* Palo Alto, CA: Mayfield Publishing Co., 1968; p. 118–119 Charts 3, 4, and 5: Astrand, P. O. and Rodahl, K. *Textbook of Work Physiology.* St. Louis: McGraw-Hill, 1986; p. 119–120 Charts 6 and 7: Cooper, K. H. *The Aerobics Program for Total Well-Being.* Toronto: Bantam Books, 1982; p. 121 Chart: Borg, G. "Psychological Bases of Perceived Exertion." *Medicine and Science in Sports and Exercise.* 14(1982):377; p. 123: © Charles B. Corbin.

Concept 9

CO9: © Paul A. Souders/Corbis; p. 130: © Leland Bobbe/Getty Images/Stone; p. 131: Courtesy of Timex®; p. 133: © Royalty-free/Corbis; p. 134: © Tim Pannell/Corbis; p. 136: © PhotoDisc/Getty Images; p. 138: © Ken Akers/First Image West.

Concept 10

CO10: © Frank Conaway/Index Stock Imagery; p. 145: © Benelux Press/Getty Images/Taxi; p. 146: © PhotoDisc/Getty Images; p. 150 Figure 4: Shier, D., Butler, J., and Lewis, R. *Hole's Human Anatomy and Physiology.* (8th ed.), St. Louis: McGraw-Hill, 2002; p. 152: Courtesy OPTP, Minneapolis, MN; p. 152: © Charles B. Corbin.

Concept 11

CO11: Jose Luis Pelaez, Inc./Corbis; p. 167 Figure 1: Shier, D., Butler, J., and Lewis, R. *Hole's Human Anatomy and Physiology.* (8th ed.), St. Louis: McGraw-Hill, 2002; p. 169: ©Sue Benett/Ad Stock; pp. 173 & 174: © Mark Ahn; p. 177: King, J. M. "The Evolution of Strength Training Equipment." *Fitness Management.* July (2001):46–51; p. 181: © David Stocklein/AdStock; p. 195: Reprinted with permission from the *Journal of Physical Education, Recreation & Dance,* January 1993, p. 89. *JOPERD* is a publication of the American Alliance for Health, Physical Education, Recreation, and Dance, 1900 Association Drive, Reston, VA 22091. p. 196: © Charles B. Corbin.

Concept 12

CO12: © Mark Ahn; p. 209: © Charles B. Corbin

Concept 13

CO13: © Fotografia, Inc./Corbis; p. 231: © MedX 96, Inc.

Concept 14

CO14: © Zeta Visual Media–Germany/Index Stock Imagery; p. 251: Corel; p. 252: © Richard Hamilton Smith/Corbis; p. 253, Table 1: Wilmore, J. H. and Costill, D. L. *Training for Sports and Activity* (2nd ed.), Dubuque, IA: Times Mirror Higher Education, 1988; p. 254: © McGraw-Hill Digital Image Library; p. 256: ©PhotoDisc/Getty Images; p. 257: Brittenham, G. "Plyometric Exercise: A Word of Caution." *Journal of Physical Education, Recreation and Dance.* January (1992): 20–23; p. 262, Table 7: Williams, M. H. "Nutritional Ergogenics and Sports Performance." *PCPFS Research Digest.* 2(10)(1998):1–8; p. 265, Chart 1: Adams, W. et al. *Foundations of Physical Activity.* Champaign, IL: Stipes, 1965, p. 111.

Concept 15

CO15: © Charles B. Corbin; p. 276 Table 2: Lohman, T. G., Houtkooper, L. H. and Going, S. B. "Body Fatness Goes High Tech." *ACSM's Health and Fitness Journal.* 1(1)(1998); p. 278: Courtesy of Tanita Corporation of America, Inc., Arlington Heights, IL.; p. 279 Figure 3: Lee, C.D., Jackson, A. A. and Blair, S. N. "Cardiorespiratory Fitness, Body Composition, and All-Cause and Cardiovascular Disease Mortality in Men."

American Journal of Clinical Nutrition, 69(3)(1999): 373–380; p. 280: © Bob Daemmrich/Stock Boston; p. 285 Table 4: Corbin, C. B. and Lindsey, R. *Fitness for Life* (4th ed.). Champaign, IL: Human Kinetics, 2002; p. 291–292 Charts 1 & 2: Baumgartner, T. A., Jackson, A. S., Mahar, M. T., and Rowe, D. A. *Measurement for Evaluation in Physical Education and Exercise Science* (7th ed.). St. Louis: McGraw-Hill, 2003.

Concept 16

CO16: © Jon Riley/Index Stock Imagery; p. 310 Figure 3: United States Department of Agriculture; p. 315: © Corbis; p. 316 Figure 6: Williams, M. *Nutrition for Fitness and Sports* (4th ed.). 1995. St. Louis: McGraw-Hill; pp. 319 & 323: © PhotoDisc/Getty Images; p. 326: Reprinted with the permission of Simon & Schuster Adult Publishing Group from EAT, DRINK, AND BE HEALTHY: The Harvard Medical School Guide to Healthy Eating by Walter C. Willett, M.D. Copyright © 2001 by President and Fellows of Harvard College.

Concept 17

CO17: © Mark Ahn; p. 335: Segway LLC Manchester, NH; p. 336: © Donna Day/Getty Images/Stone; p. 338: © ML Sinibaldi/Corbis.

Concept 18

CO18: © Brian Bailey/Getty Images/Stone; p. 349 Table 1: Kanner, A. D. et al. Comparison of Two Modes of Stress Measurement: Daily Hassles and Uplifts Versus Major Life Events." *Journal of Behavioral Medicine.* 4(1)(1981):1–39; p. 350 Figure 2: Adapted from Gallagher, R. "Survey of College Counseling Centers." University of Pittsburgh; p. 352: © Corbis; p. 356: Sarason, I. G., Johnson, J. H. and Siegel, J. M. "Assessing the Impact of Life Changes: Development of the Life Experiences Survey." 1978. *Journal of Consulting and Clinical Psychology.* 46(5):932–946.

Concept 19

CO19: © Warren Morgan/Corbis; p. 364: © Lori Adamski Peek/Getty Images/Stone; p. 367: © PhotoDisc/Getty Images; p. 369–370 Tables 5 & 6: Burns, D. D. *The Feeling Good Handbook.* New York: Plume Books, 1999.

Concept 20

CO20: © David R. Laurie; p. 387: © Gary Conner/Index Stock Imagery; pp. 388 & 389: © Mark Ahn.

Concept 21

CO21: © Bob Winsett/Corbis; p. 403: PhotoDisc/Getty Images; p. 409: Adapted from: Mitchell, T. "What's Your Excuse?" *USA Weekend.* January 4–6, 2002, page 4.

Index